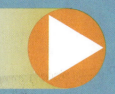

THERAPYED'S
Speech-Language Pathology: Review and Study Guide

1st EDITION

GREGORY L. LOF, PhD, CCC-SLP
ASHA Fellow
Department Chair, Professor
Department of Communication Sciences & Disorders
School of Health and Rehabilitation Sciences
MGH Institute of Health Professions
Boston, MA

ALEX F. JOHNSON, PhD, CCC-SLP
ASHA Fellow
Provost & Vice President for Academic Affairs
Professor
Department of Communication Sciences & Disorders
School of Health and Rehabilitation Sciences
MGH Institute of Health Professions
Boston, MA

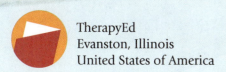

TherapyEd
Evanston, Illinois
United States of America

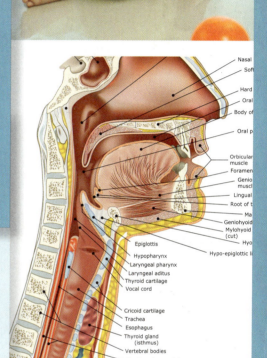
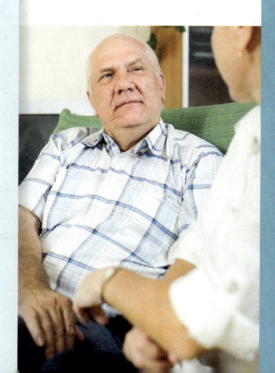

Copyright © 2015 by TherapyEd, Ltd.

"TherapyEd" is a service and trademark of TherapyEd, Ltd.

ISBN: 978-0-9904162-3-4

"ASHA" and "CCC-SLP" are registered service and trademarks of the American Speech-Language-Hearing Association. "Praxis" is a registered service and trademark of Educational Testing Services.

All marks are registered in the United States of America.

Printed in the United States of America. All rights reserved. No portion of this book or accompanying software may be reproduced, stored in a data based retrieval system or transmitted electronically or in any way without written permission from the publisher.

The authors and contributors have made a faithful attempt to include relevant summaries of current speech-language pathology practice and other information at the time of publication. It is recognized that recommended practices equipment, devices, governmental regulations, administrative procedures and other protocols and factors may change or be open to other interpretations. Readers (or SLPs) should take responsibility for being aware of technological advances, new information or conclusions available through research, new governmental regulations or ethical guidelines.

The publisher disclaims any liability or loss incurred as a result of direct or indirect use of this book. Use of this book does not guarantee successful passage of the Praxis II: Speech-Language Pathology Examination.

Copies of this book and software may be obtained from:
TherapyEd
500 Davis Street, Suite 512
Evanston, IL 60201
Telephone (847) 328-5361
Fax (847) 328-5049
www.TherapyEd.com

Preface

TherapyEd's *Speech-Language Pathology: Review and Study Guide* is designed to assist U.S. and internationally educated candidates in their preparation for the Praxis II: Speech-Language Pathology Examination. This *Review and Study Guide* provides a comprehensive overview of the depth and breadth of current speech-language pathology practice according to the field's seminal textbooks, the American Speech-Language-Hearing Association's (ASHA's) *Scope of Practice of Speech-Language Pathology*, ASHA's *Code of Ethics* and ASHA's *Practice Policy Documents*. This review text can be helpful to practitioners who are new to the field, those who are changing practice areas and/or those initiating a new role (i.e., clinical supervisor).

The text chapters cover all of the practice domains established by the most current ASHA-commissioned survey of speech-language pathology practice. While the text authors or contributors did not have access to an actual examination or to specific examination items, all chapter content and the computer-based examinations are based on the authors' critical review of recent publications and the textbooks and research articles that are likely to be foundational for the examination. Because the Speech-Language Pathology Examination items cover the entirety of the speech-language pathology profession, information that is foundational to entry-level speech-language pathology practice (i.e., anatomy, physiology, language acquisition, research methods, evidence-based practice and practice standards) is provided. This solid foundation is required to clinically reason through examination items and ensure that the exam candidate acquires what ASHA refers to as the "understanding of essential content and current practices" in speech-language pathology.

Specific methods of evaluation and intervention are provided in chapters organized according to communicative disorder diagnoses across the lifespan. Appropriate references are made across chapters when applicable, in order to provide a well-rounded approach to the field of speech-language pathology. This holistic, integrative approach allows for in-depth coverage while eliminating redundancy and reductionism. References for sources that served as the foundation for text content are provided at the end of each chapter.

Each chapter in this *Review and Study Guide* is presented in an outline format that is easy to read and provides a helpful guide for organizing a study plan. Upon reviewing each chapter's outline, the exam candidate will be able to assess his/her level of comfort with, and mastery of, each content area. Identification of areas of strength and weakness can bolster confidence and help focus studying in an efficient and effective manner. This text is not a substitute for primary resources such as classroom lectures and course textbooks. By first using this text, however, the exam candidate will not spend time extensively studying information already known. Rather, specific areas in which further knowledge is required will be identified, and appropriate study time can be planned. Strategies for effective examination preparation and successful test-taking and opportunities to practice their use via three computer-based examinations are provided.

Completion of this text's simulated examinations will help exam candidates evaluate their preparedness for the Speech-Language Pathology Examination. Consistent with the Speech-Language Pathology Examination format, this text's examination items are designed to test mastery of professional knowledge by asking the candidate to apply this knowledge to practice situations. Detailed explanations are provided to help exam candidates understand why one answer is considered the best response and the others are incorrect.

It is the authors' wish that this comprehensive review manual be of the utmost help to the reader, whether preparing for the Speech-Language Pathology Examination or transitioning into a new area of clinical practice. As speech-language pathology is always evolving, due in part to continuous efforts by many wonderful clinicians and researchers, this book shall be updated to reflect new trends and information within the field as they are revealed. By utilizing this approach, the authors hope this review book remains a constant source of information for all readers, present and future.

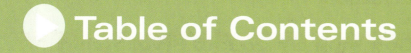
Table of Contents

Section I: Foundational Knowledge for Speech-Language Pathology Practice

Chapter 1: Anatomy and Physiology of Communication and Swallowing 3

Chapter 2: Acoustics 47

Chapter 3: Language Acquisition: Preverbal and Early Language 79

Chapter 4: Research, Evidence-Based Practice and Tests and Measurements 91

Chapter 5: The Practice of Speech-Language Pathology 103

Section II: Developmental Communication Disorders

Chapter 6: Speech Sound Disorders in Children 139

Chapter 7: Language Disorders in Young Children 167

Chapter 8: Spoken Language Disorders in School-Age Populations 193

Chapter 9: Written Language Disorders in the School-Age Population 209

Chapter 10: Autism Spectrum Disorders 225

Chapter 11: Stuttering and Other Fluency Disorders 241

Section III: Acquired Communication Disorders

Chapter 12: Acquired Language Disorders: Aphasia, Right-Hemisphere Disorders and Neurodegenerative Syndromes......255

Chapter 13: Motor Speech Disorders......299

Section IV: Structural Communication and Swallowing Disorders

Chapter 14: Cleft Palate and Craniofacial Anomalies......331

Chapter 15: Voice Disorders in Children and Adults......343

Chapter 16: Dysphagia: Swallowing and Swallowing Disorders......363

Section V: Special Considerations in Speech-Language Pathology Practice

Chapter 17: Augmentative and Alternative Communication......393

Chapter 18: Audiology and Hearing Impairment......409

Section VI: Computer Simulated Examinations

Chapter 19: Preparing for the Speech-Language Pathology Examination...439

Chapter 20: Computer Simulated Examinations......455

Examination A......456

Examination B......518

Examination C......581

Index......645

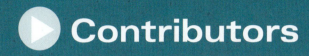
Contributors

Jean E. Andruski, PhD
Associate Professor
Department of Communication Sciences and Disorders
Wayne State University
Detroit, Michigan

Nina Capone Singleton, PhD, CCC-SLP
Associate Professor
Department of Speech-Language Pathology
Seton Hall University
South Orange, New Jersey

Derek Eugene Daniels, PhD, CCC-SLP
Associate Professor
Department of Communication Sciences and Disorders
Wayne State University
Detroit, Michigan

Sandra Laing Gillam, PhD, CCC-SLP
ASHA Fellow
Professor
Department of Communicative Disorders and Deaf Education
Utah State University
Logan, Utah

Donald M. Goldberg, PhD, CCC-SLP/A, FAAA, LSLS Cert AVT
Professor, College of Wooster
Staff Consultant, Hearing Implant Program
Head and Neck Institute–Cleveland Clinic
Cleveland, Ohio

Margaret Greenwald, PhD, CCC-SLP
Associate Professor
Department of Communication Sciences and Disorders
Wayne State University
Detroit, Michigan

Michelle Gutmann, PhD, CCC-SLP
Clinical Associate Professor
Department of Speech, Language and Hearing Sciences
Purdue University
West Lafayette, Indiana

Sue T. Hale, MCD, CCC-SLP
ASHA Fellow
Associate Professor and Director of Clinical Education
Department of Hearing and Speech Sciences
Vanderbilt University
Nashville, Tennessee

Charles W. Haynes, EdD, CCC-SLP
Professor
Department of Communication Sciences and Disorders
School of Health and Rehabilitation Sciences
MGH Institute of Health Professions
Boston, Massachusetts

James T. Heaton, PhD
Professor
Department of Communication Sciences and Disorders
School of Health and Rehabilitation Sciences
MGH Institute of Health Professions
Assistant Professor, Surgery
Harvard Medical School, Massachusetts General Hospital
Boston, Massachusetts

Pamela E. Hook, PhD
Professor Emerita
Department of Communication Sciences and Disorders
School of Health and Rehabilitation Sciences
MGH Institute of Health Professions
Boston, Massachusetts

Alex F. Johnson, PhD, CCC-SLP
ASHA Fellow
Provost and Vice President for Academic Affairs
Professor
Department of Communication Sciences and Disorders
School of Health and Rehabilitation Sciences
MGH Institute of Health Professions
Boston, Massachusetts

Gail B. Kempster, PhD, CCC-SLP
ASHA Fellow
Professor
Associate Chair, Program Director of Speech-Language Pathology
Department of Communication Disorders and Sciences
Rush University/Rush University Medical Center
Chicago, Illinois

Ann W. Kummer, PhD, CCC-SLP
ASHA Fellow
Senior Director, Division of Speech-Language Pathology
Cincinnati Children's Hospital Medical Center
Professor of Clinical Pediatrics, Professor of Otolaryngology
University of Cincinnati Medical Center
Cincinnati, OH

Gregory L. Lof, PhD, CCC-SLP
ASHA Fellow
Chair, Professor
Department of Communication Sciences and Disorders
School of Health and Rehabilitation Sciences
MGH Institute of Health Professions
Boston, Massachusetts

Craig W. Newman, PhD, CCC-A
ASHA Fellow
Section Head, Audiology
Head and Neck Institute – Cleveland Clinic
Professor
Cleveland Clinic Lerner College of Medicine of Case Western Reserve University
Cleveland, Ohio

Marjorie Nicholas, PhD, CCC-SLP
Associate Chair, Professor
Department of Communication Sciences and Disorders
School of Health and Rehabilitation Sciences
Associate Director
PhD in Rehabilitation Sciences
Center for Interprofessional Studies and Innovation
MGH Institute of Health Professions
Boston, Massachusetts

Gail J. Richard, PhD, CCC-SLP
ASHA Fellow
Director, Autism Center
Professor Emeritus
Department of Communication Disorders and Sciences
Eastern Illinois University
Charleston, Illinois

Sharon A. Sandridge, PhD
Director, Clinical Services in Audiology
Co-Director, Tinnitus Management Clinic and Audiology Research Laboratory
Cleveland Clinic
Cleveland, Ohio

Brian B. Shulman, PhD, CCC-SLP, BCS-CL, FASAHP
ASHA Fellow
Dean, School of Health and Medical Sciences
Professor of Speech-Language Pathology
Seton Hall University
South Orange, New Jersey

Vicki Simonsmeier, MS, CCC-SLP/Aud
Clinical Coordinator
Center for Persons with Disabilities
Utah State University
Logan, Utah

Zachary M. Smith, MS, CF-SLP
Speech-Language Pathologist, Clinical Fellow
Department of Communication Sciences and Disorders
School of Health and Rehabilitation Sciences
MGH Institute of Health Professions
Boston, Massachusetts

Barbara C. Sonies, PhD, CCC-SLP, BCS-S
ASHA Fellow
Dysphagia Consultant, NIH, DRM and NHGRI
Research Professor
Department of Hearing and Speech Sciences
University of Maryland
College Park, Maryland

Greg Turner, PhD, CCC-SLP
Professor
Department of Communication Disorders and Social Work
University of Central Missouri
Warrensburg, Missouri

Sofia Vallila-Rohter, PhD, CCC-SLP
Assistant Professor
Department of Communication Sciences and Disorders
School of Health and Rehabilitation Sciences
MGH Institute of Health Professions
Boston, Massachusetts

Maggie Watson, PhD, CCC-SLP
Professor
Department of Communicative Disorders
University of Wisconsin, Stevens Point
Stevens Point, Wisconsin

Amy L. Weiss, PhD, CCC-SLP, BCS-CL
ASHA Fellow
Professor, Graduate Program Coordinator
Department of Communicative Disorders
The University of Rhode Island
Kingston, Rhode Island

Margaret M. Wilson, MA, CCC-SLP
Speech Pathologist II
Division of Speech-Language Pathology
Cincinnati Children's Hospital Medical Center
Cincinnati, Ohio

Acknowledgments

In organizing and producing a comprehensive review text for speech-language pathology subject matter, it was essential to involve many valued partners. First, our team at TherapyEd has been invaluable at each step of the way. Dr. Ray Siegelman, Doug Pendry and Tom Pendry have lent their knowledge and experience from their physical therapy and occupational therapy texts to the development of this review guide, which parallels many of their great innovations in test preparation and comprehensive review books.

Our predecessors in this journey, authors Dr. Susan O'Sullivan, Dr. Ray Siegelman and Dr. Rita-Fleming-Castaldy have served as excellent role models for us. Also, most valued partners in this work have been our students, Laura Dorner and Zachary Smith. Laura helped us at the beginning of the project and became known to the contributors in the earliest phases of work. Zach has been a remarkable editor, question developer and organizer for the past 2 years. Their combined and sustained effort has been invaluable.

This book has many important contributors covering the spectrum of the discipline. How fortunate we are to have these great outstanding colleagues as collaborators.

Finally, special thanks go to those speech-language pathologists who are entering the field, preparing for the examination or using this guide to prepare for a new area of practice. You were the inspiration for this work.

GL and AJ

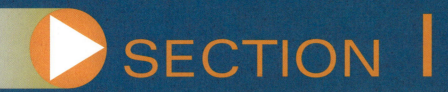

SECTION I

Foundational Knowledge for Speech-Language Pathology Practice

Section Outline

- **Chapter 1:** Anatomy and Physiology of Communication and Swallowing, 3
- **Chapter 2:** Acoustics, 47
- **Chapter 3:** Language Acquisition: Preverbal and Early Language, 79
- **Chapter 4:** Research, Evidence-Based Practice and Tests and Measurements, 91
- **Chapter 5:** The Practice of Speech-Language Pathology, 103

1

Anatomy and Physiology of Communication and Swallowing

JAMES T. HEATON, PhD
AND SOFIA VALLILA-ROHTER, PhD

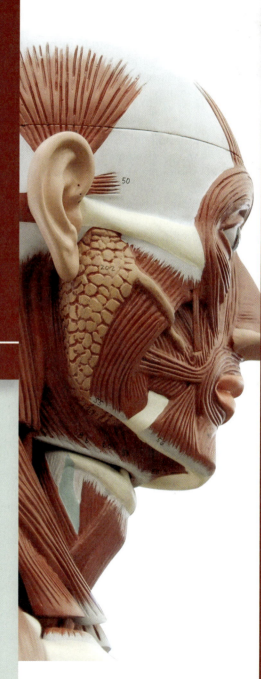

Chapter Outline

- The Study of Speech, Language, and Swallowing, 4
- Neuroanatomy and Neurophysiology for Speech, Language and Swallowing, 8
- Cerebral Blood Flow, 30
- Respiration, 32
- Anatomy of Phonation and Swallowing, 35
- References, 46

The Study of Speech, Language, and Swallowing

Areas of Study

1. Anatomy: the bodily structure of an organism and its parts.
2. Physiology: the study of normal function of bodily structure and parts.
   a. Electrophysiology: the study of the bioelectrical nature of cells.
   b. Neurophysiology: the study of the nervous system's function.
3. Kinesiology: the study of physiological, mechanical and psychological mechanisms of movement.
4. Audiology: the study of hearing disorders, evaluation, and rehabilitation.
5. Phonology: the study of how sound is used across languages to convey meaning.
6. Psychology: the study of mental processes and behavior.

Figure 1-1 Planes of Section and Directional Nomenclature

Basic Elements of Anatomy

1. There is a hierarchic organization to the body's form and function.
   a. Atoms: the basic units of matter that, it is believed, cannot be divided into smaller stable forms of matter.
   b. Molecules: two or more atoms bound together by the sharing of electrons.
   c. Tissues: integrated cells from the same developmental origin that together carry out a common function.
   d. Organs: structures made of two or more tissues that together perform a common function.
   e. Organ systems are formed by multiple organs that together perform a particular body function (e.g., muscular system, skeletal system).
      (1) Each anatomical element described is composed of contributions from earlier components of the hierarchy (e.g., tissues are made up of multiple cell types).
2. The main tissue types for animals are epithelial, connective, muscular and nervous (detailed below).

Parts of the Body

1. Planes of section and directional nomenclature (Figure 1-1).
   a. Anatomy is typically described from a particular perspective or plane of section. When examining the body as a whole, the frame of reference for planes and directional terms is the "standard anatomical position," which is the body standing upright with the arms at the sides and palms facing forward. Other planes and directional terms are in relation to the long axis of a particular structure or the relative position or movement of two or more structures.
   b. Planes of section.
      (1) Frontal (coronal) plane: divides the body vertically into anterior (front) and posterior (back) parts.
      (2) Sagittal (median) plane: divides the body vertically into right and left sides.
         (a) When the right/left dividing line is off from the midline, the plane can be called parasagittal or lateral.
      (3) Horizontal (axial) plane: divides the body along the horizon into upper and lower parts.
         (a) This is the same as the transverse plane, which divides a structure perpendicular to its long axis (e.g., cutting a loaf of bread into slices).
   c. Directional nomenclature.
      (1) Superior or cranial is toward the head, whereas inferior or caudal is toward the feet.
      (2) Anterior or ventral is toward the front, whereas posterior or dorsal is toward the back.
         (a) Rostral is similar to anterior, but means toward the front and upper part of the body, such as the location of the nose.
      (3) Medial is toward the body midline, whereas lateral is away from the midline (e.g., the big toe

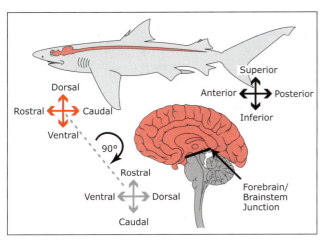

Figure 1-2 Directional Terminology for the Human Brain

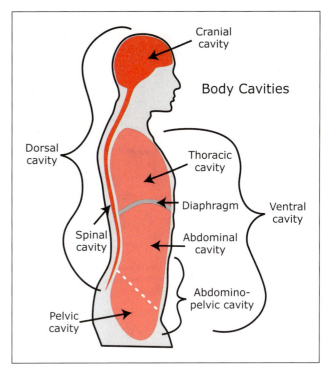

Figure 1-3 Body Cavities

is on the medial edge of the foot, and the ear is on the lateral surface of the head).
(4) Proximal is toward the trunk or origin of a part, whereas distal is away from the trunk or the origin of a part (e.g., the proximal end of the humerus bone attaches to the scapula at the shoulder, and the distal end articulates with the ulna and radius bones at the elbow).
(5) Flexing decreases a joint angle, whereas extending increases a joint angle.
　(a) For the head and neck, tucking the chin toward the sternum is flexion, and moving the back of the head toward the shoulder blades is extension.
d. Directional terminology for the human brain (Figure 1-2).
　(a) Because the forebrain is turned 90° "forward" in the skull relative to the rest of the nervous system and body, the orienting names for the brain need to be adjusted relative to the body (e.g., the dorsal surface of the brain resides at the superior aspect of the body).
2. Body cavities (Figure 1-3).
a. Major body cavities include the dorsal cavity and ventral cavity.
b. Dorsal cavity is formed by the skull and vertebral column, containing the brain and spinal cord, respectively.
c. Ventral cavity is subdivided into the thoracic and abdominal cavities, which are divided from each other by the diaphragm muscle located inferior to the lungs.
　(1) Thoracic cavity contains the heart, lungs, trachea, esophagus, large blood vessels and nerves.
　(2) Abdominal cavity contains the digestive system from the stomach to the colon, as well as the kidneys and adrenal glands.
　　(a) The inferior-most portion of the abdomen located within the pelvic skeleton is called the pelvic cavity and contains most of the urogenital system and rectum.

Tissue Types

1. Epithelial layers (Figure 1-4).
a. Epithelial layers are tightly joined cells that form coverings for the exterior body surface, as well as the interior surfaces on organs, cavities and aerodigestive tract.
b. These layers are categorized according to how many cell layers they have (single vs. multiple) and cell shape.
c. Simple epithelial layers of a single cell thickness.
　(1) Ciliated epithelium: lines the airway from the bronchi through the nasal cavities, paranasal sinuses, and false vocal folds (but not the true vocal folds).
　(2) Ciliated pseudostratified columnar epithelium: lines the trachea and the upper respiratory tract.
　　(a) Respiratory epithelium is technically a single cell layer attached to a basement membrane (which underlies all epithelial and endothelial layers). It includes multiple cell

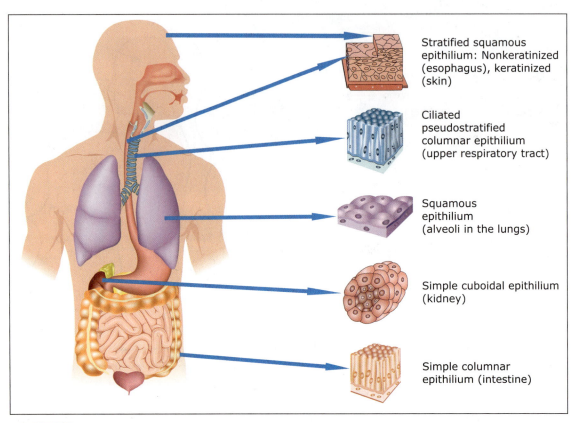

Figure 1-4 Differing Types of Epithelial Layers

types such as basal cells (for repairing damage) and goblet cells (which secrete mucus).
  (b) The upwardly (cranially) beating cilia of respiratory epithelium in the trachea transport particles caught on the epithelial surface toward our pharynx. One can then swallow or spit them out and maintain a clean airway.
 (3) Squamous epithelium: lines alveoli in the lungs and interior surface (or endothelium) of lymph and blood vessels.
 (4) Cuboidal epithelium: lines the kidney tubules and glands.
  d. Compound epithelial layers of multiple cell thickness offer more protection against friction/abrasion, microbial invasions and desiccation (drying out) than do simple epithelium.
  e. Compound epithelial layers of a multiple cell thickness.
 (1) Nonkeratinized stratified squamous epithelium ("mucosa"): lines the mouth, pharynx, esophagus, true vocal folds, rectum and some of the female reproductive tract.
 (2) Keratinized stratified squamous epithelium: forms the skin, and has an outer layer of dead cells (rich in the protein keratin) that provides a tough, waterproof barrier.
 (3) Stratified cuboidal and columnar epithelia: relatively rare and often line ducts within glands, but are found in some other locations as well.
2. Connective tissue.
  a. Connective tissue connects and supports other tissues.
  b. Loose connective tissue: contains loosely woven collagen and elastin fibers that hold organs in place while still allowing a generous range of movement.
  c. Fibrous connective tissue: contains densely packed collagen fibers that bind muscle to bone or other regions of muscle (i.e., tendons) or bind skeletal components together (i.e., ligaments) to limit range of movement.
  d. Adipose tissue (fat): stores metabolic fuel in the form of free fatty acids.
  e. Cartilage.
 (1) A pliable tissue that comes in a wide range of density and pliability to serve different purposes.
 (2) Fibrocartilage is white in color and contains a mixture of cartilage and collagen (type I).
    (a) It is found in the pubic symphysis, intervertebral discs and in some joints, including the knee and temporomandibular joint (TMJ).
 (3) Hyaline cartilage is bluish-white in color, firm and very elastic.
    (a) It helps maintain a patent airway by forming rings in the bronchi, partial rings in the trachea and most cartilages of the larynx.

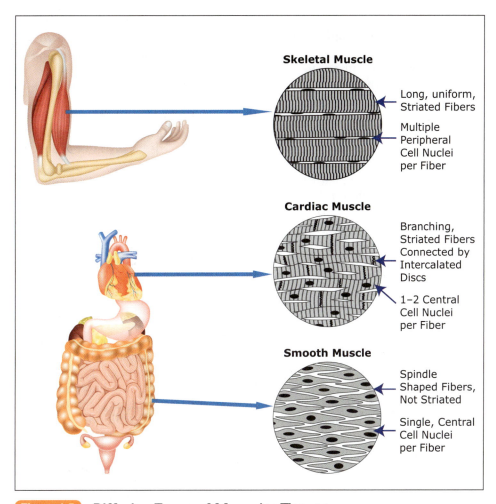

Figure 1-5 Differing Types of Muscular Tissues

      (b) It covers the articular surfaces of bones and forms the cartilaginous portions of ribs (portion attached to the sternum).
  (4) Elastic cartilage contains many yellow elastic fibers in addition to collagen (type II) and elastin, giving it great flexibility.
      (a) It is found in the epiglottis of the larynx and pinnae of the ears.
 f. Bone.
  (1) Bone is a dense tissue that is strong and hard due to crystalline minerals in compact regions.
  (2) Bone has a spongy core that also contains marrow for blood cell production.
 g. Blood.
  (1) Blood is a suspension of cells in a liquid matrix.
  (2) Transports gasses, nutrients, chemicals and waste products to/from cells throughout the body.
3. Muscular tissue (Figure 1-5).
 a. Muscular tissue is tissue composed of cells (fibers) that serve the function of movement and generation of force.
 b. Muscle cells are classified as skeletal, cardiac or smooth.
  (1) In all three classes, the cells are relatively long, with alternating layers of partially overlapping contractile filaments organized lengthwise.
 c. When stimulated, muscle cells increase the amount of filament overlap along their length, causing them to shorten.
 d. Skeletal muscle.
  (1) Is striated and under voluntary control.
  (2) Has a repeating pattern of partially overlapping filaments, giving it a striped or striated appearance when viewed under a microscope.
  (3) Is the longest muscle cell type, with uniform diameter and multiple nuclei per cell (due to the fusion of multiple cells in early development).
  (4) Is attached to the skeletal frame by tendons.
  (5) Generates voluntary body movements.
  (6) Multiple fiber types have different forms of contractile filaments, determining how quickly they contract and their relative resistance to fatigue.

e. Cardiac muscle.
  (1) Cardiac muscle is striated and contracts involuntarily.
  (2) Found in the heart wall and contracts to propel blood through the heart chambers (two atria and two ventricles).
  (3) Fibers are striated like skeletal muscle, but have only one or two nuclei and have branching patterns that fuse with one another at their ends.
  (4) Fibers are interconnected along their length by intercalated discs that pass electrical impulses from cell to cell (causing contraction).
    (a) This mechanically binds cells together, thus synchronizing the contraction of adjacent heart walls.
  (5) Specialized cardiac cells form nodes that act as internal pacemakers for the other cells, initiating about 60–100 contractions (beats) per minute without neuronal innervation.
    (a) Nervous system input can reduce (parasympathetic) or increase (sympathetic) heart rate, but is not required to generate resting heart rhythm.
f. Smooth muscle.
  (1) Smooth muscle is not striated and contracts involuntarily.
  (2) Fibers have a single nucleus and are spindle shaped (widest in the middle) with staggered patterns of overlapping filaments, making them homogenous in appearance (not striated).
  (3) Specialized for relatively slow, sustained contraction in the internal organs, blood vessels, lens and iris of the eye, and hair follicles.
  (4) Fibers contract in response to many different stimuli depending on location/function.
    (a) Hormones, endogenous chemicals and ingested chemicals/drugs.
    (b) Stretch and gasses in the airway and blood vessels.
    (c) Motoneuron input from peripheral nerves.
    (d) Via local circuit neurons intrinsic pacemaker cells for rhythmic contraction.
4. Nervous tissue.
  a. Nervous tissue comprises multiple cell types that together receive, integrate, interpret and direct the response to internal and environmental stimuli.
    (1) Neurons are cells specialized for receiving and transmitting information over long distances in the form of electrochemical impulses (action potentials [APs]).
      (a) Neurons respond to a wide range of stimuli (e.g., mechanical, noxious, chemical, thermal, light) either directly or in conjunction with transducer cells (e.g., rods/cones in retina, acoustic and vestibular hair cells, touch receptors, etc.).
      (b) Within the brain and spinal cord, neurons have multiple processes extending from their cell body, with dendrites that are highly receptive to chemical signals (input) and an axon that can extend long distances to send signals (output) to other neurons or drive the activity of glands and muscles to control behavior.
    (2) Support cells (glial cells) include multiple cell types that provide structural support, form protective barriers, clear waste materials and electrically insulate axons to facilitate AP transmission.

Neuroanatomy and Neurophysiology for Speech, Language and Swallowing

Nervous System (NS)

1. A complex information-processing system that enables interaction with the environment for survival and reproduction.

NS Cell Types

1. Neurons (Figure 1-6).
  a. Neurons are cells specialized for information reception and transmission.
    (1) Information processing, learning and memory are accomplished by changes in the strength and number of connections among neurons.
  b. Neurons have a cell body (soma) containing a single nucleus, along with one or more extensions called processes or "poles" from the soma.
    (1) Dendrites: processes specialized for receiving signals from other neurons or environmental stimuli.
    (2) Axons: processes specialized for transmitting or propagating APs in order to communicate with other neurons, contract muscle or cause glands to secrete.
      (a) APs originate at the axon's trigger zone, located at the initial segment of the axon.
  c. Neurons can be classified as multipolar, bipolar or unipolar based on how many "poles" or processes extend from their cell body.

Neuroanatomy and Neurophysiology for Speech, Language and Swallowing

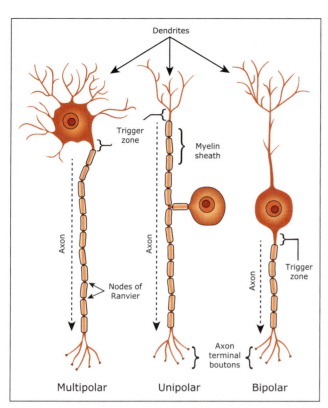

Figure 1-6 Illustration of Multiple Neuronal Types

    (1) Multipolar neurons: have multiple dendrites and a single axon extending a relatively far distance from their soma.
        (a) Are found throughout the central nervous system (CNS; brain and spinal cord).
        (b) These include motor neurons, which have axons extending sometimes several feet from the CNS to muscles via nerves in the peripheral nervous system (PNS).
    (2) Bipolar neurons: have two processes (poles) extending from the soma, with one serving as an axon and the other usually serving as a dendrite (an exception is bipolar cells of the cochlea's spiral ganglia, which have two axon extensions from their soma).
        (a) Are found in PNS sensory pathways for special senses of the head (i.e., taste, olfaction, vision, hearing and vestibular sensation).
    (3) Unipolar neurons: have a single, fused process, the distal-most portion of which serves as a dendrite, while the remainder serves as an axon.
        (a) Are found in PNS sensory pathways for senses represented throughout the body, including fine touch, vibration, proprioception, pressure, pain and temperature.
        (b) These are also called pseudounipolar neurons.
  d. Most axons are electrically insulated from surrounding tissues/fluid by a coating of glial cells called a myelin sheath.
    (1) Myelinating cells have a high lipid (fat) content, which gives a white appearance to fiber pathways (like white fat in milk).
  e. Axons terminate in a branching pattern onto their target(s), with small enlargements or swelled locations at their very ends called terminal boutons.
    (1) Boutons contain neurotransmitter for chemical signaling.
2. Glia.
  a. *Glia* is a label for multiple cells types that play supportive yet critical roles in neuronal function.
  b. Glia physically support neurons, remove metabolic waste products, and prevent toxic buildup of chemicals used in neural signaling.
  c. Glia help form the barrier between neurons and circulating blood in the CNS (blood-brain barrier) by covering the capillaries and acting as a filter.
  d. Glia also respond to neuronal injury by removing dead cells and forming neural scar tissue.
  e. One of the most important glial cell functions is the formation of myelin sheaths on axons, which provide electrical insulation and thereby increase the speed of APs (see the next section).
    (1) Oligodendrocytes myelinate axons in the CNS.
    (2) Schwann cells myelinate axons in the PNS.

Neural Signaling

1. Resting and APs.
  a. Neurons have a cell membrane that prevents the flow of particles into and out of the cell.
    (1) The membrane is a phospholipid bilayer with channels spanning across the membrane that open/close to determine the flow of particles.
  b. By controlling the flow of charged particles (ions) across the membrane, neurons are able generate electrical potentials used in neural signaling.
  c. At rest, neurons maintain a resting potential of about −65 mV on the inside of the cell compared to the outside of the cell.
    (1) This negative potential keeps the neuron prepared to "fire" or send a signal down the length of its axon.
  d. The resting potential is primarily caused by a high concentration of sodium ions (Na^+) on the outside of the neuronal membrane and negatively charged organic molecules (A^-) on the inside of the membrane.

(1) The high concentration of Na⁺ ions outside the cell relative to inside the cell leads to an inward directed concentration gradient (Na⁺ ions want to move into the cell to a region of lower Na⁺ concentration).

(2) A strong electrical gradient arises from the A⁻ ions inside the cell. Their negative charge attracts the Na+ ions toward the inside of the cell.

(3) If Na⁺ was able to flow freely, it would enter the neuron due to both concentration and electrical gradients. By default, Na⁺ channels are closed, preventing such free flow.

e. Two main types of Na⁺ channels are selectively open during neural signaling.

(1) Chemically gated sodium channels are located on the dendrites and soma of neurons.

(a) These channels act as receptors that open in response to chemical signals (neurotransmitters) released by other neurons.

(b) When chemically gated sodium channels open, it allows a brief influx of Na⁺.

(c) Because receptors are at the locations of contact between neurons, called *synapses*, this inward Na⁺ flow is called a synaptic potential (see next section).

(d) The influx of Na⁺ causes a local depolarization of the membrane away from the resting potential (i.e., the neuron becomes less negative).

(e) These synaptic potentials contribute to the overall charge of the neuron cell body. They can add up to trigger or inhibit an AP.

(2) Voltage-gated sodium channels are located on the axon membrane.

(a) Summed synaptic potentials can bring voltage-gated channels at the axon trigger zone to threshold, thus causing them to open.

(b) Once voltage-gated channels open they allow an influx of Na⁺ that causes adjacent voltage-gated channels to open.

(c) The process continues down the entire length of the axon as an AP (Figure 1-7).

(d) Most axons are electrically insulated along a vast majority of their length by a sheath of myelin.

- There are short noninsulated gaps between myelinating cells, called nodes of Ranvier where voltage-gated channels are concentrated (refer to Figure 1-6).
- This enables APs to jump along the axon from gap to gap (called saltatory conduction) at speeds much faster than nonmyelinated axons, where voltage-gated channels must sequentially open along the entire axon surface/length.

(e) Myelinated axons propagate APs at a rate of about six times the axon diameter.

- The fastest myelinated axons are about 20 μm in diameter, and transmit at 120 m/sec.
- Axons that are not myelinated tend to be small in diameter and transmit at only about 2–8 m/sec.

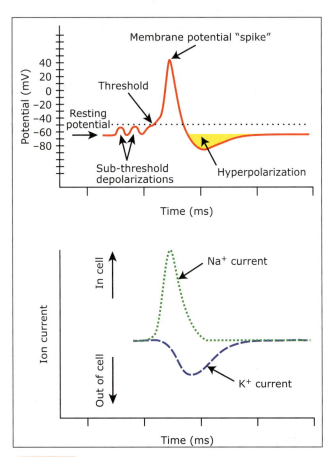

Figure 1-7 Summary of Action Potentials

f. Action potentials are all-or-none events because threshold for opening voltage-gated channels is either reached or it is not.

(1) It takes about 15 mV of depolarizing Na⁺ influx at the trigger zone to reach threshold for opening voltage-gated channels and to initiate an AP.

(2) If synaptic potentials do not adequately depolarize the neuron, then these subthreshold potentials quickly dissipate and the neuron returns to the resting potential (refer to Figure 1-7).

(3) If threshold is reached, then the strong Na⁺ influx caused by voltage-gated channel activation rapidly spreads down the axon as nearby

channels open one after the next (imagine a line of falling dominoes).
g. When an AP occurs, it causes a brief (1 ms) electrical "spike" to propagate down the axon at a uniform speed and magnitude, regardless of the input strength.
 (1) The amount of stimulation a neuron receives is therefore represented by its AP firing rate (how rapidly the APs occur back-to-back), rather than the strength of individual APs (which are all the same "size").
 (2) There is a temporal separation of APs (see below), which limits their firing rates to about 100–300 Hz.
h. The voltage-gated channels allowing Na^+ to enter the neuron during an AP are open for only a very brief amount of time (about 0.5 ms) before rapidly becoming inactivated, stopping the flow of Na^+.
 (1) Na^+ inactivation limits the duration of the AP's positive spike, and makes the AP brief in duration.
 (2) During Na^+ inactivation, it is impossible to open these voltage-gated channels, causing an absolute refractory period that forces the separation of AP from one another in time.
i. During Na^+ inactivation, there are potassium ion (K^+) channels that open and cause an outward current of K^+ from the neuron.
 (1) K^+ is driven out of the neuron by both a concentration gradient and an electrical gradient. These are the same two types of forces pushing Na^+ into the neuron during the AP spike.
 (2) This efflux of K^+ causes a brief period of hyperpolarization immediately after the action potential spike (refer to shaded area in Figure 1-7).
 (3) During this period, it is relatively more difficult to bring the neuron to threshold because of the hyperpolarized state (compared to the resting potential).
 (4) Only very strong stimuli can overcome hyperpolarization during this relative refractory period and drive neurons at their maximal firing rate.
j. After an AP, the resting potential is restored by the active transport of Na^+ to the outside and K^+ to the inside of the cell membrane by sodium-potassium pumps embedded like channels in the cell membrane.

2. Synaptic and end-plate potentials.
a. Neurons communicate with other neurons, muscles and glands via the release of chemical signals (neurotransmitters) onto the surface of their targets.
 (1) These chemical signals are released from terminal boutons into the synaptic clefts (gaps) between axon terminals and their targets, generating synaptic potentials when the signals are received by receptors.
b. Small quantities of transmitter are released by boutons when APs arrive at axon terminals.
 (1) Terminal boutons contain tiny spheres called synaptic vesicles that store neurotransmitter. They coat the inside surface of the presynaptic membrane, poised to release their neurotransmitter payload into the synaptic gap.
 (2) When an AP reaches a bouton, it opens voltage-gated calcium ion (Ca^+) channels, causing an influx of Ca^+.
 (3) In the presence of Ca^+, the synaptic vesicles fuse with the cell membrane and squirt their neurotransmitter into the synaptic gap through a process called *exocytosis*.
c. Chemically gated channels serve as receptors on the postsynaptic membrane of target cells.
 (1) Released neurotransmitters can act on these receptors as agonists that open channels, or antagonists that block channel opening.
 (2) Once a receptor channel is opened by a neurotransmitter, the result to the target cell is depolarizing (exciting), hyperpolarizing (inhibiting) or affecting the cell through second-messenger pathways, which are slower but longer lasting than the opening/closing of chemically gated channels.
  (a) Acetylcholine (ACh), is a commonly occurring neurotransmitter, which normally stimulates muscle cells to contract (excitatory).
  (b) Motor neurons (motoneurons) contact muscle cells (fibers) at specialized end-plate regions where the fibers have numerous ACh receptors. The contact points of axon terminal boutons with the muscle cell end-plates form neuromuscular junctions, where the boutons release ACh and depolarize the muscle cells, causing them to contract (shorten).
  (c) ACh receptor antagonists can be used in anesthesia, for example, to block the action of ACh and relax muscles.
  (d) Exocytosis can also be blocked in other ways. Botulinum toxin can be used as a medication to intentionally prevent exocytosis of ACh. When botulinum (Botox) is injected into a muscle, it enters the terminal boutons of the innervating motor nerve, permanently inactivates proteins critical to the process of vesicle fusion with the cell membrane, and thereby stops the release of ACh. The injected muscle is weakened or

even paralyzed for several months until new boutons have time to sprout from the axon terminals and restore ACh release.
d. Neurotransmitter rapidly clears the synaptic cleft by passive diffusion, active reuptake (by the boutons) and/or enzymatic destruction in order to prevent a prolonged effect of released transmitter (e.g., to prepare the synapse for new signal transmission).
e. The process of chemical signaling introduces a short synaptic delay of about 2 ms, the time delay between the arrival of the AP in the presynaptic neuron and the receptor response in the target cell.
f. The impact of a synaptic potential (receptor response) on the postsynaptic cell will depend on whether it is an inhibitory or excitatory response, where the input is received and what other inputs the cell receives at about the same time.
  (1) ACh released at the skeletal neuromuscular junction is always excitatory (depolarizing) and normally causes at least some contraction (twitch tension) in the targeted fibers.
     (a) Rapidly repeated ACh release may not allow the muscle fibers time to relax between twitches, causing the contractions to fuse together into a sustained tetanic contraction.
  (2) The reception of neurotransmitter from one neuron to another will cause a synaptic potential that is graded in nature, meaning that the size of the potential depends on the stimulus.
     (a) This is different from the all-or-none event of APs.
  (3) Synaptic potentials sum together in time and location across the dendrites and cell body of a neuron.
     (a) Generating an AP in the target neuron usually requires multiple, simultaneous excitatory inputs.
  (4) Excitatory synaptic potentials may generate an action potential if they bring the axon hillock (refer to "trigger zone" from Figure 1-6) to threshold, which is a depolarization of approximately 15 mV.

Central and Peripheral NS

1. In the developing embryo, a neural tube forms that eventually becomes the brain and spinal cord, referred to as the central nervous system (CNS).
   a. The PNS comprises peripheral nerves, in communication with the CNS, that stem from neural crest cells in the developing embryo. Therefore, the distinction between CNS and PNS is not arbitrary, but rather relates to their different embryological origins.

2. Two important differences between CNS and PNS include regenerative capability and exposure to blood circulation.
   a. CNS neurons have little regenerative capabilities due to their inherent tendency to retract their processes and/or die after injury rather than survive and sprout new growth. Their regeneration is actively inhibited by chemicals released from surrounding glia and glial scars.
   b. In contrast, when axons are injured in PNS motor or sensory nerves, they send numerous sprouts from the site of injury in a robust attempt to regenerate. This is actively facilitated by Schwann cells and the nerves' connective tissues.
   c. Neurons and glia within the CNS are limited in what they can receive from circulating blood due to the blood-brain barrier (BBB). The BBB is formed primarily by tight junctions between capillary endothelial cells in the CNS, which limit what molecules can diffuse from circulating blood.
   d. In contrast, neurons and glia in the PNS receive a similar diffusion of blood-borne molecules as the rest of the body.

Major Divisions of the PNS

1. Somatic and autonomic NS.
   a. The PNS can be subdivided into somatic NS and autonomic NS components (refer to Figure 1-8).
   b. The somatic NS supports sensations and motor functions of the body (soma) that are consciously perceived and volitionally controlled, respectively.
     (1) It allows one to be aware of the external environment and to act on that information.
   c. The autonomic NS (also called the visceral NS) functions mostly below conscious awareness or control, regulating visceral functions such as digestion, heart rate, blood pressure, digestion, respiration, and gland secretion. It detects and acts on the body's internal environment.
     (1) The parasympathetic division of the autonomic NS helps maintain homeostasis ("rest-and-digest") through balancing functions such as respiration, blood perfusion and food digestion in relation to metabolic needs.
        (a) The efferent (outward-flowing) signals of the parasympathetic division originate from the cranial nerves and sacral region of the spinal cord, so it is also called the craniosacral division of the autonomic NS.
     (2) The sympathetic division of the autonomic NS is activated in times of perceived threat, preparing one for fight-or-flight responses by inhibiting nonessential bodily functions (like digestion),

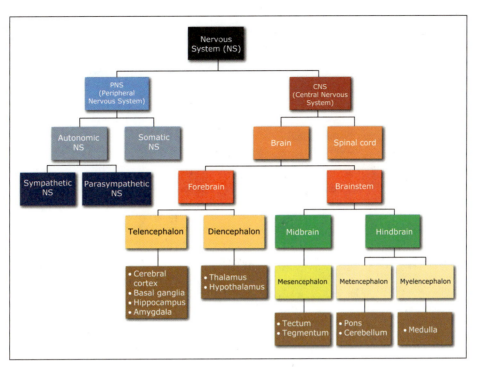

Figure 1-8 Divisions of the Human Nervous System

increasing heart rate, blood pressure, sweat production, respiratory rate, and diverting blood to the skeletal muscles in preparation for physical exertion.
   (a) The efferent signals of the sympathetic division originate from the thoracic and lumbar regions of the spinal cord, so it is also called the thoracolumbar division of the autonomic NS.
2. Cranial and spinal nerves.
   a. The CNS communicates with the body (and thereby the environment) via peripheral nerves (in the PNS), including 12 pairs of cranial nerves and 31 pairs of spinal nerves.
   b. The cranial nerves are numbered more or less according to their order of appearance on the ventral brain surface from rostral to caudal (see Figure 1-9).
   c. There are 12 pairs of cranial nerves, often referred to by Roman numerals I through XII.
   d. Cranial nerves can be composed entirely of motor axons, entirely of sensory axons, or a mixture of motor and sensory axons.
      (1) Sensory axons in cranial nerves are from bipolar or unipolar neurons with their somas clustered in peripheral ganglia at some point along on the nerve, similar to the spinal nerve dorsal root ganglia.

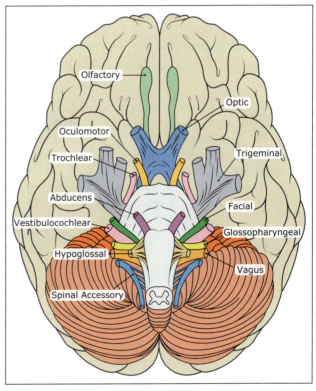

Figure 1-9 Cranial Nerves on the Ventral Surface of the Brain

Table 1-1

Cranial Nerves

		NAME	FUNCTION	SPEECH/SWALLOW CONTRIBUTION
CN I	S	Olfactory	Smell	
CN II	S	Optic	Vision	
CN III	M	Oculomotor	Eye movement, upper eyelid elevation, pupil constriction	
CN IV	M	Trochlear	Downward and lateral (midline) eye movement	
CN V	B	Trigeminal	3 major branches: ophthalmic (V1), maxillary (V2), mandibular (V3). Face sensation (V1, V2, V3), motor innervation of muscles of mastication (V3) & tensor tympani	Oral stage of swallowing: chewing, bolus sensation, dampening of internal chewing sounds
CN VI	M	Abducens	Lateral (away from midline) eye movement	
CN VII	B	Facial	Taste sensation (anterior 2/3 of tongue), motor innervation to muscles of facial expression, lacrimation, salivation	Oral stage of swallowing: taste, bolus formation. Speech: articulation
CN VIII	S	Vestibulocochlear	Hearing and vestibular sensation	Hearing, sound localization
CN IX	B	Glossopharyngeal	Taste sensation (posterior 1/3 of tongue), sensation from middle ear, upper pharynx & carotid body (blood gases and pressures), salivation (parotid), motor innervation of stylopharyngeus	Oral & pharyngeal stages of swallowing: taste, salivation pharynx elevation, gag reflex
CN X	B	Vagus	Sensation from lower pharynx, motor innervation of pharyngeal & laryngeal muscles of the soft palate, heart, lungs & digestive tract	Velum elevation, gag reflex, vocal fold tension, adduction & abduction (SLN & RLN)
CN XI	M	Spinal Accessory	Motor innervation of sternocleidomastoid and trapezius muscles	Head turning, shoulder elevation
CN XII	M	Hypoglossal	Motor innervation of intrinsic tongue muscles	Oral stage of swallowing: bolus manipulation and propulsion

(2) Motor axons in cranial nerves are from multipolar neurons clustered in the brainstem (nerves III–VII, IX, X and XII) or in the upper cervical spinal cord (nerve XI).

e. Individual cranial nerve functions are often described in terms of being afferent (sensory) vs. efferent (motor), general (body-wide) vs. special (peculiar to the head) and somatic vs. visceral (autonomic).

(1) Each cranial nerve can have several functions, including combinations of all of the above. (See Table 1-1.)

f. The spinal nerves are named in relation to the region of the vertebral column from which they exit the vertebral canal (Figure 1-10).

g. Spinal nerves all contain a mixture of motor (outward-flowing or efferent) and sensory (inward flowing or afferent) fibers at the point where they exit the vertebral column.

(1) Axons entering the spinal cord through the dorsal roots are from unipolar sensory neurons with their somas clustered in dorsal root ganglia.

(2) Axons leaving the spinal cord through the ventral roots are from multipolar lower motor neurons with their somas clustered in the ventral horns of the spinal cord.

(3) The dorsal and ventral roots converge as they travel between the vertebrae to form the 31 pairs (right and left) mixed sensory/motor spinal nerves (refer to Figure 1-10).

Central Nervous System

1. Meninges.
   a. The CNS is covered by three layers of protective membranes called the meninges (Figure 1-11).
   b. To remember these layers, think of them as protective PAD of the brain and spinal cord (pia, arachnoid, and dura mater, listed from deep to superficial).
   c. Pia mater (Latin: "tender mother"): a thin, delicate fibrous sheet that is tightly adhered to the surface of the brain and spinal cord.

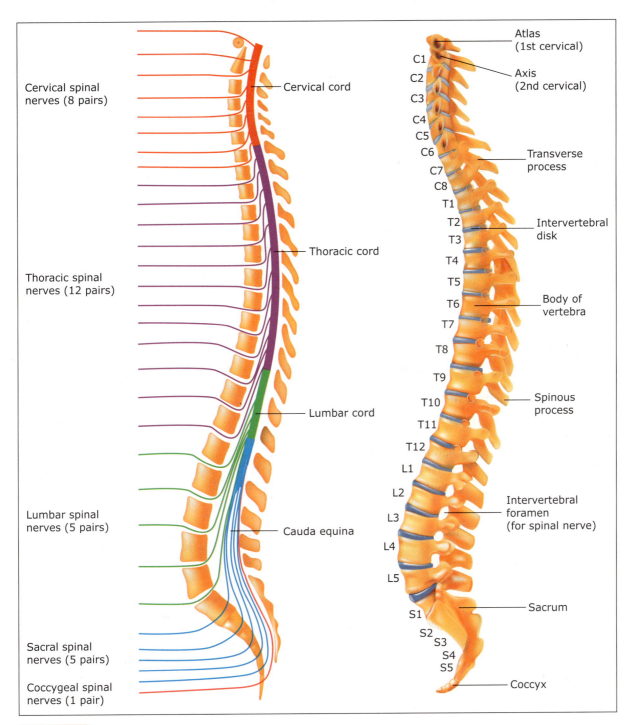

Figure 1-10 Spinal Nerves and Spinal Column

(1) The cerebrospinal fluid (CSF) flows between the outer surface of the pia and inner surface of the arachnoid.

d. Arachnoid mater: composed of a spider weblike mesh of fibers (thus the name) providing a region through which cerebral spinal fluid (CSF) can flow.

(1) The brain essentially floats in this layer of CSF, which provides an important cushion to protect the brain from mechanical injury.

e. Dura mater (Latin: "tough mother"): a tough or durable sac made of dense fibrous tissue that surrounds the entire brain and spinal cord.

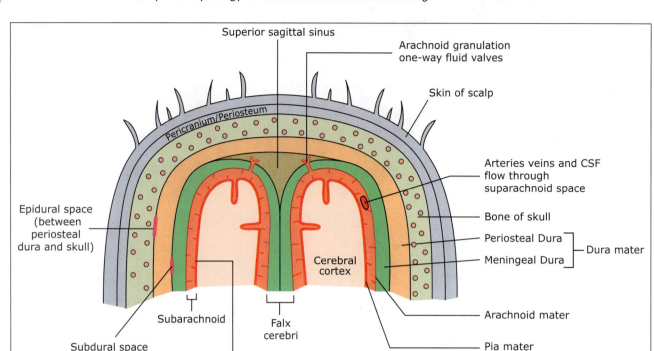

Figure 1-11 Illustration of the Meninges

(1) It has two layers that are tightly attached to one another in most locations. The outermost layer is attached to the inner surface of the skull and spinal column. The innermost surface contacts the arachnoid mater.
(2) There are specialized regions where the two layers of the dura are not attached to one another, which creates cavities or dural sinuses where deoxygenated blood from Brain's blood vessels can flow.
  (a) These sinuses converge on the right and left sides on the ventral (under) surface of the brain, and exit the skull as the jugular veins, sending the depleted blood back to the heart.
(3) The dura not only covers the brain, but also physically separates major regions of brain by extending between the right and left cerebral hemispheres (falx cerebri), between the cerebral hemispheres and the cerebellum (tentorium cerebelli), and between the cerebellar hemispheres (falx cerebelli).
  (a) These extensions act as barriers, which help protect the brain by limiting its movement within the skull.
2. Ventricular system.
  a. During early fetal development, the CNS is a fluid-filled tube. As the brain and spinal cord develop they maintain this fluid-filled core, which ultimately forms the ventricular system of the brain and the central canal of the spinal cord (Figure 1-12).
  b. CSF is a clear fluid created in the ventricular system by a highly vascular, sponge-like tissue called choroid plexus.
    (1) CSF slowly flows through the ventricular system and fills the subarachnoid space, ultimately reentering the blood stream by flowing into the dural sinus through one-way valves called arachnoid granulations (or arachnoid villi).
    (2) Standing volume of CSF in the NS is about 150 ml, which turns over about three to four times per day (daily production of about 500 ml).
    (3) If the flow of CSF through the ventricular system is blocked, it causes elevated CSF pressure in a condition known as hydrocephalus (water on the brain).
      (a) This can be treated surgically by removing the obstruction or providing an alternative route of CSF flow (shunting).
  c. There are four ventricles within the brain.
    (1) The right and left lateral ventricles at the core of the cerebral hemispheres.
    (2) The third ventricle on the midline of the brain below the corpus callosum.
    (3) The fourth ventricle at the base of the cerebellum.

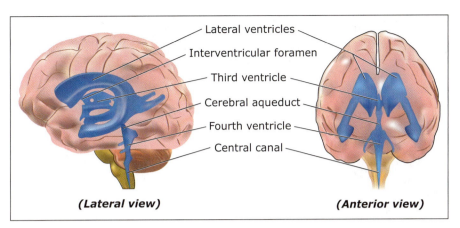

Figure 1-12 Ventricular System of the Human Brain

Adapted from "3D Rendering of Ventricles; Lateral and Anterior Views" by Bruce Blaus. Retrieved from http://en.wikipedia.org/wiki/Ventricular_system.

    (a) CSF flows between the third and fourth ventricle through the cerebral aqueduct (refer to Figure 1-12).
3. Major "encephalon" divisions.
  a. By the fifth week of embryological development, the major parts of the brain are identifiable.
  b. These include the prosencephalon (or forebrain), mesencephalon (or midbrain) and rhombencephalon (or hindbrain).
  c. The brainstem is the combined midbrain and hindbrain, minus the cerebellum.
4. Fiber connections.
  a. The CNS is an interconnected system, structurally and functionally linked through various fiber bundles, characterized as projection, association and commissural fibers.
  b. Efferent and afferent projection fibers link the cortex with the brainstem and spinal cord.
  c. Association fibers are fibers within a cerebral hemisphere and either form short connections between adjacent gyri or longer connections between lobes.
  d. Commissural fibers are transverse fibers that connect the two hemispheres of the brain.
5. Spinal cord (Figure 1-13).
  a. The division between the medulla oblongata and spinal cord occurs at the foramen magnum, which is the prominent opening in the skull at the beginning of the vertebral canal.
  b. There is continuity in much of the neuroanatomy between the brainstem and the spinal cord (i.e., it is not an abrupt distinction), but one identifying feature is that the corticospinal fibers in the pyramidal tracts cross the midline (decussate) in the medulla and then travel in the lateral corticospinal tracts within the spinal cord.
  c. Features of the spinal cord.
    (1) Extends the full length of the vertebral canal in newborns, but with growth it does not keep pace and only reaches the beginning of the lumbar vertebrae in adulthood.
    (2) It is about 18 inches long (45 cm), and varies in width from approximately ¼ inch in the thoracic region to ½ inch in the cervical and lumbar regions (which are enlarged due to the additional motor and sensory functions associated with the arms and legs, respectively).
    (3) Has a butterfly-shaped cell-rich (gray matter) central region surrounded by dense bundles of axons (white matter) carrying motor commands from the brain to motor neurons in the cord gray matter, or carrying sensory signals from the body to the brain.
    (4) Axons entering the dorsal or posterior side of the cord carry sensory signals, while axons exiting the ventral or anterior side carry motor signals.
    (5) The spinal cord has local neuronal connections (circuits) that enable it to receive incoming sensory information and respond rapidly with a motor response (i.e. withdrawal reflexes to painful stimuli, stretch reflexes, etc.).
      (a) Descending signals from the brain can modulate or even override some spinal reflexes, so a change in reflexes can indicate brain damage (i.e., when the toes flare outward instead of curling inward in response to stroking the sole of the foot: known as a positive Babinski sign).
6. Brainstem.
  a. This is a relatively conserved ("older" or less evolved) region of the brain spanning between the forebrain and the spinal cord. It serves several life-sustaining functions and is the route through which nearly all neural information travels between the body and the brain (aside from vision and olfaction).

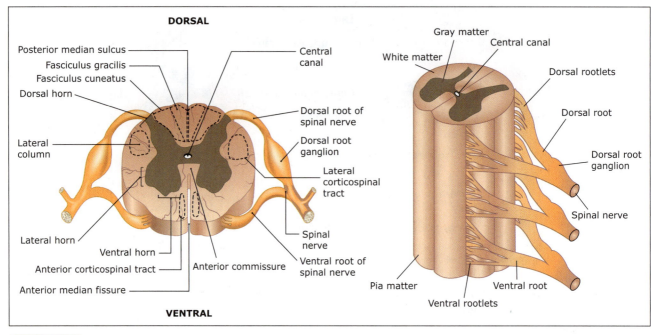

Figure 1-13 Anatomy of the Spinal Cord

b. The brainstem comprises three major segments: the medulla oblongata, the pons and the midbrain.
c. Medulla oblongata: the lowest segment of the brainstem spanning from the pons to the spinal cord.
   (1) It contains neuronal circuitry guiding several autonomic functions, including respiration, cardiac rate, vascular contraction/dilation, and integration of sensory information for reflex motor responses such as coughing, vomiting, and swallowing.
   (2) Nucleus ambiguus in the medulla contains motoneurons that innervate muscles of the larynx, pharynx and the upper esophagus via branches of nerve X (vagus nerve).
   (3) The hypoglossal motor nucleus in the medulla controls the tongue via nerve XII (hypoglossal nerve).
d. Pons: the region of brainstem with a prominent ventral bulge located immediately anterior to the cerebellum between the midbrain and the medulla.
   (1) The posterior surface contains thick bundles of axons going to/from the cerebellum called *cerebellar peduncles*.
   (2) Several cranial nerves have their associated nuclei (clusters of neuron cell bodies) located within the pons, including the motor nuclei for mastication (chewing) via nerve V, facial expressions via nerve VII, some eye movements via nerve VI, sensory nuclei for the head via nerve V, and vestibular and cochlear sensory functions via nerve VIII.
e. Midbrain: the most rostral (highest) portion of the brainstem, located just below the cerebral hemispheres and above the pons.
   (1) It has four prominent bulges on the posterior surface (two on each side), including two superior colliculi and two inferior colliculi, which process visual and acoustic information, respectively.
   (2) Just inferior to the colliculi is a cell-rich region of gray matter surrounding the cerebral aqueduct called the periaqueductal gray (PAG).
      (a) The PAG receives and processes pain information and plays a critical role in coordinating phonatory, articulatory, and respiratory movements for sound production in all vocalizing animals studied to date.
      (b) In humans, it appears that PAG lesions can cause mutism.
7. Cerebellum.
   a. Meaning "little brain" in Latin, this structure has right and left hemispheres with multiple lobes and folds of cortex similar to the cerebral hemispheres.
   b. The cerebellar cortex is thinner and much more tightly folded than the cerebrum.
   c. The cerebellum plays an important role in motor control by comparing motor intent with motor outcome, enabling it to guide ongoing movements (and improve future movements) by sending error correction information to the motor cortex of the cerebrum.

d. Lesions of the cerebellum do not cause paralysis, but disrupt the coordination and precision of motor behavior in a condition known as ataxia.
8. Reticular formation.
   a. A collection of cell columns and interconnecting networks, centered primarily in the pons, that coordinate motor functions of the body (such as posture) and of the head (such as mastication and articulation).
   b. The reticular formation is important for regulating sleep/wake cycles and actively generating both wakeful and sleeping states.
   c. It also directs attention to help us ignore repetitive stimuli but respond to novel or salient events.
   d. Connections of the reticular formation with the cerebral cortex that guide attention/arousal are part of the reticular activating system.
9. Forebrain.
   a. Telencephalon.
      (1) Consists of right and left cerebral hemispheres, divided along the midline by a longitudinal fissure.
         (a) The outer surface of each hemisphere is a convoluted (folded), cell-rich, six-layered structure called cerebral cortex.
      (2) The cortex varies in thickness from about 2 to 4 mm across the brain.
      (3) In fresh tissue, the cortex appears relatively gray due to a high cell content, whereas the deeper fiber pathways into and out of the cortex appear relatively white because of the high myelin content of the myelinated (insulated) axons.
      (4) The six horizontal layers of the cortex (Figure 1-14) have different connections, with the outer layers being primarily receptive (where incoming axons synapse), and the inner layers contain cell bodies of neurons that project to other brain areas.
         (a) Layer IV, the fourth deepest cell layer, receives sensory information from the thalamus, and is relatively thick in regions of primary sensory cortex.
         (b) Layer V contains large projection neurons (Betz cells) that send motor commands to the brainstem and spinal cord, and is relatively thick in regions of primary motor cortex.
         (c) Layer III contains neuronal cell bodies projecting to other cortical areas and is relatively thick in regions of association cortex.
      (5) Korbinian Brodmann, a German neurologist, identified 52 distinct cortical regions based on unique anatomical (e.g., layer) characteristics about 100 years ago. His anatomically numbered regions, called Brodmann's areas, are well known today because they relate to particular brain functions.
      (6) In each hemisphere, the central sulcus marks the anatomical and functional demarcation between the frontal and parietal lobes (see lobe anatomy in section below).
      (7) Each cerebral hemisphere is divided into four major lobes: frontal, parietal, temporal and occipital lobes (see Figure 1-15).
   b. Frontal lobe.
      (1) The frontal lobe is anterior to the central sulcus and superior to the lateral fissure.
      (2) The anterior-most portion of the frontal lobe, the prefrontal cortex, contributes to executive control, important for attention, monitoring, planning and decision making.
      (3) Within the prefrontal cortex is the inferior frontal gyrus, the site of Broca's area in the left hemisphere, important for language production.
      (4) Posterior to the prefrontal cortex is a region called the premotor cortex involved in the performance of skilled movements (such as those necessary for speech) and regulation of the primary motor cortex.
      (5) Posterior to the premotor cortex, is an important outward fold of cortex just anterior to the central sulcus: the precentral gyrus, site of the primary motor cortex.
         (a) This motor strip is the source of half or more of all body motor control signals (Brodmann's area four).
         (b) There is a body mapping or topography across this strip called the *homunculus* (little human). The distortions of the mapping relative to true body proportions reveals that functions requiring relatively more neural processing take up relatively more cortex. For example, precisely controlled regions of the body (like the face) have relatively large cortical representations (see Figure 1-16).
   c. Parietal lobe.
      (1) The parietal lobe is posterior to the central sulcus and superior to the lateral fissure.
      (2) The anterior-most portion of the parietal lobe, the postcentral gyrus, site of the primary somatosensory cortex.
         (a) This somatosensory strip receives body sensation (excluding the special senses such as hearing and vision).
         (b) Like the motor strip, body mapping is topographically organized across the strip with highly sensitive regions taking up relatively more cortex.
   d. Temporal lobe.

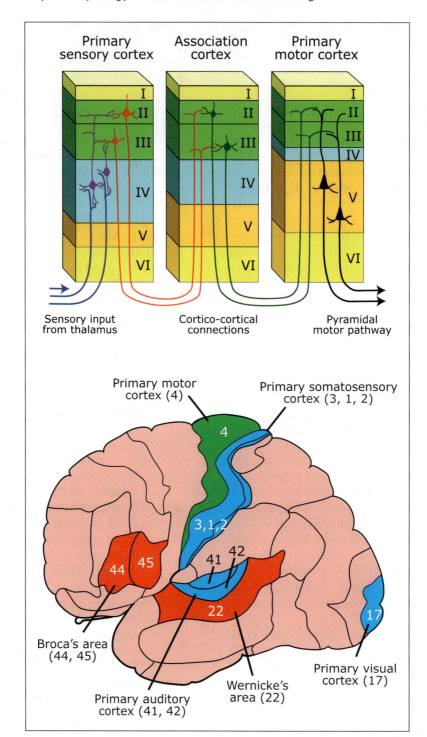

Figure 1-14   Horizontal Layers of the Cerebral Cortex

(1) The temporal lobe is inferior to the lateral sulcus, anterior to the occipital lobe, and contains three important surface gyri: the superior, middle and inferior gyri.
(2) The primary auditory cortex is located within the superior surface of the temporal lobe on a gyrus medial to the superior temporal gyrus called Heschl's gyrus.
(3) The posterior portion of the left superior temporal gyrus, adjacent to the primary auditory cortex is the site of Wernicke's area, important for language comprehension.

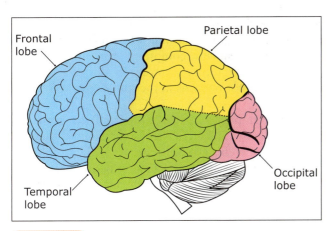

Figure 1-15 Lobes of the Cerebral Hemispheres

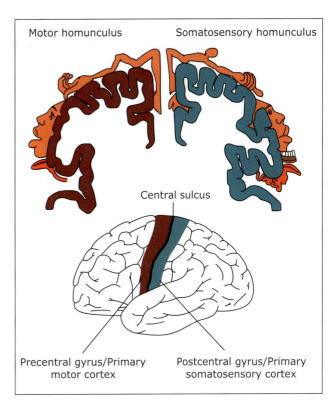

Figure 1-16 Cortical Representations of the Motor and Sensory Homunculi

e. Occipital lobe.
   (1) The occipital lobe is the most posterior lobe of the brain with no natural lateral boundary separating it from the parietal and temporal lobes.
   (2) The occipital lobe contributes to higher-order processing of visual information and is the site of the primary visual cortex and of secondary visual integration areas.
f. Limbic cortex.
   (1) The limbic cortex, sometimes referred to as the limbic *lobe* extends across portion of the temporal, parietal and occipital lobes.
   (2) This "lobe" is primarily composed of the cingulate and parahippocampal gyri, and with its interconnected structures (the hippocampus, amygdala, fornix, mammillary body and septal nuclei), makes up the limbic system important for memory, emotion, and drive-related behavior.
   (3) Limbic cortex is important for primitive behaviors and has fewer layers than a majority of our more highly evolved cortex (called neocortex).
g. Basal ganglia.
   (1) Deep in the gray and white matter of the cerebral cortex lies a collection of interconnected nuclei called the basal ganglia, or basal nuclei.
   (a) These nuclei act together to guide behavior, mostly through inhibition.
   (2) Subdivisions of the basal ganglia include the striatum, globus pallidus, substantia nigra and subthalamic nucleus.
   (3) Striatum: composed of the caudate and putamen, is functionally one structure divided by the main fiber highway into/out of the cortex called the internal capsule.
   (4) Globus pallidus (GP): comprises external and internal subdivisions.
   (5) Substantia nigra (SN): comprises two regions: the pars compacta and the pars reticulata.
      (a) Substantia nigra pars compacta (SNc): located in the midbrain and contains dopamine-producing cells that send strong projections to the striatum.
      (b) Substantia nigra pars reticulata (SNr): contains cells that produce the inhibitory neurotransmitter gamma-aminobutyric acid (GABA) that projects onto motor regions of the thalamus, which in turn project to the motor cortex.
   (6) Subthalamic nucleus (STN): nucleus that receives a projection from the external segment of the GP and projects back to the internal segment.
h. Diencephalon
   (1) Diencephalon is the region of brain spanning between the cerebral hemispheres and the midbrain (upper-most part of the brainstem).
   (2) It is divisible into four major regions: the epithalamus, the thalamus, the subthalamus and the hypothalamus.
   (3) The epithalamus contains the pineal gland (or body), as well as cellular regions and fiber pathways associated with the limbic system.

(a) These structures play a role in the regulation of sleep/wake cycles, stress responses and emotions.
(b) Atrophy of the epithalamus has been found in cases of severe depression.
(4) The thalamus surrounds the third ventricle (see above) on the brain midline below the corpus callosum. It contains many subdivisions that process sensory and motor information.
   (a) Almost all sensory information reaching the cerebral hemispheres that we consciously perceive is relayed through (and is processed by) the thalamus.
   (b) Motor pathways of the basal ganglia and cerebellum travel through motor subdivisions of the thalamus en route to the motor cortex.
   (c) Some movement disorders are treated by placing deep brain stimulator electrodes into motor regions of the thalamus.
(5) The subthalamus contains the subthalamic nucleus, which is an important component of the basal ganglia motor control circuit (see section on subthalamic nucleus [STN] above).
(6) The hypothalamus is located on the floor of the diencephalon between the optic chiasm to the mammillary bodies (about the size of an almond).
   (a) It communicates with the pituitary gland through a stalk of neural and vascular tissue, and interacts with the pituitary to maintain body homeostasis of metabolic and endocrine (hormonal) functions such as body temperature, thirst, hunger, fatigue, circadian rhythms and sleep/wake cycles.

Neural Pathways

1. Neural pathways connect portions of the nervous system.
2. As previously described, nerve impulses, or APs, are generated at cell bodies or sensory nerve endings, and information is then rapidly conveyed to other parts of the brain or body through axons.
3. APs are all or none electrochemical impulses that code information via their frequency, connections and receptor types.
4. Our nervous system contains important descending and ascending neural pathways that contribute to our movement and sensation, respectively.
   a. Damage to these pathways can occur from trauma, disease, toxins or restricted blood supply, affecting nerve activity and impacting the way we regulate and respond to our internal and external environment.
5. Direct motor pathway.
   a. The direct motor pathway, often referred to as the pyramidal system, comprises axons that descend from upper motor neurons in the cerebrum to lower motor neurons in the spinal cord and brainstem.
   b. Nerve impulses carried away from the brain are described as efferent signals or simply efferents (Hint: *efferents ex*it the brain).
   c. The function of the direct motor pathway is to control skilled, voluntary movements of our extremities.
   d. The corticospinal tract is one of two major tracts (pathways) of the pyramidal system. It is further subdivided into two pathways: the lateral corticospinal tract and the anterior corticospinal tract (described later in further detail).
   e. Corticospinal tract (Figure 1-17).
      (1) Upper motor neurons of the corticospinal tract originate from the primary and premotor cortex, as well as from supplementary motor areas and the parietal lobe.
      (2) Approximately 3% of these cortical motor neurons are exceptionally large cells (called Betz cells) that look like inverted pyramids, giving rise to the name *pyramidal tract*.
      (3) Corticospinal tract fibers descend through the internal capsule, a thick layer of white matter located above the midbrain carrying ascending and descending axons that connect the cortex with the brainstem and spinal cord.
      (4) Fibers then descend into the midbrain with many other axons in a white matter bundle called the cerebral peduncles.
      (5) In the brainstem, fibers descend through the ventral portion of the pons to the ventral surface of the medulla in pyramid-shaped fiber bundles called the medullary pyramids (thus reinforcing the name *pyramidal tract*).
      (6) When the descending pyramidal tract fibers reach the transition point from the brainstem to spinal cord (cervicomedullary junction), 85% of all corticospinal tract fibers cross over in the pyramidal decussation and control muscles on the opposite (contralateral) side of the body.
      (7) Fibers that decussate form the main subdivision of the corticospinal tract called the lateral corticospinal tract whose primary function is contralateral, fine, rapid limb control.
         (a) Axons of the lateral corticospinal tract synapse with lower motor neurons (or nearby interneurons that then synapse with lower motor neurons) in the gray matter of the anterior horn of the spinal cord (also called the ventral horn).

Neuroanatomy and Neurophysiology for Speech, Language and Swallowing

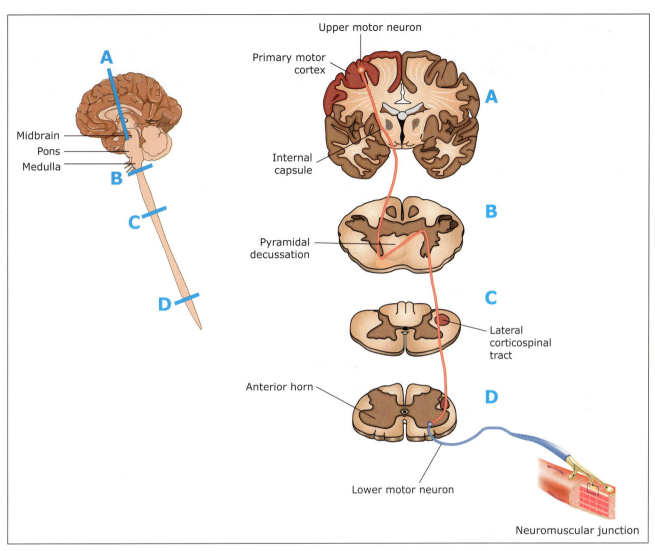

Figure 1-17 Corticospinal Motor Pathways

(b) Axons that project from lower motor neurons contact striated muscle and are often referred to as the final common pathway, damage to which results in paresis (partial paralysis) or paralysis, muscle atrophy, fibrillations (random, spontaneous contractions) from denervated muscle cells, fasciculations (whole motor unit twitches) from spontaneous axon discharges, and decreased reflexes (hyporeflexia).

(8) The 15% of corticospinal fibers that *do not* decussate in the pyramidal decussation form the anterior corticospinal tract. These axons synapse contralaterally or bilaterally in the spinal cord anterior horns at the level of an action and are involved in the control of midline (trunk) musculature.

f. Corticobulbar tract.
  (1) The corticobulbar tract, whose axons course from upper motor neurons in the cerebrum to lower motor neurons in the brainstem, is the other major tract of the direct motor pathway.
  (2) The function of the corticobulbar tract is to control muscles of the face, head and neck.
  (3) Upper motor neurons of the corticobulbar tract originate from a lateral portion of the motor cortex close to the Sylvian fissure.
  (4) Similar to the corticospinal tract, fibers of the corticobulbar tract descend ipsilaterally through the internal capsule and then through the ventral portion of the midbrain cerebral peduncles.

Table 1-2

Summary of the Indirect Motor Pathway

EXTRAPYRAMIDAL MOTOR SYSTEM		CONTROL CIRCUITS: MODULATE DESCENDING MOTOR OUTPUT		
CORTICORETICULAR	**RUBROSPINAL**	**BASAL GANGLIA**		**CEREBELLUM**
Inputs: from the premotor, motor and sensory cortices	Inputs to red nucleus (midbrain): from cerebellum and motor cortex	Inputs to striatum: from motor cortex and substantia nigra pars compacta		Inputs to cerebellum: cerebral cortex sensory systems, brainstem, spinal cord
Outputs: to reticular formation of the brainstem	Outputs: to spinal cord	Outputs: to motor systems of cortex and brainstem		Outputs: to motor systems of cortex and brainstem
		Direct Pathway	**Indirect Pathway**	
Function: contributes to regulation of somatic motor control, automatic gait movements and automatic posturing, controls proximal and axial extensors of the upper extremities.	Function: contributes to movement of extremities, automatic gait movements (arm swinging) and automatic posturing, controls flexors of the upper extremities.	Function: tends to facilitate movement	Function: tends to inhibit movement	Function: coordination (limbs, trunk), balance, motor planning
		Associated Disorders		
Damage can lead to decorticate posturing: hyperflexion of upper extremities.	Damage can lead to decerebrate posturing: hyperextension of upper extremities.	Parkinson's disease: loss of dopamine net inhibition of movement Huntington's disease: caudate and putamen neuron degeneration, less inhibition of thalamus, early stage hyperkinetic movement		Ataxia: uncoordinated movement

(5) Within the pons and medulla, axons of the corticobulbar tracts project contralaterally or bilaterally onto cranial nerve motor nuclei.

(6) Axons from the motor nuclei then exit the brainstem ipsilaterally at various levels, forming the motor components of the cranial nerves.

(7) Projections of the corticobulbar tract onto brainstem motor nuclei can be both bilateral and contralateral. Typically, corticobulbar control is bilateral, with the exception of contralateral control to the lower face (via CN VII) and tongue (via CN XII).

6. Indirect motor pathways.
   a. The motor system also contains descending pathways that are indirect, forming part of the extrapyramidal system. (See Table 1-2.)
      (1) The cortex projects onto multiple brainstem motor centers, which then project onto lower motor neurons to exert their control (hence, the indirect motor pathway).
      (2) These targets include the tectum (corticotectal), red nucleus (corticorubral), and reticular formation (corticoreticular).
   b. The indirect activation pathway is involved in reflexes and coordination of multiple muscle groups, as well as in the modulation and regulation of posture, balance, tone, and some voluntary movements.
   c. Rubrospinal tract.
      (1) Rubrospinal tract fibers originate in the red nucleus of the midbrain and descend into the lateral column of the spinal cord.
      (2) This tract is relatively rudimentary in humans and contributes to postural control through its regulation of muscle tone and inhibition of extensor movement.
   d. Reticulospinal tract.
      (1) Medial and lateral reticulospinal tracts receive inputs from the cortex through the corticoreticular tract and also have origins in the reticular formation of the pons and medulla.
      (2) These tracts play a role in the control of autonomic function as well as in the regulation of somatic motor control.
   e. Vestibulospinal tract.
      (1) The vestibulospinal tract originates in the vestibular nuclei of the lower pons and medulla.
      (2) This tract contributes to body and limb adjustments related to balance.
7. Extrapyramidal system control circuits.
   a. Cerebellar control circuits.

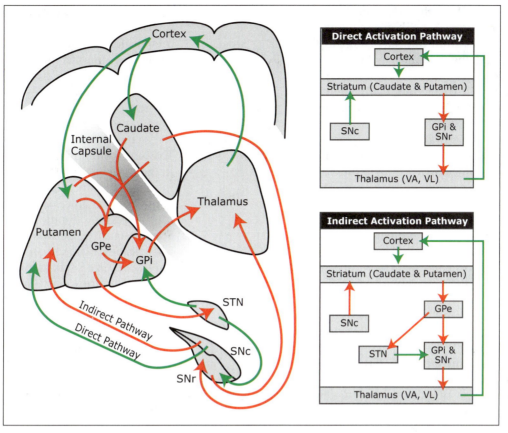

Figure 1-18 Basal Ganglia Control Circuits

GPe = globus pallidus (external segment); GPi = globus pallidus (internal segment); STN = subthalamic nucleus; SNc = substantia nigra pars compacta; SNr = substantis nigra pars reticulata; VA = ventral anterior nucleus; VL = ventral lateral nucleus

(1) As previously noted, the cerebellum contributes to planning, coordination, timing and precision of movements as well as to motor learning.
(2) The cerebellum integrates afferent and efferent inputs from the brain and spinal cord.
(3) Through this process of integration, the cerebellum compares motor intent with actual motor execution such that motor programs can be altered to most accurately match output goals.
(4) Damage to cerebellar control circuits can lead to incoordination, intention tremor, limb ataxia, hypotonia, disequilibrium, dysarthria and dysmetria.

b. Basal ganglia control circuits (Figure 1-18).
(1) The basal ganglia contain multiple interconnected loops, sending projections between basal ganglia nuclei and the cortex (via the thalamus) as well as to the brainstem, which are critical to the regulation of motor activity (these loops serve additional functions related to cognition, emotion and motivation).
(2) The basal ganglia do not exert direct motor control; instead, circuits contribute inhibitory or facilitatory input to the cortex, modulating cortical output on a time scale of hundreds of milliseconds.
(3) When functioning correctly, the basal ganglia refine movements, increasing precision and form while reducing extraneous activity.
(4) Most cortical, thalamic and brainstem inputs to the basal ganglia are glutamatergic and are excitatory to the striatum.
(5) The SNc provides an important dopaminergic input to the striatum of the basal ganglia (which is lost in Parkinson's disease).
(6) The neurotransmitter dopamine is both excitatory and inhibitory to the striatum, depending on which particular cells receive the transmitter.
(7) Within the basal ganglia, inhibitory projections exist between:
   (a) The striatum to the GP (internal and external).
   (b) The striatum to the SNr.
   (c) The globus pallidus external (GPe) to the STN.
   (d) The GPi to the thalamus.

(8) Projections from the STN to the SNr and globus pallidus internal (GPi) are excitatory.
(9) Projections from the cerebellum to the thalamus and the thalamus to the cortex are also excitatory.
(10) There are two predominant pathways within the basal ganglia: the direct pathway and the indirect pathway.
(11) The direct pathway projects outputs to the cortex and brainstem from the striatum via the GPi or the SNr, which then project to the thalamus.
  (a) The net result of excitatory input to this pathway is excitatory (facilitation of movement).
  (b) Dopaminergic input from the SNc to the direct pathway is excitatory.
(12) The indirect pathway first projects to the GPe, then to the STN and the GPi, and finally to the thalamus.
  (a) The net result of excitatory input to this pathway is inhibitory (inhibition of movement).
  (b) Dopaminergic input from the SNc to the indirect pathway is inhibitory.
(13) Interruption of either of these pathways leads to movement disorders of initiation or muscle tone, each with different manifestations based on the location of damage. These include, but are not limited to:
  (a) Tremors: rhythmic alternating contraction of opposing muscles.
  (b) Athetosis: slow, repetitive writhing movements.
  (c) Ballism: sudden, jerky flinging movements.
  (d) Chorea: rhythmic, repetitive jerking movements.
8. Ascending pathways.
  a. Overview of sensory systems.
    (1) Sensory pathways convert environmental stimuli into neural signals that the brain interprets as particular sensations based on where they go in the brain.
    (2) They are called ascending pathways because sensory signals typically ascend as they enter the CNS and get processed by progressively higher and higher brain regions.
    (3) Sensory signals are called afferent signals (Hint: *afferents arr*ive) because information propagates from the body's periphery *to* the brain.
    (4) Afferent signals originate from nerve endings found throughout the body (except in the brain itself) that are either "bare" or that contact specialized transducer cells (sensory receptors).
      (a) Bare nerve endings respond to change in temperature (thermoreception), mechanical stimulation (deep or crude touch), and can detect tissue trauma (pain) when intracellular fluid is released into the extracellular fluids during cell injury.
      (b) The axons of bare nerve endings are not myelinated in their pathway from the PNS to the CNS, but sensory and motor pathways in the PNS and CNS are typically otherwise myelinated.
      (c) The most common sensory transducer cells found throughout our body surface and cavities are mechanoreceptors, specialized for detecting mechanical stimulation (forms of touch, pressure, vibration, etc.).
      (d) Some sensory pathways are "special" because they are found only in the head and have specialized transducer cells responding to chemicals (taste and smell), light (vision), head rotation/gravity (vestibular sensation), and acoustic waves (hearing).
  b. Major somatosensory pathways.
    (1) Somatosensory pathways (*soma-* means "body") convey sensation received throughout the body (excluding the special sense of the head described in the next section), including touch, vibration, pain, temperature, and our body's relative position in space (proprioception).
    (2) We have two major ascending pathways: the anterolateral pathway and the posterior column-medial lemniscal system.
      (a) Both pathways use three synapses (or three points of neural connection) to transmit information from the periphery to the cerebrum, but the particular location of these first-, second-, and third-order neurons differ somewhat (detailed below).
    (3) The anterolateral system (Figure 1-19).
      (a) The anterolateral system is the ascending pathway that conveys the sensations of pain and temperature as well as crude or non-localizable touch.
      (b) It comprises the spinothalamic tract, the spinoreticular tract and the spinotectal tract.
      (c) First-order neurons of the anterolateral system are pseudounipolar, with a single axonal extension from each neuron that branches into a distal and proximal process (refer to Figure 1-6).
        • Cell bodies of the first-order neurons are located in the dorsal root ganglia (refer to Figure 1-13).
        • Their distal processes collectively extend throughout the body via the PNS and terminate within tissues as bare nerve endings.

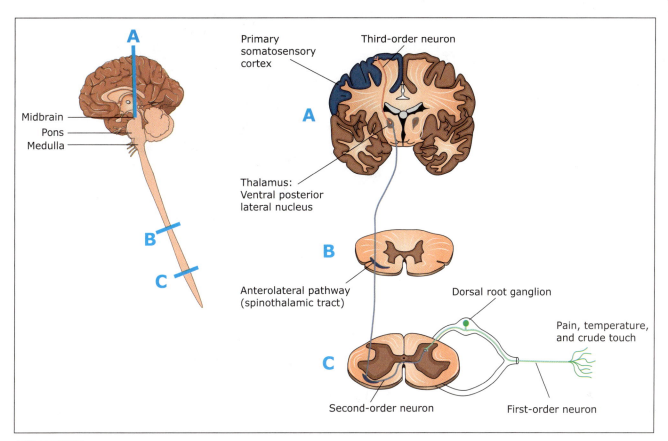

Figure 1-19 Anterolateral Pathway

- Their proximal processes enter the spinal cord through the dorsal roots and synapse onto sensory neurons located within the dorsal horns (or posterior horn).
(d) Second-order neurons of the anterolateral system have cell bodies located within the dorsal (or posterior) horns, with axons that cross over to the contralateral spinothalamic tract through the anterior white commissure located just below the central canal. They also synapse with local motoneurons and interneurons bilaterally within the spinal cord ventral horns to generate reflexive responses to pain.
  - Second-order neuron axons travel up the spinal column, with lateral fibers transmitting pain and temperature sensation (lateral spinothalamic tract) and anterior fibers carrying information about crude touch (anterior spinothalamic tract).
(e) Finally, axons of the spinothalamic tract synapse with third-order neurons located in the ventral posterolateral (VPL) nucleus of the thalamus, from which axons project to the primary somatosensory cortex via the internal capsule.
(f) Sensations of pain, temperature and crude touch from the head and face are carried in the cranial equivalent of the spinothalamic tract: the spinal trigeminal pathway.
(g) The spinoreticular tract follows a similar course as the spinothalamic tract, only instead of being in the thalamus, its third-order neurons terminate in the medullary-pontine reticular formation. From the reticular formation, axons project and synapse in the thalamus before projecting to the cerebral cortex.
(h) Finally, some fibers of the spinothalamic tract project to the periaqueductal gray (PAG) of the midbrain, a region of gray matter that modulates pain responses. Fibers that project to the PAG are described as spinomesencephalic because of their termination in the mesencephalon (midbrain) where the PAG is located.
(4) The posterior column-medial lemniscal system (Figure 1-20).
  (a) Another major ascending sensory fiber tract is the posterior column-medial lemniscal system.

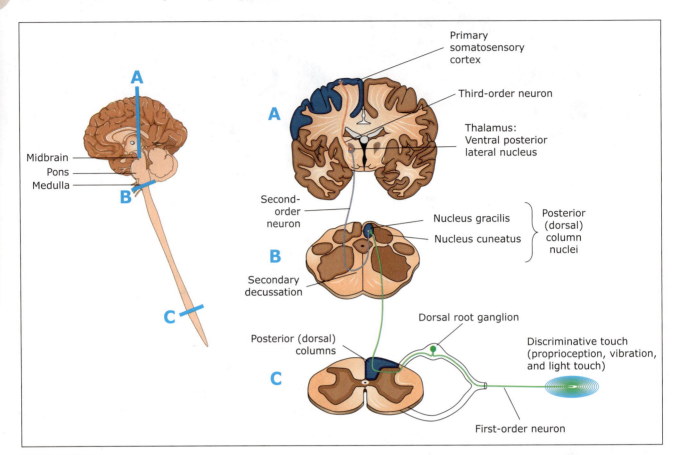

Figure 1-20 Posterior Column-Medial Lemniscal System

(b) The posterior column-medial lemniscal system carries information about pressure, vibration and fine touch.

(c) There are four major receptor types that contribute to this ascending system. These are described as discriminatory receptors.
- Meissner's corpuscles are sensory receptors found just below the epidermis. Meissner's corpuscles are rapidly adapting and only produce APs when a force is first applied. These receptors respond to deformations of the skin and low frequency vibrations.
- Pacinian corpuscles are found subcutaneously (deep under the skin), giving them a large receptive field. Like Meissner's corpuscles, Pacinian corpuscles are rapidly adapting. They sense high-frequency vibratory pressure.
- Ruffini endings/corpuscles are also subcutaneous receptors. These receptors contain long, collagenous fibers that run parallel to the surface of the skin. They sense stretch and are slowly adapting, meaning that APs continue to fire throughout a stretch.
- Merkel receptors are found just below the epidermis and sense sustained touch, pressure and textures. These receptors help perceive the edges and forms of objects.

(d) Similar to the spinothalamic tract, first-order neurons of the posterior column-medial lemniscus are pseudounipolar with a discriminatory receptor as the distal process, a cell body in the dorsal root ganglion and a proximal process that enters the dorsal horn of the spinal cord.

(e) Distinct from the spinothalamic tract, proximal axons immediately ascend ipsilaterally through the spinal column forming the gracile fasciculus and the cuneate fasciculus.
- The gracile fasciculus, located medially, carries information from the lower extremities (legs) and trunk.
- The cuneate fasciculus, located laterally, carries information from upper extremities (arms and neck).

- This somatotopic organization is maintained for second-order neurons found in the nucleus gracilis and nucleus cuneatus at the level of the medulla oblongata.
(f) Axons of second-order neurons decussate and travel through the medial lemniscus, a white matter pathway that ascends through the brainstem.
  - Note that the point of decussation for the posterior column-medial lemniscus (carrying discriminative touch) is within the brainstem, whereas decussation of the spinothalamic tract (carrying pain/temperature) is within the spinal cord.
(g) Third-order neurons located in the VPL of the thalamus have axons that project through the internal capsule to the primary somatosensory cortex.
(h) A trigeminal equivalent of the posterior column-medial lemniscus carries pressure, vibration and fine touch sensation from the face. Third-order neurons of this pathway synapse in the ventral posterior medial nucleus (VPM) of the thalamus adjacent to the VPL.

c. Proprioception.
  (1) An additional body sense called proprioception is mediated by a distinct set of receptors and informs the brain about the musculoskeletal system movement and orientation.
  (2) These receptors include muscle spindles, Golgi tendon organs and joint receptors.
  (3) Muscle spindles are long, thin, complex somatosensory receptors found in the majority of striated muscles of the body.
    (a) Muscle spindles contribute to reflexive regulation of skeletal muscle stretch by detecting the magnitude and rate of stretch in muscles.
    (b) This function is achieved by way of intrafusal muscles, small muscle fibers within muscle spindles that run parallel to standard muscle fibers (extrafusal muscle fibers). Whenever a standard muscle is stretched, an intrafusal muscle within a muscle spindle is also stretched.
    (c) The stretching of intrafusal muscles generates a receptor potential, triggering an action potential that is transmitted to sensory neurons within the dorsal horn of the spinal cord. These sensory neurons in turn form synapses with lower motor neurons and cause a reflexive muscle contraction.
    (d) Muscle spindles must adjust when voluntary contractions are made (contraction of a muscle releases tension in intrafusal muscle fibers thereby reducing their sensitivity to stretch). This adjustment is provided through gamma motor neurons, small motor neurons that supply intrafusal fibers to restore tension and sensitivity.
  (4) Golgi tendon organs are receptors composed of encapsulated, interwoven collagen bundles located between muscles and tendons that provide information about muscle tension, or load.
  (5) Joint receptors, Ruffini endings and Pacinian corpuscles found in joints are thought to contribute to proprioception by detecting joint angle. Muscle receptors (muscle spindles and Golgi tendon organs), however, likely play a larger role in proprioception than joint receptors.

d. Special senses of the head.
  (1) Sensory pathways for pain, temperature and discriminative touch from the head are described as part of the somatosensory pathways in the section above because these modalities (forms of sensation) are found throughout the body.
  (2) Sensory modalities associated with specialized sensory epithelia (or organs) found only in the head are considered "special" senses, and do not always follow the general pattern of having first-, second- and third-order sensory neurons from the PNS to the cerebral cortex as described for somatosensation.
  (3) Special senses include olfaction (CN I), vision (CN II), gustation (CN VII, IX, X), and hearing and balance (CN VIII).
  (4) Specialized sensory transducers for these sensations include olfactory receptor cells for smell, rods and cones for vision, taste buds for gustation, and acoustic and vestibular hair cells for hearing and balance, respectively.
  (5) Most special senses project bilaterally to the cerebral cortex via dedicated regions of the thalamus (except for olfaction, which projects directly to the telencephalon).
    (a) The lateral geniculate nucleus (or body) of the thalamus is specialized for vision.
    (b) The medial geniculate nucleus (or body) of the thalamus is specialized for hearing.
    (c) Olfaction and gustation are processed in a region adjacent to VPM (where other head sensations are received).
    (d) Vestibular sensation has only a minor projection through the thalamus to the cortex. Rather, it plays a critical role in the brainstem and spinal cord for guiding eye movements, posture and balance.

Cerebral Blood Flow

Arteries

1. Arteries deliver oxygen and nutrient-rich blood to the body.
2. Arteries branch into smaller and smaller vessels (arterioles) in order to reach all tissues of the body, including the nervous system.
3. Arteries ultimately branch down to a very small vessel size called capillaries, where gas and nutrient exchange occurs with surrounding tissues.
4. Capillaries progressively fuse to form veins, which lead back to the heart and lungs.

Veins

1. Veins carry deoxygenated, waste-laden blood from the body back to the heart and lungs.
2. Veins are relatively thin walled and lower in blood pressure than arteries, so they are not prone to rupture.
3. Because of their low pressure, most veins contain one-way valves to ensure that blood flows in the correct direction.

Blood Flow from the Heart to the Brain

1. The anterior blood supply to the brain originates from left and right carotid arteries (see Figure 1-21).
2. The posterior blood supply to the brain originates from the left and right subclavian arteries.

Carotid Arteries

1. Left and right carotid arteries originate from the arch of the aorta and ascend from the thorax to the neck.
   a. At the level of the hyoid bone, they both divide into internal and external branches, which themselves branch into smaller arteries.
2. Internal carotid arteries (anterior supply): divide into two principal branches after entering the skull.
   a. Anterior cerebral arteries (ACA).
      (1) Supply medial surfaces of cortex from frontal to parietal lobes.
      (2) Supply regions deep to lobes (e.g., basal ganglia).
   b. Middle cerebral arteries (MCA).
      (1) Supply lateral frontal lobe.
      (2) Supply lateral temporal lobes.
      (3) Supply portions of lateral parietal lobe.
      (4) Supply regions deep to lobes (e.g., basal ganglia).
3. External carotid arteries: supply the head and dura, not the brain.

Subclavian Arteries

1. Left subclavian artery originates from the arch of the aorta.
   a. Right subclavian artery stems from the brachiocephalic trunk. The subclavian arteries give rise to the vertebral arteries (Figure 1-21).
2. Vertebral arteries (posterior supply): ascend in the neck along the cervical vertebrae before entering the skull through the foramen magnum (exit point for the spinal cord).
   a. Left and right vertebral arteries send off branches that supply the anterior spinal cord and posterior cerebellum.
      (1) Anterior spinal artery.
      (2) Posterior inferior cerebellar arteries.
   b. Left and right vertebral arteries then join together to form the basilar artery.
3. Basilar artery: travels on the ventral midline of the brainstem (Figure 1-22).
   a. Sends off branches that supply portions of the medulla, pons and cerebellum.
      (1) Anterior inferior cerebellar arteries.
      (2) Superior cerebellar arteries.
   b. At the level of the midbrain, the basilar artery splits into the right and left posterior cerebral arteries.
      (1) Posterior cerebral arteries (PCA).
         (a) Supply occipital lobes and inferior and medial temporal cortices.
         (b) Supply regions deep to lobes (e.g., thalamus).

Cerebral Blood Flow

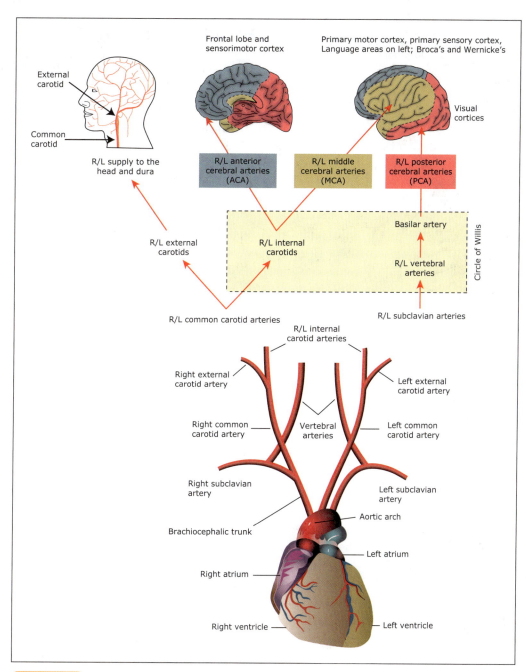

Figure 1-21 Cerebral Blood Flow from the Heart

Circle of Willis

1. The internal carotid and vertebral artery supplies converge at the level of the ventral midbrain through relatively small communicating arteries that form a circle.
   a. These bring together the anterior/posterior and right/left blood supplies (see Figure 1-22).
2. Posterior communicating arteries ipsilaterally join the middle cerebral and PCAs (anterior/posterior connection).
3. Anterior communicating arteries join the right and left ACA (right/left connection).
4. Communicating arteries allow for compensatory blood flow should flow be restricted at some point near the arterial circle.

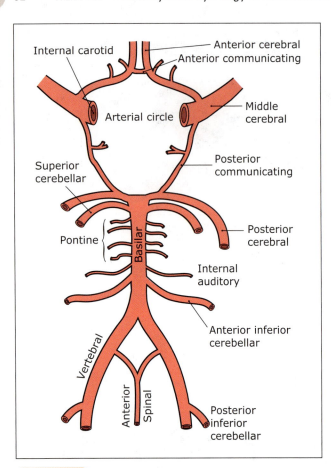

Figure 1-22 Circle of Willis

Blood Supply and the Brain

1. Although the brain represents only around 2% of a human's body mass, it consumes approximately 20% of the body's oxygen and glucose, and is very susceptible to cell death (anoxia) in the absences of an adequate blood supply.
   a. It is important to understand the vessel pathways that provide blood supply to the brain, because interruption of this supply is the largest cause of neurologic deficit (and communication/swallowing disorders) worldwide, and the location of vessel hemorrhage and/or occlusion will have particular functional impacts.

Respiration

Gas Exchange with the Environment

1. Respiration supports cellular metabolism.
2. Breathing plays an essential role in vocalization and must be coordinated with swallowing.
3. Respiratory abnormalities can contribute to speech and swallowing disorders.

Critical Respiratory Anatomy

1. The lungs: organs containing alveoli for gas exchange.
   a. Left and right lungs are located within the thorax, separated by the heart and midline structures (see Figure 1-23).
      (1) The left lung is slightly smaller and has only two lobes compared with the three lobes of the right lung.
      (2) Based on the angle with which the bronchi enter lungs, aspiration is more common into the right lung.
      (3) The internal thoracic wall and lungs are coated in connective tissue called pleural linings.
         (a) Pleural linkage: surface tension between the wet pleural linings draw the lungs to the rib cage and diaphragm.
         (b) Without the pleural linkage, the lungs would collapse and the chest wall would expand.
      (4) The volume of these connected structures at rest (relaxation volume) is a compromise between the uncoupled volume of the lungs and chest wall.
2. The chest and rib cage: due to the pleural linkage between the lungs and the chest wall, movements of the chest and rib cage passively or actively contribute to adjustments of breathing.

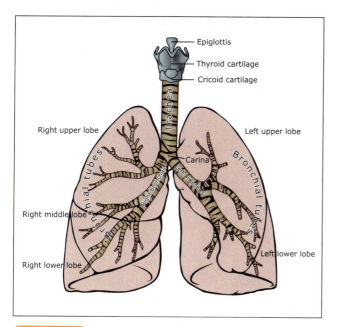

Figure 1-23 Critical Respiratory Anatomy

3. The trachea.
   a. Colloquially referred to as the *windpipe*, the trachea is a tube composed of fibrous and cartilaginous tissue (fibrocartilage) that extends from the inferior larynx to the bronchi of the lungs.
   b. The fibrous portion of the trachea lends it a flexible quality, while hyaline cartilage rings support the trachea and help maintain its opening.
   c. The cartilaginous rings of the trachea are incomplete posteriorly, where the trachea is composed of smooth muscle that abuts the esophagus, which runs adjacent (deep) to the trachea.
   d. Due to the proximal anatomy of the trachea and esophagus, it is critical that airway protection be well timed and coordinated during a swallow.
   e. The trachea has an average diameter of 2.5 cm in adult humans, and is approximately 10–16 cm long.
   f. At the level of the sternal angle, the trachea divides into right and left bronchi.
4. In addition, four major groups of muscles are involved in respiration: the diaphragm, abdominals and external and internal intercostals.
5. The sternocleidomastoid and the scalene muscles are considered important accessory muscles of inspiration.

Quiet Breathing (Automatic/Metabolic/Involuntary/Passive)

1. Autonomic function is responsible for regulating gas levels in the blood.
2. The brainstem, in particular the medulla, is critical to the process of passive breathing.
3. Areas of the brainstem monitor blood gas levels, respiratory system pressures, and respiratory anatomy position/contractions.
   a. Chemical monitoring: chemoreceptors in the medulla monitor O_2, CO_2 and pH levels of the blood, both directly and through special sensors in arteries.
   b. Mechanical monitoring: mechanoreceptors in the lung, airway, thoracic wall and abdominal wall detect and respond to:
      (1) Changes in lung or abdominal wall volumes.
      (2) Changes in the force exerted by inspiratory and expiratory muscles.
      (3) The presence of aggravating substances such as dust, smoke or cold air.
   c. Proprioceptors in respiratory system muscles and associated joints:
      (1) Inform brainstem respiratory centers about body position and muscle movement.
4. The integration of chemical and mechanical information paired with emotional and cognitive factors help guide respiratory efforts.

Inspiration during Quiet Breathing

1. Medulla sends signals to the diaphragm to contract.
   a. Signals are sent via motor axons from cervical spinal nerves 3-5, which converge to form the right and left phrenic nerves.
   b. Contraction lowers/flattens the diaphragm, vertically enlarging the thoracic cavity and thereby expanding the lungs.
   c. Expansion of the lungs increases volume and generates negative pressure.
   d. Negative pressure draws air inward (inhalation).
2. Medulla sends signals to the external intercostals (rib cage muscles) to contract.
   a. Signals are sent to contract via thoracic spinal nerves.
   b. Contraction causes rib cage elevation and horizontal expansion, further distending the lungs.
   c. Contraction contributes to negative lung pressures that cause inhalation.
   d. Air rushes into the lungs until the pressures inside and outside of the lungs are equal.

Expiration during Quiet Breathing

1. In the expiratory phase of breathing, the lungs, chest wall, and rib cage return to their relaxed (nondistended) position due to:

a. Elastic recoil of the distended lungs and rib cage.
b. Gravitational pull on the elevated rib cage.
2. The diaphragm returns to its resting (domed) position.
3. These changes compress the lungs and cause alveolar pressure to rise.
4. Air is passively pushed out of the lungs until the relaxation volume is reached.
5. For each cycle of quiet respiration:
   a. The inspiratory phase accounts for 40% of the breathing cycle.
   b. The expiratory phase accounts for 60% of the breathing cycle.

Speech Breathing (Volitional/Active)

1. During speech, airflow is actively controlled to maintain sufficient and constant pressure for sustained phonation.

Inspiration during Speech Breathing

1. Larger volumes of air are inspired during speech breathing than during passive breathing.
2. Inspiration takes place faster than during passive breathing.
3. The inspiratory phase accounts for 10% of the breathing cycle (instead of 40%).
4. Primary muscles used in quiet breathing also initiate inspiration during speech breathing.
   a. Diaphragm.
   b. External intercostals.
5. To allow for greater volumes of air to be inspired rapidly, accessory muscles of the rib cage wall and abdominal wall may also contract.

Expiration during Speech Breathing

1. Larger volumes of air are expired than during quiet breathing.
2. Expiration is prolonged relative to inspiration during speech.
3. The expiratory phase accounts for 90% of the breathing cycle.
4. In contrast to passive breathing where expiration is passive, during speech breathing expiration must be actively controlled in order to support long phrase lengths and steady phonation.
5. Expiration is controlled/slowed by:
   a. Valving of expired air by the glottis (contact point of the vocal folds) during phonation.

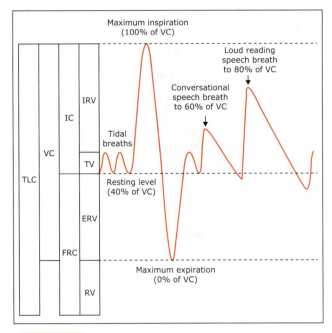

Figure 1-24 Respiratory Volumes and Capacities

TLC = total lung capacity; VC = vital capacity; IC = inspiratory capacity; FRC = functional residual capacity; IRV = inspiratory reserve volume; TV = tidal volume; ERV = expiratory reserve volume; RV = residual volume

   b. Contraction of muscles of inspiration to counteract gravitational pull and tissue recoil forces (when lung volume is greater than the relaxation level).
6. Primary muscles that can induce forced expiration such as during coughing include:
   a. Abdominal muscles.
   b. Internal intercostals.

Respiratory Volumes/Capacities

1. Air within the respiratory system is often described in terms of four discrete (nonoverlapping) volumes, as well as in terms of combined volumes, referred to as capacities (see Figure 1-24).
2. Discrete, nonoverlapping volumes.
   a. Tidal volume (TV): average volume of air exchanged in a cycle of passive breathing.
      (1) Represents approximately 10% of a person's vital capacity (see capacities).
   b. Inspiratory reserve volume (IRV): the maximal volume of air that can be inspired above the level of tidal inspiration.
   c. Expiratory reserve volume (ERV): the maximum volume of air that can be expired below relaxation volume.
   d. Residual volume (RV): the volume of air that remains in the lungs after a maximum exhalation.

e. This volume changes over the course of healthy aging, as people use less of their total lung capacity during breathing.
3. Capacities/combined volumes.
   a. Vital capacity (VC): volume of air exchanged between a maximum inspiration and a maximum expiration.
      (1) Approximately 4 L in women, 5 L in men.
      (2) Vital capacity = IRV + TV + ERV.
   b. Functional residual capacity (FRC)/resting/relaxation volume: volume of air in the lungs at the end of the expiratory phase of tidal breathing.
      (1) Functional residual capacity = ERV + RV.
   c. Inspiratory capacity (IC): maximum volume of air that can be inspired.
      (1) Inspiratory capacity = TV + IRV.
   d. Total lung capacity (TLC): = IRV + TV + ERV + RV.

Anatomy of Phonation and Swallowing

Speech Breathing

1. Controlled in a manner that allows one to maintain constant pressure for phonation.
2. Pressure and airflow create the aerodynamic forces that drive phonation (voice production).
3. Respiration/phonation must be coordinated with swallowing.

The Larynx

1. An organ critical to airway protection and phonation (Figure 1-25).
   a. Located in the neck, at the level of C3–C6.
   b. Connects the oropharynx and laryngopharynx to the trachea.
2. Comprises cartilages, connective tissues, epithelia, nerves and muscles.
   a. The larynx has prominent folds of tissue (vocal folds or cords) that can be positioned to interact with the flow of air from the trachea and generate sound, or squeezed together to act as a sphincter that closes off the airway for protection or when generating high thoracic/abdominal pressures for heavy lifting, defecation, childbirth, etc.
   b. Multiple pairs of muscles attach to the cartilages of the larynx, which enable one to control vocal fold position, length, and tension to manipulate vocal frequency and amplitude (in conjunction with the respiratory system).
3. The larynx also plays a critical role in airway protection during swallowing.

Laryngeal Cartilages

1. The larynx has a framework of single midline cartilages (thyroid, cricoid, and epiglottis) and smaller right/left cartilage pairs (arytenoid, corniculate, cuneiform).
   a. These cartilages, and the muscles that move them, maintain an open airway for respiration and enable one to control the flow of air and prevent aspiration (food/liquid entering the trachea and lungs).
2. Thyroid cartilage.
   a. The largest cartilage of the larynx, the thyroid is formed by two hyaline plates that join at the front of the neck in a shape like a shield and are open in the back.
   b. Laryngeal prominence: an anterior projection where left and right thyroid plates fuse.
      (1) Often called the Adam's apple because it is larger and more visible in males.
      (2) The angle of fusion is more acute in males (90°) than in females (120°), causing greater anterior projection in males.
   c. Superior horns: superior extensions or cornu (Latin for horn) from the thyroid plates that attach to the hyoid bone via the hyothyroid ligaments.
   d. Inferior horns: smaller, inferior extensions from the thyroid plates that form joints with the cricoid cartilage.
3. Cricoid cartilage.
   a. A complete ring of cartilage attached to the superior end of the trachea that forms the base of the larynx.
   b. Connects to the first tracheal semicircular ring.
   c. Has a signet shape whereby the anterior height (arch in front) is about 7 mm tall but the posterior portion is three times as tall. The relatively narrow anterior height can be felt with your fingertip by pressing into the cricothyroid membrane (connecting the cricoid and thyroid cartilages) at the front of your neck.
   d. Posterior lamina: large, flattened posterior portion of the cricoid. The superior edge has right and left facets on which the arytenoid cartilages sit and articulate (rock back/forth and slide front/back).

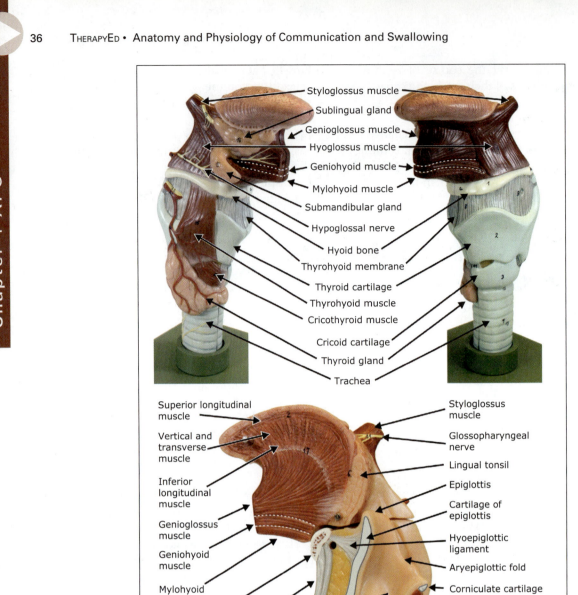

Figure 1-25 Anatomy of the Larynx and Tongue

4. Arytenoid cartilages.
  a. Two small cartilages that articulate on saddle-shaped joints located on the laminar (posterior) surface of the cricoid.
  b. Pyramid or cone-shaped.
  c. Muscular process: projection at the lateral base of each arytenoid.

    (1) The muscular process is the connection point for:
      (a) Posterior cricoarytenoid muscle.
      (b) Lateral cricoarytenoid muscle.
      (c) Thyroarytenoid muscle.
  d. Vocal process: projection at the anterior base of each arytenoid.

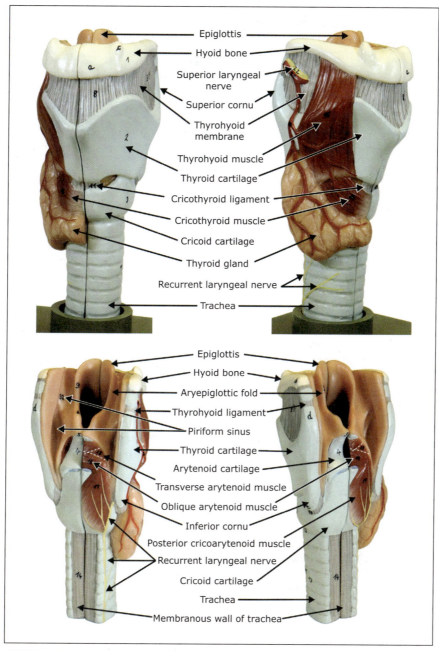

Figure 1-25 Anatomy of the Larynx and Tongue (*Continued*)

   (1) Vocal process is the connection point for the vocal folds and is a part of the posterior ⅓ ("cartilaginous") portion of the vocal folds.
5. Epiglottis.
   a. Mucous membrane covered elastic cartilage that originates just below the thyroid notch and extends upward toward the hyoid bone.
   b. Tear-drop shaped (inverted).
   c. Made of highly flexible, perforated elastic cartilage.
   d. Aryepiglottic folds: folds made up of connective tissue and muscle that extend posteriorly between the lateral sides of the epiglottis and the arytenoid cartilages.
      (1) The aryepiglottic folds form a division between the laryngeal opening and the pyriform sinuses.
      (2) Contraction of the muscle of the aryepiglottic folds inverts the epiglottis.
   e. The coordinated anterior and superior motion of the hyoid and larynx during swallowing leads to epiglottic inversion, protecting the airway.

Table 1-3

Intrinsic Muscles of the Larynx

VOCALIS MUSCLES[a]	THYROARYTENOIDS [TA]
Action: Form vibrational mass of vocal folds Function: Change thickness/tense vocal folds, change vocal tone Motor Innervation: CN X–RLN	Action: Draw arytenoids cartilages forward Function: Tense, shorten vocal folds Motor Innervation: CN X–RLN
CRICOTHYROIDS [CT]	**LATERAL CRICOARYTENOIDS [LCA]**
Action: Tilt thyroid cartilage down, stretching vocal folds Function: Work with the TA muscles to raise pitch Motor Innervation: CN X–SLN	Action: Medially rotate arytenoid cartilages Function: Adduct vocal folds Motor Innervation: CN X–RLN
TRANSVERSE AND OBLIQUE INTERARYTENOIDS (IA)	**POSTERIOR CRICOARYTENOIDS [PCA]**
Action: Draw arytenoids together Function: Adduct vocal folds Motor Innervation: CN X - RLN	Action: Externally rotate arytenoid cartilages Function: Abduct vocal folds Motor Innervation: CN X–RLN

[a] Often considered a subdivision of the TA muscles
RLN = recurrent laryngeal nerve, SLN = superior laryngeal nerve

Hyoid Bone

1. A free-floating bone anchored by muscle and ligament connections to the tongue, jaw, skull, pharynx, laryngeal cartilages, sternum and scapula.
2. Horseshoe-shaped.
3. Not technically part of the larynx, but an important contributor to laryngeal and tongue positioning.

Intrinsic Muscles of the Larynx

1. Muscles that span between two or more laryngeal cartilages. (See Table 1-3.)
2. The primary function of two of the intrinsic laryngeal muscles is to control vocal fold length and tension.
3. Thyroarytenoid muscles (TA).
   a. Make up the body of the vocal folds (along with the vocal ligament).
   b. Span from the interior surface of the thyroid cartilage to the vocal and muscular processes of the arytenoids.
   c. Sometimes described in terms of two muscular divisions:
      (1) Thyromuscularis: lateral division.
      (2) Thyrovocalis/vocalis: medial division.
   d. Contraction typically draws the arytenoid cartilages forward.
   e. Contraction shortens and tenses the body of the vocal folds.
4. Cricothyroid muscles (CT).
   a. Span from the anterior/superior surface of the cricoid cartilage to the inferior edge and inferior horns of the thyroid cartilage.
   b. Two subdivisions:
      (1) Pars rectus: medial division.
      (2) Pars oblique: lateral division.
   c. Contraction typically draws the cricoid and thyroid cartilages together anteriorly.
   d. Contraction rocks the cricoid cartilage backward at the location of the arytenoid cartilages, which stretches the vocal folds and contributes to raising pitch.

Vocal Fold Adductors

1. Lateral cricoarytenoid muscles (LCA).
   a. Span from the lateral/superior surface of the cricoid cartilage to the muscular process of the arytenoids (anterior surface).
   b. Contraction draws the muscular processes of the arytenoids forward and medially (together), adducting the vocal folds.
2. Transverse and oblique interarytenoid muscles (IA).
   a. Span from the posterior surfaces of the arytenoid cartilages to the opposite posterior arytenoid cartilage surface.
   b. Fibers of the single midline transverse muscle run horizontally.
   c. Right and left oblique muscles have fibers that cross diagonally and either attach to the apex of

the contralateral arytenoid cartilage or continue beyond the arytenoid and reach the epiglottis within the aryepiglottic fold (forming the aryepiglottic muscle).
  d. Contraction rotates the arytenoids forward, drawing them together and adducting the vocal folds. Contraction of the oblique interarytenoid and aryepiglottic fibers narrows the laryngeal inlet and draws the epiglottis posteriorly to protect the airway during swallowing.

Vocal Fold Abductors

1. Posterior cricoarytenoid muscles (PCA).
  a. Span from the cricoid laminae (posterior surface) to the muscular processes of the arytenoids (posterior surface).
  b. Contraction pulls the muscular processes of the arytenoids posteriorly. From a superior view, contraction of the PCA can be seen to rotate the left arytenoid cartilage counterclockwise and the right arytenoid clockwise, abducting the vocal folds.

Motor Innervation of Intrinsic Laryngeal Muscles

1. All laryngeal muscles are innervated by branches of the vagus nerve (cranial nerve X).
2. The cricothyroid (CT) muscles receive motor innervations through the external branch of the superior laryngeal nerve (eSLN).
3. All remaining intrinsic laryngeal muscles receive motor innervations via the recurrent laryngeal nerve (RLN). (See Figure 1-26.)

Extrinsic Muscles of the Larynx

1. Muscles connected to the hyoid bone or laryngeal cartilage that vertically positions and supports the hyolaryngeal complex.
  a. The hyoid bone and thyroid cartilage of the larynx are attached via the thyrohyoid ligament and thyrohyoid membrane, so they tend to move as a unit, or complex. (See Table 1-4.)
2. Suprahyoid muscles.
  a. Contribute to hyoid elevation, and their action may raise the larynx, tensing the vocal folds and contributing to increased pitch.
  b. Help widen the pharynx and esophageal opening during swallowing.
  c. Mylohyoid.
    (1) Spans from the mandible to the hyoid.
    (2) Flat muscle that forms a majority of the floor of mouth.
    (3) Contraction elevates the hyoid bone and draws it forward or lowers the jaw if the hyoid bone is fixed (held stable by other muscles).
    (4) Motorically innervated by the mandibular nerve, a division of the trigeminal (CN V).
  d. Geniohyoid.
    (1) Spans from the mandible to the hyoid.
    (2) Cylindrical muscle that lies superior to the mylohyoid.
    (3) Contraction elevates the hyoid bone and draws it forward.
    (4) Motorically innervated by the hypoglossal nerve (CN XII).
  e. Stylohyoid.
    (1) Spans from the styloid process of the temporal bone to the hyoid.
    (2) Cylindrical muscle that is identifiable near its attachment to the hyoid bone because the posterior digastric pierces through the middle of the muscle.
    (3) Contraction elevates the hyoid bone and draws it backward.
    (4) Motorically innervated by the facial nerve (CN VII).
  f. Digastric muscle.
    (1) Comprises two parts: anterior belly and posterior belly, with a common tendon attached to the hyoid bone.
      (a) Anterior belly of the digastric.
        • Originates from the mandible.
        • Motorically innervated by the mandibular nerve, a division of the trigeminal (CN V).
      (b) Posterior belly of the digastric.
        • Longer than the anterior belly.
        • Originates from the mastoid process of the temporal bone.
        • Motorically innervated by the digastric nerve, a branch of the facial nerve (CN VII).
    (2) Anterior and posterior bellies join at an intermediate tendon.
    (3) The intermediate tendon passes through a fibrous sling connected to the hyoid bone.
    (4) The fibrous sling allows the tendon to slide forward and backward.
    (5) Contraction elevates and steadies the hyoid bone.
    (6) Contraction may also draw the hyoid bone forward (anterior belly) or backward (posterior belly).
3. Infrahyoids (strap muscles).
  a. The infrahyoid muscles (strap muscles) contribute to hyolaryngeal depression.
  b. Sternohyoid.

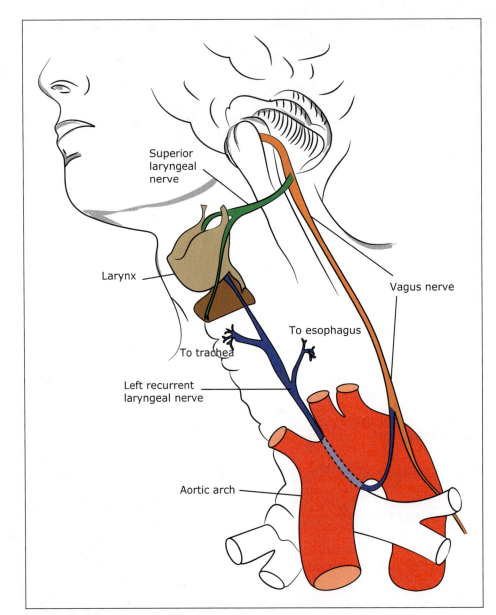

Figure 1-26 Motor Innervation of the Laryngeal Musculature

Adapted from "Laryngeal Nerve" by Truth-Seeker2004. Retrieved from http://en.wikipedia.org/wiki/Recurrent_laryngeal_nerve.

(1) Spans from the sternum and inner clavicle to the lower edge of the hyoid bone.
(2) Long, flat, vertically coursing muscle.
(3) Contraction lowers the hyoid bone or steadies the hyoid bone in the context of opposing contractions.
(4) Motorically innervated by the ansa cervicalis, which is a nerve arising from motor axons of spinal nerves C1, C2 and C3.
  c. Omohyoid.
    (1) From the scapula (shoulder blade) to the lower edge of the hyoid bone.

(2) Comprises two parts: anterior and posterior.
(3) Anterior and posterior portions connect at an intermediate tendon, passing through a fascial sling.
(4) The fascial sling is attached to the clavicle, maintaining the tendon's positioning.
(5) Contraction lowers the hyoid bone and draws it backward and steadies the hyoid bone in the context of opposing contractions.
(6) Motorically innervated by the ansa cervicalis.
  d. Thyrohyoid.
    (1) Spans from the thyroid cartilage to the lower edge of the hyoid bone.

Table 1-4

Extrinsic Muscles of the Larynx	
SUPRAHYOID MUSCLES—CONTRIBUTE TO HYOID ELEVATION	
Mylohyoid Action: Elevates hyoid, tenses floor of mouth Innervation: CN V	**Stylohyoid** Action: Elevates and retracts hyoid bone, lengthens floor of mouth Innervation: CN VII
Geniohyoid Action: Elevates and advances hyoid widening pharynx during swallow, shortens floor of mouth Innervation: CN XII	**Digastric** Action: Elevates hyoid, supports hyoid during swallow, depresses mandible Anterior belly innervation: CN V Posterior belly innervation: CN VII
INFRAHYOID (STRAP) MUSCLES—CONTRIBUTE TO HYOID/THYROID DEPRESSION	
Sternohyoid Action: Depresses hyoid bone, helps steady hyoid Innervation: C1–C3 (ansa cervicalis)	**Sternothyroid** Action: Depresses hyoid bone and larynx Innervation: C1-C3 (ansa cervicalis)
Thyrohyoid Action: Depresses hyoid or elevates larynx toward hyoid bone for airway protection during swallow Innervation: CN XII	**Omohyoid** Action: Depresses, retracts and steadies hyoid bone during speaking and swallowing Innervation: C2, C3 (ansa cervicalis)

(2) Contraction lowers the hyoid bone and elevates the larynx.
(3) Motorically innervated by ansa cervicalis.
e. Sternothyroid.
  (1) Spans from the manubrium of the sternum to an oblique line across the anterior surface of the thyroid cartilage.
  (2) Runs over portions of the thyroid gland and may limit thyroid gland expansion.
  (3) Contraction lowers the larynx or steadies the larynx in the context of opposing contractions.
  (4) Motorically innervated by ansa cervicalis.

The Vocal Folds

1. Two pliable mucous membranes within the larynx that extend from the anterior thyroid cartilage to the vocal process of the arytenoids (Figure 1-27).
2. The vocal folds are a layered structure, covered in a nonkeratinized stratified squamous epithelium (see section "The Study of Speech, Language, and Swallowing" above).
3. Vocal fold layers (from internal to external structures).
   a. Vocalis muscle/thyrovocalis (internal/medial division of the TA muscle).
   b. Lamina propria (LP): thin layer of connective tissue that, together with the epithelium, forms a mucous membrane.
      (1) Deep (DLP): primarily collagen fibers.
      (2) Intermediate (ILP): primarily elastic fibers.
      (3) Superficial (SLP): few elastic and collagenous fibers.
   c. Epithelium: external tissue that covers the entire body of the vocal folds.
4. The glottis: term used to describe the space between the right and left vocal folds.
5. The vocal folds are often described in terms of the *body* and *cover*.
   a. The body comprises the thyroarytenoid muscle, the deep LP and the intermediate LP.
   b. The cover is highly gelatinous and pliable; comprises the superficial LP and epithelium.
   c. The body is stiffer than the cover.
6. Factors such as radiation therapy or vocal fold pathologies such as nodules and polyps may affect stiffness and pliability.

Myoelastic Aerodynamic Theory

1. A theory that describes the driving force and process of vocal fold vibration in terms of three major components.
2. *Myo-* means "muscle."
   a. Muscle contractions of intrinsic and extrinsic laryngeal muscles affect the tension and positioning of the vocal folds.
   b. Vocal folds are drawn together, or medialized, during voicing.
   c. Vocal folds are drawn apart during breathing and for the production of voiceless phonemes.

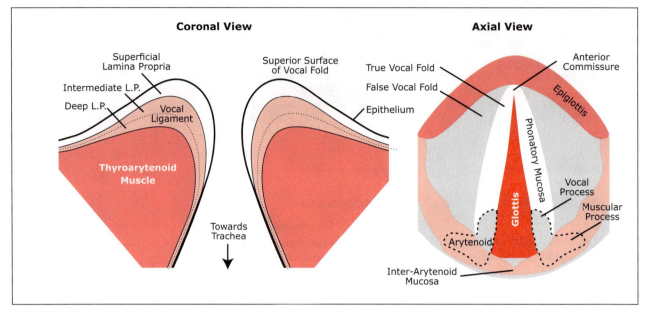

Figure 1-27 The Vocal Folds

3. Elastic.
   a. Refers to the elastic, pliable property of the LP.
   b. The elastic nature of superficial vocal fold layers leads to vibration that is wavelike, rather than rigid.
   c. Vocal fold vibration produces a mucosal wave.
   d. Contraction of the intrinsic and extrinsic laryngeal muscles will impact the stiffness of the cover.
4. Aerodynamic.
   a. Vocal fold vibration depends on vocal fold tension and positioning as well as on airflow.
   b. Air pressure and airflow provide the forces that drive phonation.
5. Typical cycle of voicing.
   a. The vocal folds are adducted, closing the glottis.
   b. Subglottal air pressure (pressure below the vocal folds) builds up.
   c. Air pressure eventually blows open the vocal folds.
      (1) Inferior portions open before superior portions, producing a wavelike motion from bottom to top.
      (2) Described as a mucosal wave.
   d. As explained by the Bernoulli principle, as air rushes through the glottis, pressure decreases.
   e. The decrease in pressure, paired with the pliable nature of the vocal folds, closes the vocal folds.
   f. With the vocal folds closed, pressure once again builds up leading to another cycle of vibration.
6. Glottal pulse: each puff of air that is emitted as vocal folds blow apart.
   a. Glottal pulse rate determines a person's fundamental frequency (F0).
   b. Glottal pulse rate/fundamental frequency (F0) varies across individuals.
      (1) A typical male F0 is around 125 Hz while a typical female F0 is around 210 Hz.

Muscles of Mastication

1. There are four primary muscles of mastication responsible for vertical and lateral motion of the jaw. Movement of the mandible is critical to the oral preparatory stage of swallowing and for speaking (Figure 1-28).
   a. Masseter muscles.
      (1) Contribute to mandible elevation.
   b. Temporal muscles.
      (1) Contribute to mandible elevation.
      (2) Contraction of posterior fibers of the temporal muscles retracts the mandible.
   c. The medial (or internal) pterygoid muscles.
      (1) Contribute to mandible elevation.
   d. The lateral (or external) pterygoid muscles.
      (1) Responsible for depressing and protruding the mandible.
      (2) The suprahyoid muscles assist in mandible depression.
   e. Alternating contraction of the medial and lateral pterygoid muscles produces side-to-side motion of the jaw.
2. All muscles of mastication are paired, meaning that there is a left and right muscle.
3. The muscles of mastication are innervated by the mandibular division of the trigeminal nerve.

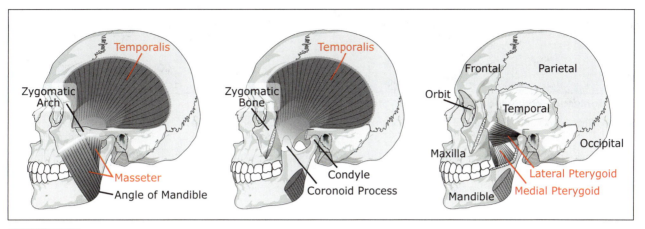

Figure 1-28 **Muscles of Mastication**

4. The temporomandibular joint (TMJ).
   a. The TMJ, a small hinge joint located at the boundary of the temporal bone and the mandible makes jaw motion in three planes of direction possible (lateral, vertical and anterior-posterior).
   b. The TMJ is divided into two parts by the articular disc, a piece of small fibrocartilaginous tissue.
      (1) There is a superior joint that connects the temporal bone with the articular disc, and an inferior joint that connects the articular disc with the mandible.
   c. The TMJ is involved in speech, chewing and swallowing and is susceptible to dysfunction or dislocation.

The Tongue

1. The tongue is a large mass of muscles extending from the oropharynx to the oral cavity and covered by a mucous membrane.
   a. This muscular hydrostat, so called because of its primarily muscular composition without skeletal support, is capable of making highly complex, controlled movements important for speech, chewing, swallowing and, to some degree, dental hygiene.
2. The tongue is also important for taste, containing small prominences on its surface that contain taste receptors.
3. The tongue comprises multiple parts: a root, body, apex, dorsum and inferior surface.
   a. The anterior and posterior portions of the tongue are separated by a V-shaped groove called the terminal groove.
4. On the inferior surface of the tongue there is a small fold of mucous membrane called the lingual frenulum that attaches the undersurface of the tongue to the floor of the mouth.
5. Blood is supplied to the tongue through the lingual artery, a branch of the external carotid artery.
6. The tongue is composed of eight major muscles, divided into two groups: the intrinsic and the extrinsic muscles.
7. All of the muscles of the tongue receive innervation from CN XII, the hypoglossal nerve, with the exception of the palatoglossus (see below).

Tongue Muscles

1. Intrinsic muscles (Table 1-5).
   a. There are four intrinsic muscles of the tongue, grouped together because they are not attached to any bone and therefore only exist within the tongue.
   b. These muscles, whose contraction leads to shape changes of the tongue, are: the superior longitudinal, the inferior longitudinal, transverse and vertical muscle (Figure 1-25).
      (1) Superior longitudinal muscles: contain fibers that run anteriorly to posteriorly underneath the mucous membrane of the tongue dorsum.
         (a) Contraction of the superior longitudinal muscles shortens the tongue or elevates the tongue tip and/or sides of the tongue.
      (2) Inferior longitudinal muscles: a narrow band of fibers that course along the inferior surface of the tongue whose contraction shortens the tongue or causes the apex of the tongue to curl down.
      (3) Transverse muscles: course deeper than the superior longitudinal muscles and contain fibers that originate in the median plane of the tongue and extend laterally.
         (a) Contraction of these muscles narrows and elongates the tongue.
      (4) Vertical muscles: run top to bottom in the tongue and flatten the tongue when contracted.

Table 1-5
Intrinsic and Extrinsic Muscles of the Tongue

MUSCLES	ORIENTATIONS/CONNECTIONS	ACTION	CONTRIBUTIONS TO SPEECH AND SWALLOWING
Intrinsic Muscles–Within the Tongue (all innervated by CN XII)			
Superior longitudinal	Superficial antero–posterior fibers	Tongue shortening, tongue tip elevation, lateral edge elevation	Intrinsic tongue muscles produce fine lingual shape changes important to speech articulation, mastication and swallowing
Inferior longitudinal	Deep antero–posterior fibers	Tongue shortening, tongue tip depression	
Transverse	Side-to-side fibers, interwoven with vertical muscles	Tongue narrowing and elongation	
Vertical	Top-to-bottom fibers, interwoven with transverse muscles	Tongue flattening	
Extrinsic Muscles–From Tongue to Other Structures (almost all innervated by CN XII)			
Genioglossus	Body of mandible to root, dorsum, blade and tip of tongue. Bulk of tongue	Tongue protrusion/anterior movement, side-to-side movement	Extrinsic muscles contribute to gross positioning and movements of the tongue important for mastication, swallow initiation and swallowing
Hyoglossus	Greater horn of hyoid to inferior sides of tongue	Tongue body lowering, backward movement	
Styloglossus	Styloid process to sides of tongue	Tongue retraction, shortening, lateral edge elevation	
Palatoglossus*	Soft palate to sides of tongue, forms anterior faucial pillars	Posterior tongue elevation, soft palate depressionn	

* Palatoglossus innervated by CN IX and X via the pharyngeal plexus

2. Extrinsic muscles (Table 1-5).
   a. The four extrinsic muscles of the tongue originate from bone and extend into the tongue. Contraction of these muscles primarily contributes to tongue motion and positioning.
      (1) Genioglossus: a large, fan-shaped muscle that constitutes the majority of the tongue body.
         (a) Originates in the mental spine (posterior midline) of the mandible and inserts into the hyoid bone and tongue dorsum.
         (b) Contraction of the genioglossus protrudes the tongue and can also produce side-to-side movement of the tongue when contracted unilaterally.
      (2) Hyoglossus: a thin, square-shaped muscle that courses from the body and greater horn of the hyoid to each side of the tongue.
         (a) Contraction of the hyoglossus pulls the tongue edges down and helps shorten the tongue.
      (3) Styloglossus: runs from the lower end of the styloid process to the sides and inferior aspects of the tongue.
         (a) Contraction of the styloglossus shortens the tongue and curls the edges up, helping create a narrow trough in the tongue center through which a bolus can cohesively move during deglutition.
      (4) Palatoglossus: a narrow muscle joining the posterior border of the hard palate (the palatine aponeurosis) with the posterolateral tongue.
         (a) Some fibers of the palatoglossus pass deeply into the tongue and intermingle with the intrinsic transverse muscles.
         (b) Contraction of the palatoglossus lowers the soft palate or elevates the posterior tongue. Contraction of the palatoglossus is essential for swallowing in order to constrict the isthmus of fauces, a constricted space that connects the mouth and the pharynx.
         (c) The palatoglossus is the only tongue muscle not innervated by CN XII (it is innervated by CN IX and X via the pharyngeal plexus).

Muscles of the Face

1. Several facial muscles are critical to speech production and swallowing, in addition to producing facial expressions used in nonverbal communication.
2. Orbicularis oris: comprises intertwined fibers, forms a ring around the lips, and when contracted, contributes to opening and closing of the lips, puckering, and vertical or lateral movements of the lips.

3. Buccinator: a broad muscle with horizontally coursing fibers that originate from several locations, including the outer alveolar processes of the maxilla and mandible (above and below the cheek wall, respectively) as well as the pterygomandibular ligament that separates it from the superior pharyngeal constrictor posteriorly.
   a. Inserts into the upper and lower lip.
   b. Forms part of the cheek wall, and contraction produces tension that pulls the cheek against the teeth.
4. Risorius: sometimes referred to as the "laughter muscle," is a narrow bundle of horizontally coursing fibers that originates from the masseter muscle and insert at the angle of the mouth.
   a. Contraction retracts the angle of the mouth.
5. Five paired muscles contribute to the raising or lowering of the lips.
   a. The levator labii superioris, levator labii superioris alaeque nasi and the zygomatic minor insert into the upper lip and contribute to elevating or everting (turning it outward) the upper lip. Contraction of the zygomatic minor also pulls the corners of the mouth upward.
   b. The zygomatic major originates from the zygomatic bone and inserts into the corner of the mouth. Contraction draws the corners of the mouth backward, simultaneously lifting and pulling the corners of the mouth sideways.
   c. The depressor labii inferioris is a flat muscle that originates from the anterior surface of the mandible, coursing upward to insert into the lower lip. Contraction depresses and turns the lower lip outward.
6. Mentalis: originates from the mandible inferior to the incisor teeth and courses downward into the chin.
   a. This muscle is often referred to as the "pouting muscle" due to its contraction, which forces a curling of the lower lip.
7. Paired levator anguli oris and depressor anguli oris muscles draw the corners of the mouth up and down, respectively. Contraction of each of these muscles can also draw the lips together.
8. Beneath the levator anguli oris and depressor oris are the incisivus labii superioris and incisivus labii inferioris. Contraction of these muscles pulls the corners of the mouth upward toward the midline or downward toward the midline.
9. Platysma: a broad, superficial muscle with infra- and supraclavicular origins that courses medially and obliquely up the neck, inserting into the lower edge of the mandible and into muscles of the lower face.
   a. Contraction of the platysma can depress the lower lip and corners of the mouth or produce a vertical wrinkling of the skin of the neck as the skin of the neck is drawn toward the mandible.

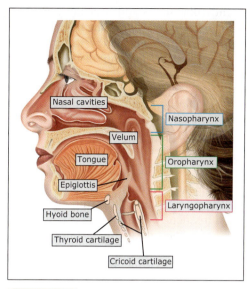

Figure 1-29 Major Cavities of the Supralaryngeal System

Systems Involved in Speech Production

1. Three major systems contribute to speech production: the respiratory system, the laryngeal system and the supralaryngeal system.
2. The respiratory system provides the driving force behind voice production and other articulated sounds of speech.
3. The laryngeal system, located on top of the trachea, acts as a valve for airway protection, closing like a sphincter during swallowing to prevent aspiration, and generating voice with specialized vocal folds or cords when powered by the respiratory system.
   a. Periodic vocal fold vibration is the principle sound source of speech.
4. The supralaryngeal system comprises articulators and cavities that filter and shape phonation and glottal aspiration sounds.
5. The three major cavities of the supralaryngeal system are the pharyngeal cavity, the oral cavity and the nasal cavity (Figure 1-29).
   a. The pharynx, a cavity that can be divided into the nasopharynx, the oropharynx and the laryngopharynx, is a tube of tendon and muscle that extends from the base of the skull to behind the larynx where it is continuous with the esophagus.
   b. The oral cavity, or mouth cavity, is bounded by the palate, the oropharynx and the cheeks and lips.
      (1) The anterior portion of the palate, the hard palate, is bony, while the posterior portion, the soft palate, consists of fleshy mucous membrane,

muscular fibers and mucous glands. Together, these form the roof of the mouth.
   (2) The velum consists of the soft palate and uvula (a fleshy tissue and muscle extension of the soft palate in the back of the throat).
   (3) Paired contraction of the tensor veli palatini and the levator veli palatini elevates the velum and draws it backward, making contact with the posterior pharyngeal wall.
  c. Contact between the velum and the posterior pharyngeal wall stops the passage of air through the nasal cavity, the large air-filled space behind the nose.
6. These cavities act as resonating tubes that amplify and dampen frequencies that radiate through them.
  a. These amplified resonant frequencies produce the formants that are used to describe and recognize vowels.
7. In order to articulate consonants and vowels, fine motor movements are made with the lips, tongue, mandible and glottis to further shape sound as it resonates through the supralaryngeal cavities.
  a. The lower lip, tongue and glottis move during the production of speech and are considered active speech articulators.
  b. Active articulators approach or make contact with structures such as the upper lip, teeth, alveolar ridge, hard palate, soft palate, uvula and pharynx, which remain fixed during speech and are considered passive articulators.
8. Often, the interaction of these systems is described by source filter theory, an acoustic theory that describes speech production based on two fundamental processes: sound production and sound filtering.

References

Barnett, M. W., & Larkman, P. M. (2007). The action potential. *Practical Neurology*, 7(3), 192–197.

Bhatnagar, S. C. (2013). *Neuroscience for the Study of Communicative Disorders*, 4th ed. Philadelphia, PA: Wolters Kluwer Health/Lippincott Williams & Wilkins.

Blumenfeld, H. (2010). *Neuroanatomy through Clinical Cases*, 2nd ed. Sunderland, MA: Sinauer Associates.

Burdett, E., & Mitchell, V. (2011). Anatomy of the larynx, trachea and bronchi. *Anaesthesia and Intensive Care Medicine*, 12(8), 335–339.

Colton, R. H., Casper, J. K., & Leonard, R. (2011). *Understanding Voice Problems: A Physiological Perspective for Diagnosis and Treatment*, 4th ed. Philadelphia, PA: Wolters Kluwer Health/Lippincott Williams & Wilkins.

Davis, M. C., Griessenauer, C. J., Bosmia, A. N., Tubbs, R. S., & Shoja, M. M. (2014). The naming of the cranial nerves: a historical review. *Clinical Anatomy*, 27(1), 14–19.

Fuller, D. R., Pimentel, J. T., & Peregoy, B. M. (2012). *Applied Anatomy & Physiology for Speech-Language Pathology & Audiology*. Philadelphia, PA: Wolters Kluwer/Lippincott Williams & Wilkins Health.

Gray, H., Standring, S., Ellis, H., & Berkovitz, B. K. B. (2005). *Gray's Anatomy: The Anatomical Basis of Clinical Practice*, 39th ed. Edinburgh, UK: Elsevier Churchill Livingstone.

Hixon, T. J., Weismer, G., & Hoit, J. D. (2014). *Preclinical Speech Science: Anatomy, Physiology, Acoustics, Perception*, 2nd ed. San Diego, CA: Plural Publishing.

Hodgkin, A. L., & Huxley, A. F. (1952). Propagation of electrical signals along giant nerve fibers. *Proceedings of the Royal Society of London. Series B: Biological Sciences*, 140(899), 177–183.

Kandel, E. R. (2013). *Principles of Neural Science*, 5th ed. New York, NY: McGraw-Hill Medical.

Mildner, V. (2006). *The Cognitive Neuroscience of Human Communication*. Mahwah, NJ: Lawrence Erlbaum Associates.

Moon, J., & Alipour, F. (2013). Muscular anatomy of the human ventricular folds. *Annals of Otology, Rhinology and Laryngology*, 122(9), 561–567.

Myers, P. S. (1999). *Right Hemisphere Damage: Disorders of Communication and Cognition*. San Diego, CA: Singular Publishing.

Osborn, A. G., Jacobs, J. M., & Osborn, A. G. (1999). *Diagnostic Cerebral Angiography*, 2nd ed. Philadelphia, PA: Lippincott-Raven.

Seikel, J. A., King, D. W., & Drumright, D. G. (2010). *Anatomy & Physiology for Speech, Language, and Hearing*, 4th ed. Clifton Park, NY: Delmar Cengage Learning.

Titze, I. R. (2006). *The Myoelastic Aerodynamic Theory of Phonation*. Iowa City, IA: National Center for Voice and Speech.

Van Den Berg, J. (1958). Myoelastic-aerodynamic theory of voice production. *Journal of Speech and Hearing Research*, 1(3), 227–244.

Zeitels, S. M., & Healy, G. B. (2003). Laryngology and phonosurgery. *New England Journal of Medicine*, 349(9), 882–892.

2
Acoustics

JEAN ANDRUSKI, PhD

Chapter Outline

- Nature of Sound, 48
- Graphical Representations of Sounds, 50
- Types of Sounds and Their Graphical Representations, 52
- Periodic Complex Sounds in Speech, 55
- Aperiodic Complex Sounds in Speech, 56
- The Source-Filter Theory of Speech Production, 57
- Acoustic Characteristics of the Supralaryngeal Vocal Tract (SLVT), 59
- How Sounds Resonate in the Vocal Tract, 60
- Acoustic Characteristics of Resonant Sounds, 61
- Acoustic Characteristics of Obstruent Sounds, 65
- Acoustic Cues to Consonant Place of Articulation, 68
- Acoustic Measurement of Vocal Fold Vibration, 73
- References, 77

Nature of Sound

Pressure Wave

1. Sound propagates through air or another medium.
   a. It cannot propagate through a vacuum.

Vibration

1. Sound is produced by vibration.
   a. Molecules in a propagating medium are set in motion by a vibrating object.
   b. Molecules collide with other molecules, passing on the vibrational pattern.
   c. Sound produces alternating areas of high and low molecular density.
      (1) Areas of higher density and pressure are called areas of condensation.
      (2) Areas of lower density and pressure are called areas of rarefaction.

Frequency

1. A sound's frequency (f) is a count of the number of repetitions of a cyclic pattern in 1 second.
2. Most common measurement units of sounds are Hertz (Hz) and kilohertz (kHz).
   a. Periodic sounds have a frequency but aperiodic sounds do not.

Pitch

1. f is *perceived* as pitch.
   a. Equal changes in f do not correspond to equal changes in pitch.

2.
3. Perceptual scales for pitch include Mels and semitones (Table 2-1).
   a. Mels: pitch *units* that listeners judge to be equally distant from one another.
      (1) 1000 Mels = 1000 Hz.
   b. Semitones: intervals between sounds (Table 2-2).
      (1) 1 semitone change is always perceptually equal.
      (2) 12 semitones = 1 octave.
      (3) Octave: a doubling of f (Hz).
   c. Semitones must be expressed relative to some baseline frequency, e.g., 100 Hz.
      (1) When f is below the baseline, the semitone value will be negative, e.g., 89 Hz is −2 ST re: 100 Hz.

Period

1. Period (T): duration of 1 cycle.
   a. f and T have an inverse relationship, for example:
      (1) $T = 1/f$; e.g., if f = 100 Hz, $T = 1/100 = 0.01$ sec.
      (2) $f = 1/T$; e.g., if $T = 0.005$ sec, $T = 1/0.005 = 200$ Hz.

Amplitude

1. Amplitude (A): physical measure of extent of vibrational change from resting position.
2. Amplitude measurement methods that are regularly used in speech science.
   a. Peak amplitude—the maximum pressure reached by the pressure wave.
   b. Root mean square amplitude (RMS amplitude)—the average amplitude of a sound over some period of time.

Table 2-1

Examples of Perceptually Equal Changes in Pitch, as Measured in Mels and in Hertz

PITCH	100 MELS	200 MELS	300 MELS	400 MELS	500 MELS	600 MELS	700 MELS	800 MELS	900 MELS	1000 MELS	1100 MELS
FREQUENCY	65 HZ	136 HZ	213 HZ	298 HZ	391 HZ	492 HZ	603 HZ	724 HZ	855 HZ	1000 HZ	1158 HZ
Increase in *pitch* (Mels) vs. **frequency** (Hz) from preceding column	n/a	100 71	100 77	100 85	100 93	100 101	100 111	100 121	100 131	100 155	100 158

Table 2-2

Examples of Octave Intervals Relative to Baselines of 100, 125 and 150 Hz						
Example 1	**100 Hz**	200 Hz	400 Hz	800 Hz	1600 Hz	3200 Hz
Example 2	**125 Hz**	250 Hz	375 Hz	500 Hz	625 Hz	750 Hz
Example 3	**150 Hz**	300 Hz	600 Hz	1200 Hz	2400 Hz	4800 Hz
# of semitones above baseline	n/a	12	24	36	48	60
# of octaves above baseline	n/a	1	2	3	4	5

The interval from each column to the next is always 1 octave.

Intensity

1. Intensity (I): power of a sound over a particular area.
   a. Measured in watts per unit area, usually W/cm^2 or W/m^2.
2. $I = A^2$.
   a. A and I are both measured in decibels (dB).
      (1) Decibels are logarithmic units.
   b. Allows large range of intensities to be expressed more easily, i.e., using a smaller range of numbers.
   c. Also corresponds better with amplitude/intensity perception than linear scales.
   d. dB express a ratio of a sound's amplitude or intensity relative to a reference.
      (1) Reference level is typically threshold of human hearing for a 1000 Hz sinusoid.
      (2) 0 dB is the quietest sound that can be heard.
      (3) A is measured in decibels sound pressure level (dB-SPL).
   e. Reference level—20 µPa RMS, i.e., 20 micro Pascals root mean square amplitude.
      (1) Pascals—units of pressure.
3. I is measured in decibels intensity level (dB-IL).
   a. Reference level is 10^{-12} W/m^2, i.e., 10^{-12} watts per square meter.
      (1) Watts—units of power.

Loudness

1. Physical measures of A and I perceived as loudness.
2. Perception of A/I affected by factors including the sound's:
   a. f (frequency).
   b. Duration.
   c. Energy distribution across the frequency spectrum.
   d. Bandwidth.

3. Human hearing is most sensitive to sounds between 2 and 4 kHz.
   a. Measurement scales used for *perceived* loudness of sounds include phons and sones.

Duration

1. Duration—length of time a sound continues.
   a. Often measured in milliseconds (ms).
   b. 1 ms = 1/1000 sec.

Wavelength

1. Wavelength (λ): distance travelled by a sound during a single cycle (Figure 2-1).
   a. $\lambda = v/f$, where v is the velocity of sound travel.
   b. λ depends on the medium through which a sound is travelling.
      (1) For example, sound travels faster in helium than in air, resulting in a shorter λ.

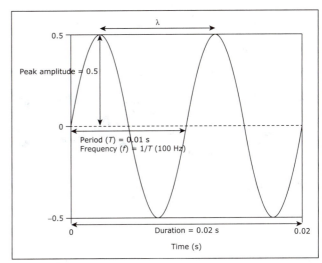

Figure 2-1 Waveform showing the peak amplitude, duration, period, frequency and wavelength of a sinusoid.

50 THERAPYED • Acoustics

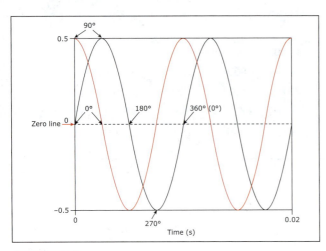

Figure 2-2 Two 100 Hz sinusoids that are 90° out of phase.

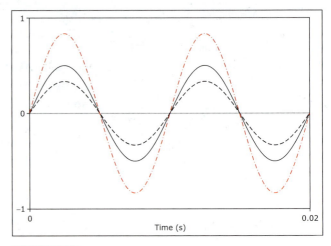

Figure 2-3 Two 100 Hz sine waves that are in phase (black lines) and their sum (red line).

Phase

1. Phase: location of a particular point in a waveform cycle relative to the zero line.
   a. Measured in degrees of a circle (Figure 2-2).
   b. Important in determining how sounds interact and resonate.
   c. Adding 2 sinusoids with same phase and f gives a sinusoid with same f and higher A (Figure 2-3).
   d. Adding 2 sinusoids with same f but 180° out of phase gives a sinusoid with same f and lower amplitude (Figure 2-4).

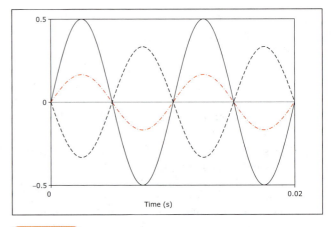

Figure 2-4 Two 100 Hz sine waves that are 180° out of phase (black lines) and their sum (red line).

Graphical Representations of Sounds

Waveforms

1. Waveforms—show variations in amplitude, pressure or intensity of a sound over time.
   a. X-axis is time.
   b. Y-axis may be amplitude, pressure or intensity.
2. Waveform use.
   a. Finding the exact fundamental frequency (F_0).
   b. Measuring time-related cues such as voice onset time (VOT).
   c. Determining whether a signal is periodic or aperiodic.
   d. Other analyses based on waveforms.
   e. Pitch contours.
   f. Voice quality analyses that relate to periodicity.

Spectrograms

1. Spectrograms—show regions of high-amplitude energy and changes over time.
   a. X-axis is time.
   b. Y-axis is frequency.

Table 2-3

Summary of Most Common Graphical Representations of Speech and Their Characteristics

TYPE OF ANALYSIS	X-AXIS	Y-AXIS	NOTES
Waveform	Time	Amplitude or a related measure	Frequency can be measured indirectly, by finding the period (T) and taking the inverse ($f = 1/T$), e.g., if $T = 0.005$ sec, $f = 1/0.005$, or 200 Hz. Provide information on manner of articulation, e.g., whether a sound resonant (periodic) or obstruent (aperiodic). Also helpful for time-related measurements such as VOT.
Spectrum	Frequency	Amplitude or a related measure	No time axis. Always averaged over some period of time. Used to measure harmonic amplitude, verify formant locations, measure noise characteristics such as center of gravity. To clearly see harmonics, F_0 and vowel quality must be held steady.
Spectrogram	Time	Frequency	Amplitude shown by level of darkness; darker regions have higher amplitude. Most useful analysis for examining speech sounds. Narrowband: precise frequency detail. Broadband: precise time detail.

(1) Level of detail on the Y- (frequency) axis can be adjusted by changing analysis bandwidth.
   (a) Broadband—averages amplitude across a wide band of frequencies, e.g., 300 Hz. Details can be seen along time axis but not the frequency axis.
   (b) Narrowband—averages amplitude across a narrow band of frequencies, e.g., 60 Hz. Details can be seen along the frequency axis but not the time axis.
c. Darkness dimension on a spectrogram shows amplitude or intensity at different frequencies.
   (1) No scale is provided to interpret this dimension.
d. Most frequently used tool in speech analysis.
2. Spectrogram use.
  a. Broadband (Figure 2-5).
    (1) Finding different sounds by manner of articulation and voicing.
    (2) Measuring time-related cues such as VOT.
    (3) Measuring frequency-related cues such as formant frequencies.
  b. Narrowband (Figure 2-6).
    (1) Checking pitch contour accuracy by comparing it with harmonic contours.
    (2) Estimating periodicity by examining number of harmonics that are clearly visible.

Amplitude Spectra

1. Amplitude spectra—show amplitude of individual sinusoids present in a sound (Figure 2-7).
  a. X-axis is frequency.
  b. Y-axis is amplitude, pressure or intensity.

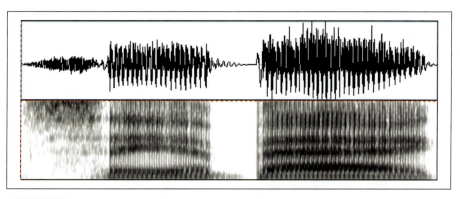

Figure 2-5 Waveform and broadband spectrogram of "say a bag."

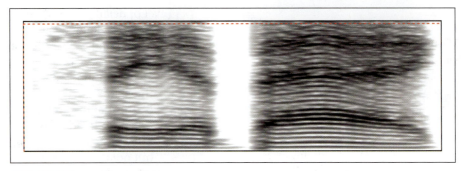

Figure 2-6 Narrowband spectrogram of "say a bag."

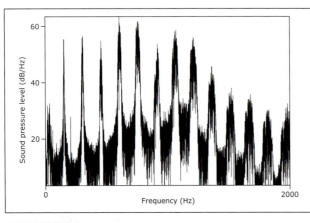

Figure 2-7 Amplitude spectrum for a sustained /ɑ/ (a complex periodic sound). Produced by a male speaker, showing harmonics from 0 to 2000 Hz.

2. Amplitude spectra use.
   a. Measure amplitude of individual harmonics.
   b. Measure the highest-amplitude harmonic within a formant.
   c. Examine how energy is distributed across the frequency spectrum in aperiodic sounds such as fricatives and stop bursts.

Types of Sounds and Their Graphical Representations

Sinusoids

1. Sinusoids consist of a single frequency.
   a. Called simple sounds or pure tones.
   b. Exhibit simple harmonic motion (SHM).
      (1) Examples of SHM.
         (a) Motion of a pendulum.
         (b) Motion of a weight attached to a spring.
   c. Adding sinusoids of the same frequency gives another sinusoid with the same frequency.
   d. Adding sinusoids of different frequencies gives a complex sound.

Waveforms of Sinusoids

1. Waveforms of sinusoids show simple repetitive patterns (Figure 2-8).
   a. Cycle of a sinusoid—simple, symmetrical up-and-down motion around the 0 axis.
   b. Number of oscillations (cycles) per second is the frequency of the sinusoid.
   c. Greatest distance of sinusoid from 0 axis is its peak amplitude.
   d. Peak amplitude always occurs at 90° and 270° of a sinusoid's cycle.
2. Amplitude spectrum of a sinusoid consists of a single vertical line (Figure 2-9).
   a. X-axis—top of the line gives peak amplitude.
   b. Y-axis—line location gives sinusoid's frequency.
   c. Sinusoids can be completely described by A and f or by A and T.
      (1) Since T can be calculated from f and vice-versa, only one of these two numbers is needed.
3. Spectrograms are not needed to examine sinusoids.
   a. Contain only 1 f that does not change over time.
4. Complex sounds: produced by adding sinusoids of *different* frequencies (Figure 2-10).
   a. May be periodic or aperiodic.
   b. Vocal fold vibration is a complex sound.

(1) Often referred to as periodic, but is never perfectly periodic.
(2) More accurately referred to as quasi-periodic (somewhat periodic).

5. Periodic complex sounds—each sinusoidal frequency is an integer multiple of a greatest common denominator (*GCD*).
   a. *GCD*—largest whole number (integer) that can be multiplied to give the frequencies of all sinusoids present in the sound.
      (1) Called the *fundamental* frequency (F_0) of the sound.
      (2) As with f, F_0 of a complex periodic sound is the inverse of T.
   b. Sinusoids in a periodic complex sound are said to be in a harmonic relationship with F_0.
      (1) Each is an integer multiple of F_0.
      (2) Referred to as harmonics (Table 2-4).

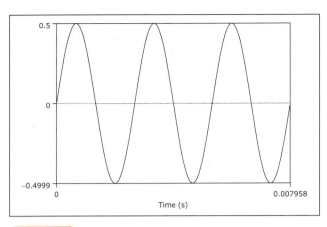

Figure 2-8 Waveform showing three cycles of a sinusoid.

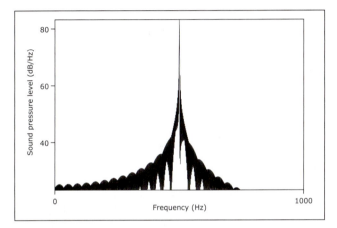

Figure 2-9 Spectrum of a 500 Hz sinusoid with a peak amplitude of 82 dB-SPL.

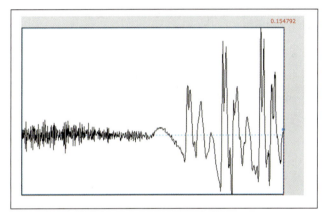

Figure 2-10 Waveform showing two complex speech sounds. Left: aperiodic complex sound (a fricative). Right: periodic or quasi-periodic complex sound (a vowel).

Table 2-4

Frequency of Harmonics and the Related Greatest Common Denominator

FREQUENCY (HZ) OF THE FIRST FOUR HARMONICS IN A SOUND				THE GREATEST COMMON DENOMINATOR GCD (INTEGER MULTIPLES THAT ARE PRESENT)	NOTES
H1	H2	H3	H4		
100	200	300	400	100 (1 × 100, 2 × 100, 3 × 100, 4 × 100)	In these sounds, the *GCD* and H1 have the same *f*. Another way of saying this is that H1 = F_0 = *GCD*. Every integer multiple of the *GCD* is present. This kind of harmonic sequence is produced by the human voice: H1 is the *GCD* and every multiple of the *GCD* is present.
200	400	600	800	200 (1 × 200, 2 × 200, 3 × 200, 4 × 200)	
500	750	1000	1250	250 (2 × 250, 3 × 250, 4 × 250, 5 × 250)	In these sounds, H1 is *not* the *GCD*. The "real" H1 is missing. This is deliberately done for telephone signals (frequencies < ~300 Hz and > ~3.5 kHz are filtered out). As a result, H1 is usually not present in a telephone signal. Although H1 is absent, F_0 is still equal to the *GCD*. In addition, we still *perceive* F_0 to be the *GCD*.
300	450	600	750	150 (2 × 150, 3 × 150, 4 × 150, 5 × 150)	
100	300	500	700	100 (1 × 100, 3 × 100, 5 × 100, 7 × 100)	In these sounds, only the *odd multiples* of the *GCD* are present. When only the odd multiples are present, result is a square wave. The human voice does not produce this type of signal. Signals of this type are often used in digital circuits.
150	450	750	1050	150 (1 × 150, 3 × 150, 5 × 150, 7 × 150)	

(3) Look at the first four harmonics listed for each sound and find the *GCD*. Most, but not all of these harmonic sequences could be found in recordings of the human voice.
6. Waveforms of complex periodic sounds show a repetitive pattern (the cycle) that is more complex than a sinusoid (Figure 2-11).

7. Amplitude spectrum of a periodic complex sound—always has more than one line since more than one sinusoidal frequency is present.
   a. Each line represents a harmonic.
   b. Harmonics are regularly spaced since they occur at integer multiples of F_0.
   c. In the human voice, harmonics are infinite in number (Figure 2-12).
8. Narrowband spectrograms of complex periodic sounds show individual harmonics and how their frequencies change over time.
9. Aperiodic complex sounds—the sinusoidal frequencies are *not* integer multiples of any common denominator other than 1.
   a. Relationship between sinusoidal frequencies is random.
   b. Individual sinusoids are *not* harmonics.
   c. Aperiodic sounds are often referred to as noises.

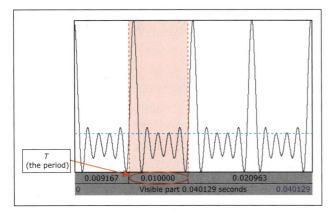

Figure 2-11 Waveform of a perfectly periodic complex sound.

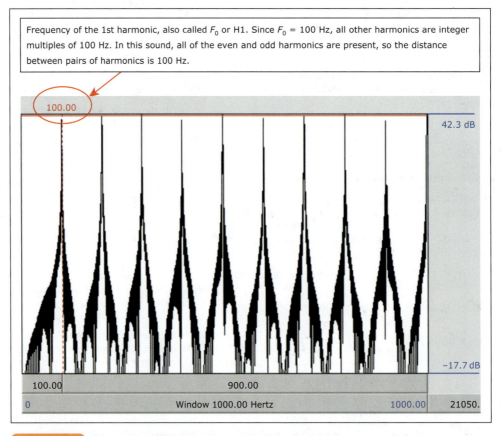

Figure 2-12 Amplitude spectrum of a perfectly periodic complex sound, showing 10 harmonics between 0 and 1000 Hz.

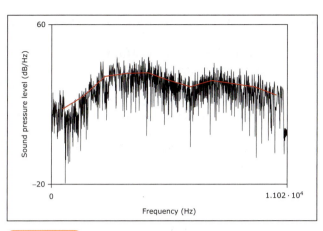

Figure 2-13 Amplitude spectrum of an aperiodic complex sound (a fricative).

10. Waveforms of aperiodic complex sounds—do not show a repetitive pattern, i.e., do not have a cycle.
    a. Since there is no cycle, aperiodic sounds do not have F_0.
11. Amplitude spectra of aperiodic sounds: show average amplitude of sinusoids across the frequency spectrum.
    a. Individual sinusoids not usually visible (Figure 2-13).

Table 2-5

Summary Information on Sound Type and Associated Characteristics

SOUND TYPE	NUMBER OF FREQUENCIES PRESENT	RELATIONSHIP BETWEEN COMPONENT FREQUENCIES	NOTES ON FINDING FREQUENCY
Sinusoid *Speech example:* individual harmonics of the human voice.	1	n/a	Count number of cycles in 1 second on a waveform. Find T and take the inverse, e.g., if $T = 0.01$ sec, $f = 1/0.01$, or 100 Hz. T = Period (time to complete 1 cycle). Measure f of the single line that is present in an amplitude spectrum.
Complex periodic *Speech examples:* vowels, resonant consonants.	>1 to an infinite number. Complex periodic speech sounds contain an infinite number of sinusoids.	Harmonic, i.e., all component sinusoids are integer multiples of a fundamental frequency. In speech, all integer multiples (odd and even) are present unless the signal has been filtered, e.g., during a telephone call.	Count number of cycles in 1 second on a waveform. Find T and take the inverse. Measure f of any two harmonics in an amplitude spectrum or narrowband spectrogram and find the interval between them; e.g., if H5 = 1000 Hz and H6 = 1200 Hz, F_0 = 1200−1000 = 200 Hz. Measure f of any harmonic and divide by its harmonic number; e.g., if H10 = 1000 Hz, $F_0 = 1000/10 = 100$ Hz.
Complex aperiodic *Speech examples:* fricatives, stops.	>1 to an infinite number. Complex aperiodic speech sounds contain an infinite number of sinusoids.	Random	N/A: Aperiodic sounds do not have a frequency. To have a period and frequency, sounds must have a cycle. Aperiodic sounds do not have a cycle.

Periodic Complex Sounds in Speech

Glottal Source

1. Glottal source—complex periodic sound produced by vocal fold vibration.
   a. Also referred to as phonation or voicing.
   b. Source of sound energy for voiced sounds, e.g., vowels and resonant consonants.
      (1) Although all voiced sounds have some vocal fold vibration, vocal folds often do not vibrate continuously during voiced obstruents.
   c. A *quasi*-periodic sound, often called periodic.
      (1) Vocal folds do not vibrate in a perfectly periodic pattern.
   d. Contains an infinite number of harmonics.
   e. Harmonic amplitude decreases as harmonic frequency increases.
      (1) For each octave increase in frequency, harmonic amplitude decreases by ~12 dB.
      (2) Sometimes referred to as spectral roll-off (Figure 2-14).

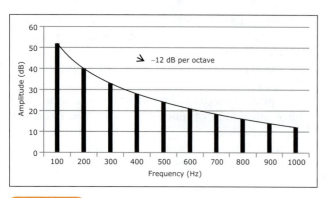

Figure 2-14 Spectrum showing spectral roll-off of the glottal source (–12 dB per octave).

2. Determines vocal pitch and voice quality.
   a. Vocal pitch—determined by rate of vocal fold vibration.
      (1) Changes in F_0 perceived as intonation.
         (a) Intonation is an important element of prosody.
   b. Languages use vocal pitch in different ways.
      (1) Intonation contributes to perception of emotions and attitudes in all languages.
      (2) In English, F_0 contributes to perception of word and sentential stress.
         (a) F_0 typically rises on stressed syllables and words.
      (3) In many East Asian and African languages, pitch is phonemic, i.e., it can change word meaning.
         (a) Referred to as tone languages, e.g., Mandarin Chinese and all other Chinese languages.
         (b) Tones are classified by pitch height and contour, e.g., Mandarin Chinese has four tones—high level, a mid-rising, a low dipping and high-falling.
      (4) Some languages have a restricted tonal system called pitch accent, e.g., some Scandinavian languages and Japanese.
         (a) Pitch accent systems usually have only two tones, high and low.
         (b) Mode of vocal fold vibration and degree of regularity or irregularity in the glottal cycle are perceived as voice quality.
   c. Languages use voice quality in different ways.
      (1) In some tone languages, both pitch and voice quality are phonemic
         (a) For example, in Hmong languages of southeast Asia, using modal vs. breathy or creaky voice may change word meaning.
      (2) Amplitude of the glottal source determines overall loudness of the voice.

Aperiodic Complex Sounds in Speech

Production and Types

1. Produced by impeding or obstructing airflow.
2. Impulse noises—very brief aperiodic sounds (Figure 2-15).
   a. Can be produced by suddenly releasing air pressure that has built up behind a blockage.
      (1) For example, stop consonant bursts.
   b. Can be produced by sucking the tongue against the roof of the oral cavity, then pulling it away to produce a click.
      (1) In English, clicks are not speech sounds, but can still have a meaning.
      (2) For example, lateral click is used to mean "giddy-up" to a horse.
      (3) Clicks are used as phonemes of speech in some African languages.
3. Turbulent noises—have longer duration than impulse noises.
   a. Molecules set into turbulent motion by forcing air through a narrow channel or against an obstruction such as the teeth.
      (1) For example, continuant obstruents (fricatives) (Figure 2-16).

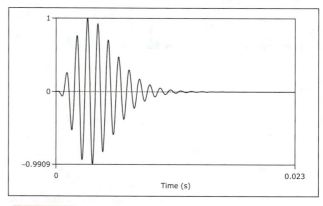

Figure 2-15 Waveform of an impulse noise (duration = 0.01 sec).

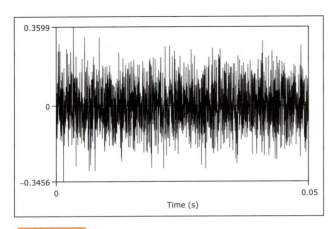

Figure 2-16 Waveform of a turbulent noise (duration = 0.05 sec).

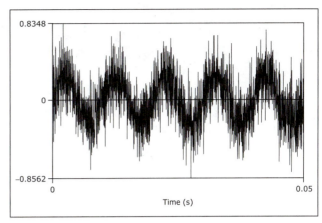

Figure 2-17 Waveform of an amplitude modulated noise (i.e., turbulent noise plus a periodic sound). In this case, the noise is white noise and the periodic sound is a 100 Hz sinusoid.

4. Obstruent sounds always include aperiodic noise as a sound source.
   a. Voiceless obstruents—aperiodic noise is the only sound source.
   b. Voiced obstruents—aperiodic noise combined with vocal fold vibration.
5. Adding turbulent noise to a periodic sound results in amplitude modulated noise (Figure 2-17).

The Source-Filter Theory of Speech Production

Acoustic Theory of Speech Production

1. Also called the acoustic theory of speech production (Figure 2-18).
2. States that speech is produced by passing a sound source through a sound filter.
3. Mathematically, source filter theory can be expressed as $U(f) \times T(f) \times R(f) = P(f)$.
   a. $U(f)$ = the source function.
      (1) Most common sound source is vocal fold vibration.
      (2) Turbulent and impulse noises also act as sound sources for speech.
   b. $T(f)$ = the filter (or transfer) function.
      (1) Supralaryngeal vocal tract (SLVT) acts as a filter and modifies sound input.
         (a) The filter changes amplitudes of sinusoids in the sound source.
         (b) Some component sinusoids in the source resonate in the SLVT and gain amplitude as they pass through the filter.
         (c) Other component sinusoids lose amplitude as they pass through the filter.

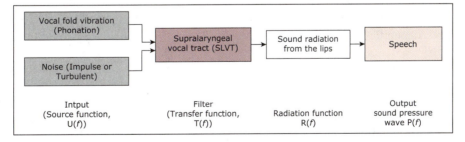

Figure 2-18 The source-filter theory of speech production states that speech (the output) is produced by passing a sound source (the input) through the supralaryngeal vocal tract, which acts as a filter. The output contains the component sinusoids from the input, but their amplitudes now match the amplitude envelope of the filter.

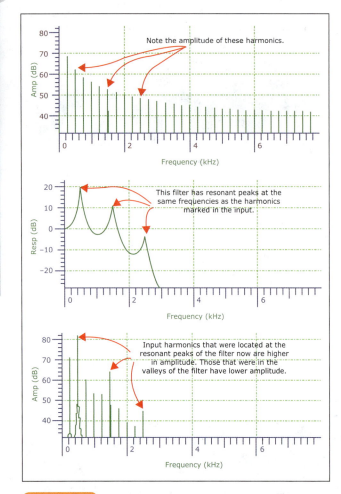

Figure 2-19 Amplitude spectra for a source function (the input), a filter function and the output that results from passing the source through the filter.

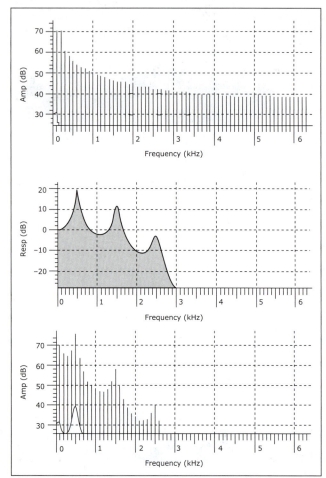

Figure 2-20 Top spectrum: source function (input sound). Middle spectrum: filter function. Bottom spectrum: output.

    c. $R(f)$ = effect of sound radiating outward from the lips.
      (1) Sounds gains about 6 dB per octave in amplitude as they radiate from the lips.
    d. $P(f)$ = speech output.
4. Combining different source functions with different filter functions produces all of the sounds of speech (Figure 2-19).
5. Mathematically, a function is a relation in which the output changes, depending on the input, for example, x^2.
    a. Source and filter functions change continuously in speech.
      (1) Source function changes.
        (a) Sometimes periodic, sometimes aperiodic.
        (b) Harmonics in the glottal source change as a function of F_0.
      (2) Filter function.
        (a) Oral and pharyngeal cavities change size and shape.
        (b) Sometimes includes airflow through nasal cavities.
        (c) Frequencies that resonate in the SLVT cavities are a function of cavity size.
        (d) Larger cavities have deeper resonating frequencies.
        (e) Smaller cavities have higher resonating frequencies.
    b. Speech output changes as a function of changes in the sound source and SLVT filter.
    c. Effect of the SLVT filter—changes amplitude of sinusoids that pass through it.
      (1) Sinusoids that exit the SLVT have exactly the same frequencies as sinusoids in the input.
      (2) SLVT filter cannot add, delete or change the frequencies of component sinusoids (Figure 2-20).
6. Shape of the SLVT filter.
    a. Resonant sounds—filter envelope shows peaks and valleys.
      (1) For example, vowels, resonant consonants.

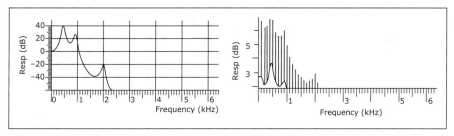

Figure 2-21 Spectra showing the amplitude envelope of a filter and how harmonic amplitudes in the output conform to the shape of the envelope.

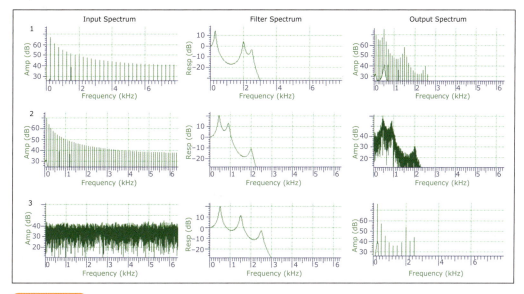

Figure 2-22 Match the inputs and filters to arrive at appropriate output spectrums (Answers: Output 1 = Input 2 + Filter 3; Output 2 = Input 3 + Filter 2; Output 3 = Input 1 + Filter 1).

(2) Peaks are located at resonant frequencies of the SLVT.
   (a) Location of resonant frequencies is a function of SLVT shape.
(3) Resonant frequencies are called formants.
   (a) Sinusoids at or near formant peaks gain amplitude as they pass through the filter.
(4) Sinusoids within valleys of the filter function lose amplitude as they pass through the filter.

   b. Obstruent sounds—filter envelope may be a high-pass or band-pass filter.
      (1) For example, frication noise, stop bursts, aspiration noise.
7. The amplitude envelope of the filter is superimposed on input sounds as they pass through (Figures 2-21 and 2-22).

Acoustic Characteristics of the Supralaryngeal Vocal Tract (SLVT)

Neutral Position

1. In this position, the SLVT acts like a uniform tube.
   a. Uniform tube—tube that has an equal diameter throughout.
   b. Approximately the shape for the vowel schwa.
2. It is open at one end and closed at the other.
   a. Glottis—closed end of the uniform tube.
   b. Lips—open end of the uniform tube.

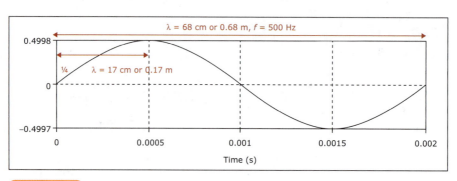

Figure 2-23 Waveform of a 500 Hz sinusoid.

Quarter Wave Resonator

1. Lowest frequency that resonates has a wavelength (λ) 4 times as long as the tube, i.e., the tube is ¼ of the wavelength of its lowest resonating frequency (Figure 2-23).
2. ¼ wave resonators have additional filter peaks at every odd multiple of the lowest resonating frequency.
   a. For example, a 17-cm-long vocal tract with F1 = 500 Hz would have:
      (1) F2 at *3 × 500 Hz = 1500 Hz*
      (2) F3 at *5 × 500 Hz = 2500 Hz*
   b. Other speech sounds require different vocal tract shapes, which give different formant frequencies.

Variable Shape

1. SLVT shape can be changed.
   a. Amplitude envelope of the filter varies as a function of SLVT shape.
   b. SLVT is therefore a *variable filter*.

2. Soft tissues of the vocal tract dampen or absorb some sound energy.
   a. Result is that sound output dies away immediately when the sound source stops.
   b. SLVT is therefore a *heavily damped filter*.
3. Soft tissues allow the SLVT to react to a range of frequencies near peaks of the filter function.
   a. The SLVT is therefore a *broadly tuned filter*.
4. Filter function of the SLVT has an infinite number of resonant peaks.
   a. The SLVT has an infinite number of formant frequencies.
   b. Formants that are most important for speech perception are F1, F2 and, to a lesser extent, F3.

How Sounds Resonate in the Vocal Tract

Amplitude Gain

1. Sinusoids at or near filter peaks (i.e., formant frequencies) gain amplitude as they pass through the vocal tract.
   a. Sinusoids in a complex wave travel from the glottis towards the lips.
   b. At the lips, a portion of each sinusoid passes to the surrounding air and a portion is reflected back to the glottis.
   c. The wave travelling from glottis to lips (the incident wave) meets the wave that is reflected back toward the glottis (the reflected wave).
      (1) The incident and reflected waves add together.
      (2) Referred to as interference, i.e., addition of two waves that come from the same source.
   d. Reflected sinusoid that falls within a resonant peak of the vocal tract filter undergoes constructive interference.
      (1) Incident and reflected waves are in phase or nearly in phase (Figure 2-24).
         (a) Resultant wave is higher in amplitude than the original (input) sinusoid.
         (b) These sinusoids resonate in the SLVT.
      (2) Resultant wave appears to stand still rather than move through the SLVT.

Acoustic Characteristics of Resonant Sounds

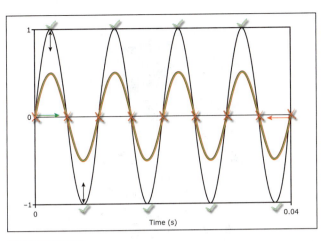

Figure 2-24 Waveform of an incident sinusoid and a reflected sinusoid that are in phase.

(a) Called a standing wave.
(b) Standing waves have nodes (regions of minimal air motion) and antinodes (regions of maximal air motion).

e. Reflected sinusoids that fall outside peaks of the vocal tract filter undergo *destructive interference*.
  (1) Incident and reflected waves are out of phase or nearly out of phase.
   (a) Resultant wave is lower in amplitude than the original (input) sinusoid.
   (b) These sinusoids are "filtered out."
   (c) SLVT is broadly tuned and has an infinite number of formants.
  (2) Many sinusoids gain some amplitude as they travel through the vocal tract (Figure 2-25).

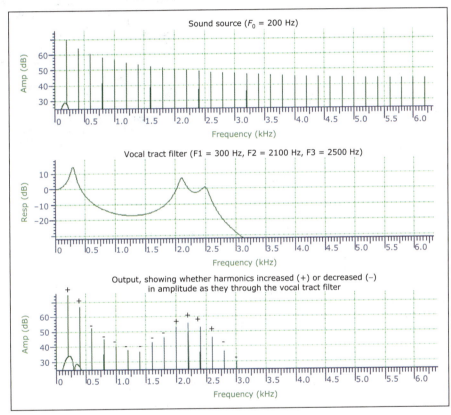

Figure 2-25 Spectra for an input sound (top), a vocal tract filter (middle) and the output sound (bottom).

 Acoustic Characteristics of Resonant Sounds

Letters, Shapes and Sounds

1. Includes vowels and resonant consonants (nasals, liquids and glides).
2. SLVT shape is relatively open.
   a. Vowels have most open vocal tract shape.
3. No aperiodic noise is produced during articulation of resonant sounds.
   a. Default sound source is vocal fold vibration.
   b. Characterized by presence of formants.
     (1) F1, F2 and F3 most important for perceiving and identifying resonant sounds.

(2) F1, F2 and F3 have a characteristic relationship with one another.
(3) Actual formant frequencies will vary, depending on factors such as:
   (a) Speaker gender and size.
   (b) Speaking situation (e.g., informal or formal).
   (c) Rate of speech.
   (d) Phonetic context.
   (e) Word frequency.
   (f) Placement of stress within sentences.
c. Formant frequencies depend on size of pharynx and oral cavity and location of constrictions in SLVT.
d. F1—most closely associated with pharynx size.
   (1) Pharynx size varies with tongue height.
   (2) Size of the air pocket in the pharynx increases as the tongue is pulled up towards the roof of the mouth.
      (a) The larger the air pocket, the lower the resonating frequency.
      (b) High vowels and glides have highest tongue position.
      (c) High vowels and glides have a low F1 frequency.
   (3) When the tongue is low, it occupies space in the pharynx, leaving only a small air pocket.
      (a) The smaller the air pocket, the higher the resonating frequency.
      (b) Low vowels have lowest tongue position.
      (c) Low vowels have a high F1 frequency (Figure 2-26).
e. F2—most closely associated with oral cavity size.
   (1) Oral cavity size varies with tongue advancement.
   (2) Size of the air pocket in the oral cavity decreases as the tongue moves forward.
      (a) The smaller the air pocket, the higher the resonating frequency.
      (b) Front vowels have the most forward tongue position.
      (c) Front vowels have a high F2 frequency.
   (3) When the tongue is at the back of the mouth, it leaves a larger air pocket in the oral cavity.
      (a) The larger the air pocket, the lower the resonating frequency.
      (b) Back vowels have the farthest-back tongue position.
      (c) Back vowels have a low F2 frequency.
f. F3—important for distinguishing the retroflexed vowels /ɝ/ and /ɚ/ and the consonant /r/ in English.
   (1) Vocal tract constrictions for these sounds result in a low F3.
      (a) Retroflex sounds typically have constrictions at the lips, towards the back of the hard palate and near the epiglottis.
      (b) Constricting the vocal tract, these locations lower F3 (Figure 2-27).
      (c) Spectrogram of four front vowels produced by a male speaker, with F1, F2 and F3 marked.

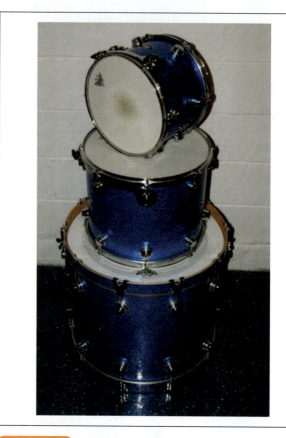

Figure 2-26 Each drum has an air cavity in which a range of frequencies resonate. As the drums get progressively larger, the frequencies that will resonate in the air cavity become increasingly lower in pitch. The same is true of vocal tract cavities.

- F1 rises from /i/ to /æ/.
- F2 moves towards the middle of its range as we go from /i/ to /æ/.
- F3 moves very little—it is near 3000 Hz for all presented vowels.

g. As the mouth opens, the tongue tends to move to a more central position in the mouth.
   (1) Since this movement relates to tongue advancement, it is reflected in the frequency of F2.
      (a) As the mouth opens, F2 values tend to move towards the middle of the F2 scale.
      (b) For front vowels, this means that F2 drops.
      (c) For back vowels, this means that F2 rises.
h. The exact F1–F2 frequencies of any vowel cannot be predicted, but when F1–F2 values for a speaker are averaged across many tokens, vowels will always appear in the same position relative to one another on an F1–F2 plot.
   (1) For example, /i/ and /u/ will have the lowest F1 values, /i/ will have the highest F2 value and /u/ will have the lowest F2 value (Figure 2-28).

Acoustic Characteristics of Resonant Sounds 63

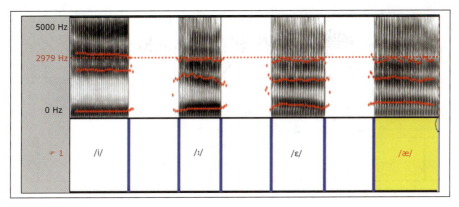

Figure 2-27 Spectrogram of four front vowels produced by a male speaker, with F1, F2 and F3 marked.

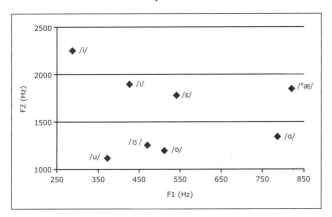

Figure 2-28 An F1-F2 plot of selected vowels for an English speaker from Michigan. The high vowels /i/ and /u/ have low F1 values because the tongue is pulled up toward the roof of the mouth, leaving a large air pocket in the pharynx. In contrast, the low vowels /æ/ and /ɑ/ have a high F1 because the tongue leaves only a small air pocket in the pharynx. Mid vowels have intermediate F1 values. The front vowels /i, ɪ, ɛ/ and /æ/ have high F2 values because the tongue is near the front of the oral cavity, leaving a small air pocket. The back vowels /u, ʊ, o/ and /ɑ/ have low F2 values because the tongue is near the back of the oral cavity, leaving a large air pocket.

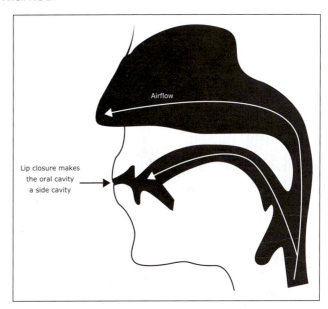

Figure 2-29 An example of nasal consonant articulation: When the lips close for /m/, the oral cavity is not directly connected with the open air. It acts as a side cavity, which results in zeros, or anti-resonances, in the speech output.

Vocal Tract Constriction

1. For resonant consonants, the vocal tract is more constricted than for vowels but less constricted than for obstruent consonants.
   a. As the degree of constriction increases, sound amplitude is reduced.
      (1) As a result, resonant consonants tend to be lower in amplitude than vowels.
   b. Tongue position for resonant consonants can produce a "side cavity" that is not directly connected with the open air (Figure 2-29).
      (1) Resonances from side cavities are absorbed by the side cavity—they do not show up in the output speech signal.
         (a) In the output signal, these appear as zeros or "anti-resonances."
         (b) A zero is the opposite of a formant.
         (c) In a spectrogram, a zero will appear as white space or, if it is near a formant frequency, as a sudden reduction in formant amplitude.

Nasal Consonants

1. Nasal consonants have a complete closure at some location in the oral cavity.
   a. In English, the closure may be at the lips, the alveolar ridge or the velum.

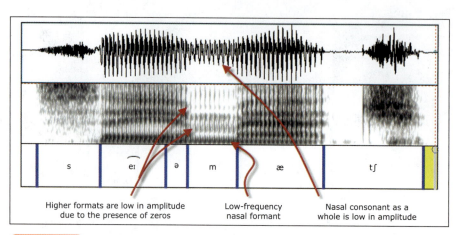

Figure 2-30 Waveform and spectrogram for the phrase "say a match," showing a bilabial nasal consonant between two vowels.

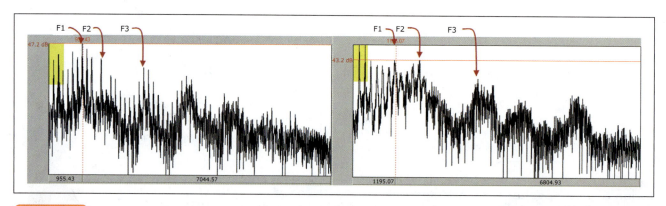

Figure 2-31 Spectra for the vowel /ɑ/ produced by a normal female speaker (left) and a child with cleft palate (right). As a low vowel, /ɑ/ has a high F1. In the female speaker's /ɑ/, harmonics in the region of F1 have the highest amplitude in the spectrum. However, in the child's /ɑ/, H1 and H2 (highlighted in yellow in both spectra) are highest in amplitude. This is an indication that H1 and H2 are resonating in the child's nasal cavity.

b. When the closure is formed, the oral cavity acts as a side cavity that is not directly connected with the open air.
   (1) Nasal consonants are therefore characterized by the presence of zeros in the output.
c. Air flows through the nose and resonates in the nasal cavity.
   (1) The nasal cavity is a large pocket of air which resonates at a low frequency.
      (a) As a result, nasal consonants have a low frequency formant, often called a nasal formant (Figure 2-30).
      (b) Nasalized vowels and nasal speech in general are also characterized by the presence of a low-frequency nasal formant and higher formants that tend to be low in amplitude (Figure 2-31).
      (c) In nasalized vowels, air flows out of the oral cavity as well as the nasal cavity.

Liquids and Glides

1. Liquids and glides involve a constriction in the vocal tract that does not produce turbulent airflow.
   a. As a result, liquid and glide articulation does not produce aperiodic noise.
   b. Acoustically, each English liquid and glide resembles an English vowel.
      (1) Liquids and vowels together are often referred to as semivowels.
      (2) Formant frequencies for liquids and glides are similar to their vocalic counterparts (Table 2-6).
   c. Because the vocal tract is more constricted than for vowels, semivowel amplitude tends to be lower than for vowels.
   d. The tongue shape for /l/ produces a side air pocket behind the tip of the tongue, which introduces zeros into the spectrum for /l/.

Table 2-6

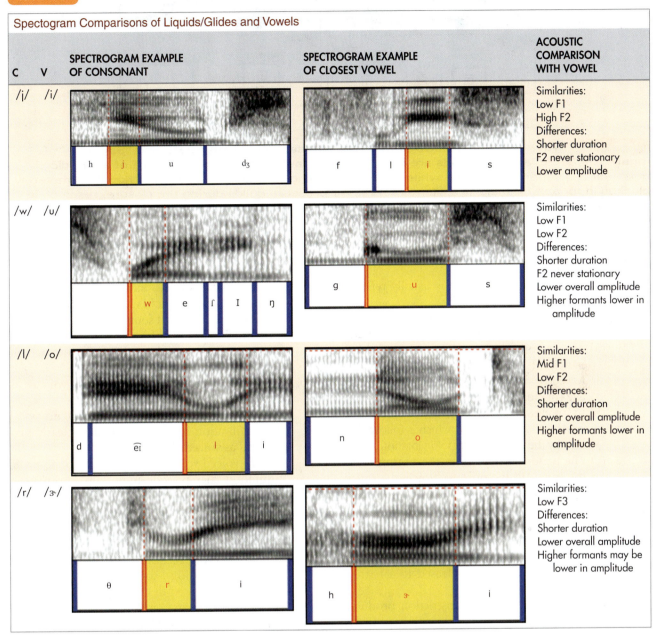

Spectogram Comparisons of Liquids/Glides and Vowels

Acoustic Characteristics of Obstruent Sounds

Vocal Tract

1. The obstruent sounds of English include stops, fricatives and affricates.
2. For all obstruent sounds, the vocal tract is relatively constricted.

a. The presence of a narrow constriction somewhere in the vocal tract results in turbulent airflow.
b. When airflow becomes turbulent, *aperiodic noise* is produced.
   (1) In fricatives, airflow through the constriction is continuous, i.e., airflow is never completely blocked.

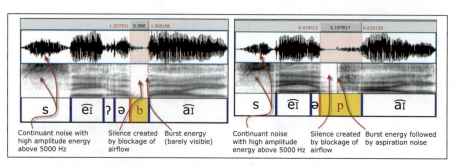

Figure 2-32 Waveform and spectrogram of the phrases "Say a buy" (left) and "Say a pie" (right). The /s/, /b/ and /p/ sounds are obstruents characterized by the presence of aperiodic noise. /s/ is a continuant sound, while /b/ and /p/ are non-continuants. When airflow is completely blocked in /b/ and /p/ there is a silent interval. Air pressure builds during the closure, resulting in a burst when the blockage is released. After the burst, word-initial voiceless stops in English are characterized by a period of aspiration.

(a) As a result, fricatives are characterized by *continuant* noise.
- This continuant noise is usually referred to as *frication noise*.

(2) In stops, airflow is completely blocked for a brief period of time, i.e., they are noncontinuant sounds.
(a) As a result, stops are characterized by a period of *silence* during the blockage, followed by a *burst* of energy when the blockage (or closure) is released.
(b) In voiceless stops, the burst may be followed by *aspiration underscore noise*, which is followed in turn by the onset of vocal fold vibration.
(c) The period of time from the beginning of the burst till the onset of voicing is called *voice onset time* or *VOT*.

(3) Affricates combine the features of stops and fricatives.
(a) In affricates, airflow is briefly blocked, producing a period of silence.
(b) The blockage is then released to a narrow constriction.
(c) Airflow through the constriction produces frication noise.

Waveforms and Spectrograms

1. In a waveform, aperiodic noise is characterized by the lack of a repeating pattern.
2. In a spectrogram, aperiodic noise tends to be distributed over a range of frequencies and is often higher in amplitude in certain parts of the frequency spectrum (Figure 2-32).

Voiced and Voiceless Cognates

1. In English, all obstruents have voiced and voiceless cognates (Table 2-7).

a. Aperiodic noise can serve as the only sound source for obstruents.
(1) Because all obstruents have aperiodic noise as a sound source, vocal fold vibration is not required to produce an output sound.
(2) Obstruents can therefore be voiceless, whereas for resonant sounds, voicing is the default sound source.

b. In English voiced obstruent sounds, voicing is rarely continuous throughout the sound.
(1) Voiced obstruents sometimes show no vocal fold vibration but are nevertheless clearly perceived as voiced.
(2) In all voiced-voiceless obstruent cognate pairs, duration cues provide important information about voicing.
(a) Voiced obstruents are characterized by shorter durations than voiceless obstruents.

c. In obstruents, the section of the vocal tract that is in front of the noise source acts as an acoustic filter.
(1) As with any sound, air pocket size determines how noise source is filtered.
(2) When the constriction is near the front of the vocal tract, high-frequency components of the noise source are enhanced.
(3) When the constriction is near the back of the vocal tract, lower-frequency components of the noise source are enhanced.
(4) As the constriction location moves back in the vocal tract, the air pocket in front of the constriction gets larger.
(a) For example, the air pocket in front of the alveolar ridge for the sound /s/ is smaller than the air pocket in front of the palate for /ʃ/.
(b) As a result, /s/ has more energy at higher frequencies than /ʃ/.

Acoustic Characteristics of Obstruent Sounds

Table 2-7

A Comparison of Voiced and Voiceless Cognate Pairs for Stops, Fricatives and Affricates

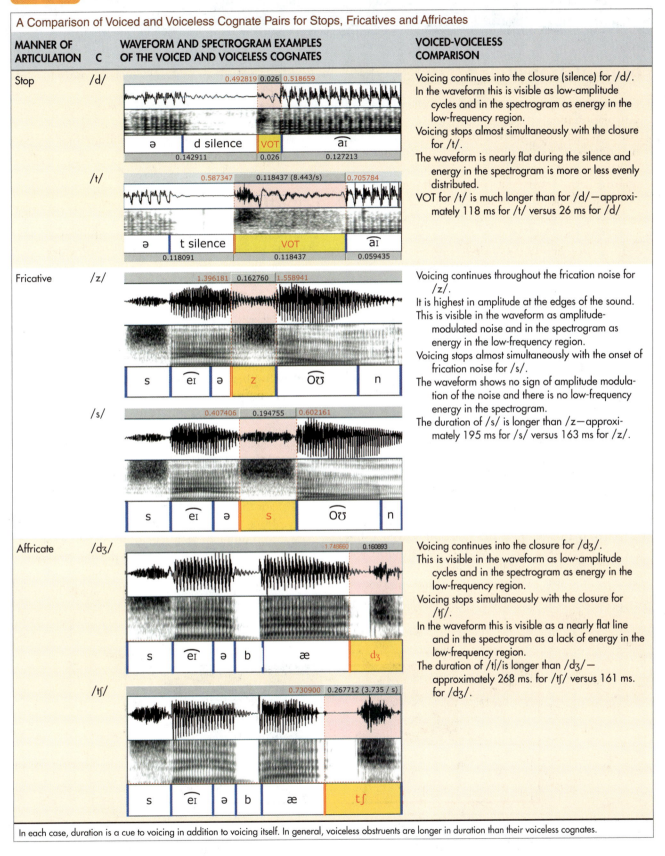

MANNER OF ARTICULATION	C	WAVEFORM AND SPECTROGRAM EXAMPLES OF THE VOICED AND VOICELESS COGNATES	VOICED-VOICELESS COMPARISON
Stop	/d/		Voicing continues into the closure (silence) for /d/. In the waveform this is visible as low-amplitude cycles and in the spectrogram as energy in the low-frequency region. Voicing stops almost simultaneously with the closure for /t/. The waveform is nearly flat during the silence and energy in the spectrogram is more or less evenly distributed. VOT for /t/ is much longer than for /d/—approximately 118 ms for /t/ versus 26 ms for /d/
	/t/		
Fricative	/z/		Voicing continues throughout the frication noise for /z/. It is highest in amplitude at the edges of the sound. This is visible in the waveform as amplitude-modulated noise and in the spectrogram as energy in the low-frequency region. Voicing stops almost simultaneously with the onset of frication noise for /s/. The waveform shows no sign of amplitude modulation of the noise and there is no low-frequency energy in the spectrogram. The duration of /s/ is longer than /z/—approximately 195 ms for /s/ versus 163 ms for /z/.
	/s/		
Affricate	/dʒ/		Voicing continues into the closure for /dʒ/. This is visible in the waveform as low-amplitude cycles and in the spectrogram as energy in the low-frequency region. Voicing stops simultaneously with the closure for /tʃ/. In the waveform this is visible as a nearly flat line and in the spectrogram as a lack of energy in the low-frequency region. The duration of /tʃ/ is longer than /dʒ/—approximately 268 ms. for /tʃ/ versus 161 ms. for /dʒ/.
	/tʃ/		

In each case, duration is a cue to voicing in addition to voicing itself. In general, voiceless obstruents are longer in duration than their voiceless cognates.

Acoustic Cues to Consonant Place of Articulation

Formant Transitions

1. Formant transitions are an important cue to place of articulation for all consonants.
2. Formant transitions are regions of relatively rapid formant movement that indicate rapid movement of the articulators.
   a. Articulator movement for diphthongal vowels also results in formant movement, but movement within vowels tends to be slower than CV and VC transitions.
3. Formant transitions have characteristic shapes that indicate where the consonant constriction is being formed (Figure 2-33).
   a. In English, F1 transitions always move downward as you look from the vowel toward the consonant.
   b. F2 transitions provide the most information about consonant place of articulation.
      (1) For bilabial consonants, F2 moves downward as the bilabial constriction is formed and upward as it is released.
      (2) For alveolar consonants, F2 tends to move towards a frequency of about 1800 Hz.
         (a) If a vowel on either side of the alveolar has a high F2 frequency, the F2 transition will point downward as you look from the vowel towards the alveolar consonant. For example, this would be the case for high front vowels.
         (b) If a vowel on either side of the alveolar has a low F2 frequency, the F2 transition will move upward as you look from the vowel towards the alveolar consonant. For example, this would be the case for high back vowels.
      (3) For velar consonants, F2 tends to move towards F3 forming a "velar pinch."
4. Formant transitions tend to be most easily seen for voiced consonants.
   a. For voiceless consonants, transitions may be partially voiceless.

Fricatives

1. In fricatives, the amplitude and distribution of noise energy across the frequency spectrum provides information about the fricative's place of articulation.
   a. Amplitude of frication noise distinguishes sibilant (sometimes called strident) fricatives from nonsibilant fricatives.
      (1) The sibilant fricatives /s, z, ʃ/ and /ʒ/ have higher amplitude noise than the nonsibilant fricatives /f, v, θ, ð/ and /h/ (Figures 2-34 and 2-35).
2. As with other sounds, the size of the resonating cavity in front of the frication noise source determines which frequency components in the noise will resonate.
   a. Labiodental and interdental fricatives are articulated so far forward that the vocal tract in front of the noise source has relatively little effect on the frication noise.
      (1) For these nonsibilant fricatives, formant transitions appear to be the best source of information on place of articulation.
         (a) Visual cues are also useful, when available.
   b. Sibilant fricatives show a dramatic effect of resonating cavity size on their frication noise characteristics.

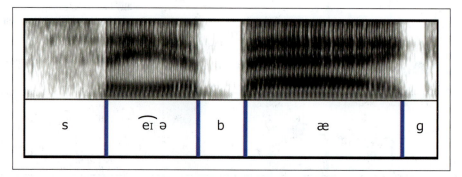

Figure 2-33 The phrase "say a bag" showing examples of formant transitions for alveolar, bilabial and velar consonants (/s /, /b/ and /g/ respectively).

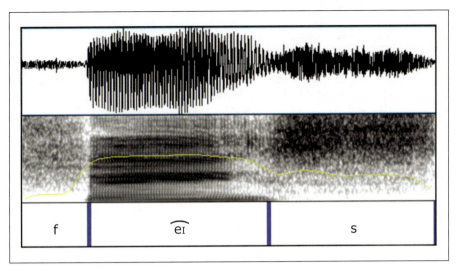

Figure 2-34 Waveform, spectrogram and intensity contour of the word "face" produced by a female speaker.

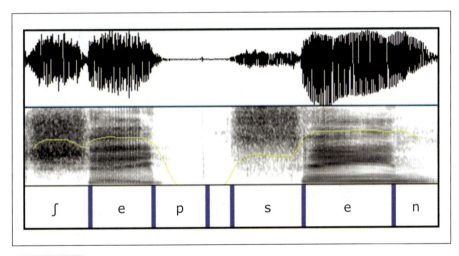

Figure 2-35 Waveform, spectrogram and intensity contour of the words "shape" and "sane" produced by a female speaker.

(1) Most of the noise energy for /s/ is at frequencies above 4000 Hz since the resonating cavity in front of the alveolar ridge is very small.
   (a) For women's and children's voices, the highest amplitude energy may be at frequencies near 8000 Hz.
   (b) To see the noise energy for /s/ on a spectrogram, it may be necessary to raise the upper limit for frequency on the vertical axis.
(2) The average frequency of frication noise for /s/ is typically at least 2500 Hz higher than for /ʃ/.

Acoustic Characteristics of Frication Noise

1. The acoustic characteristics of frication noise can be measured and described using spectral moments.
   a. Spectral moments can be used to describe the shape of the noise spectrum for a fricative in numerical terms (Table 2-8).
      (1) Center of gravity (COG) is the average frequency of the spectrum, weighted by the amplitude of the noise at different frequencies.
      (2) Standard deviation (SD) is the dispersion of energy around the COG.

Table 2-8

Comparison of the Spectral Moment Characteristics of Nonsibilant and Sibilant Fricatives

SUMMARY OF SPECTRAL MOMENTS	
1. COG	Center of gravity—Location of the average energy concentration.
2. SD	Standard deviation—How widely energy is distributed around the COG.
3. Skewness	Degree of symmetry around the COG. *Zero*—energy distribution is symmetrical; *Negative*—energy concentrated above the COG; *Positive*—energy concentrated below the COG.
4. Kurtosis	Flatness of shape. *Negative*—the spectrum is flat; *Positive*—the spectrum has clearly defined peaks.

EXAMPLES OF NONSIBILANT FRICATIVE SPECTRA	LABIODENTAL: /f/ IN "FACE"	INTERDENTAL: /θ/ IN "THEME"
	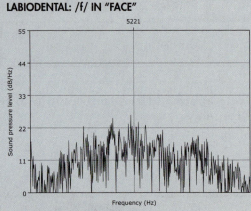	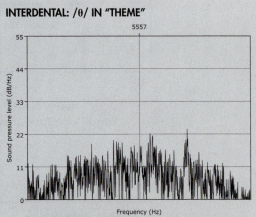
COG	5221	5557
SD	2002	2174
Skewness	0.217	−0.216
Kurtosis	−0.013	−0.379

Summary: For nonsibilants, the COG is in the middle of the spectrum; the SD indicates that energy is widely distributed in comparison with sibilants; the spectrum is quite symmetrical around the COG (skewness is near 0); there are no clear peaks (kurtosis is negative). In addition, overall amplitude is low in comparison with sibilants.

EXAMPLES OF SIBILANT FRICATIVE SPECTRA	ALVEOLAR: /s/ IN "SANE"	PALATAL: /ʃ/ IN "SHAPE"
	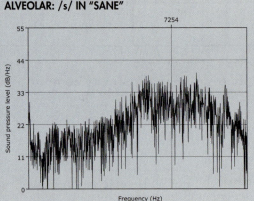	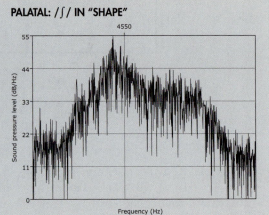
COG	7254	4550
SD	1416	1241
Skewness	−0.872	1.332
Kurtosis	2.934	2.050

Summary: For sibilants, the COG is off-center (high for /s/, low for /ʃ/); the SD indicates that energy is concentrated in a compact region of the spectrum in comparison with nonsibilants; the spectrum is quite asymmetrical around the COG (skewness is negative for /s/ = energy is concentrated above the COG and positive for /ʃ/ = energy is concentrated below the COG); the spectrum is peaked rather than flat (kurtosis is positive). In addition, overall amplitude is high in comparison with nonsibilants.

All words were produced by a female speaker.

(3) Skewness is the degree to which the energy on either side of the COG is distributed symmetrically or asymmetrically.
(4) Kurtosis is the degree to which the noise spectrum is flat or shows clearly defined peaks.
b. Information provided by spectral moments is interrelated, since the presence of a resonating cavity in front of the noise source increases the amplitude of some frequencies and reduces others.

(1) The COG shifts away from the center of the spectrum towards the resonant peak.
(2) As a result, the spectrum is asymmetrical and energy is concentrated in a relatively compact area rather than being evenly distributed across the spectrum.

Table 2-9

Examples of Stop VOTs by Place of Articulation

BILABIALS: SHORT VOT

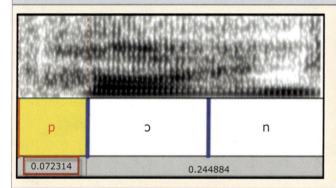
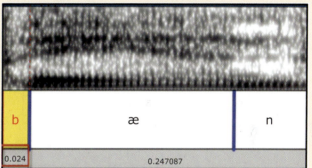

ALVEOLARS: SHORT TO INTERMEDIATE VOT

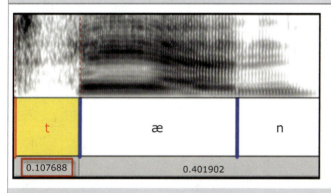
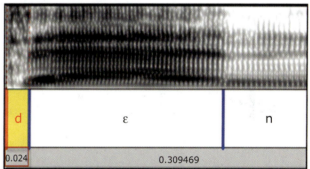

VELARS: LONG VOT

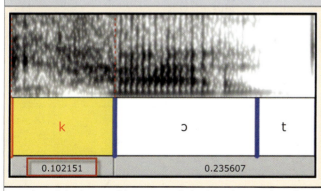
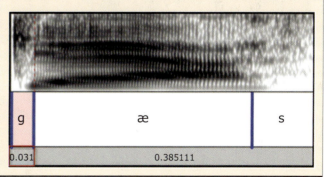

In each word, the duration of the VOT is marked with a red rectangular outline.

(Continued)

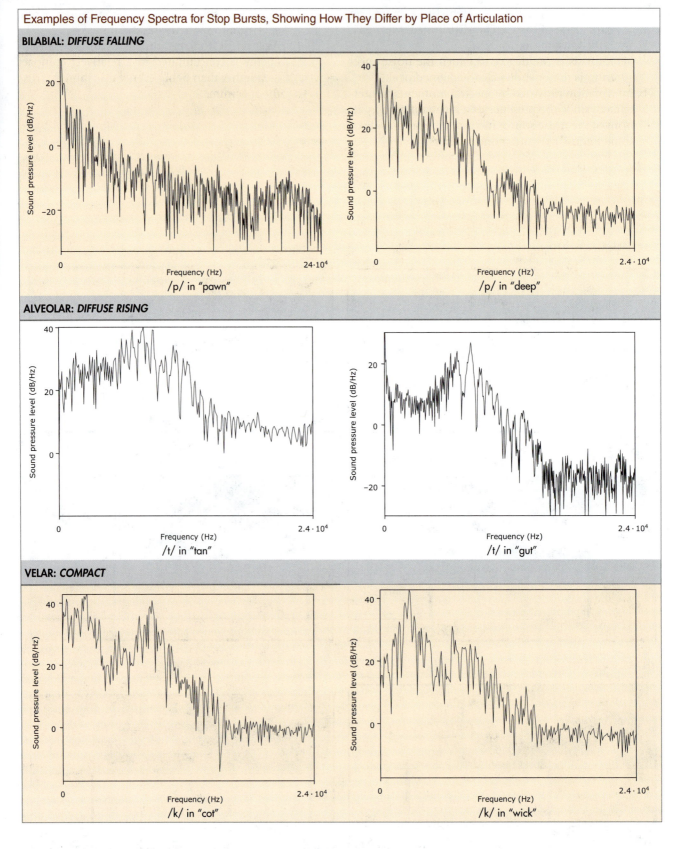

Examples of Frequency Spectra for Stop Bursts, Showing How They Differ by Place of Articulation

BILABIAL: *DIFFUSE FALLING*

ALVEOLAR: *DIFFUSE RISING*

VELAR: *COMPACT*

Stop Consonants

1. In stop consonants, VOT duration and the frequency characteristics of burst noise also provide cues to place of articulation.
   a. VOT duration tends to increase as the place of articulation moves back in the mouth (Table 2-9).
      (1) Bilabial stops tend to have shorter VOTs than other stops with the same voicing.
      (2) Velar stops tend to have longer VOTs than bilabial and alveolar stops with the same voicing.
      (3) Alveolar stops tend to have either short VOTs like bilabials, or VOTs that are intermediate between bilabials and velars.

Stop Bursts

1. The shape of the frequency spectrum for stop bursts also provides information about place of articulation.
   a. In bilabial stops the burst spectrum tends to be flat or falling and to have no noticeable peaks.
      (1) This is described as a "diffuse flat" or "diffuse falling" spectrum.
   b. In alveolar stops, the burst spectrum tends to rise gradually, especially in the region up to about 5000 Hz (higher for women and children).
      (1) This is described as a "diffuse rising" spectrum.
   c. In velar stops, the burst spectrum tends to have peaks in the region of F1 and F2 for the adjacent vowel.
      (1) This is described as a "compact" spectrum.

Acoustic Measurement of Vocal Fold Vibration

Frequency

1. Frequency, stability and manner of vocal fold vibration are perceived as pitch and voice quality.
2. Frequency of vocal fold vibration (F_0) is most often measured from a waveform or pitch contour.
   a. From a waveform, select exactly one cycle and find its period (T).
      (1) Calculate F_0 as $1/T$.
      (2) F_0 measurements are very accurate, providing a cycle can be detected (Figure 2-36).
      (3) Although changes in F_0 are visible in waveforms, waveforms are not convenient for analyzing pitch over time (Figure 2-37).
   b. Pitch contours are the best display for examining F_0 over time.
      (1) To create an accurate pitch contour, acoustic analysis software must detect the cycle.
      (2) This can be difficult or impossible in disordered voices.
         (a) Pitch contour accuracy should be checked even in healthy voices.
         (b) Accuracy is most easily checked by showing a narrowband spectrogram behind the pitch contour.
         (c) If accurate, pitch contour shape will closely resemble the curves of the harmonics.
      (3) Pitch contour measurements are an average of cycles around the measurement point.
         (a) Measurements may not perfectly match waveform measurements at the same location (Figure 2-38).
   c. It may not be possible to create an accurate pitch contour for some disordered voices (Figure 2-39).
      (1) Estimates of F_0 may be obtainable from the waveform or narrowband spectrogram.

Summary Statistics

1. Summary statistics on F_0 across time can assist in objectively evaluating vocal health (Table 2-10).
   a. Results can be compared with published values for the speaker's sex and age group.
      (1) F_0 units must be the same as published values (e.g., semitones RE: 100 Hz) and should opti-mally be made from the same type of vocal sample.

Stability

1. Stability of vocal fold vibration.
   a. Jitter is cycle-to-cycle variability in frequency.
   b. Shimmer is cycle-to-cycle variability in amplitude.

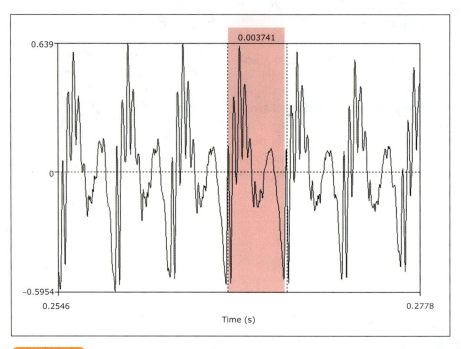

Figure 2-36 A section of a vowel waveform in which a single cycle can be accurately selected. The period of the highlighted cycle is 0.003741 seconds, therefore F_0 at this location in the vowel is 1/0.003741 or approximately 267 Hz.

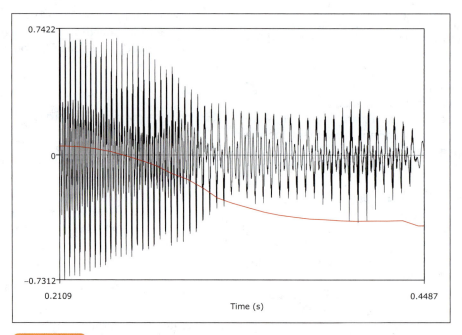

Figure 2-37 Waveform of a vowel with its pitch contour superimposed in red. In the waveform, the drop in pitch can be seen by comparing the distance between cycle peaks on the left vs. the right.

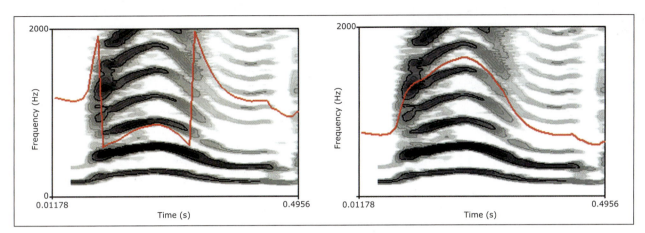

Figure 2-38 An incorrect pitch contour (left) and the corrected version (right). Both contours are superimposed on a narrowband spectrogram of the sound. The harmonics in the narrowband spectrogram show a smooth rising-falling curve. Since each harmonic is an integer multiple of F_0, the pitch contour should have the same general shape as the harmonics. The contour on the left shows an octave error, i.e., the pitch found in the center of the sound is an octave lower than the actual pitch.

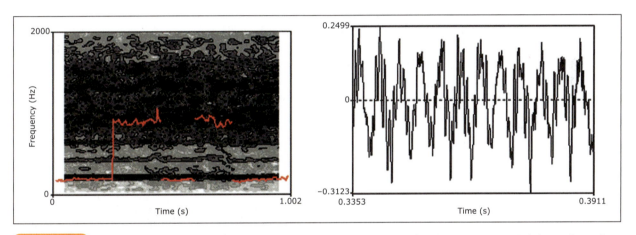

Figure 2-39 Pitch contour and narrowband spectrogram (left) for a sustained /ɑ/ produced by a speaker with a disordered voice. Harmonics are not clearly visible except at the bottom of the narrowband spectrogram, indicating that the voice is relatively aperiodic. The pitch contour (red) appears to be inaccurate. A section of the vowel's waveform, on the right, shows the irregularity of the cycle. Given the lack of clear periodicity, it may not be possible to correct the pitch contour. However, the clinician may be able to estimate F_0 by measuring harmonics in the narrowband spectrogram or attempting to find a cycle in the waveform.

Table 2-10

F_0 Statistics and the Vocal Samples Used to Obtain Them	
F_0 STATISTIC	**TYPICAL VOCAL SAMPLE**
Average speaking fundamental frequency (SFF)	Mean F_0 from a read passage or conversational speech
F_0 SD	SD of F_0 from a read passage or conversational speech
Speaking F_0 range	Distance between the minimum and maximum F_0 values in a read passage or conversation
Maximum phonational frequency range (MPFR)	Distance between the minimum and maximum F_0 values from an /ɑ/ that glides from a comfortable pitch to the highest pitch a speaker can reach and an /ɑ/ that glides from a comfortable pitch to the lowest pitch a speaker can reach
Cycle-to-cycle frequency variability (Jitter)	A sustained /ɑ/
Cycle-to-cycle amplitude variability (Shimmer)	A sustained /ɑ/

Table 2-11

A Comparison of Different Voice Qualities

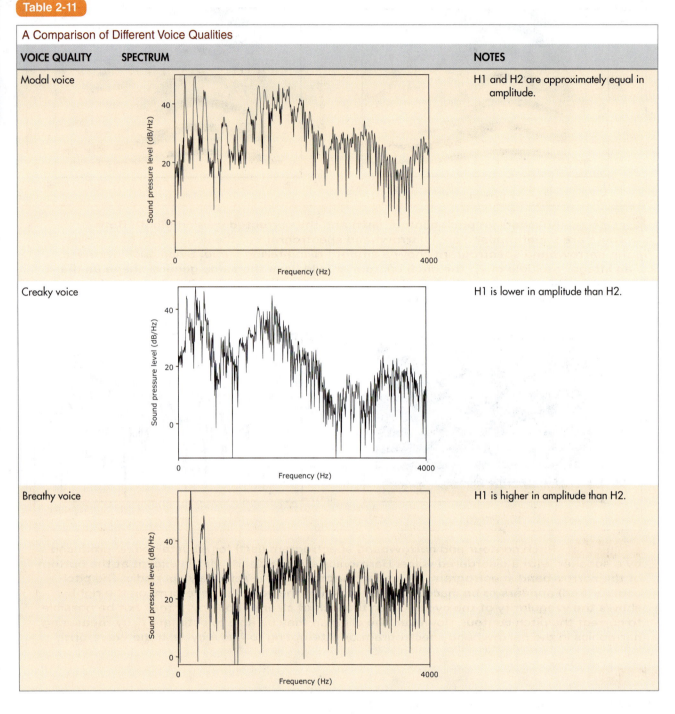

VOICE QUALITY	SPECTRUM	NOTES
Modal voice		H1 and H2 are approximately equal in amplitude.
Creaky voice		H1 is lower in amplitude than H2.
Breathy voice		H1 is higher in amplitude than H2.

    c. Jitter and shimmer should be measured from a sustained /a/.
       (1) Healthy speakers can voluntarily produce voice qualities that appear disordered.
       (2) It is important to have the speaker produce /a/ in the "clearest" voice he/she can generate.
    d. Calculations of jitter, frequency or amplitude of each cycle in the recorded sample is compared with one, two or three cycles on either side.

       (1) To accurately determine the amount of jitter and shimmer, acoustic analysis software must accurately find the cycles.
       (2) Only the user can determine whether or not the software has accurately found the individual cycles in the speech sample.
    e. Jitter and shimmer measurements can be compared with published thresholds for disorder.

Voice Quality

1. Often divided into modal voice, creaky voice and breathy voice.
   a. Modal voice is the typical voice quality produced by a healthy speaker.
   b. In creaky voice, the vocal folds pulse irregularly and often at a very low frequency.
   c. In breathy voice, the vocal folds never completely close, resulting in airflow even at maximal closure.
2. Changes in mode of vocal fold vibration correlate with changes in spectral tilt.
   a. Spectral tilt can be measured by comparing H1 and H2 amplitude or by comparing H1 amplitude with the highest-amplitude harmonic in the second or third formant (F2 or F3).
   b. In modal voice, H1 and H2 are approximately equal in amplitude.
   c. In creaky voice, H1 is lower in amplitude than H2.
   d. In breathy voice, H1 is higher in amplitude than H2.
3. Voice quality can be voluntarily changed by healthy speakers (Table 2-11).
   a. Some languages use voice quality phonemically, i.e., it can change word meaning.
   b. To ensure that voluntary changes are not interpreted as disorder, speakers need to produce a sustained /ɑ/ in the "clearest" voice they can generate.
   c. Harmonics-to-noise ratio (HNR) is a measurement of the amount of periodic versus aperiodic energy in a voice (Figure 2-40).
      (1) HNR is measured from a sustained /ɑ/.
      (2) The inverse of HNR is noise-to-harmonics ratio.
      (3) Healthy speakers should be able to produce about 99% periodic energy, or a harmonics-to-noise ratio of 20 dB.
      (4) Voluntary changes in voice quality can decrease HNR but do not indicate disorder.

```
Time range of SELECTION
   From 0.014563 to 0.495589 seconds (duration: 0.481026 seconds)
Pitch:
   Median pitch: 202.452 Hz
   Mean pitch: 221.672 Hz
   Standard deviation: 51.189 Hz
   Minimum pitch: 157.597 Hz
   Maximum pitch: 300.909 Hz
Pulses:
   Number of pulses: 106
   Number of periods: 105
   Mean period: 4.520652E−3 seconds
   Standard deviation of period: 1.033685E−3 seconds
Voicing:
   Fraction of locally unvoiced frames: 0 (0 / 48)
   Number of voice breaks: 0
   Degree of voice breaks: 0 (0 seconds / 0.481026 seconds)
Jitter:
   Jitter (local): 1.759%
   Jitter (local, absolute): 79.540E−6| seconds
   Jitter (rap): 0.639%
   Jitter (ppq5): 0.649%
   Jitter (ddp): 1.916%
Shimmer:
   Shimmer (local): 4.694%
   Shimmer (local, dB): 0.556 dB
   Shimmer (apq3): 1.339%
   Shimmer (apq5): 1.951%
   Shimmer (apq11): 3.835%
   Shimmer (dda): 4.016%
Harmonicity of the voiced parts only:
   Mean autocorrelation: 0.924791
   Mean noise-to-harmonics ratio: 0.090310
   Mean harmonics-to-noise ratio: 13.927 dB
```

Figure 2-40 Example of a voice report from the Praat acoustic analysis program, showing F_0 summary statistics, jitter, shimmer and harmonics to noise ratio information for a sustained vowel.

References

Behrman, A. (2012). *Speech and Voice Science*, 2nd ed. San Diego: Plural Publishing.

Durrant, J. D., & Lovrinic, J. H. (1995). *Bases of Hearing Science*, 3rd ed. Baltimore: Williams & Wilkins.

Johnson, K. (2011). *Acoustic & Auditory Phonetics*, 3rd ed. Hoboken, NJ: Wiley-Blackwell.

Kent, R. D., & Ball, M. J. (2000). *Voice Quality Measurement*. San Diego: Singular/Thomson Learning.

Kent, R. D., & Read, C. (2001). *Acoustic Analysis of Speech*, 2nd ed. Stamford: Cengage Learning.

Ladefoged, P. (1996). *Elements of Acoustic Phonetics*, 2nd ed. Chicago: University of Chicago Press.

Ladefoged, P., & Disner, S. F. (2012). *Vowels and Consonants*, 3rd ed. Hoboken, NJ: Wiley-Blackwell.

Laver, J. (1994). *Principles of Phonetics*. New York: Cambridge University Press.

Moore, B. C. J. (2003). *An Introduction to the Psychology of Hearing*, 5th ed. San Diego: Academic Press.

Mullin, W. J., Gerace, W. J., Mestre, J. P., & Velleman, S. L. (2003). *Fundamentals of Sound with Applications to Speech and Hearing Science*. Boston: Pearson.

Stevens, K. N. (1998). *Acoustic Phonetics*. Cambridge, MA: MIT Press.

3

Language Acquisition: Preverbal and Early Language

NINA CAPONE SINGLETON, PhD
AND BRIAN B. SHULMAN, PhD

Chapter Outline

- Language, 80
- Pragmatics, 80
- Phonology, 82
- Semantics, 83
- Morphology, 86
- Syntax, 89
- References, 90

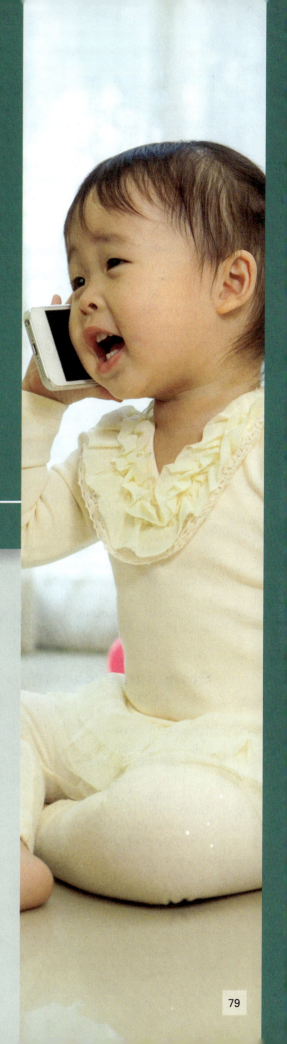

Language

Symbols and Parameters

1. A complex and dynamic system of conventional symbols that is used in various modes for thought and communication.
   a. Language evolves within specific historical, social and cultural contexts.
   b. Language is rule-governed behavior.
2. Language parameters (domains).
   a. Language domains characterize the form (phonologic, morphologic, syntactic), content (semantic) and use (pragmatic) of language.

Learning and Use

1. Language learning and use are determined by the interaction of biological, cognitive, psychosocial and environmental factors.
2. Effective use of language to communicate requires a broad understanding of human interaction, including nonverbal cues, motivation and sociocultural roles.
3. The spoken modality can be understood and produced.
   a. Receptive language or comprehension is the understanding of language.
   b. Expressive language is the production of language or what is written or signed.

Pragmatics

Function, Competence and Social Interaction

1. The domain of language that governs communication to be functional and socially appropriate within a given context.
2. Pragmatics refers to communicative competence.
3. Pragmatic rules guide the use of language in social interactions in a variety of contexts.

Stages of Pragmatic Development

1. Perlocutionary stage.
   a. Birth–8 months.
   b. Adults infer communicative intent from unintentional, vegetative behaviors such as the infant's cough or burp.
2. Illocutionary stage.
   a. 8 months–12 months.
   b. The use of gestures and vocalizations but no words to express intentions to communicate.
   c. Infants show objects and shortly after give objects over to adults to initiate interaction.
   d. Infants also use ritual request gestures to request action or attention.
      (1) For example, touching the adult's arm and making eye contact.
   e. Pointing to objects emerges as the infant approaches the first birthday.
   f. Pointing precedes and predicts first words in hearing children and first signs in hearing-impaired children exposed to sign language.
3. Locutionary stage.
   a. 12 months–lifespan.
   b. The use of words to express intentions to communicate.
   c. Gesture and other nonverbal behaviors become integrated with spoken language.

Communicative Behaviors

1. Nonverbal behaviors (e.g., eye contact, gestures, proxemics).
2. Intention expressed in spoken and nonverbal communication.
3. Discourse-related skills.
4. Theory of Mind.

Pragmatic Skills in Infancy

1. Pragmatic skills present in infancy that are the foundation for the social use of language.
   a. Eye contact.
   b. Turn-taking.
   c. Joint attention.

Children's Communicative Intentions

1. Children express their intentions using gestures, vocalizations or words.
   a. Intention refers to how language and other behaviors accomplish things in the world.
   b. Communicative intentions (also referred to as speech acts) expressed by infants and toddlers.
      (1) Requesting action.
      (2) Naming or labeling.
      (3) Protesting.
      (4) Greeting.
      (5) Repeating.
      (6) Calling.
      (7) Practicing.
      (8) Answering.
   c. Communicative intentions expressed by preschoolers.
      (1) Requesting permission.
      (2) Acknowledging.
      (3) Asking questions.
      (4) Making jokes.
      (5) Relating a story.
      (6) Suggesting.
      (7) Indirect requesting.
   d. Analyses of early pragmatic development.
      (1) Dore's Primitive Speech Acts.
      (2) Dore's Conversational Acts.
      (3) Martlew's Conversational Moves.

Children's Use of Gestures

1. Children use gestures to communicate.
   a. Children express intentions via gesture and vocalizations before words (e.g., pointing to guide adult attention).
   b. Iconic gestures (sticking tongue out to represent frog) and conventional gestures (nodding head, wave) emerge at the time of first words.
   c. Gestures are initially produced in isolation but gradually become integrated with spoken language by 2 years of age.

Longer Linguistic Units

1. Engaging in longer linguistic units of discourse is a pragmatic skill that requires the integration of all five domains of language.
   a. A narrative is a decontextualized monologue that conveys a story, personal recount or retelling of book or movie told to a listener with little support for the speaker.
      (1) Narratives are rule-governed in their organization.
         (a) Establish the central event.
         (b) Sequence events that are related to each other.
         (c) Specify the outcome.
      (2) Narratives reflect the culture of the speaker and the listener.
      (3) Two-year-old children tell proto-narratives characterized by related utterances that do not require sequencing.
      (4) Children gradually chain-link events to one another in an additive manner.
      (5) Children accurately describe a sequence of events in late preschool.
   b. A conversation is a dialogue between two communicative partners that emerges in toddlerhood and is refined through the preschool years.
      (1) Initiating a topic of conversation, maintaining a topic, transitioning to related topics, turn-taking and clarifying misunderstandings given verbal and/or nonverbal cues by the listener are skills that characterize a competent conversationalist.
      (2) Two-year-olds engage in short dialogues with few interruptions; however, these changes are highly scaffolded by the caregiver who explicitly requests clarifications.
      (3) Preschoolers engage in conversations that refer to the immediate context or specific past events.
   c. A monologue other than a narrative is characterized by self-conversation during focused, goal-directed activities, with no desire to involve others.
      (1) Emerges in preschool years.
   d. Expository discourse is an academic discourse device that develops in school-age children.
   e. Cohesion devices make communication efficient early in preschool.
      (1) Pronouns (me, mine, you, he, she, they).
      (2) Conjunctions (and, because).
   f. Ellipsis and deixis refer to the omission of redundant information in discourse.
      (1) Ellipsis refers to deleting already said information even if it results in an ungrammatical sentence (e.g., Did Mary eat the cookie? Yes, she did [ellipsis]).
      (2) Deixis devices are words or gestures that rely on context to glean meaning, such as pointing and using personal or other pronouns (this, that, here, there).
      (3) At least one deixis term is present in the first 50-word vocabulary but mastery continues through school-age years.
   g. The style of speech varies by speaker and context.
      (1) Dialect differences and register changes related to ethnicity, gender, region and generation.

(2) Preschool children use *motherese* when talking with younger children and take on various roles in play.
(3) Appropriate volume and tone of voice when communicating.
(4) Politeness (e.g., please, thank you).

Theory of Mind

1. Ability to take the listener's point of view including what they may believe, know or feel.
2. Must be taken into account to convey sufficient and accurate information to a listener.
   a. For example, providing the referent for subsequent pronoun use or providing all background or introduction information to establish a topic of discourse.

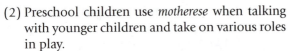

Phonology

System of Sound

1. Sound system of a language and the rules that govern the sound combinations.
2. The smallest linguistic unit that signals a difference in word meaning is the phoneme.
   a. C = consonant
   b. V = vowel
3. Phonemes are transcribed using the International Phonetic Alphabet (IPA).

Phonological Rules

1. Phonological rules govern the form of phonemes.
   a. *Place of articulation* refers to where the articulators approximate each other to create a sound source for consonants.
   b. *Manner of articulation* refers to how the sound is modified along the vocal tract for consonants.
   c. *Voicing* refers to whether or not there is vocal fold vibration during sound production for consonants.
      (1) /b/
         (a) Place of articulation is bilabial.
         (b) Manner of articulation is stop.
         (c) The phoneme is voiced.
      (2) /h/
         (a) Place of articulation is glottal (vocal fold level).
         (b) Manner of articulation is fricative.
         (c) The phoneme is voiceless (no vocal fold vibration).
   d. Vowels are characterized by lingual (tongue) height and anterior-posterior lingual posture in the oral cavity.
      (1) Vowels are high, mid or low in lingual height.
      (2) Vowels are front, central or back in lingual posture.
         (a) Vowel /i/ is a high, front vowel.
         (b) Vowel /a/ is a low, back vowel.
      (3) Vowels are also characterized by tension (/i, u, e, o/) and rounding (/u, ʊ, o, ɑ/).
   e. Vowels are always voiced.
2. Phonological rules govern how phonemes are sequenced in syllables.
   a. Phonotactic probability is the frequency with which certain sound sequences occur in a language.
      (1) Established through experience with the ambient language.
      (2) Sound sequences comprised of common phonotactic probability sequences occur often.
      (3) Sound sequences comprised of rare phonotactic probability sequences occur infrequently.
      (4) Common sequences are perceived and produced more quickly than rare sequences.
      (5) Awareness of phonotactic probabilities emerges at approximately 9 months of age.
3. Phonological rules govern how syllables are structured.
   a. Syllables require a V and can have a variety of C and V configurations.
      (1) Examples of syllable structures are V (a), VC (in), CV (to), CVC (cat), CVCV (baby), CVCC (walk) and CCVC (stop).

Phonological Development

1. Early phonological development is fairly consistent across children.
   a. First words consist of a single CV syllable, single V and CVCV syllables.
   b. Early sound repertoire includes phonemes /p, b, t, d, g, k, h, m, w, n/.
   c. Production of phonemes is variable.
   d. Children are more likely to attempt to say new words that contain phonemes already in their phonological repertoire.
   e. Phonological development is initially holistic but the child is eventually able to segment phonemes within a word.

2. When children reach a threshold of vocabulary they begin to evince phonological processes.
   a. A phonological process is a pattern of speech production in which a child simplifies the adult form of a production.
   b. Phonological processes have a typical course of use and resolution.
      (1) For example, reduplication, such as saying "baba" for bottle.
      (2) For example, final consonant deletion, such as saying "ca" for cat.
   c. An analysis of the phonological processes used by the child is used to evaluate the timeliness of resolution.

3. In the preschool years, children emerge with awareness that words can be deconstructed into phonological parts (sounds, syllables); this is referred to as phonological awareness.
   a. Development of phonological awareness begins by early preschool and continues into the school-age years.
   b. Phonological awareness skills begin as rhyming and evolve to identifying the first sound of words, sound comparison between words and segmentation of words into smaller units.
   c. Phonological awareness is strongly correlated with reading and writing skills development.

Semantics

System of Meanings

1. System that governs the meanings of words and sentences.
   a. Semantics encompasses the rules for learning and using words, word combinations and higher-level meaning units (e.g., idioms, metaphors and other types of figurative language in the school-age years).
   b. Children store words in long-term semantic memory, also referred to as the *lexicon*.

Word Learning

1. Word learning encompasses mapping the word form or label (lexical representation), word meaning (semantic representation) and grammatical specifications (word class information), in addition to making connections between the various phonological representations and articulatory representations.
2. Word learning is a gradual and long-term process that begins with fast mapping a sketch of the word and subsequently slow mapping the details of the word.
   a. Fast mapping happens when the initial association or link between the word label and meaning is made and stored in memory.
      (1) QUick Incidental Learning (QUIL) reflects the more naturally occurring word learning situations that offer minimal support in ongoing scenes.
   b. Slow mapping refers to the learning that occurs during the protracted period of word learning after fast mapping has occurred.
      (1) Enrichment of semantic and lexical representations occurs during slow mapping.
         (a) Richer representations result from more frequent experience and high-quality experience.
   c. Words that are more frequently heard in the ambient language are learned more quickly.
   d. Nouns are more easily learned than other word classes.
      (1) Verbs take more exposure to learn than nouns most likely because a more subtle inference needs to be made about verbs from ongoing events.
      (2) In Korean and German, where cultural practice or structure of the language promotes verb over noun learning, nouns predominate in early lexicons.
   e. Phonological, lexical and semantic representations of the word itself influence word learning.
      (1) Phonological representations refer to sound representations.
         (a) Infants produce more words comprised of rare phonotactics than common phonotactics.
      (2) Lexical representations refer to word label representations.
         (a) Neighborhood density of a word refers to the number of possible words (i.e., neighbors) that differ by one phoneme from it.
            • For example, the word "cat" resides in a high density neighborhood because it has several neighbors, including "sat," "pat," "cab," "rat," "coat," "cute," and "can."

(b) Infants produce more words that are short and from dense neighborhoods (with many neighbors) than long words from sparse neighborhoods.
(3) Semantic representations refer to meaning or conceptual representations.
(a) Richness of knowledge and connections.
(b) Infants produce more words with many interconnected semantic neighbors and strong connections.
f. Neighborhood density is a lexical representation variable that influences word learning.
(1) A word that resides in a dense neighborhood may be easier to learn because it has many connections between words, but it may be more difficult to perceive or retrieve that word for production because of interference activation from those same neighbors.
g. Enriching the quality of word exposure hastens fast and slow mapping.
(1) Richer semantic representations support word retrieval to name words.
(2) Weaker semantic representations may support recognition of the word but they are often associated with errors when the child attempts to name it.

The Phonological Loop

1. The capacity of the phonological loop is the component of working memory that is strongly associated with word learning.
   a. The phonological loop encodes, maintains and manipulates speech-based (i.e., phonological) information.
   b. The gold standard measure of the phonological loop is nonword repetition.
   c. Children who are better at repeating nonwords tend to have larger vocabularies.

Semantic Hierarchy

1. The semantic system is hierarchically organized with superordinate (animal), ordinate (dog), and subordinate (poodle, boxer, schnoodle) words.
   a. Semantically related words are linked more closely in the lexicon.
   b. Children's first words are ordinate terms.

Retrieval Errors

1. Words that are fast mapped or infrequently encountered are weakly represented in memory and therefore vulnerable to retrieval errors when naming.
   a. Word retrieval errors are often logically related to the target word.
      (1) Phonologically related, such as saying "chicken" for "kitchen."
      (2) Semantically related, such as saying "key" for "door."
      (3) Phonologically and semantically related, such as "elevator" for "escalator."
   b. Indeterminate errors such as saying "thing," "I don't know" or giving no response are common and related to lack of semantic knowledge.
   c. Perseverative responding occurs when the child uses the same word to label different objects within a set time interval of having said the erred word correctly.
   d. Visual misperception errors such as saying "lollipop" for "balloon" are less common.
   e. Semantically related and indeterminate errors are the most common error types that occur.
   f. Children with and without language impairments make the same types and patterns of word retrieval errors, but children with language impairments make many more errors overall.

Spoken Language

1. Spoken language emerges at a lexical level.
   a. The infant spends one year preparing for the first word.
      (1) Infants vocalize predominately vowel-like sounds before 4 months of age.
      (2) Between 4 and 6 months of age infants string together C-V combinations that eventually become more complex in structure.
         (a) Complex babble is referred to as variegated babble.
         (b) Variegated babble is thought to be continuous with first words in that sounds heard in variegated babble tend to also occur in first words.
      (3) Jargon emerges at approximately 10 months of age when intentional communication begins.
      (4) At 10 months of age infants understand (receptive vocabulary) approximately 10 words.
   b. First words emerge around the first birthday but can emerge earlier or later.
   c. Initial vocabulary growth, from 12 to 18 months, is slow with stops and starts.
   d. The expressive lexicon is approximately 10 words in size by 15 months.
   e. Children slowly acquire 50 words in their expressive vocabulary (mean age of 19 months) but have, on average, 100–300 words by 24 months of age.
   f. Early noun vocabulary includes words from the animal category, food category, and toy category.

g. Once the child acquires 50 words in their lexicon, word learning accelerates and the child begins combining words.
   (1) Word learning acceleration is referred to as the "word spurt."
   (2) Early word combinations include "more cookie," "mommy eat" and "go bye-bye."
      (a) Word combinations are preceded by gesture + word combinations, such as pointing to a dog and saying "dog" or pointing to a cookie and saying "eat."
   (3) During the word spurt, word retrieval errors accelerate because the child is mapping many new but weak lexical-semantic representations.
   (4) Children overextend and underextend words as they are acquiring the boundaries of each word's meaning.
h. Overgeneralization and undergeneralization errors are semantic errors that predominate in the child's early vocabulary development.
   (1) Overgeneralization, such as saying "ball" for "moon," indicates a child thinks a word's meaning is more broadly applied.
      (a) Occurs because of a perceptual or functional similarity between the word said and the referent.
   (2) Undergeneralization, such as only saying the child's "dog" is a "dog" but not other dogs, indicates a child thinks a word's meaning is too restricted or narrow.
i. Children invent a word when there is a gap in their lexicon, such as saying "spooning" for "stirring," and bilingual children will mix a word from one language with another language to fill a lexical gap.
j. Bilingual children have vocabularies in each of their languages that minimally overlap, referred to as few word equivalents.
   (1) A word equivalent is a word from each language that refers to the same referent.

Nouns

1. A universal semantic feature of language is that nouns make up the largest proportion of the early vocabulary.
   a. Children who follow this pattern of having a preponderance of nouns in their vocabulary are referred to as referential.
   b. Those who do not follow this pattern are referred to as expressive.
   c. Referential children have:
      (1) Larger vocabularies.
      (2) Reach morphological and syntactic milestones sooner.
      (3) Have greater growth of verb vocabulary at 20 months of age.
      (4) Have more productive control over function words by 28 months.
      (5) Use words in a context flexible way (i.e., decontextualized).
         (a) Decontextualization refers to the gradual distancing of a symbol from its original referent or learning context and is a skill that is later required for written language development.
   d. Expressive children:
      (1) Have nominal accounting for less than half their lexicons.
      (2) Show a slow and steady pace in word learning with no word spurt.
      (3) Learn and use language as holistic chunks or phrases initially.
      (4) Later produce use of function words than for referential children.

Verbs, Relational Terms and Double-Function Words

1. At approximately 24 months of age children begin acquiring many more verbs.
   a. A threshold number of verbs in the child's lexicon is thought to drive morphological development.
2. After 24 months of age, the lexicon expands significantly to include relational terms (on, under, next to), interrogative terms (what, who, how, why), temporal relationship terms (when, before), physical relations (big, little, wide, narrow) and kinship terms (son, parent, aunt, nephew).
3. A variety of word classes continue to expand in the preschool years and children are learning the concrete or physical definitions of double-function words such as "cold."
   a. In the preschool years, children continue to have an easier time learning nouns in fewer exposures than other word classes.

Biological and Environmental Factors

1. Biological and environmental factors influence word learning.
   a. Factors that may negatively impact language development include chronic otitis media with effusion, motor speech problems, socioeconomic status, exposure to television and international adoption.
   b. Vocabulary size is positively related to maternal language use and education.
      (1) Motherese refers to modifications made in an adult's speech when it is directed toward young children.

(2) Motherese is characterized by utterances that are:
   (a) Shorter in length.
   (b) Simpler in grammatical complexity.
   (c) Slower in rate of speech.
   (d) Less diverse and more concrete vocabulary.
   (e) Contextually redundant.
   (f) Perceptually salient.
   (g) Speech that has a higher fundamental frequency, exaggerated stress, a wider range of intonation, and with more pausing.
(3) Motherese is not used to the same extent in all cultures throughout the world.
(4) Young children attend to and use other salient social cues by caregivers to learn words, including pointing to and directing eye gaze toward referents while labeling or talking about them.

c. Children come equipped with innate skills and biases to learn words.
(1) Bootstrapping refers to use of language to infer the meaning of words they do not know.
   (a) Syntactic bootstrapping when s/he uses morpho-syntactic structures s/he knows to infer the word class of a novel word (e.g., "gorping" is a verb but "the gorp" is a noun).
(2) Early word learning biases make word learning and use efficient.
   (a) Help children determine what referent is being labeled.
   (b) The principle of reference refers to the belief that words but not other sounds label objects, actions and events.
   (c) The novel-name-nameless category principle (N3C) refers to the belief that a novel word will be taken as the name for a previously unnamed object.
   (d) The principle of mutual exclusivity refers to the belief that a referent cannot have more than one word label.
   (e) The whole-object bias refers to the belief that words refer to an entire object and not just a part, an attribute or its motion.
   (f) The principle of extendability refers to the belief that a word refers to a category of objects, events or actions if they share similar properties, namely shape or function.
   (g) The shape bias refers to the belief that a word refers to a category of objects that are defined by sharing the same shape.

Late Talkers

1. Toddlers who do not meet early word learning milestones in a timely manner are referred to as late talkers.
   a. Most outgrow their early language delay (late bloomers) but a small percentage persists in their language delay beyond the preschool years.
   b. Defined by a small vocabulary and no two-word combinations.
   c. Those with more words show stronger language learning than those with the smallest vocabularies.

Morphology

System of Structure

1. System that governs the structure of words and the construction of word forms.
2. A morpheme is the smallest unit of language that carries meaning.
   a. The meaning of a word changes by modifying its morphemes.
   b. Morphemes specify syntactic relationships.
3. Morphemes are free of or bound to other morphemes.
   a. Free morphemes are those that stand alone and carry meaning.
      (1) Examples of free morphemes are tree, house, dog, milk, shake, run, pretty, of, in.
   b. Bound morphemes must be combined to a free morpheme to be meaningful.
      (1) Examples of bound morphemes are plural –s, possessive –s, present progressive –ing verb form, suffix –er, suffix –est, prefix dis–, prefix re–.

Morphological Construction

1. Morphological construction is the creation of new words using affixes.
   a. Affixes are prefixes and suffixes.
      (1) Affixes can be inflectional.
         (a) For example, third-person singular –s (e.g., He walks).
         (b) Inflectional morphology is mastered by 6 years of age.
      (2) Affixes can be derivational.

(a) For example, New Yorker is derived by adding the suffix –er to New York.
(b) Knowledge of derivational morphology is closely related to reading and spelling ability in school-age children.
(c) Derivational morphology develops throughout the school-age years, adolescent years and adulthood.

Compounding and Combinations

1. Compounding refers to the formation of a new word by combining two lexical morphemes without the use of affixes (e.g., sunshine).
2. Children mark syntactic relations early in development first by word combinations and later with morphemes.
   a. For example, "mommy shoe" later becomes "mommy's shoe."

Morphemes in Early Development

1. During early development, the length and complexity of utterances increases by use of morphemes.
   a. Discernable advances in utterance complexity is captured by calculating the Mean Length of Utterance (MLU).
   b. MLU is the average length of an utterance based on free and bound morphemes (not words).
   c. MLU is a good indicator of grammatical development before 6 years of age.
   d. Calculation of the MLU is taken from the middle 50–100 utterances of a sample of spontaneous language that was elicited in a natural environment.
      (1) Tally the individual free and bound morphemes in each utterance (Table 3-1).

Table 3-1

Brown's (1973) Stages and MLU

BROWN'S STAGE	AGE IN MONTHS	MLU-M	MLU-M RANGE	MORPHOLOGICAL STRUCTURE	EXAMPLES
Stage I	15–30	1.75	1.5–2.0	combine basic words	that car more juice give it
Stage II	28–36	2.25	2.0–2.5	present progressive (-ing endings on verbs)	it go**ing** fall**ing** off
				in	**in** box
				on	**on** tree
				-s plurals (regular plurals)	my car**s**
Stage III	36–42	2.75	2.5–3.0	irregular past tense	me **fell** down you **sat** on
				-s possessives	doggie**'s** bone
				uncontractible copula (the full form of the verb "to be" when it is the only verb in a sentence)	Are they there? Is she coming?
Stage IV	40–46	3.5	3.0–3.7	articles	a book the book
				regular past tense (-ed endings on verbs)	she jumped he laughed
				third person regular present tense	he swims she goes
Stage V	42–52+	4.0	3.7–4.5	third person irregular	she has he does
				uncontractible auxiliary (the full form of the verb "to be" when it is an auxiliary verb in a sentence)	**Are** they swimming? **Is** she going?
				contractible copula (the shortened form of the verb "to be" when it is the only verb in a sentence)	She**'s** ready. They**'re** here. I**'m** here.
				contractible auxiliary (the shortened form of the verb "to be" when it is an auxiliary verb in a sentence)	They**'re** coming. He**'s** going. I**'m** done.

Table 3-2

The Age of Acquisition Order for Grammatical Morphemes (Early Years 3–5)

MORPHEMES	AGE OF ACQUISITION IN MONTHS	EXAMPLES
1. Present Progressive	19–28	I eating
2&3. Prepositions in, on	27–30	Ball in box, car on table
4. Plural –s	24–33	Toys
5. Irregular Past Tense	25–46	Ate, ran
6. Possessive –s	26–40	Kayla's doll
7. Uncontractible Copula –is	27–39	This is cold
8. Articles –a, the	28–46	This is a car, put in the box
9. Regular Past Tense –ed	26–48	He jumped
10. 3rd Person Present Tense –s (regular)	26–46	She dances
11. 3rd Person Present Tense (irregular)	28–50	He does not
12. Uncontracible Auxiliary	29–49	Kayla is dancing
13. Contractible Copula –'s	29–49	She's nice
14. Contractible Auxiliary –'s	30–50	She's dancing

(2) Sum the number of free and bound morphemes from all utterances.
(3) MLU = total number of free and bound morphemes/total number of utterances.
e. MLU roughly corresponds to a child's age from 1 to 5 years; however, children produce utterances that are far longer than their MLU would indicate.
(1) The child's longest utterance is referred to as the Upper Bound Length (UBL).
f. MLU corresponds to Brown's stages of grammatical development.

Brown's Grammatical Morphemes

1. Roger Brown (1973) studied the development of a subset of English morphemes that were easily identified for obligatory context in a spontaneous speech sample (Table 3-2).
    a. Analysis of Brown's 14 grammatical morphemes examines whether or not children have mastery over each morpheme.
        (1) Mastery is defined as 90% use of a given Brown's morpheme given all obligatory contexts for that morpheme in a spontaneous language sample.
        (2) To calculate the percentage of use for each of Brown's 14 grammatical morphemes, sum all obligatory contexts for each morpheme separately and then sum the number of those obligatory contexts in which the child used the morpheme.
            (a) Percent mastery = sum of morpheme use/number of obligatory contexts.

Mastering Morphemes

1. Children with Specific Language Impairment (SLI) have particular difficulty with mastery of verb inflections that indicate tense and agreement.
    a. It is suggested that difficulty with verb inflections is a clinical marker of SLI.
2. The WUG Test (Berko, 1958) is a well-known experimental procedure that elicits production of the following morphemes: plural –s, possessive –s, present progressive -ing tense, third-person singular present tense, and past tense.
3. The order in which morphemes are acquired is highly similar between children.
4. Present progressive tense (–ing), in, on, and plural –s are the earliest to be mastered.
5. Copula and auxiliary verb TO BE are the last to be mastered.
6. Children go through a period in development during which they make predictable errors in morpheme production.
    a. Optional infinitive stage occurs when children treat verb tense and agreement markers as optional.
        (1) Gradually declines around age 3 years in English.
        (2) Children learning rich inflectional languages such as Italian or Spanish do not show an optional infinitive stage.
        (3) Children with SLI in rich inflectional languages tend to have fewer verb tense errors than those in American English.
    b. Overgeneralization of past tense –ed to irregular verbs (e.g., saying "runned" instead of "ran") and overgeneralization of plural –s to nouns with irregular plurals (e.g., saying "mouses" instead of "mice").

Syntax

System of Word Order and Combination

1. System governing the order and combination of words to form sentences, and the relationships among the elements within a sentence.
2. Words are combined in a systematic, rule-governed way.
3. The theory of universal grammar and the government and binding theory by Noam Chomsky describe the learning and use of syntax.
   a. There are two levels of representation: deep structure (what is conceptualized) and surface structure (what is said).
   b. At the deep structure, phrases and sentences are constructed according to phrase structure rules and information contained about individual words in the lexicon.
   c. The surface structure is constructed according to thematic roles assigned by the verb and transformational rules that guide how words change order from deep to surface structure.
      (1) Transformational rules are responsible for a variety of sentences and questions to be formed from a single deep-structure representation.
      (2) A language uses a variety of sentence types to efficiently and succinctly convey a speaker's intended meaning.
   d. Syntactic categories are the inflection category (Infl), which dictates tense of the clause or sentence it governs, and the complementizer (Comp), which is used to embed a clause into another clause using words like "that" and "whether."
   e. A Language Acquisition Device (LAD) in the brain was responsible for the development of syntax in young children.
      (1) The child sets language-specific parameters for grammar by hearing the ambient language.

Syntactic Construction and Combination

1. The length of a child's sentences in morphemes is a good measure of syntactic development.
2. Sentences are constructed of content words (open-classed words such as nouns and verbs) and function words (closed-class words such as prepositions, articles, conjunctions, pronouns).
3. Early sentences are telegraphic and characterized by content word combinations that often contain a pivot word or phrase (e.g., more, I want).
4. A universal feature of early word combinations is that a small set of semantic relations are expressed with a consistent word order.
   a. Examples of prevalent semantic relations include agent + action (mommy eat), action + object (eat cookie), possessor + possession (mommy shoe), and entity + location (cookie table).
   b. Characteristic of Brown's Stage I of grammatical development.
5. Producing simple sentences, questions, negatives and imperatives characterize Brown's Stages II and III of grammatical development.
6. Grammatical development in toddlers is closely tied to vocabulary development and, in particular, that of verbs.
7. Passive sentences (a noncanonical form used to highlight the object of a sentence), coordinated sentences (with conjunctions) and embedded relative clauses characterize syntactic developments of Brown's Stage IV and V of grammatical development.
   a. A passive sentence is reversible if both the subject and object are animate, requiring the use of syntax to understand them.
   b. Reversible passive sentences are one of the last sentences to be understood in the preschool years.
   c. Coordinating sentences with conjunctions expresses complex propositions between phrases or sentences.
   d. Embedded relative clauses are infrequently produced spontaneously, but older preschoolers (Brown's Stage IV) are capable of producing them under experimental conditions.

Syntactic Development

1. Noun phrase elaboration begins by combining words in isolation and gradually evolves to the sentence level and the use of determiners, adjectives, possessive pronouns and other modifiers (e.g., prepositional phrases, embedded clauses).
2. Verb phrase elaboration occurs through the development of verb tense and agreement morphemes, the use of auxiliary verbs, verb particles (e.g., pick up), infinitive forms of verbs, negation and gerund phrases (e.g., using "running" as a noun).
   a. Semi-infinitives, such as "wanna," develop before true infinitives such as "want to."

3. Expansion of sentence types includes declaratives, interrogatives, imperatives, negatives.
   a. Subject-verb-object declarative sentences emerge by 30 months of age and gradually increase in length to include verb phrase components and indirect objects.
   b. Interrogatives develop from the use of rising intonation on one-word utterances and gradually increase the syntactic complexity of them by including semantically specific wh-question words and auxiliary inversion.
      (1) "What," "where" and "who" questions emerge first, and in the preschool years children ask "why," "how" and "when" questions at a time when the cognitive skills related to them (e.g., time) are also developing.
      (2) Tag questions and negative interrogatives are the last to develop.
   c. Imperatives appear between 2 and 3 years of age.
   d. Negative sentences evolve from just the use of "no" to the negative being embedded within the verb phrase.
      (1) Contracted forms such as "don't" and "can't" occur first and are learned as a holistic form.
4. Complex sentences are those with subordinated clauses and coordinated clauses and sentences.
   a. Subordinate clauses are initially used with an holistic phrase, such as "I know" or "I think," followed by an object complement, and verbs "look" or "see," and eventually subordinating conjunctions are used (e.g., that, when).
   b. Subordinate clauses can fill a sentence position or can modify a noun.
   c. Coordination emerges with "and" to list things and later a series of related events around 3 years of age, and then "because" emerges.
   d. Other conjunctions to appear are "if," "but," "that's why" and "so."

References

AAC Institute (2009). *Brown's Stages of Morphological Development.* 2009. Pittsburgh, PA. Retrieved from: http://www.aacinstitute.org/Resources/ParentsCorner/2009June3.JPG.

American Speech-Language-Hearing Association (1982). Language [Relevant Paper]. Available from www.asha.org/policy.

American Speech-Language-Hearing Association (1993). Definitions of Communication Disorders and Variations [Relevant Paper]. Available from www.asha.org/policy.

Berko-Gleason, J., & Bernstein Ratner, N. (2009). *The Development of Language*, 7th ed. Boston: Pearson.

Capone, N. C., & Sheng, L. (2010). "Individual Differences in Word Learning: Implications for Clinical Practice" in *Perspectives on Individual Differences Affecting Therapeutic Change in Communication Disorders*. NY: Taylor & Francis.

Owens, R. E. (2012). *Language Development: An Introduction.* Boston: Pearson.

Retherford, K. S. (2000). *Guide to Analysis of Language Transcripts*, 3rd ed. Eau Claire, WI: Thinking Publications.

Shulman, B. B., & Capone, N.C. (2010). *Language Development. Foundations, Processes, and Clinical Applications.* Sudbury, MA: Jones and Bartlett Publishers.

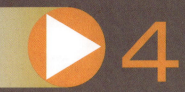

4

Research, Evidence-Based Practice and Tests and Measurements

MARGARET GREENWALD, PhD

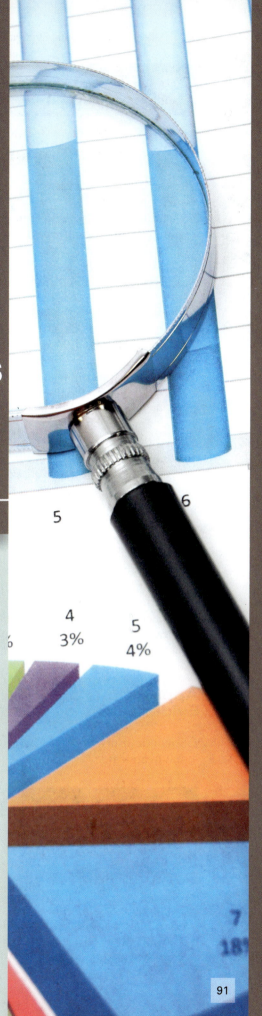

Chapter Outline

- Research Principles and the Speech-Language Pathologist, 92
- Evidence-Based Practice (EBP), 92
- Interpreting Research Articles, 93
- Treatment Efficacy Studies and Evidence-Based Practice, 99
- Interpreting Tests and Measurements, 100
- Cultural Diversity in Evidence-Based Practice, 100
- References, 100

Research Principles and the Speech-Language Pathologist

The Research Process

1. Research is a process of asking and answering questions.
2. Scientific principles guide the research process in communication sciences and disorders.
   a. Testability—it is better to ask specific research questions than vague questions because specific ones can be evaluated and answered.
   b. Replication—reproducing the findings of one research study in a second research study is valuable.
   c. Objectivity—research questions and findings should be addressed and interpreted without bias, and alternative interpretations should be considered.
3. Types of research questions.
   a. A descriptive research question, such as "What is?" or "What exists?"
   b. A difference research question, such as "What is the difference?"
   c. A relationship research question, such as "What is the relationship?"
4. A hypothesis is a prediction about how the research question will be answered.
5. The null hypothesis is about what will happen if the hypothesis does not come true.
6. Examples of a hypothesis and its corresponding null hypothesis.
   a. The hypothesis: "X will be greater than Y."
   b. The null hypothesis: "X will not be greater than Y."
7. Research involves generating hypotheses and testing them.

Applications of Research in Evidence-Based Practice

1. Scientific principles are the basis of effective diagnosis and treatment.
2. Diagnostic and treatment hypotheses are tested systematically through impartial efforts to collect and score speech, language or swallowing performance data.
3. Client performance is described along with any differences and relationships among the data.
4. Tentative conclusions are drawn about the diagnosis or treatment.

ASHA'S Code of Ethics and Research Ethics

1. The American Speech-Language-Hearing Association (ASHA) Code of Ethics reflects 4 principles and 44 rules.
2. This code is modified by ASHA as needed to reflect the evolution of the professions of speech-language pathology, audiology and speech-language-hearing sciences.
3. The four principles in the ASHA Code of Ethics involve:
   a. The welfare of persons.
   b. Professional competence and performance.
   c. Responsibilities to the public.
   d. Responsibilities to the profession.
4. Statements about research ethics in the ASHA Code of Ethics coincide with other documents describing the Responsible Conduct of Research (RCR).
   a. The welfare of persons and animals must be protected.
   b. Persons participating in research must give voluntary informed consent.
   c. The privacy and confidentiality of subjects and participants must be protected.
5. The ASHA Code of Ethics reflects the value placed on clinical research and evidence-based practice for:
   a. Providing high-quality service.
   b. Evaluating the effectiveness of services and products.

Evidence-Based Practice (EBP)

Definition and Process

1. EBP involves basing clinical decisions on the integration of best current research evidence, clinical expertise, and the needs, abilities and perspectives of the client and his/her family.
2. The process of EBP begins with a specific and answerable question.
   a. For example, a PICO-format question.
      (1) Population of interest (or, the patient or problem identified).
      (2) Intervention.

(3) Comparison.
(4) Outcomes.
b. A sample PICO-format question: In stroke survivors with verbal anomia (P), does training in the use of gesture (I) as compared to no gesture (C) facilitate word retrieval (O)?

Collect the Best Available Evidence

1. Sources could be external evidence from the scientific literature, clinical practice guidelines or expert opinion from SLP clinicians.
2. The SLP searches the literature. The SLP who is information-literate is proficient in the research process and able to find appropriate information.

Evaluate the External Evidence

1. The external evidence is critically evaluated using strict criteria.
   a. Does the study have good internal validity?
      (1) Internal validity is how well the study is testing or describing what it purports to be testing or describing.
      (2) Internal validity depends on the methods and procedures used to answer the research question(s).
   b. Does the study have good external validity?
      (1) External validity is the generalizability of results.
         (a) Results should not be generalized across populations, settings, measurements or treatments until there is evidence to show that the results are valid beyond the confines of one study.
         (b) External validity can be extended by replication. Replication can provide consistent results across populations, settings, measurements or treatments.
   c. What is the level of evidence of the study?
      (1) There are several hierarchies that have been used to rank treatment studies according to scientific quality and rigor.
      (2) The credibility of the level of evidence is ranked based on:
         (a) Convergence of evidence.
         (b) Adequacy of experimental control.
         (c) Reduction of researcher bias.
         (d) Size of treatment effect.
         (e) Relevance.
      (3) The strongest treatment evidence comes from meta-analyses that are well designed and based on multiple randomized controlled clinical studies and also from systematic reviews. This is discussed further below in the section "Treatment Efficacy Studies and Evidence-Based Practice."
2. The SLP assesses the impact of the evidence on clinical practice and comes to an informed clinical decision.
   a. The SLP focuses on the client. The environment and stakeholders are also considered.
   b. Environment includes the context and place of treatment, as well as communication partners.
   c. Stakeholders include the client's family member(s) and level of motivation.

Interpreting Research Articles

The "Introduction" Section

1. Includes the review of the literature, statement of the problem and rationale for the study.
2. Leads to the research questions and hypotheses.

The "Methods" Section

1. Sufficient detail should be included so that the study can be replicated.
2. Subjects.
   a. Subjects in communication sciences and disorders (CSD) research are typically human participants but may include other subjects such as models or specimens.
   b. Subject selection criteria should be clearly defined.
   c. Usually it is not feasible for researchers to study an entire population of interest; therefore, a sample of subjects is studied.
   d. The subject sample size should be sufficient for the purposes of the study. Sufficient sample size is affected by the study design and the variability of the data in that particular study.

e. In random sampling, each individual in a population of interest has an equal chance of being selected for the study.
f. The generalizability of the study results is enhanced when the subject sample is large and randomly selected from the population of interest. However, many studies in communicative disorders do not use large random samples because they can be difficult to obtain.
3. Materials.
   a. Should be adequate to generate and/or measure the variables studied.
      (1) The independent variable can be described as a condition that can change behavior.
      (2) The dependent variable can be described as the behavior that may change.
      (3) Examples of independent and dependent variables:
         (a) Research question: "What is the difference in a participant's ability to recognize speech under conditions of high versus low noise level?"
         (b) Independent variable: Noise level.
         (c) Dependent variable: Ability to recognize speech.
      (4) Extraneous (i.e., nuisance) variables—other factors that can alter the dependent variable, making it difficult to understand the relationship between the independent variable and the dependent variable.
         (a) Samples of such extraneous variables include the participant's level of attention, medications, prior treatment and comprehension of test instructions.
   b. Levels of measurement defined by four characteristics. The simplest level (nominal) has one characteristic and the most complex level (ratio) has all four characteristics:
      (1) Identity—attributes are categorized into mutually exclusive groups, such as Broca's aphasia versus Wernicke's aphasia type (nominal level).
      (2) Identity and magnitude—attributes are put into a relative ranking from least to most, such as the persons ranked third, second or first in production of reading errors (ordinal level).
      (3) Identity, magnitude and equality of an interval—there are equal intervals between the attributes that are ranked from least to most, such as air temperature readings (interval level).
      (4) Identity, magnitude, equality of an interval and a true zero—it is possible that the attribute is absent and equal to zero, for example, number of spelling errors or sound intensity (ratio level).
      (5) More statistical operations are allowed with the more complex levels of measurement; therefore, the most complex level of measurement possible should be used.
   c. Reliability of measurement refers to how much we can depend on a measure.
      (1) The reliability of a measurement can be evaluated in a variety of ways.
         (a) Stability of measurement (e.g., using the test-retest method).
         (b) Equivalence of measurement (e.g., comparing performance on alternate or parallel forms of a test).
         (c) Internal consistency of measurement (e.g., the split-half method, in which performance on one half of a test is compared to performance on the other half of items from the same test).
      (2) A measurement can be evaluated for its precision and also for its accuracy.
         (a) A measurement that is precise remains relatively stable if it is repeated with the same research subject under similar conditions.
         (b) A measurement that is precise may not always be accurate.
         (c) The accuracy of a measurement reflects the level of error that is present.
         (d) There are many potential sources of errors.
            - Systematic errors such as those resulting from poor equipment calibration.
            - Unsystematic errors that occur unpredictably, such as from intermittent equipment malfunction.
            - Day-to-day changes in the characteristics of the person being measured.
            - The behavior of the researcher.
      (3) Standard error of measurement—indicates the expected variability of a subject's score if the measurement were repeated several times. A small standard error suggests higher reliability.
      (4) Two ways of estimating measurement error associated with the researcher/observer:
         (a) Interobserver agreement is how consistent two or more researchers are in making a particular measurement.
         (b) Intraobserver agreement is how consistent one researcher is when making the same measurement more than once.
         (c) Agreement coefficients can be calculated to determine the level of interobserver or intraobserver agreement.
         (d) These coefficients do not tell whether the measure itself is accurate or precise.
   d. Validity of measurement—how well it measures what it purports to measure.

(1) Content validity refers to how well the test items measure the characteristics or behaviors of interest.
(2) Criterion validity refers to how well the measure correlates with an outside criterion that is known to be a good indicator of the characteristic or behavior of interest.
(3) Construct validity refers to how well the measure reflects a theoretical construct of the characteristic or behavior of interest.

4. Procedure.
   a. How did the researchers address possible threats to internal validity?
      (1) Subject selection procedures may be biased.
      (2) History—extraneous event(s) occurring between the initial measurement and subsequent measurement(s) may contaminate the results.
      (3) Reactive pretest—scores on a posttest may be influenced by administration of a pretest.
      (4) Statistical regression—if subjects are selected based on extreme scores, their scores on subsequent administrations of the same measure may be closer to the average score even with no treatment.
      (5) Researcher bias—the researcher's preconceived notions may influence the way data are interpreted.
      (6) The test environment (e.g., noise level) may affect results.
      (7) Subject performance may be influenced by the subject's awareness that they are in a research study and how they perceive the consequences of their behavior in the study. This is known as the Hawthorne effect.
   b. How did the researchers address possible threats to external validity?
      (1) The subjects selected may not represent the population to which the researcher is generalizing.
      (2) The experimental arrangement (e.g., setting) may influence the study results, thus limiting generalizability of study results to other people who have not experienced the same arrangement.
      (3) If multiple sequences or numbers of treatments are studied, the study results may only generalize to other people who have received the same sequences and numbers of treatments.

5. Research design.
   a. Research studies can be quantitative, qualitative or a combination of the two.
   b. In quantitative research, data are obtained using numerical measures.
      (1) It is expected that there is no subjective bias of the researcher during data collection or interpretation.
   c. Quantitative research can be experimental, descriptive or mixed experimental–descriptive.
      (1) In experimental research, the researcher manipulates one or more independent variables and observes the effect on the dependent variable(s). The researcher also attempts to control the effects of extraneous variables on the dependent variable.
         (a) In experimental research, there can be two levels of the independent variable (e.g., high vs. low noise) or more than two levels (e.g., high, medium, low noise).
         (b) An experiment can be designed to study the simultaneous effects of more than one independent variable (e.g., diet and exercise) on the dependent variable (e.g., weight loss). This is called a *parametric experiment*.
      (2) In descriptive research, it is not possible for the researcher to manipulate the independent variable because it is a subject characteristic (e.g., type of speech disorder, age or history).
      (3) In descriptive research, the researcher observes the relations between a subject characteristic (i.e., an attribute) and the dependent variable.
         (a) Example: The researcher may observe group differences between children with or without dyslexia on measures of phonological awareness.
      (4) Mixed experimental–descriptive research is often used in speech-language pathology.
         (a) For example, in a study measuring the dependent variable of oral reading accuracy, the descriptive component may be the comparison of two groups based on subject attributes (e.g., dyslexic versus nondyslexic) and the experimental component may be the manipulation of an independent variable (e.g., rapid vs. slow presentation of written words).
   d. Quantitative research can involve groups or a single subject.
      (1) Group research design can involve between-subject group or within-subject group comparisons, or both.
         (a) Between-subjects design involves comparisons of two or more groups of subjects.
         (b) It is critical that extraneous variables be controlled when subjects are assigned to a group, to reduce the possible effects of these factors on the dependent variable. Two ways to match subjects across group are:
            • Overall matching of averages across the groups (e.g., average age).
            • Pairwise matching of each subject to another subject on the extraneous

variables (e.g., age, education, gender). This method is particularly effective when followed by random assignment of one member of the pair to each group.

(c) Between-group designs can be used with either experimental or descriptive research. However, subject attributes (e.g., dyslexic or nondyslexic) in descriptive research do not allow random assignment of subjects to a group. This makes it more difficult to infer cause–effect relationships in descriptive studies than in experimental studies.

(d) In within-subjects design, the behavior of the same subjects is studied under different conditions. Within-subjects designs can be used with either experimental or descriptive research.
- In experimental research, the same subjects receive all levels of the independent variable. For example, speech perception in the same subjects may be compared in the context of high, moderate and low levels of noise.
- All conditions of the independent variable should be equivalent except for the one that is being manipulated, to control for extraneous factors affecting the dependent variable.
- In within-subjects experimental research, possible sequence effects must be controlled.
  - An order effect (i.e., potential change from beginning to end of an experiment due to factors such as fatigue or familiarity).
  - A carryover effect (e.g., the first treatment condition could affect subject performance in the second treatment condition).
- Ways to attempt to control sequence effects.
  - Randomizing the order of treatment conditions.
  - Counterbalancing, in which all possible orders of the treatments are identified first; then subjects are randomly assigned to receive one of these sequences.
- If within-subjects design is used in descriptive research, the same subjects are observed under different conditions, such as in longitudinal developmental studies.

(e) A study can involve both between-group and within-group design elements.

(2) Single-subject research is focused on the individual, and may involve only one subject or may involve a few subjects whose performance is reported individually.
  (a) Withdrawal designs.
   - An individual's performance is compared when the treatment is present versus absent (i.e., withdrawn).
   - Examples are a simple A-B-A design (representing baseline, treatment and withdrawal segments) and more complex A-B-A-B-A design or A-B-A-C-A design (in which B and C represent different treatments that are subsequently withdrawn).
  (b) Multiple-baseline designs.
   - Withdrawal or reversal of treatment is not necessary with this design. Stable baseline performance is established, followed by a treatment or sequence of treatments.
   - If applied across behaviors, a stable baseline is established for each behavior prior to treatment and the ongoing effect of intervention on several behaviors can be studied concurrently.

e. Qualitative research involves exploration of factors that may underlie behavior (e.g., an individual's values, thoughts, perceptions and attitudes).
  (1) Hypotheses emerge from observation and interpretation; new hypotheses are generated as the study is underway.
  (2) The researcher's experiences and biases are expected to influence how the data are interpreted.
  (3) Data collection occurs in real-world contexts, and behavior is described and interpreted.
  (4) Multiple and varied methods may be used for data collection in one qualitative research study.
   (a) Examples include observations, semistructured or unstructured interviews, narratives and case study techniques.
   (b) Focused on a group or groups, or on a single subject.

f. Both quantitative and qualitative research methods can be used in the same study (i.e., mixed methods research).

6. Data analysis.
 a. The "Methods" section of the research study should include a description of the methods to be used for data organization and analysis.
 b. In qualitative research, descriptive ways to focus the data are used to identify emerging themes. In quantitative research, numerical analyses allow for objective descriptions that can be analyzed statistically.

c. Depending upon the research question(s), it may be appropriate to describe the data using only descriptive statistics. Other studies include statistical analyses to further define the data.
d. The appropriate statistical tests depend upon whether nominal, ordinal, interval or ratio measurement is used. Other important factors are the sample type, number of observations and shape of the data distribution.

The "Results" Section

1. The results should be reported in relation to the research problem and the hypotheses.
2. For quantitative research, data distributions are reported.
3. For nominal or interval measurement data, it is usually sufficient to report numbers per category or rankings.
4. Interval or ratio measurement data may be described in terms of the following.
   a. Central tendency—the average score for a group.
   b. Three measures of central tendency:
      (1) Mean—the arithmetic average.
      (2) Median—the middle score of the distribution.
      (3) Mode—the most commonly occurring score.
   c. Variability—how much the scores vary from the average.
   d. Measures of variability:
      (1) Range—the lowest score to the highest score.
      (2) Variance—how far each score in the distribution varies from the mean score.
      (3) Standard deviation (SD)—the average amount that all the scores in the distribution deviate from the mean. A small SD indicates more homogeneity.
   e. Skewness—the lack of symmetry of the distribution of scores, which can be skewed positively or negatively.
   f. Kurtosis—the general shape of the distribution of scores (i.e., the peak in relation to the tails of the distribution).
5. A normal distribution of the data (i.e., the normal curve model) results when the middle scores occur most often and the lower and higher scores do not occur often. When graphed, the data distribution forms a bell shape.
6. If there is a normal distribution of the data, then parametric statistics can be used. However, nonparametric statistical procedures (i.e., not based on a normal curve model) would be used if the data are not normally distributed.
   a. Parametric statistics are more powerful than nonparametric. Several assumptions should be met.
      (1) Normal distribution of the data.
      (2) Interval or ratio level of measurement.
      (3) If two or more data distributions will be analyzed and compared, their variances should be similar.
      (4) Large sample size; usually 30 or more per group.
   b. Nonparametric statistics are used when one or more of the above assumptions is not met.
7. Statistical significance testing involves testing the null hypothesis in the context of the data. The null hypothesis is either rejected or accepted based on the statistical test.
   a. The researcher can make two types of errors.
      (1) Type I (a true null hypothesis is rejected).
      (2) Type II (a false null hypothesis is accepted).
   b. The level of significance is the probability of making a Type 1 error.
   c. When the level of significance is small, then the researcher usually decides to reject the null hypothesis and therefore, to decide that the hypothesis is probably true.
      (1) Example: For the hypothesis "X and Y are different" where the null hypothesis is "X and Y are not different," the researcher who rejects the null hypothesis would be deciding that the hypothesis is true and that X and Y are different.
   d. A level of significance of .05 or less ($p < .05$) indicates that the difference between X and Y could have resulted from chance only 5 times in 100.
      (1) This number is usually considered small enough to reject the null hypothesis.
   e. The nature of the hypothesis often determines what type of statistical test is done.
      (1) If the hypothesis is directional (e.g., "X is greater than Y"), then the statistical test is one-tailed; whereas if the hypothesis is nondirectional (e.g., "X and Y are different"), then a two-tailed test is done.
      (2) Two-tailed tests are stricter than one-tailed tests, so some researchers do not use one-tailed tests.
   f. The degrees of freedom (df) in the data should be reported so that the results can be interpreted. Generally, $df = n - 1$, when n represents the total number of scores in the data distribution.
8. Data analysis techniques can be correlational or inferential.
   a. Correlational statistics evaluate relationships among data.
      (1) Relationships are often described using correlation coefficients.
      (2) Examples:
         (a) Pearson product-moment correlation (r) coefficient (parametric)—used with interval or ratio level data.

(b) Spearman rank-order correlation (ρ) coefficient (nonparametric)—used with ordinal level data.
(3) A perfect positive relationship between two variables is indicated by 1.0, a perfect negative relationship is indicated by –1.0 and the absence of a relationship is indicated by zero.
(4) A small number indicates a weak relationship between two variables, either in a positive or negative direction (e.g., +0.12 or –0.12).
(5) A large number indicates a strong relationship between two variables, either in a positive or negative direction (e.g., +0.89 or –0.89).
(6) The square of the correlation coefficient (r^2) is used to assess its practical meaning.
   (a) For example, a squared correlation coefficient of $+0.40^2$ equals .16, meaning that 84% of the variance is remaining. This much variance indicates that the variables are not strongly correlated.
   (b) Variables that are correlated can be described as varying together, but there may be no cause–effect relationship.
b. Presenting the results of correlational statistics.
   (1) Regression analyses may be reported along with correlational analyses. Regression analyses measure the degree to which the value of one variable can be predicted from the value of other variables.
   (2) Correlational and regression analyses can be used in bivariate analyses (i.e., analyzing the relationship between two variables) or in multivariate analyses (i.e., analyzing the relationships among more than two variables).
   (3) For nominal level data, associations between variables can be presented in a contingency table (i.e., a two-dimensional table in which the frequencies of attribute variables are cross-referenced with other variables).
      (a) The level of significance of any relationship among the nominal variables can be examined using chi-square (X^2) or the contingency coefficient (C).
      (b) Chi-square does not indicate the strength of the relationship, whereas the contingency coefficient does measure the strength of the relationship.
c. Inferential statistics evaluate differences among data, either between-subjects or within-subjects.
   (1) When there is a single dependent variable, differences between two sets of data can be analyzed using:
      (a) Parametric procedures.
         • z ratio—when samples are 30 or more.
         • t-test—when samples are less than 30.
            – Independent t-test—used to compare two different groups.
            – Dependent t-test—used for within-group comparisons.
      (b) Nonparametric procedures.
         • Mann-Whitney U Test—for differences between groups; for ordinal level data.
         • Wilcoxon matched-pairs signed-ranks tests—for examining changes within a group over time.
   (2) When there is a single dependent variable, but more than two sets of data being compared between-groups or within-groups, differences are analyzed using parametric or nonparametric methods.
      (a) Parametric procedures include:
         • ANOVA (analysis of variance)—allows simultaneous comparisons of several means; yields an F ratio.
         • A one-way ANOVA is used when there is only one independent or classification (attribute) variable.
         • A two-way ANOVA is used when there are two independent or classification variables. The researcher examines:
            – The effect of each independent variable.
            – The interaction between each combination of independent variables.
      (b) Nonparametric procedures include:
         • Kruskal-Wallis one-way ANOVA by ranks (for ordinal level data in a between-subjects comparison).
         • Cochran Q Test (for nominal level data from related samples).
         • Friedman two-way ANOVA by ranks (for ordinal level data in a within-subjects comparison).
         • Chi-square test for independent samples (for nominal level data).
   (3) When there is more than one dependent variable, and one or more independent variables, analysis procedures used are:
      (a) MANOVA—multivariate analysis of variance.
      (b) ANCOVA—analysis of covariance.
      (c) Sometimes multiple t-tests can be used; however, an adjustment such as the Bonferroni correction may be needed.
d. Effect size estimates can help the SLP to understand the practical significance of data in a research study.
   (1) This estimate is independent from statistical significance. Rather than reflecting whether the null hypothesis is false, effect size estimates the degree to which it is false. A finding can be statistically significant and yet not important in practical terms, especially for a very large sample size.

(2) Various effect size estimators are used depending on the research design or statistical analysis method.
(3) One common effect size estimate is *Cohen's d*, used to compare the means of two or more groups.

e. A power analysis is often completed to measure the probability of rejecting a null hypothesis when the null hypothesis is false.
(1) Generally, a minimum value of .80 is an acceptable measure of power.

Treatment Efficacy Studies and Evidence-Based Practice

Efficacy, Effectiveness and Fidelity

1. "Treatment efficacy" research is aimed at demonstrating the benefits of treatment through well-controlled studies with internal validity, statistical significance and practical significance.
2. "Treatment effectiveness" is demonstrated when there is clinical improvement from the treatment when applied in real-world context.
3. "Treatment fidelity" is the degree to which actual implementation of the treatment in the real world is consistent with the prototype treatment administered in the controlled conditions of the treatment efficacy study.

National Outcomes Measurement System

1. ASHA developed the National Outcomes Measurement System (NOMS) as one way to collect data on clinical outcomes in speech-language pathology and audiology.

Treatment Efficacy

1. A variety of experimental designs are used for studying treatment efficacy.
   a. Studies including a control group are stronger designs generally than studies involving only one group, particularly when the control group is well matched to the experimental group.
   b. Time-series designs include repeated baseline measures prior to treatment.
      (1) They typically include systematic ongoing measurement of participant performance on the dependent variable during the course of treatment.
      (2) Time-series studies can be strengthened by including control subjects, a second baseline segment after treatment or multiple alternating treatment and baseline segments.
   c. Randomization of treatment across matched control groups is a stronger design than nonrandomized application of treatment.
   d. The strongest evidence of treatment efficacy comes from:
      (1) Meta-analyses, particularly when well designed and based on multiple randomized controlled clinical studies.
         (a) In a meta-analysis, accumulated evidence from multiple studies is analyzed statistically to evaluate the consistency of results and effect sizes across studies.
      (2) Systematic reviews, which are objective and comprehensive overviews of research focused on a particular clinical issue. To promote objectivity, strict criteria are used in selecting and reviewing relevant studies.
      (3) The use of meta-analyses and systematic reviews in SLP is limited by the few randomized controlled studies available.
   e. Clinical practice guidelines (CPGs) relate to identifying best practices for clinical care.
      (1) They are formed by a group of experts and communicated in terms of strength of recommendation.
      (2) In addition to factors noted above in the section "Evidence-Based Practice," the CPG is one factor the clinician considers in arriving at a clinical decision.

Interpreting Tests and Measurements

Test Interpretation

1. The process of EBP assists the SLP in test interpretation.
2. Well-designed and controlled research studies can provide evidence about test sensitivity and specificity.
   a. Sensitivity refers to how well the test detects that a condition (e.g., dysphagia) is present when the condition actually is present (i.e., the proportion of true positives correctly identified by the test).
   b. Specificity refers to how well the test detects that a condition (e.g., dysphagia) is not present when the condition actually is not present (i.e., the proportion of true negatives correctly identified by the test).
3. The relationship among clinical signs elicited by different clinical tests and measurements can be quantified in a variety of ways.
   a. Positive predictive value—the number of true positives divided by the combined true and false positives.
   b. Negative predictive value—the number of true negatives divided by the combined true and false negatives.
   c. Positive and negative predictive values should only be calculated from studies reflecting the actual prevalence of the condition or disease in the population of interest at that time because these values are dependent on prevalence.

Cultural Diversity in Evidence-Based Practice

Ethnic Minority Groups

1. Evidence-based practice considers how research outcomes data may apply differently to ethnic minority groups that were not included in the research studies.
   a. The SLP can obtain information about client preferences and values through a cultural assessment (e.g., interview questions).
   b. Knowledge of the client's culture supports the SLP in shared clinical decision-making with the client and his/her family.

Values, Beliefs and Customs

1. Cultural values, beliefs and customs shape the perspectives of the client, his/her family and the SLP toward health, illness and communication.

References

American Speech-Language-Hearing Association (2003). *National Outcomes Measurement System (NOMS): Adult Speech-Language Pathology User's Guide.* Rockville, MD. Available from www.asha.org.

American Speech-Language-Hearing Association. (2010). *Code of Ethics.* [Ethics]. Available from www.asha.org/policy.

Deviant, S. (2010). *The Practically Cheating Statistics Handbook, The Sequel,* 2nd ed. Jacksonville, FL: Kenrose Media.

Dollaghan, Christine A. (2007). *The Handbook for Evidence-Based Practice in Communication Disorders.* Baltimore, MD: Paul H. Brookes Publishing Co., Inc.

Graziano, A. M., & Raulin, M. L. (2010). *Research Methods: A Process of Inquiry,* 7th ed. Boston, MA: Pearson/Allyn & Bacon.

Horner, J., & Minifie, F. D. (2011a). Research Ethics I: Responsible Conduct of Research (RCR)—Historical and contemporary issues pertaining to human and animal experimentation. *Journal of Speech, Language and Hearing Research,* 54, S303–S329.

Hulme, P. (2010). Cultural considerations in evidence-based practice. *Journal of Transcultural Nursing*, 21(3), 271–280.

Kaderavek, J. N., & Justice. L. M. (2010). Fidelity: An essential component of evidence-based practice in speech-language pathology. *American Journal of Speech-Language Pathology*, 19, 369–379.

Nail-Chiwetalu, B. J., & Bernstein Ratner, N. (2006). Information literacy for speech-language pathologists: A key to evidence-based practice. *Language, Speech, and Hearing Services in Schools*, 37, 157–167.

Richardson, W., Wilson, M., Nishikawa, J., & Hayward, R. (1995). The well-built clinical question: A key to evidence-based decisions. *American College of Physicians Journal Club*, 123, A12–13.

Robey, R. R. (2004b). Levels of evidence. *The ASHA Leader*, 9(7), 5.

Sackett, D. L., Straus, S. E., Richardson, W. S., Rosenberg, W., & Haynes, R. B. (2000). *Evidence-Based Medicine: How to Practice and Teach EBM*. Edinburgh: Churchill Livingstone.

Schiavetti, N., Metz, D. E., & Orlikoff, R. F. (2011). *Evaluating Research in Communicative Disorders*, 6th ed. Boston: Pearson Education, Inc.

Stevens, S. S. (1946). On the theory of scales of measurement. *Science*, 103, 677–680.

Tompkins, C. A., Scott, A. G., & Scharp, V. (2008). "Research Principles for the Clinician." In R. Chapey (Ed.), *Language Intervention Strategies in Aphasia and Related Neurogenic Communication Disorders*, 5th ed. Philadelphia: Lippincott, Williams & Wilkins, pp. 163–185.

5

The Practice of Speech-Language Pathology

SUE T. HALE, M.C.D.

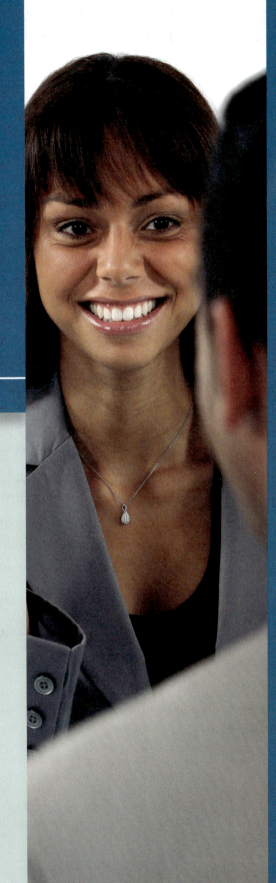

Chapter Outline

- History of Speech-Language Pathology, 104
- Scope of Practice, 104
- Credentialing, 105
- Professional Organizations, 107
- Ethical Issues, 108
- Workforce Issues and Employment, 110
- Health Care Environment, 110
- Educational Service Delivery, 111
- Early Intervention, 113
- Professional Liability and Responsibility, 113
- Policies and Procedures, 114
- Serving Multicultural Populations, 114
- Supervision, 115
- Telepractice, 115
- Evidence-Based Practice (EBP), 116
- References, 116
- Appendix A, 117
- Appendix B, 129
- Appendix C, 132

History of Speech-Language Pathology

First Organizational Meeting

1. 1925 meeting of the National Association of Teachers of Speech (NATS).
   a. Organized by Carl Seashore and Lee Edward Travis of the University of Iowa.
   b. 25 charter members.
2. Ultimately evolved into today's American Speech-Language-Hearing Association (ASHA).

Disorders Addressed in the Early History

1. 1920s and 1930s: stuttering (Lee Edward Travis, Wendell Johnson and others).
   a. Members of the early group were interested in fluency disorders.
   b. Wanted to protect the public from spurious treatments.
2. Late 1930s and 1940s: adult neurological disorders and motor speech (Karl Goldstein, Norman Geschwind).
3. 1943: childhood aphasia (Mildred Berry, Jon Eisenson).
4. Early and mid-1940s: aphasia and hearing loss from war injuries (Jon Eisenson and Joseph Wepman).

Professional Development

1. Original group became the American Speech Correction Association (ASCA) in 1934.
2. A Code of Ethics was written for the ASCA in 1935.
3. The *Journal of Speech Disorders* was first published in 1936.
4. The ASCA became the American Speech and Hearing Association (ASHA) in 1947.
5. The first standards for clinical certification were established in 1952.
6. Throughout the rest of the century, the scope of practice, name and activities of the organization and research publications continued to expand exponentially.

Scope of Practice

Focus

1. Areas of professional practice for typical and atypical communication and swallowing.
   a. Speech-sound production, including articulation, apraxia of speech, dysarthria, ataxia and dyskinesia.
   b. Resonance, including hypernasality, hyponasality, cul de sac and mixed resonance.
   c. Voice related to phonation quality, pitch, loudness and respiration.
   d. Fluency, including stuttering and cluttering.
   e. Language comprehension and expression, including phonology, morphology, syntax, semantics, pragmatics, literacy, prelinguistic communication and paralinguistic communication.
   f. Cognition related to attention, memory, sequencing, problem solving and executive functioning.
   g. Feeding and swallowing, including all phases of swallowing, orofacial myology and oral-motor functions.
2. Clinical services.
   a. Prevention and pre-referral.
   b. Screening.
   c. Assessment/evaluation.
   d. Consultation.
   e. Diagnosis.
   f. Treatment, intervention, management.
   g. Counseling.
   h. Collaboration.
   i. Documentation.
   j. Referral.
3. Inform others (health care providers, teachers, other professionals, consumers, payers, regulators and the public) about speech-language pathology services.
   a. Promoting healthy lifestyle practices to prevent communication and swallowing disorders.
   b. Presenting primary prevention information to at-risk individuals or groups.
   c. Providing early identification/intervention services.
   d. Advocating for individuals and families.

e. Advising regulatory and legislative agencies.
   f. Promoting and marketing professional services.
   g. Advocating for better administrative and governmental policies.
   h. Advocating for research funding.
   i. Participating in professional organizations.
4. Support for the provision of evidence-based services and conduct of clinical research.
   a. Improving the quality of life by optimizing individuals' ability to communicate and swallow and in accordance with the World Health Organization International Classification of Functioning, Disability and Health Resources (ICF, 2001).
      (1) Impairments of body functions and structures.
      (2) Activity limitations.
      (3) Participation restrictions.
      (4) Barriers created by contextual factors.
   b. Competently delivering services or conducting research with a culturally and linguistically diverse population.
   c. Basing clinical decisions on best available evidence.
   d. Exchanging professional knowledge and information nationally and internationally.
5. Guidance for the training of speech-language pathologists.
   a. Hold the ASHA Certificate of Clinical Competence in Speech-Language Pathology (CCC-SLP).
      (1) Master the designated skills and knowledge and achieve a master's, doctoral or other recognized post-baccalaureate degree from a program accredited by the Council on Academic Accreditation (CAA) of ASHA.
      (2) Complete a supervised, postgraduate, professional experience equivalent to 36 weeks of full-time employment.
      (3) Pass a national examination (PRAXIS administered by ETS).
      (4) Demonstrate continuing professional development to maintain the certificate of 3 CEUs (30 clock hours) for every 3-year period.
6. The recognition that an individual speech-language pathologist does not practice in all areas of the field.
   a. Must have adequate training for the disorders treated.
   b. Must provide all services within the scope of individual competence.
7. Must have previous supervised experience.
8. Supported by other related documents including the Code of Ethics and other practice guidelines.
9. The *Scope of Practice* does not exclude emerging areas of practice within the dynamic and evolving profession of speech-language pathology.
   a. See the complete document, Appendix A of the ASHA *Scope of Practice in Speech-Language Pathology* from which the above information is excerpted at the end of this chapter on page 117.

Credentialing

Certificate of Clinical Competence (CCC)

1. National credential administered by the Council for Clinical Certification (CFCC) of ASHA.
2. Considered "gold-standard" credential for speech-language pathologists and required of employees in virtually all clinical/medical settings and many educational settings.
3. Reciprocal credential for state licensure since most state licensure laws parallel CCC requirements.
4. Universally required for supervising students-in-training who are seeking the CCC credential.
5. Students from a graduate program accredited by the Council on Academic Accreditation (CAA) applying less than 3 years postgraduation complete only the demographic and attestation portions of the CCC application.
6. New standards are in effect as of 2014.
7. Requirements:
   a. Master's, doctoral or other graduate degree.
   b. 75 semester credit hours (sch) of study focused on the knowledge and skills pertinent to the field of speech-language pathology, at least 36 sch at the graduate level.
   c. Graduate coursework and clinical practicum completed in a CAA-accredited program.
   d. Prerequisite knowledge (one course each) in biological science, statistics, social science and either physics or chemistry.
   e. Knowledge of the bases of human communication and swallowing processes, including:
      (1) Biological.
      (2) Neurological.
      (3) Acoustic.
      (4) Psycholinguistic.
      (5) Linguistic.
      (6) Cultural.

f. Knowledge of the nature of communication disorders, differences and swallowing disorders in the ("Big 9") areas of:
   (1) Articulation.
   (2) Fluency.
   (3) Voice and resonance, including respiration and phonation.
   (4) Receptive and expressive language (phonology, morphology, syntax, semantics and pragmatics) in speaking, listening, reading, writing and manual modalities.
   (5) Hearing, including the impact on speech and language.
   (6) Swallowing (oral, pharyngeal, esophageal and related functions, including oral function for feeding; orofacial myofunction).
   (7) Cognitive aspects of communication (attention, memory, sequencing, problem-solving and executive functioning).
   (8) Social aspects of communication (including challenging behavior, ineffective social skills and lack of communication opportunities).
   (9) Communication modalities (including oral, manual, augmentative and alternative communication techniques and assistive technologies). See Appendix B, Speech-Language Pathology Clinical Fellowship (SLPCF) Report and Rating Form at the end of this chapter on page 129.
g. Knowledge of prevention, assessment, and intervention for the disorders listed in (f) above.
h. Knowledge of ethical standards.
i. Knowledge of research principles and integrating those principles into evidence-based practice.
j. Knowledge of contemporary professional issues.
k. Knowledge about national, state and specialty credentialing.
l. Skills in assessment, intervention and interaction across disorders and the lifespan and with clients from all backgrounds.
m. Skills in oral and written communication sufficient for professional practice.
n. Clinical experience during the educational program of at least 400 clock hours (25 in observation and 375 direct contact); 325 clock hours must be obtained at the graduate level and experience must be obtained with clients:
   (1) Across the lifespan.
   (2) With a variety of disorders.
   (3) From diverse backgrounds.
   (4) While being supervised by an individual who holds the CCC.
o. Ongoing assessment of student skills and knowledge must be conducted throughout the graduate program.
p. Must pass a national examination.
   (1) PRAXIS II in speech-language pathology, administered by the Educational Testing Service (ETS).
q. After graduation, complete the equivalent of 36 weeks of full-time employment with periodic assessment and recommendation for certification by a mentor holding the CCC-SLP.
   (1) View the entire certification standards from which this is excerpted at http://www.asha.org/certification/slp_standards/. See Appendix B for the SLPCF Report and Rating form.

State Licensure

1. Legal requirement to practice as an SLP in all 50 states and the District of Columbia.
2. Defines the minimum qualifications for practicing in the state (often the same as ASHA CCC requirements, but not always).
3. State grants an individual the right to practice in a defined scope of practice (may be narrower than the ASHA Scope of Practice).
4. Licensure laws are typically designed to protect the public health and welfare, not to protect/preserve/uplift the profession.
5. Most laws prohibit unlicensed persons from using the title of speech-language pathologist and doing so is a violation of the law.
6. May exempt certain individuals from the licensure requirement, including:
   a. Individuals practicing in the schools with a teaching license.
   b. Federal employees.
7. Most boards require evidence of continuing education to maintain the license.
8. Clinical fellowship may be administered through registration or temporary license prior to full licensure depending on state statute.
9. Typically allow some level of reciprocity from state to state.
10. Holding the CCC makes the holder eligible for state licensure.
11. Typically administered by a board of examiners through a state board of health.
    a. Members of the board are often appointed by the governor or other elected official.
    b. May be recommended by the state speech-language-hearing association to the person making appointments, but official may not be bound to act on the recommendations.

Teacher Licensure

1. All states regulate practice in educational settings through teacher licensure requirements.

2. Administered by state departments of education.
3. Practicing in schools may require state license from board of health in addition to teacher license or only teacher license; varies from state to state.
4. Requires bachelor's or master's degree depending on state regulations.
5. Usually valid for serving children Kindergarten through 12th grade.

Specialty Recognition

1. Voluntary program recognizing advanced knowledge in a given specialty area.
2. Awarded in addition to basic credential, such as the CCC.
3. ASHA has four specialty recognition credentials:
   a. Child Language.
   b. Fluency Disorders.
   c. Swallowing and Swallowing Disorders.
   d. Intraoperative monitoring.
4. Academy of Neurologic Communication Disorders and Sciences (ANCDS) grants board certification for expertise in neurologic communication disorders (BC-NCD) of children, adults or children and adults (dual).

Professional Organizations

American Speech-Language-Hearing Association (ASHA)

1. Largest and oldest scientific and professional association representing both speech-language pathology and audiology.
2. Home office is in Rockville, MD.
3. Vision—"Making effective communication a human right, accessible and achievable for all."
4. Mission—"Empowering and supporting speech-language pathologists, audiologists and speech, language and hearing scientists."
   a. Advocating on behalf of persons with communication and related disorders.
   b. Advancing communication science.
   c. Promoting effective human communication.
      (1) Vision and Mission quoted directly from ASHA Strategic Pathway to Excellence, 2011.
5. Membership.
   a. As of the end of 2013, 160,905 certified members, noncertified members, international affiliates and nonmember certificate holders who are speech-language pathologists, audiologists and speech, language and hearing scientists. Almost 13,000 others are student members or affiliated support personnel.
   b. Approximately 95% of members/certificate holders are female.
   c. Slightly more than 7% of members/certificate holders are members of ethnic or racial minorities.
6. Standards.
   a. The Council for Clinical Certification (CFCC) reviews and establishes standards for practice and competence for individual members.
   b. The Council on Academic Accreditation (CAA) determines standards for academic training programs.
7. Examples of member services supported by work clusters within the ASHA national office.
   a. Membership.
   b. Public relations, communication and marketing.
   c. Professional education and materials.
   d. Governmental relations and public policy.
   e. State-national relations.
   f. Science, research and evidence-based practice.
   g. Scholarly and professional publications.
   h. Academic affairs and accreditation.
   i. Practices.
   j. Certification and specialty recognition.
   k. Ethics.
   l. Special interest groups (SIGs).
   m. International relationships/affiliations.
   n. Multicultural affairs.
   o. General and financial operations.
8. Special interest groups (SIGs).
   a. Established within ASHA to promote knowledge and skills in targeted areas.
   b. Currently 18 SIGs.
   c. Divisions are comprised of members with similar interests/expertise with access to educational programs, research, publications and dialogue.
   d. Examples of SIGs include fluency disorders, voice disorders, administration and supervision, school-based issues, augmentative and alternative communication, etc.
9. Authority for conducting the business of the association is vested in an elected Board of Directors.

State Organizations

1. Often affiliated with a larger national organization with similar purposes and structure.
2. Many state associations for speech-language pathologists and audiologists are recognized affiliates of ASHA.
3. ASHA provides information, advocacy and sometimes monetary support to affiliated state organizations for legislation, licensure and other state-focused issues.
4. State organizations are influential in practice issues, regulations, funding decisions and other aspects of practice for a specific locale.

National Student Speech-Language-Hearing Association (NSSLHA)

1. Student organization for speech-language pathology students and audiology students.
2. As of 2011, NSSLHA was integrated into ASHA. NSSLHA remains a student-led organization within the larger association, and its national advisor holds a position on the ASHA Board of Directors.
3. Membership is targeted to students with an interest in normal and disordered human communication who are enrolled in a training program (graduate or undergraduate) in communication sciences.
4. Local chapters allow for leadership development, volunteerism, philanthropic work and professional networking.
5. Members of NSSLHA receive reduced fees for membership and convention attendance at state and national professional meetings.

International Organizations

1. International Association of Logopedics and Phoniatrics (IALP) provides membership and education opportunities for speech-language pathologists worldwide.
2. Many countries have national organizations for the profession of speech-language pathology with similar missions/visions to ASHA.

Related Professional Organizations

1. Organizations for individuals who have specialized research, clinical or educational interests not addressed within the scope of ASHA or state organizations.
2. May be of interest to the student or professional in areas not included in the array of Special Interest Groups.

Ethical Issues

Considerations

1. Professionals have special expertise and render services to individuals in the area(s) of expertise.
2. Highly specialized skills create an obligation to serve individuals in a highly competent manner.
3. Professionals abide by legally specified standards and also a code of ethics.
4. Codes of ethics are developed by the profession itself, and the standards of conduct exceed legal standards.
5. As a member of a profession, one agrees to uphold the principles of the code of ethics.
6. Ethical behavior is constant across employment settings and different clients.

Five Philosophical Concepts Underlying Ethical Standards

1. Utilitarian approach: What action will do the most good and the least harm?
2. The rights approach: What action best respects the rights of all stakeholders?
3. Fairness/justice approach: Which option treats people equally or proportionally?
4. Common good approach: What action best serves the whole community and not just some members?
5. Virtue approach: Which option causes me to act as the sort of person I want to be?

Three Components of Codes of Ethics (from General to Specific)

1. Preamble or Introduction—the vision statement and audience to whom it applies.
2. Principles—the goals to be maintained.
3. Rules—more specific "dos and don'ts" of each principle.

ASHA Code of Ethics

1. Preamble.
   a. To discharge obligations responsibly, the highest standards of integrity and ethical principles must be set forth.
   b. All individuals who are ASHA members, certificate holders, applicants for membership or Clinical Fellows must abide by the code.
2. The code is both aspirational and inspirational in nature.
3. Principles of ethics and rules govern responsibility to:
   a. Persons served.
      (1) Hold paramount the welfare of the persons served.
      (2) Hold true for clients and research subjects and extends to humane research with animals.
   b. To achieving and maintaining high levels of professional competence and performance.
      (1) Hold the CCC for the area in which services are provided.
      (2) Engage in activities within the scope of practice.
      (3) Maintain competence through lifelong learning.
      (4) Supervise staff and maintain clinical equipment responsibly.
   c. The public.
      (1) Promoting public understanding of the professions.
      (2) Supporting the development of services to fulfill unmet needs.
      (3) Providing accurate information in communicating about the professions.
   d. The professions and relationships with colleagues, students and other professionals.
      (1) Maintain the dignity and autonomy of the profession.
      (2) Practice with honesty and integrity.
      (3) Adhere to guidelines in scholarly work.
      (4) Adhere to principles of nondiscrimination in professional relationships.
      (5) Comply fully with policies of the Board of Ethics and report suspected violations of others.

Note: The Code of Ethics of the American Speech-Language-Hearing Association (2010) is contained in Appendix C at the end of this chapter on page 132.

Issues in Ethics Statements

1. Provide additional guidance concerning specific issues of ethical conduct.
2. Intended to increase sensitivity and awareness.
3. Assist in self-guided ethical decision-making.
4. Statements currently cover confidentiality, conflicts of interest, cultural competence, reimbursement, supervision of students, support personnel, client abandonment and other areas.

Violations of the Code of Ethics

1. All members are responsible for adhering to the Code of Ethics and reporting when others violate the Code.
2. Reasons for sanctioning.
   a. Penalize the person in violation.
   b. Educate and rehabilitate.
   c. Inform other members that the Code is enforced and that penalties are enforced.
3. Types of sanctions that can be imposed by the Board of Ethics (BOE).
   a. Reprimand—privately to the person who made a minor or inadvertent violation and to the complainant.
   b. Censure—public reprimand, published to the membership.
   c. Revocation—for serious violations; membership and certification can be revoked for a year, multiple years or life; published to the membership; must seek reinstatement at the end of the revocation period from Board of Ethics.
   d. Suspension—for serious violations but membership and certification are revoked for a shorter period, typically 6 months; reinstatement at the end of the suspension can be addressed directly to ASHA and does not need BOE approval; published to the members.
   e. Withholding—for Clinical Fellows in violation; may withhold ability to apply for the CCCs for a period of years up to life; published to the members.
   f. Cease and Desist—BOE may specify a particular action that must stop immediately and failure to do so is also a violation of the Code.

Workforce Issues/Employment

Settings

1. Clinical/medical settings—approximately 40% of employed SLPs.
   a. Acute care hospitals.
   b. Rehabilitation hospitals.
   c. Community clinics.
   d. Private practice.
   e. University-based clinics.
   f. Long-term care facilities.
2. Educational settings—approximately 53% of employed SLPs.
   a. Public schools.
   b. Private schools.
   c. Colleges and universities.

Service Delivery Models

1. Multidisciplinary—client is seen by multiple professionals with some communication between disciplines in regard to referral and follow-up; little cooperative service delivery; independent assessment and treatment by all disciplines.
2. Interdisciplinary—client is seen by multiple professionals who communicate regarding treatment and share information about overall status; independent assessment by all disciplines.
3. Transdisciplinary—professionals cooperate in service delivery and communicate frequently; assessment and treatment are often delivered by multiple professionals in a more natural environment.

General Laws Governing Nondiscriminatory Employment and Practice

1. Title VII of the Civil Rights Act of 1964—prohibits employment discrimination based on race, color, sex, religion, national origin and prohibits sexual harassment.
2. The Age Discrimination and Employment Act of 1967—prohibits discrimination against persons from 40 to 70 years of age in any area of employment.
3. The 1973 Rehabilitation Act—prohibits discrimination based on disability in any facility receiving federal support, including Medicare and Medicaid.
4. The Americans with Disability Act (ADA), 1990—prevents discrimination against individuals with disabilities and ensures their integration into mainstream American life; requires reasonable accommodations in the work place.

Health Care Environment

Regulations

1. Health care is highly regulated, mostly by laws at the state and federal levels.
2. Legal regulations are set by the Centers for Medicare and Medicaid Services (CMS) of the U.S. Department of Health and Human Services.
3. SLPs must conform to the laws and regulations for billing and reimbursement in order to be paid for services.

Health Care Legislation

1. Social Security Act Amendments, 1965–1996.
   a. Title XVIII of the Social Security Act, Medicare.
      (1) Provides health insurance for individuals age 65 and older.
      (2) Provides health insurance for disabled individuals, notably those with kidney failure, under the age of 65.
      (3) Part A covers patients in hospitals, skilled nursing facilities and hospice care.
      (4) Part B covers physician visits and outpatient services.
      (5) Each patient pays a monthly premium.
      (6) Does not cover all medical expenses.
      (7) Physician must prescribe SLP services covered under Medicare.
   b. Title XIX of the Social Security Act, Medicaid.
      (1) A joint state and federal program.
      (2) Provides health care services to the poor, elderly and disabled regardless of age who do not receive Medicare.
      (3) Benefits vary from state to state.

(4) Preauthorization is needed by a physician before SLP can treat.
c. Social Security Act Amendments of 1982, 1983—eliminated reimbursement to hospitals for direct costs and provided strong incentives for efficient services.
   (1) Impact on SLPs was reduction in inpatient services.
   (2) Shift from language-based inpatient services to dysphagia.
d. Technology-Related Assistance for Individuals with Disabilities Act of 1988 (and reauthorization of 1998).
   (1) Provided assistive technology devices and services, including augmentative and alternative communication (AAC) devices prescribed by SLPs.
   (2) Reauthorization included provisions for low-interest loans for purchasing assistive technology.
e. Health Insurance Portability and Accountability Act (HIPAA) of 1996.
   (1) Protects availability of health insurance coverage for workers when they move from one employer to another.
   (2) Strong emphasis on protection of confidentiality for medical records, especially targeting record storage and transmission.
2. Omnibus Budget Reconciliation Acts—change in payment systems in order to cut costs and reduce waste.
3. Social Security Act Amendments of 1993.
   a. Defined speech-language pathology services and speech-language pathologist for the first time.
      (1) Speech-language services—speech, language and related function assessment and rehabilitation services furnished by a qualified speech-language pathologist.
      (2) Qualified speech-language pathologist—an individual with a master's or doctoral degree in speech-language pathology who is licensed by the state in which services are furnished or who meets equivalent qualifications if providing services in a state that does not license SLPs.
      (3) Health care coding.
         (a) Charges for services in SLP required under HIPAA.
- Reporting of diseases and disorders is required using the *International Classification of Disease,* 9th edition, *Clinical Modification.*
- Procedures must be identified using *Current Procedural Terminology* (CPT) codes.
4. Balanced Budget Act of 1997—imposed an annual cap on SLP (and physical therapy) services to outpatients of $1500; subsequent actions by Congress have placed a continuing moratorium on the therapy caps.
5. Patient Protection and Affordable Care Act of 2010.
   a. Provides more health care coverage to more individuals.
   b. Of importance to SLPs, the act provides coverage for "habilitative" care (issues associated with developmental delays) and not restricted to "rehabilitative" care (issues that are acquired).
   c. The Affordable Care Act's implementation continues to affect and define health care and is subject to changes through legislative, judicial and executive action.

SLP Roles in the Medical Setting

1. Assessment and treatment of disorders of swallowing and communication as a result of a medical condition.
2. Providing counseling regarding surgery that may impact communication or swallowing.
3. Collaborating with medical and other health care staff in treating patients.
4. Use of all modes of service delivery, including those that are technology based.
5. Participation in the evaluation and selection and use of assistive devices or voice prostheses.
6. Participation in the continuum of health care, including prevention.
7. Counseling patients, families and caregivers regarding assessment and treatment.
8. Consulting with other professionals and agencies regarding patient management.

Educational Service Delivery

Regulations

1. Education policy has directed SLP service delivery in the schools.
2. Students must be identified and ruled eligible to receive services, all decisions and services must be documented and dismissal must be warranted based on achievement.

3. Positive effects of federal legislation on SLP services include team approach to management, the use of outcomes measurement, evidence-based practice and inclusion of literacy in service delivery.

Legislation and Legal Decisions Affecting SLP Services in Schools

1. Brown vs. the Board of Education, 1954—eliminates segregated education.
2. Section 504 of the Rehabilitation Act of 1973—all agencies receiving federal support cannot discriminate against persons on the basis of a handicap (precursor to PL 94-142).
3. PL 94-142—The Education for All Handicapped Children Act of 1975.
   a. All children have the right to a free and appropriate public education (FAPE).
   b. Their rights and the rights of their parents are protected by due process.
   c. States and local school districts are to receive federal support for providing the services.
   d. Effectiveness of education programs are to be assessed.
   e. An Individualized Education Program (IEP) is to be the written record of the commitment to meet a student's goals as determined by school personnel and the child's parents.
   f. Defines special education and mandates a process to include handicapped children in regular schools and in the least restricted environment.
   g. Has a pervasive and profound effect on public school speech-language and hearing programs.
   h. Defines the categories of children to be served in special education and related services.
   i. Speech-language therapy is defined as a related service for most children.
4. PL 99-457—Education for the Handicapped Act Amendments of 1986.
   a. Requires states to use qualified personnel to provide special education and related services.
5. PL 101-476—Individuals with Disabilities Education Act (IDEA), 1990.
   a. Replaces the word *handicap* in previous legislation with the word *disability*.
   b. Expands the original law to include instruction in all settings.
   c. Adds categories of treatment for children, including autism and traumatic brain injury (TBI).
   d. Reauthorizations of this act have changed the scope or requirements for documenting efficacy over time.
   e. Most significant change to IDEA came in 2004, which sought to improve the original act, particularly improving outcomes for special education and to make IDEA consistent with No Child Left Behind (NCLB).
6. PL 107-110—The No Child Left Behind Act of 2001.
   a. Sought to improve outcomes through:
      (1) Highly qualified teachers and paraprofessionals.
      (2) Use of accommodations, modifications and alternative assessments for children with disabilities.
      (3) Assessment of English-language learners.
      (4) Sanctions for schools identified as in need of improvement.
      (5) Requires accountability and adequate yearly progress.
   b. As an unfunded mandate, NCLB has resulted in dissatisfaction with excessive reliance on achievement test outcomes and conflicts with IDEA.

Role of the SLP in the School Setting

1. Identification of eligible children—typically by referral from parents, teachers and outside agencies.
2. Evaluation—if children fail screening, the SLP must have informed consent signed by the parents giving permission to evaluate.
3. Determining eligibility—the evaluation must determine eligibility for special education and related services as well as educational needs.
4. Developing the IEP—developed by the IEP team for all children age 3 or older who qualify for speech-language services and is developed to meet each child's individual needs.
5. IEP implementation—with parental consent, the IEP's goals and objectives are implemented through a program of therapy.
6. Dismissal—the IEP team must agree that goals have been achieved and termination is warranted.
7. Language-learning connection to literacy has received prominent attention in recent years.
   a. SLPs now participate in literacy/reading intervention.
   b. Literacy/reading intervention often occurs in the classroom.
   c. Children who are not achieving are often seen by SLPs in services referred to as Response to Intervention (RTI)—essentially trial therapy or classroom support to determine if difficulties can be overcome without resorting to special education services.
8. Caseload/workload may be mandated by state regulations or local district guidelines and includes indirect and direct services; caseloads are often so high that quality of services can be affected.

Early Intervention

Regulation

1. Governed by IDEA 1997 (PL 105-17); Part C recognizes an urgent need to:
   a. Enhance the development of infants and toddlers with disabilities.
   b. Reduce educational costs by minimizing later special education needs.
   c. Minimize need for institutionalization and maximize potential for independent living.
   d. Enhance families' capacities to meet the needs of their infants and toddlers with disabilities.
   e. Enhance the capacity of education agencies and service providers to identify, evaluate and manage young children from underrepresented groups.
   f. Provide services to children age 3 years and younger with special needs.

Role of the SLP

1. Developmental screening—requires states to have policies and procedures to identify infants and toddlers with developmental delays.
2. Evaluation—timely, comprehensive and multidisciplinary evaluation.
3. Assessment of results—must delineate appropriate services to meet the child's special needs.
4. Individualized Family Service Plan (IFSP)—goals and objectives for the child and family, services to be provided, preservice levels, plan for intervention and evaluation of services/outcomes.
5. Work with the service coordinator and other members of the service delivery team to provide competent and comprehensive services.

Guiding Principles for Early Intervention Services

1. Services are family-centered and culturally and linguistically responsive.
2. Services are developmentally supportive and promote children's participation in their natural environments.
3. Services are comprehensive, coordinated and team based.
4. Services are based on the highest quality evidence that is available.
   a. American Speech-Language-Hearing Association's (2008) *Roles and Responsibilities of Speech-Language Pathologists in Early Intervention: Guidelines*.

Professional Liability and Responsibility

Autonomy Entails Responsibilities, Duties and Liabilities

1. Liabilities arise from promises made to abide by standards of practice and codes of ethics.
2. Lapses in professional judgment, lack of care in evaluation or treatment methods or failure to use best practices or conform to applicable law create situations in which the SLP may be liable for professional misconduct.
3. Licensure laws protect the health, safety and welfare of its citizens.
4. Citizens or others may enter a complaint to the licensure board regarding professional misconduct, and the licensure board must investigate the allegation.
5. Professionals manage risks by adhering to scope of practice and practice guidelines, by participation in continuing education and by having a commitment to quality improvement.
6. SLPs should carry professional liability insurance coverage provided by their employer or obtained from an insurance company.
7. Professional liability insurance covers errors in judgment but not willful or intentional acts of malfeasance.
8. Errors in judgment should immediately be reported and guidance sought as to how to correct or limit the result of the error.
9. Errors in judgment should never be covered up or ignored.

Policies and Procedures

Typical Policies and Procedures

1. Some policies and procedures are typical from setting to setting and SLPs will expect to find such requirements in place wherever they work. It is typical for each unit in a facility to have a policies and procedures handbook that contains institutional, departmental and programmatic policies including:
   a. Applicable accrediting and regulatory requirements.
   b. Legal considerations.
   c. Infection control—universal precautions that prevent the spread of disease through the use of barriers (gloves), good hygiene (hand washing) and sterilization of materials.
   d. Continuous Quality Improvement program—parameters for developing and implementing.

Rules and Regulations

1. Dress code.
2. Attendance/leave policies.
3. Procedures to institute in case of emergency.
4. Patient admission and discharge procedures.
5. Confidentiality for protected patient information.
6. Ethics.
7. Taking/reporting disciplinary actions.
8. Roles of professionals in the unit.
9. Evaluation and treatment protocols.
10. Continuing education and student training requirements.
11. Patient safety.

Serving Multicultural Populations

Providing Services in a Multi-ethnic Society

1. Far fewer SLPs (7%) come from culturally and linguistically diverse (CLD) backgrounds than the number of patients to be seen.
2. SLPs are required to provide services competently (by Code of Ethics).
3. This requirement includes cultural competence or humility.
4. CLD populations have traditionally included Native, Hispanic, African, and Asian Americans.
5. Also includes diversity related to age, gender, race, ethnicity, language, religion, politics, sexual orientation and socioeconomic status, according to ASHA.
6. Caseloads in all settings reflect a growing diversity.

Issues Associated with CLD Populations

1. Bilingualism or second-language acquisition—may be addressing a primary language in the home and English as the second language (ESL) in the school environment.
2. Respect for the culture of the home and assisting acculturation in the environment.
3. Interactions of testing and treatment may affect clinical outcomes.
4. Use of interpreters may affect clinical decisions and outcomes.
5. Test instruments may lack sensitivity to cultural diversity and result in invalid data.
   a. Modification of test instruments may be necessary to eliminate bias.
   b. Dynamic assessment in the client's environment may reveal better information than standardized testing.
   c. Cultural differences may include perception of gender roles.
   d. Advice regarding cultural differences and competence in addressing them should be sought in order to provide services competently.
   e. Clinicians should develop therapeutic relationships with clients and their families in order to increase understanding and success.

Supervision

Types of Supervision

1. Students must be supervised by someone who holds the CCC-SLP in order for the hours to count toward certification requirements. Allowing clock hours to count when students are supervised by individuals in other professions is part of the current discussion associated with interprofessional practice.
2. SLPs often supervise students in externships but also supervise Clinical Fellows in real-world settings. The goal is to assist the learner in becoming an independent practitioner.
   a. Goal of supervision is for both supervisor and supervisee to experience professional growth resulting in better client outcomes.
   b. Skills for effective supervision for students and CFs:
      (1) Relinquish control without feeling threatened.
      (2) Promote problem solving and critical thinking.
      (3) Teach clinical competence in assessment, intervention and documentation.
      (4) Good interpersonal communication.
      (5) Conduct effective supervisory conferences.
      (6) Evaluate growth of the supervisee.
      (7) Clinical acumen that serves as a role model to the learner.
      (8) Ability to model and teach professional and ethical behavior.
      (9) Assist the student/CF to achieve clinical independence.
3. SLPs supervise speech-language pathology assistants (SLPAs), who work under the direction of the SLP and are not intending to become independent practitioners.
   a. Appropriate use of SLPAs—SLP should be knowledgeable of state regulations and appropriate policy documents. Training for SLPAs varies from state to state.
   b. Role of the SLPA—to increase the availability, frequency and efficiency of services. The SLPA may, at the direction of the SLP:
      (1) Assist with screenings without making interpretations.
      (2) Assist with documentation as directed.
      (3) Follow treatment plans or protocols developed by the SLP.
      (4) Document client performance through charts or tables.
      (5) Assist with assessment.
      (6) Assist with preparing materials, scheduling or clerical duties.
      (7) Check and maintain equipment.
      (8) Provide support for projects or training programs conducted by the SLP.
      (9) Assist with departmental operations.
      (10) Collect data for quality improvement projects.
      (11) Comply with regulations and job responsibilities.

Telepractice

Definition

1. An encounter with real-time audio and video connection between client(s) and a clinician, similar to an in-person session.
   a. May also utilize software or other digital media as accompaniment to live interaction.
   b. Live events may be supplemented with other contacts (phone, e-mail, etc.).
   c. May include any service delivery venue where the technology is available.
   d. Must conform to professional standards of ethics and best clinical practices and should be evaluated for efficacy and quality on an ongoing basis.
   e. All rules for privacy and confidentiality of patient information must be followed.
   f. Variability of licensure rules exists; however, many states currently require the telepractitioner to be licensed in the state where the services are delivered.
   g. States and other professional groups are working on assistance with the licensure issue such as limited license.
   h. Telepractice has the potential to improve access to SLP services.
   i. Research is needed as to the efficacy of telepractice in comparison to direct knee-to-knee services.

Evidence-Based Practice (EBP)

Definition

1. "...The conscientious, explicit, and judicious use of current best evidence in making decisions about the care of individual patients... [by] integrating individual clinical expertise with the best available external clinical evidence from systematic research" (Sackett et al., 1996).
   a. Evidence must be supplemented with clinical expertise and patient values while identifying and making use of the best evidence available.
   b. Practitioners should gain evidence from their own study but look for efficiencies by going to "high-yield" sources.
   c. Knowledge is continually changing, so reference scholarly journals available online or from evidence compilers such as professional organizations.
   d. ASHA has the National Center for Evidence-Based Practice (NCEP) in addition to journals—sources that provide relevant evidence across a wide range of disorders/areas of practice.
   e. NCEP conducts several comprehensive, systematic reviews each year for the benefit of members and practitioners in SLP.
   f. The ASHA website provides all published material in ASHA publications, including the scholarly journals, by search topic.
   g. Other specialty organizations and Special Interest Groups have focused information as well.
   h. Practitioners must assess evidence critically to determine if it is pertinent and of sufficient strength and quality.
   i. Questions the practitioner might ask:
      (1) Were there significant differences between treated and untreated groups?
      (2) Were outcome measures reliable and valid?
      (3) Were patients randomly assigned to groups?
      (4) Were investigators blind to group assignment?
      (5) Were group differences acceptable?
   j. EBP offers a means by which practitioners can improve as clinicians.

References

American Speech-Language-Hearing Association (2013). *2013 ASHA Member Counts:* Available from http://www.asha.org/uploadedFiles/2013-Member-Counts-Year-End-Highlights.pdf#search=%22member%22.

American Speech-Language-Hearing Association (2011). *ASHA Strategic Pathway to Excellence.* Available from http://www.asha.org/uploadedFiles/ASHAPublicPathwayHandout.pdf#search=%22mission%22.

American Speech-Language-Hearing Association (2010). *Code of Ethics* [Ethics]. Available from www.asha.org/policy.

American Speech-Language-Hearing Association (2010). *Professional Issues in Telepractice for Speech-Language Pathologists* [Professional Issues Statement]. Available from www.asha.org/policy.

American Speech-Language-Hearing Association (2007). *Scope of Practice in Speech-Language Pathology* [Scope of Practice]. Available from www.asha.org/policy.

Colorado Department of Education, Special Education Services Unit (2004). Fast Facts: Speech-Language Pathology Assistants (SLPA). Available from www.cde.state.co.us.

Dollaghan, C. (2004). Evidence-based practice: Myths and realities. *The ASHA Leader,* April 13, 2004. Available from http://www.asha.org/Publications/leader/2004/040413/f040413al.htm.

Duchan, J. F. (2002). What do you know about your professions' history and why it is important? *The ASHA Leader,* December 24, 2002. Available from http://www.asha.org/Publications/leader/2002/021224/021224a.htm.

Lubinski, R., Golper, L., & Frattali, C. (2007). *Professional Issues in Speech-Language Pathology and Audiology,* 3rd ed. Clifton Park, NY: Thomson Delmar Learning.

Lusis, I. (2010). New health care law brings changes. *The ASHA Leader,* April 27, 2010. Available from http://www.asha.rg/Publications/leader/2010/100427/New-Health-Care-Law.htm.

Markula Center for Applied Ethics (2009). A framework for thinking ethically. Santa Clara University. Available from http://www/scu/edu/ethics/practicing/decision/framework/html.

McCready, V. (2007). Supervision of speech-language pathology assistants: A reciprocal relationship. *The ASHA Leader,* May 8, 2007. Available from http://www.asha.org/Publications/leader/2007/070508/f070508b/.

Sackett, D. L., Rosenberg, W. M. C., Gray, J. A. M., Haynes, R .B., & Richardson, W. S. (1996). Evidence-based medicine: What it is and what it isn't. Article based on an editorial from the *British Medical Journal, 312,* 71–72.

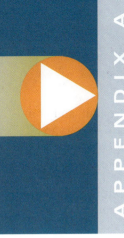

APPENDIX A

Scope of Practice in Speech-Language Pathology

About This Document

This scope of practice document is an official policy of the American Speech-language-Hearing Association (ASHA) defining the breadth of practice within the profession of speech-language pathology. This document was developed by the ASHA Ad Hoc Committee on the Scope of Practice in Speech-Language Pathology. Committee members were Kenn Apel (chair), Theresa E. Bartolotta, Adam A. Brickell, Lynne E. Hewitt, Ann W. Kummer, Luis F. Riquelme, Jennifer B. Watson, Carole Zangari, Brian B. Shulman (vice president for professional practices in speech-language pathology), Lemmietta McNeilly (ex officio), and Diane R. Paul (consultant). This document was approved by the ASHA Legislative Council on September 4, 2007 (LC 09-07).

Introduction

The *Scope of Practice in Speech-Language Pathology* includes a statement of purpose, a framework for research and clinical practice, qualifications of the speech-language pathologist, professional roles and activities, and practice settings. The speech-language pathologist is the professional who engages in clinical services, prevention, advocacy, education, administration, and research in the areas of communication and swallowing across the life span from infancy through geriatrics. Given the diversity of the client population, ASHA policy requires that these activities are conducted in a manner that takes into consideration the impact of culture and linguistic exposure/acquisition and uses the best available evidence for practice to ensure optimal outcomes for persons with communication and/or swallowing disorders or differences.

As part of the review process for updating the *Scope of Practice in Speech-Language Pathology*, the committee made changes to the previous scope of practice document that reflected recent advances in knowledge, understanding, and research in the discipline. These changes included acknowledging roles and responsibilities that were not mentioned in previous iterations of the *Scope of Practice* (e.g., funding issues, marketing of services, focus on emergency responsiveness, communication wellness). The revised document also was framed squarely on two guiding principles: evidence-based practice and cultural and linguistic diversity.

Statement of Purpose

The purpose of this document is to define the *Scope of Practice in Speech-Language Pathology* to:

1. Delineate areas of professional practice for speech-language pathologists;
2. Inform others (e.g., health care providers, educators, other professionals, consumers, payers, regulators, members of the general public) about professional services offered by speech-language pathologists as qualified providers;
3. Support speech-language pathologists in the provision of high-quality, evidence-based services to individuals with concerns about communication or swallowing;
4. Support speech-language pathologists in the conduct of research;
5. Provide guidance for educational preparation and professional development of speech-language pathologists.

This document describes the breadth of professional practice offered within the profession of speech-language pathology. Levels of education, experience, skill, and proficiency with respect to the roles and activities identified within this scope of practice document vary among individual providers. A speech-language pathologist typically does not practice in all areas of the field. As the ASHA Code of Ethics specifies, individuals may practice only in areas in which they are competent (i.e., individuals' scope of competency), based on their education, training, and experience.

In addition to this scope of practice document, other ASHA documents provide more specific guidance for practice areas. Figure A-1 illustrates the relationship between the ASHA Code of Ethics, the *Scope of Practice*, and specific practice documents. As shown, the ASHA Code of Ethics sets forth the fundamental principles and rules considered essential to the preservation of the highest standards of integrity and ethical conduct in the practice of speech-language pathology.

Speech-language pathology is a dynamic and continuously developing profession. As such, listing specific areas within this *Scope of Practice* does not exclude emerging areas of practice. Further, speech-language pathologists may provide additional professional services (e.g., interdisciplinary work in a health care setting, collaborative service delivery in schools, transdisciplinary practice in early intervention settings) that are necessary for the well-being of the individual(s) they are serving but are not addressed in this *Scope of Practice*. In such instances, it is both ethically and legally incumbent upon professionals to determine whether they have the knowledge and skills necessary to perform such services.

This scope of practice document does not supersede existing state licensure laws or affect the interpretation or implementation of such laws. It may serve, however, as a model for the development or modification of licensure laws.

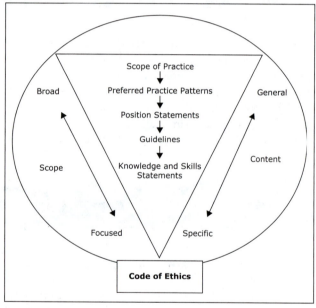

Figure A-1 Conceptual Framework of ASHA Practice Documents

Framework for Research and Clinical Practice

The overall objective of speech-language pathology services is to optimize individuals' ability to communicate and swallow, thereby improving quality of life. As the population profile of the United States continues to become increasingly diverse (U.S. Census Bureau, 2005), speech-language pathologists have a responsibility to be knowledgeable about the impact of these changes on clinical services and research needs. Speech-language pathologists are committed to the provision of culturally and linguistically appropriate services and to the consideration of diversity in scientific investigations of human communication and swallowing. For example, one aspect of providing culturally and linguistically appropriate services is to determine whether communication difficulties experienced by English language learners are the result of a communication disorder in the native language or a consequence of learning a new language.

Additionally, an important characteristic of the practice of speech-language pathology is that, to the extent possible, clinical decisions are based on best available evidence. ASHA has defined evidence-based practice in speech-language pathology as an approach in which current, high-quality research evidence is integrated with practitioner expertise and the individual's preferences and values into the process of clinical decision making (ASHA, 2005). A high-quality basic, applied, and efficacy research base in communication sciences and disorders and related fields of study is essential to providing evidence-based clinical practice and quality clinical services. The research base can be enhanced by increased interaction and communication with researchers across the United States and from other countries. As our global society is becoming more connected, integrated, and interdependent, speech-language pathologists have access to an abundant array of resources, information technology, and diverse perspectives and influence (e.g., Lombardo, 1997). Increased national and international interchange of professional knowledge, information, and education in communication sciences and disorders can be a means to strengthen research collaboration and improve clinical services.

The World Health Organization (WHO) has developed a multipurpose health classification system known as the International Classification of Functioning, Disability and Health (ICF; WHO, 2001). The purpose of this classification system is to provide a standard language and framework for the description of functioning and health. The ICF framework is useful in describing the breadth of the role of the speech-language pathologist in the prevention, assessment, and habilitation/rehabilitation, enhancement, and scientific investigation of communication and swallowing. It consists of two components:

- Health Conditions
  - Body Functions and Structures: These involve the anatomy and physiology of the human body. Relevant examples in speech-language pathology include craniofacial anomaly, vocal fold paralysis, cerebral palsy, stuttering, and language impairment.
  - Activity and Participation: Activity refers to the execution of a task or action. Participation is the involvement in a life situation. Relevant examples in speech-language pathology include difficulties with swallowing safely for independent feeding, participating actively in class, understanding a medical prescription, and accessing the general education curriculum.
- Contextual Factors
  - Environmental Factors: These make up the physical, social, and attitudinal environments in which people live and conduct their lives. Relevant examples in speech-language pathology include the role of the communication partner in augmentative and alternative communication, the influence of classroom acoustics on communication, and the impact of institutional dining environments on individuals' ability to safely maintain nutrition and hydration.
  - Personal Factors: These are the internal influences on an individual's functioning and disability and are not part of the health condition. These factors may include, but are not limited to, age, gender, ethnicity, educational level, social background, and profession. Relevant examples in speech-language pathology might include a person's background or culture that influences his or her reaction to a communication or swallowing disorder.

The framework in speech-language pathology encompasses these health conditions and contextual factors. The health condition component of the ICF can be expressed on a continuum of functioning. On one end of the continuum is intact functioning. At the opposite end of the continuum is completely compromised functioning. The contextual factors interact with each other and with the health conditions and may serve as facilitators or barriers to functioning. Speech-language pathologists may influence contextual factors through education and advocacy efforts at local, state, and national levels. Relevant examples in Speech-language pathology include a user of an augmentative communication device needing classroom support services for academic success, or the effects of premorbid literacy level on rehabilitation in an adult post brain injury. Speech-language pathologists work to improve quality of life by reducing impairments of body functions and structures, activity limitations, participation restrictions, and barriers created by contextual factors.

Qualifications

Speech-language pathologists, as defined by ASHA, hold the ASHA Certificate of Clinical Competence in Speech-Language Pathology (CCC-SLP), which requires a master's, doctoral, or other recognized postbaccalaureate degree. ASHA-certified speech-language pathologists complete a supervised postgraduate professional experience and pass a national examination as described in the ASHA certification standards. Demonstration of continued professional development is mandated for the maintenance of the CCC-SLP. Where applicable, Speech-language pathologists hold other required credentials (e.g., state licensure, teaching certification).

This document defines the scope of practice for the field of speech-language pathology. Each practitioner must evaluate his or her own experiences with preservice education, clinical practice, mentorship and supervision, and continuing professional development. As a whole, these experiences define the scope of competence for each individual. Speech-language pathologists may engage in only those aspects of the profession that are within their scope of competence.

As primary care providers for communication and swallowing disorders, Speech-language pathologists are autonomous professionals; that is, their services are not prescribed or supervised by another professional. However, individuals frequently benefit from services that include speech-language pathologist collaborations with other professionals.

Professional Roles and Activities

Speech-language pathologists serve individuals, families, and groups from diverse linguistic and cultural backgrounds. Services are provided based on applying the best available research evidence, using expert clinical judgments, and considering clients' individual preferences and values. Speech-language pathologists address typical and atypical communication and swallowing in the following areas:

- Speech sound production
  - Articulation
  - Apraxia of speech
  - Dysarthria
  - Ataxia
  - Dyskinesia
- Resonance
  - Hypernasality
  - Hyponasality
  - Cul-de-sac resonance
  - Mixed resonance
- Voice
  - Phonation quality
  - Pitch
  - Loudness
  - Respiration
- Fluency
  - Stuttering
  - Cluttering
- Language (comprehension and expression)
  - Phonology
  - Morphology
  - Syntax
  - Semantics
  - Pragmatics (language use, social aspects of communication)
  - Literacy (reading, writing, spelling)
  - Prelinguistic communication (e.g., joint attention, intentionality, communicative signaling)
  - Paralinguistic communication
- Cognition
  - Attention
  - Memory
  - Sequencing
  - Problem solving
  - Executive functioning
- Feeding and swallowing
  - Oral, pharyngeal, laryngeal, esophageal
  - Orofacial myology (including tongue thrust)
  - Oral-motor functions

Potential etiologies of communication and swallowing disorders include:

- Neonatal problems (e.g., prematurity, low birth weight, substance exposure);

- Developmental disabilities (e.g., specific language impairment, autism spectrum disorder, dyslexia, learning disabilities, attention deficit disorder);
- Auditory problems (e.g., hearing loss or deafness);
- Oral anomalies (e.g., cleft lip/palate, dental malocclusion, macroglossia, oral-motor dysfunction);
- Respiratory compromise (e.g., bronchopulmonary dysplasia, chronic obstructive pulmonary disease);
- Pharyngeal anomalies (e.g., upper airway obstruction, velopharyngeal insufficiency/incompetence);
- Laryngeal anomalies (e.g., vocal fold pathology, tracheal stenosis, tracheostomy);
- Neurological disease/dysfunction (e.g., traumatic brain injury, cerebral palsy, cerebral vascular accident, dementia, Parkinson's disease, amyotrophic lateral sclerosis);
- Psychiatric disorder (e.g., psychosis, schizophrenia);
- Genetic disorders (e.g., Down syndrome, fragile X syndrome, Rett syndrome, velocardiofacial syndrome).

The professional roles and activities in speech-language pathology include clinical/ educational services (diagnosis, assessment, planning, and treatment), prevention and advocacy, and education, administration, and research.

Clinical Services

Speech-language pathologists provide clinical services that include the following:

- Prevention and pre-referral
- Screening
- Assessment/evaluation
- Consultation
- Diagnosis
- Treatment, intervention, management
- Counseling
- Collaboration
- Documentation
- Referral

Examples of these clinical services include:

1. Using data to guide clinical decision making and determine the effectiveness of services;
2. Making service delivery decisions (e.g., admission/eligibility, frequency, duration, location, discharge/dismissal) across the lifespan;
3. Determining appropriate context(s) for service delivery (e.g., home, school, telepractice, community);
4. Documenting provision of services in accordance with accepted procedures appropriate for the practice setting;
5. Collaborating with other professionals (e.g., identifying neonates and infants at risk for hearing loss, participating in palliative care teams, planning lessons with educators, serving on student assistance teams);
6. Screening individuals for hearing loss or middle ear pathology using conventional pure-tone air conduction methods (including otoscopic inspection), otoacoustic emissions screening, and/or screening tympanometry;
7. Providing intervention and support services for children and adults diagnosed with speech and language disorders;
8. Providing intervention and support services for children and adults diagnosed with auditory processing disorders;
9. Using instrumentation (e.g., videofluoroscopy, electromyography, nasendoscopy, stroboscopy, endoscopy, nasometry, computer technology) to observe, collect data, and measure parameters of communication and swallowing or other upper aerodigestive functions;
10. Counseling individuals, families, coworkers, educators, and other persons in the community regarding acceptance, adaptation, and decision making about communication and swallowing;
11. Facilitating the process of obtaining funding for equipment and services related to difficulties with communication and swallowing;
12. Serving as case managers, service delivery coordinators, and members of collaborative teams (e.g., individualized family service plan and individualized education program teams, transition planning teams);
13. Providing referrals and information to other professionals, agencies, and/or consumer organizations;
14. Developing, selecting, and prescribing multimodal augmentative and alternative communication systems, including unaided strategies (e.g., manual signs, gestures) and aided strategies (e.g.,

speech-generating devices, manual communication boards, picture schedules);
15. Providing services to individuals with hearing loss and their families/caregivers (e.g., auditory training for children with cochlear implants and hearing aids; speechreading; speech and language intervention secondary to hearing loss; visual inspection and listening checks of amplification devices for the purpose of troubleshooting, including verification of appropriate battery voltage);
16. Addressing behaviors (e.g., perseverative or disruptive actions) and environments (e.g., classroom seating, positioning for swallowing safety or attention, communication opportunities) that affect communication and swallowing;
17. Selecting, fitting, and establishing effective use of prosthetic/adaptive devices for communication and swallowing (e.g., tracheoesophageal prostheses, speaking valves, electrolarynges; this service does not include the selection or fitting of sensory devices used by individuals with hearing loss or other auditory perceptual deficits, which falls within the scope of practice of audiologists; ASHA, 2004);
18. Providing services to modify or enhance communication performance (e.g., accent modification, transgender voice, care and improvement of the professional voice, personal/professional communication effectiveness).

Prevention and Advocacy

Speech-language pathologists engage in prevention and advocacy activities related to human communication and swallowing. Example activities include:

1. Improving communication wellness by promoting healthy lifestyle practices that can help prevent communication and swallowing disorders (e.g., cessation of smoking, wearing helmets when bike riding);
2. Presenting primary prevention information to individuals and groups known to be at risk for communication disorders and other appropriate groups;
3. Providing early identification and early intervention services for communication disorders;
4. Advocating for individuals and families through community awareness, health literacy, education, and training programs to promote and facilitate access to full participation in communication, including the elimination of societal, cultural, and linguistic barriers;
5. Advising regulatory and legislative agencies on emergency responsiveness to individuals who have communication and swallowing disorders or difficulties;
6. Promoting and marketing professional services;
7. Advocating at the local, state, and national levels for improved administrative and governmental policies affecting access to services for communication and swallowing;
8. Advocating at the local, state, and national levels for funding for research;
9. Recruiting potential speech-language pathologists into the profession;
10. Participating actively in professional organizations to contribute to best practices in the profession.

Education, Administration, and Research

Speech-language pathologists also serve as educators, administrators, and researchers. Example activities for these roles include:

1. Educating the public regarding communication and swallowing;
2. Educating and providing in-service training to families, caregivers, and other professionals;
3. Educating, supervising, and mentoring current and future speech-language pathologists;
4. Educating, supervising, and managing speech-language pathology assistants and other support personnel;
5. Fostering public awareness of communication and swallowing disorders and their treatment;

6. Serving as expert witnesses;
7. Administering and managing clinical and academic programs;
8. Developing policies, operational procedures, and professional standards;
9. Conducting basic and applied/translational research related to communication sciences and disorders, and swallowing.

Practice Settings

Speech-language pathologists provide services in a wide variety of settings, which may include but are not exclusive to:

1. Public and private schools;
2. Early intervention settings, preschools, and day care centers;
3. Health care settings (e.g., hospitals, medical rehabilitation facilities, long-term care facilities, home health agencies, clinics, neonatal intensive care units, behavioral/mental health facilities);
4. Private practice settings;
5. Universities and university clinics;
6. Individuals' homes and community residences;
7. Supported and competitive employment settings;
8. Community, state, and federal agencies and institutions;
9. Correctional institutions;
10. Research facilities;
11. Corporate and industrial settings.

References

American Speech-Language-Hearing Association. (2004). *Scope of practice in audiology.* Available from www.asha.org/policy.

American Speech-Language-Hearing Association. (2005). *Evidence-based practice in communication disorders* [Position statement]. Available from www.asha.org/policy.

Lombardo, T. (1997, Spring). The impact of information technology: Learning, living, and loving in the future. *The Labyrinth: Sharing Information on Learning Technologies. 5* (2). Available from www.mcli.dist.maricopa.edu/LF/Spr97/spr97L8.html.

U.S. Census Bureau. (2005). *Population profile of the United States: Dynamic version. Race and Hispanic origin in 2005.* Available from www.census.gov.

World Health Organization. (2001). *International classification of functioning, disability and health.* Geneva, Switzerland: Author.

American Speech-Language-Hearing Association. (2005). *Standards for the certificate of clinical competence in speech-language pathology.* Available from www.asha.org/about/membership-certification/handbooks/slp/slp_standards.htm.

General Service Delivery Issues

Admission/Discharge Criteria
American Speech-Language-Hearing Association. (2004). *Admission/discharge criteria in speech-language pathology* [Guidelines]. Available from www.asha.org/policy.

Autonomy
American Speech-Language-Hearing Association. (1986). *Autonomy of speech-language pathology and audiology* [Relevant paper]. Available from www.asha.org/policy.

Culturally and Linguistically Appropriate Services
American Speech-Language-Hearing Association. (2002). *American English dialects* [Technical report]. Available from www.asha.org/policy.

American Speech-Language-Hearing Association. (2004). *Knowledge and skills needed by speech-language pathologists and audiologists to provide culturally and linguistically appropriate services* [Knowledge and skills]. Available from www.asha.org/policy.

Resources

ASHA Cardinal Documents

American Speech-Language-Hearing Association. (2003). *Code of ethics (Revised).* Available from www.asha.org/policy.

American Speech-Language-Hearing Association. (2004). *Preferred practice patterns for the profession of speech-language pathology.* Available from www.asha.org/policy.

Definitions and Terminology

American Speech-Language-Hearing Association. (1982). *Language* [Relevant paper]. Available from www.asha.org/policy.

American Speech-Language-Hearing Association. (1986). *Private practice* [Definition]. Available from www.asha.org/policy.

American Speech-Language-Hearing Association. (1993). *Definition of communication disorders and variations* [Definition]. Available from www.asha.org/policy.

American Speech-Language-Hearing Association. (1998). *Terminology pertaining to fluency and fluency disorders* [Guidelines]. Available from www.asha.org/policy.

Evidence-Based Practice

American Speech-Language-Hearing Association. (2004). *Evidence-based practice in communication disorders: An introduction* [Technical report]. Available from www.asha.org/policy.

American Speech-Language-Hearing Association. (2005). *Evidence-based practice in communication disorders: An introduction* [Position statement]. Available from www.asha.org/policy.

Private Practice

American Speech-Language-Hearing Association. (1990). *Considerations for establishing a private practice in audiology and/or speech-language pathology* [Technical report]. Available from www.asha.org/policy.

American Speech-Language-Hearing Association. (1991). *Private practice* [Technical report]. Available from www.asha.org/policy.

American Speech-Language-Hearing Association. (1994). *Professional liability and risk management for the audiology and speech-language pathology professions* [Technical report]. Available from www.asha.org/policy.

American Speech-Language-Hearing Association. (2002). *Drawing cases for private practice from primary place of employment* [Issues in ethics]. Available from www.asha.org/policy.

Professional Service Programs

American Speech-Language-Hearing Association. (2005). *Quality indicators for professional service programs in audiology and speech-language pathology* [Quality indicators]. Available from www.asha.org/policy.

Speech-Language Pathology Assistants

American Speech-Language-Hearing Association. (2001). *Knowledge and skills for supervisors of speech-language pathology assistants* [Knowledge and skills]. Available from www.asha.org/policy.

American Speech-Language-Hearing Association. (2004). *Guidelines for the training, use, and supervision of speech-language pathology assistants* [Guidelines]. Available from www.asha.org/policy.

American Speech-Language-Hearing Association. (2004). *Support personnel* [Issues in ethics]. Available from www.asha.org/policy.

American Speech-Language-Hearing Association. (2004). *Training, use, and supervision of support personnel in speech-language pathology* [Position statement]. Available from www.asha.org/policy.

Supervision

American Speech-Language-Hearing Association. (1985). *Clinical supervision in Speech-language pathology and audiology* [Position statement]. Available from www.asha.org/policy.

American Speech-Language-Hearing Association. (2004). *Clinical fellowship supervisor's responsibilities* [Issues in ethics]. Available from www.asha.org/policy.

American Speech-Language-Hearing Association. (2004). *Supervision of student clinicians* [Issues in ethics]. Available from www.asha.org/policy.

Clinical Services and Populations

Apraxia of Speech

American Speech-Language-Hearing Association. (2007). *Childhood apraxia of speech* [Position statement]. Available from www.asha.org/policy.

American Speech-Language-Hearing Association. (2007). *Childhood apraxia of speech* [Technical report]. Available from www.asha.org/policy.

Auditory Processing

American Speech-Language-Hearing Association. (1995). *Central auditory processing: Current status of research and implications for clinical practice* [Technical report]. Available from www.asha.org/policy.

American Speech-Language-Hearing Association. (2005). *(Central) auditory processing disorders* [Technical report]. Available from www.asha.org/policy.

American Speech-Language-Hearing Association. (2005). *(Central) auditory processing disorders—the role of the audiologist* [Position statement]. Available from www.asha.org/policy.

Augmentative and Alternative Communication (AAC)

American Speech-Language-Hearing Association. (1998). *Maximizing the provision of appropriate technology services and devices for students in schools* [Technical report]. Available from www.asha.org/policy.

American Speech-Language-Hearing Association. (2001). *Augmentative and alternative communication: Knowledge and skills for service delivery* [Knowledge and skills]. Available from www.asha.org/policy.

American Speech-Language-Hearing Association. (2004). *Roles and responsibilities of speech-language pathologists with respect to augmentative and alternative communication* [Position statement]. Available from www.asha.org/policy.

American Speech-Language-Hearing Association. (2004). *Roles and responsibilities of speech-language pathologists with respect to augmentative and alternative communication* [Technical report]. Available from www.asha.org/policy.

Aural Rehabilitation

American Speech-Language-Hearing Association. (2001). *Knowledge and skills required for the practice of audiologic/aural rehabilitation* [Knowledge and skills]. Available from www.asha.org/policy.

Autism Spectrum Disorders

American Speech-Language-Hearing Association. (2006). *Guidelines for speech-language pathologists in diagnosis, assessment, and treatment of autism spectrum disorders across the life span* [Guidelines]. Available from www.asha.org/policy.

American Speech-Language-Hearing Association. (2006). *Knowledge and skills needed by speech-language pathologists for diagnosis, assessment, and treatment of autism spectrum disorders across the life span* [Knowledge and skills]. Available from www.asha.org/policy.

American Speech-Language-Hearing Association. (2006). *Principles for speech-language pathologists in diagnosis, assessment, and treatment of autism spectrum disorders across the life span* [Technical report]. Available from www.asha.org/policy.

American Speech-Language-Hearing Association. (2006). *Roles and responsibilities of speech-language pathologists in diagnosis, assessment, and treatment of autism spectrum disorders across the life span* [Position statement]. Available from www.asha.org/policy.

Filipek, P. A., Accardo, P. J., Ashwal, S., Baranek, G. T., Cook, E. H., Dawson, G., et al. (2000). Practice parameter: Screening and diagnosis of autism—report of the Quality Standards Subcommittee of the American Academy of Neurology and the Child Neurology Society *Neurology, 55,* 468–479

Cognitive Aspects of Communication

American Speech-Language-Hearing Association. (1990). *Interdisciplinary approaches to brain damage* [Position statement]. Available from www.asha.org/policy.

American Speech-Language-Hearing Association. (1995). *Guidelines for the structure and function of an interdisciplinary team for persons with brain injury* [Guidelines]. Available from www.asha.org/policy.

American Speech-Language-Hearing Association. (2003). *Evaluating and treating communication and cognitive disorders: Approaches to referral and collaboration for speech-language pathology and clinical neuropsychology* [Technical report]. Available from www.asha.org/policy.

American Speech-Language-Hearing Association. (2003). *Rehabilitation of children and adults with cognitive-communication disorders after brain injury* [Technical report]. Available from www.asha.org/policy.

American Speech-Language-Hearing Association. (2005). *Knowledge and skills needed by speech-language pathologists providing services to individuals with cognitive-communication disorders* [Knowledge and skills]. Available from www.asha.org/ policy.

American Speech-Language-Hearing Association. (2005). *Roles of speech-language pathologists in the identification, diagnosis, and treatment of individuals with cognitive-communication disorders:* [Position statement]. Available from www.asha.org/policy.

Deaf and Hard of Hearing

American Speech-Language-Hearing Association. (2004). *Roles of speech-language pathologists and teachers of children who are deaf and hard of hearing in the development of communicative and linguistic competence* [Guidelines]. Available from www.asha.org/policy.

American Speech-Language-Hearing Association. (2004). *Roles of speech-language pathologists and teachers of children who are deaf and hard of hearing in the development of communicative and linguistic competence* [Position statement]. Available from www.asha.org/policy.

American Speech-Language-Hearing Association. (2004). *Roles of speech-language pathologists and teachers of children who are deaf and hard of hearing in the development of communicative and linguistic competence* [Technical report]. Available from www.asha.org/policy.

Dementia

American Speech-Language-Hearing Association. (2005). *The roles of speech-language pathologists working with dementia-based communication disorders* [Position statement]. Available from www.asha.org/policy.

American Speech-Language-Hearing Association. (2005). *The roles of speech-language pathologists working with dementia-based communication disorders* [Technical report]. Available from www.asha.org/policy.

Early Intervention

American Speech-Language-Hearing Association. *Roles and responsibilities of Speech-language pathologists in early intervention* (in preparation). [Position statement, Technical report, Guidelines, and Knowledge and skills].

National Joint Committee on Learning Disabilities (2006). *Learning disabilities and young children: Identification and intervention* Available from www.ldonline.org/article/11511?theme=print.

Fluency

American Speech-Language-Hearing Association. (1995). *Guidelines for practice in stuttering treatment* [Guidelines]. Available from www.asha.org/policy.

Hearing Screening

American Speech-Language-Hearing Association. (1997). *Guidelines for audiologic screening* [Guidelines]. Available from www.asha.org/policy.

American Speech-Language-Hearing Association. (2004). *Clinical practice by certificate holders in the profession in which they are not certified* [Issues in ethics]. Available from www.asha.org/policy.

Language and Literacy

American Speech-Language-Hearing Association. (1981). *Language learning disorders* [Position statement]. Available from www.asha.org/policy.

American Speech-Language-Hearing Association and the National Association of School Psychologists (1987). *Identification of children and youths with language learning disorders* [Position statement]. Available from www.asha.org/policy.

American Speech-Language-Hearing Association. (2000). *Roles and responsibilities of speech-language pathologists with respect to reading and writing in children and adolescents* [Guidelines]. Available from www.asha.org/policy.

American Speech-Language-Hearing Association. (2000). *Roles and responsibilities of speech-language pathologists with respect to reading and writing in children and adolescents* [Position statement]. Available from www.asha.org/policy.

American Speech-Language-Hearing Association. (2000). *Roles and responsibilities of speech-language pathologists with respect to reading and writing in children and adolescents* [Technical report]. Available from www.asha.org/policy.

American Speech-Language-Hearing Association. (2002). *Knowledge and skills needed by speech-language pathologists with respect to reading and writing in children and adolescents* [Knowledge and skills]. Available from www.asha.org/policy.

Mental Retardation/Developmental Disabilities

American Speech-Language-Hearing Association. (2005). *Knowledge and skills needed by speech-language pathologists serving persons with mental retardation/developmental disabilities* [Knowledge and skills]. Available from www.asha.org/policy.

American Speech-Language-Hearing Association. (2005). *Principles for speech-language pathologists serving persons with mental retardation/developmental disabilities* [Technical report]. Available from www.asha.org/policy.

American Speech-Language-Hearing Association. (2005). *Roles and responsibilities of speech-language pathologists serving persons withmental retardation/developmental disabilities* [Guidelines]. Available from www.asha.org/policy.

American Speech-Language-Hearing Association. (2005). *Roles and responsibilities of speech-language pathologists serving persons withmental retardation/developmental disabilities* [Position statement]. Available from www.asha.org/policy.

Orofacial Myofunctional Disorders

American Speech-Language-Hearing Association. (1989). *Labial-lingual posturing function* [Technical report]. Available from www.asha.org/policy.

American Speech-Language-Hearing Association. (1991). *The role of the speech-language pathologist in assessment and management of oral myofunctional disorders* [Position statement]. Available from www.asha.org/policy.

American Speech-Language-Hearing Association. (1993). *Orofacial myofunctional disorders* [Knowledge and skills]. Available from www.asha.org/policy.

Prevention

American Speech-Language-Hearing Association. (1987). *Prevention of communication disorders* [Position statement]. Available from www.asha.org/policy.

American Speech-Language-Hearing Association. (1987). *Prevention of communication disorders tutorial* [Relevant paper]. Available from www.asha.org/policy.

Severe Disabilities

National Joint Committee for the Communication Needs of Persons With Severe Disabilities. (1991). *Guidelines for meeting the communication needs of persons with severe disabilities.* Available from www.asha.org/docs/html/GL1992-00201.html.

National Joint Committee for the Communication Needs of Persons With Severe Disabilities (2002). *Access to communication services and supports: Concerns regarding the application of restrictive "eligibility" policies* [Technical report]. Available from www.asha.org/policy.

National Joint Committee for the Communication Needs of Persons With Severe Disabilities (2003). *Access to communication services and supports: Concerns regarding the application of restrictive "eligibility" policies* [Position statement]. Available from www.asha.org/policy.

Social Aspects of Communication

American Speech-Language-Hearing Association. (1991). *Guidelines for speech-language pathologists serving persons with language, socio-communicative and/or cognitive-communicative impairments* [Guidelines]. Available from www.asha.org/policy.

Swallowing

American Speech-Language-Hearing Association. (1992). *Instrumental diagnostic procedures for swallowing* [Guidelines]. Available from www.asha.org/policy.

American Speech-Language-Hearing Association. (1992). *Instrumental diagnostic procedures for swallowing* [Position statement]. Available from www.asha.org/policy.

American Speech-Language-Hearing Association. (2000). *Clinical indicators for instrumental assessment of dysphagia* [Guidelines]. Available from www.asha.org/policy.

American Speech-Language-Hearing Association. (2001). *Knowledge and skills needed by speech-language pathologists providing services to individuals with swallowing and/or feeding disorders* [Knowledge and skills]. Available from www.asha.org/policy.

American Speech-Language-Hearing Association. (2001). *Knowledge and skills for speech-language pathologists performing endoscopic assessment of swallowing functions* [Knowledge and skills]. Available from www.asha.org/policy.

American Speech-Language-Hearing Association. (2001). *Roles of speech-language pathologists in swallowing and feeding disorders* [Position statement]. Available from www.asha.org/policy.

American Speech-Language-Hearing Association. (2001). *Roles of speech-language pathologists in swallowing and feeding disorders* [Technical report]. Available from www.asha.org/policy.

American Speech-Language-Hearing Association. (2004). *Guidelines for speech-language pathologists performing videofluoroscopic swallowing studies* [Guidelines]. Available from www.asha.org/policy.

American Speech-Language-Hearing Association. (2004). *Knowledge and skills needed by speech-language pathologists performing videofluoroscopic swallowing studies* Available from www.asha.org/policy.

American Speech-Language-Hearing Association. (2004). *Role of the speech-language pathologist in the performance and interpretation of endoscopic evaluation of swallowing* [Guidelines]. Available from www.asha.org/policy.

American Speech-Language-Hearing Association. (2004). *Role of the speech-language pathologist in the performance and interpretation of endoscopic evaluation of swallowing* [Position statement]. Available from www.asha.org/policy.

American Speech-Language-Hearing Association. (2004). *Role of the speech-language pathologist in the performance and interpretation of endoscopic evaluation of swallowing* [Technical report]. Available from www.asha.org/policy.

American Speech-Language-Hearing Association. (2004). *Speech-language pathologists training and supervising other professionals in the delivery of services to individuals with swallowing and feeding disorders* [Technical report]. Available from www.asha.org/policy.

Voice and Resonance

American Speech-Language-Hearing Association. (1993). *Oral and oropharyngeal prostheses* [Guidelines]. Available from www.asha.org/policy.

American Speech-Language-Hearing Association. (1993). *Oral and oropharyngeal prostheses* [Position statement]. Available from www.asha.org/policy.

American Speech-Language-Hearing Association. (1993). *Use of voice prostheses in tracheotomized persons with or without ventilatory dependence* [Guidelines]. Available from www.asha.org/policy.

American Speech-Language-Hearing Association. (1993). *Use of voice prostheses in tracheotomized persons with or without ventilatory dependence* [Position statement]. Available from www.asha.org/policy.

American Speech-Language-Hearing Association. (1998). *The roles of otolaryngologists and speech-language pathologists in the performance and interpretation of strobovideolaryngoscopy* [Relevant paper]. Available from www.asha.org/policy.

American Speech-Language-Hearing Association. (2004). *Evaluation and treatment for tracheoesophageal puncture and prosthesis* [Technical report]. Available from www.asha.org/policy.

American Speech-Language-Hearing Association. (2004). *Knowledge and skills for speech-language pathologists with respect to evaluation and treatment for tracheoesophageal puncture and prosthesis* [Knowledge and skills]. Available from www.asha.org/policy.

American Speech-Language-Hearing Association. (2004). *Roles and responsibilities of speech-language pathologists with respect to evaluation and treatment for tracheoesophageal puncture and prosthesis* [Position statement]. Available from www.asha.org/policy.

American Speech-Language-Hearing Association. (2004). *Vocal tract visualization and imaging* [Position statement]. Available from www.asha.org/policy.

American Speech-Language-Hearing Association. (2004). *Vocal tract visualization and imaging* [Technical report]. Available from www.asha.org/policy.

American Speech-Language-Hearing Association. (2005). *The role of the speech-language pathologist, the teacher of singing, and the speaking voice trainer in voice habilitation* [Technical report]. Available from www.asha.org/policy.

American Speech-Language-Hearing Association. (2005). *The use of voice therapy in the treatment of dysphonia* [Technical report]. Available from www.asha.org/policy.

Health Care Services

Business Practices in Health Care Settings

American Speech-Language-Hearing Association. (2002). *Knowledge and skills in business practices needed by speech-language pathologists in health care settings* [Knowledge and skills]. Available from www.asha.org/policy.

American Speech-Language-Hearing Association. (2004). *Knowledge and skills in business practices for speech-language pathologists who are managers and leaders in health care organizations* [Knowledge and skills]. Available from www.asha.org/policy.

Multiskilling

American Speech-Language-Hearing Association. (1996). *Multiskilled personnel* [Position statement]. Available from www.asha.org/policy.

American Speech-Language-Hearing Association. (1996). *Multiskilled personnel* [Technical report]. Available from www.asha.org/policy.

Neonatal Intensive Care Unit

American Speech-Language-Hearing Association. (2004). *Knowledge and skills needed by speech-language pathologists providing services to infants and families in the NICU environment* [Knowledge and skills]. Available from www.asha.org/policy.

American Speech-Language-Hearing Association. (2004). *Roles and responsibilities of speech-language pathologists in the neonatal intensive care unit* [Guidelines]. Available from www.asha.org/policy.

American Speech-Language-Hearing Association. (2004). *Roles and responsibilities of speech-language pathologists in the neonatal intensive care unit* [Position statement]. Available from www.asha.org/policy.

American Speech-Language-Hearing Association. (2004). *Roles and responsibilities of speech-language pathologists in the neonatal intensive care unit* [Technical report]. Available from www.asha.org/policy.

Sedation and Anesthetics

American Speech-Language-Hearing Association. (1992). *Sedation and topical anesthetics in audiology and speech-language pathology* [Technical report]. Available from www.asha.org/policy.

Telepractice

American Speech-Language-Hearing Association. (2004). *Speech-language pathologists providing clinical services via telepractice* [Position statement]. Available from www.asha.org/policy.

American Speech-Language-Hearing Association. (2004). *Speech-language pathologists providing clinical services via telepractice* [Technical report]. Available from www.asha.org/policy.

American Speech-Language-Hearing Association. (2005). *Knowledge and skills needed by speech-language pathologists providing clinical services via telepractice* [Technical report]. Available from www.asha.org/policy.

School Services

Collaboration

American Speech-Language-Hearing Association. (1991). *A model for collaborative service delivery for students with language-learning disorders in the public schools* [Relevant paper]. Available from www.asha.org/policy.

Evaluation

American Speech-Language-Hearing Association. (1987). *Considerations for developing and selecting standardized assessment and intervention materials* [Technical report]. Available from www.asha.org/policy.

Facilities
American Speech-Language-Hearing Association. (2003). *Appropriate school facilities for students with speech-language-hearing disorders* [Technical report]. Available from www.asha.org/policy.

Inclusive Practices
American Speech-Language-Hearing Association. (1996). *Inclusive practices for children and youths with communication disorders* [Position statement]. Available from www.asha.org/policy.

Roles and Responsibilities for School-Based Practitioners
American Speech-Language-Hearing Association. (1999). *Guidelines for the roles and responsibilities of the school-based speech-language pathologist* [Guidelines]. Available from www.asha.org/policy.

"Under the Direction of" Rule
American Speech-Language-Hearing Association. (2004). *Medicaid guidance for Speech-language pathology services: Addressing the "under the direction of" rule* [Position statement]. Available from www.asha.org/policy.

American Speech-Language-Hearing Association. (2004). *Medicaid guidance for Speech-language pathology services: Addressing the "under the direction of" rule* [Technical report]. Available from www.asha.org/policy.

American Speech-Language-Hearing Association. (2005). *Medicaid guidance for Speech-language pathology services: Addressing the "under the direction of" rule* [Guidelines]. Available from www.asha.org/policy.

American Speech-Language-Hearing Association. (2005). *Medicaid guidance for Speech-language pathology services: Addressing the "under the direction of" rule* [Knowledge and skills]. Available from www.asha.org/policy.

Workload
American Speech-Language-Hearing Association. (2002). *Workload analysis approach for establishing speech-language caseload standards in the schools* [Guidelines]. Available from www.asha.org/policy.

American Speech-Language-Hearing Association. (2002). *Workload analysis approach for establishing speech-language caseload standards in the schools* [Position statement]. Available from www.asha.org/policy.

American Speech-Language-Hearing Association. (2002). *Workload analysis approach for establishing speech-language caseload standards in the schools* [Technical report]. Available from www.asha.org/policy.

Ad Hoc Committee on the Scope of Practice in Speech-Language Pathology
© Copyright 2007 American Speech-Language-Hearing Association. All rights reserved.
Disclaimer: The American Speech-Language-Hearing Association disclaims any liability to any party for the accuracy, completeness, or availability of these documents, or for any damages arising out of the use of the documents and any information they contain.

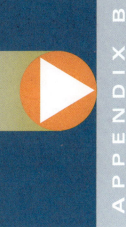

APPENDIX B
Speech-Language Pathology Clinical Fellowship (SLPCF) Report and Rating Form

 About This Document

The Speech-Language Pathology Clinical Fellowship (SLPCF) Report and Rating Form is part of an application for membership and certification to be obtained from the American Speech-Language-Hearing Association (ASHA). This document requests the clinical fellow's name and contact information, the mentor's name and account number, the facility name and location where the fellowship took place, the duration of fellowship, a breakdown of the fellowship activities, the mentor's rating of the clinical fellow's skills, the mentor's recommendations and verification, and the signatures of both mentor and clinical fellow at the completion of the fellowship.

SPEECH-LANGUAGE PATHOLOGY CLINICAL FELLOWSHIP (SLPCF) REPORT AND RATING FORM
2005 CERTIFICATION STANDARDS

INSTRUCTIONS:
- ► An application for Membership and Certification must be submitted at this time if you have not already done so.
- ► A separate SLPCF Report and Rating Form must be submitted for each change in mentor, location, or regularly scheduled hours worked per week.
- ► All blanks and boxes must be filled in. Incomplete Report & Rating forms will be returned and will delay the processing of your application.
- ► A full-time SLPCF consists of a minimum of 35 hours worked per week and equals 1,260 hours throughout the 36-week SLPCF. The SLPCF must consist of at least 36 mentoring activities, including 18 hours of on-site direct client contact observations and 18 other monitoring activities.
- ► Professional experience of less than 5 hours per week **cannot** be used to meet the SLPCF requirement.
- ► Use **black ink only** when completing this form. Print all information clearly.

Section 1. Speech-Language Pathology Clinical Fellow Information

Name _____   _____
       Last   First   Middle   Maiden/Former

Home Address _____
              Street   City   State   Zip Code

Home Phone Number (____)_____   Social Security Number _____-____-_____

I understand that it is my responsibility to verify my SLPCF Mentor holds and maintains current ASHA certification in speech-language pathology throughout the CF experience in order for the experience to be accepted as meeting standards.

_____   _____   _____
Signature of SLP Clinical Fellow   Date   ASHA Account #

Section 2. SLPCF Mentor Information

Name _____   Mentor's ASHA Account Number _____

I verify that I hold current ASHA certification in speech-language pathology and understand that I must maintain this certification throughout the SLPCF experience in order for the experience to be accepted as meeting standards.

_____   _____
Signature of SLPCF Mentor   Date

Section 3. SLPCF Setting Information

Facility Name _____   Phone Number (____)_____

Address _____
         Street   City   State   Zip Code

Section 4. SLPCF Duration (beginning and ending dates)

► The beginning date of this SLPCF is ____/____/____   The ending date of this SLPCF is ____/____/____

► Total number of weeks for this SLPCF _____

Section 5. SLPCF Activity Information (How many hours per week did you work in direct clinical contact?)

- ► At least 80% of the SLPCF work week must be in direct clinical contact (assessment/diagnosis/evaluation, screening, treatment, report writing, family/client consultation, and/or counseling) related to the management process of individuals who exhibit communication difficulties.
- ► Do not include travel or lunch hours.
- ► Do not enter percentages or ranges of time.
- ► If the number of hours you work per week varies, you may estimate the number of hours you work in a typical week. Work weeks that consist of less than 5 hours cannot be counted towards the clinical fellowship experience.
- ► Indicate the number of hours per week you spent in each of the following activities:

    _____ Assessment/diagnosis/evaluation
    _____ Screening
    _____ Treatment (direct and indirect services)
    _____ Activities related to client management (report writing, family/client consultation, and/or counseling, etc.)
    _____ Other (includes in-service training and presentations)

    _____ Total hours per week

Appendix B   131

SLP Clinical Fellow's Name _____ (please print)

Section 6. SLPCF Skills Rating Chart Instructions for the SLPCF Mentor
▶ Circle the rating that corresponds to each skill. See the Clinical Fellowship Skills Inventory for a description of each skill.
▶ Rate the clinical fellow on 18 skills, using the N/A (Not Applicable) rating only for skills 13 and 18.
▶ Discuss the ratings with the SLP Clinical Fellow.
▶ Ensure each segment is equal to one-third of the CF experience. *The core skills for SLP are 2-5, 8-11, and 14-17.

SEGMENT 1	SEGMENT 2	SEGMENT 3
Beginning date _____ Ending date _____	Beginning date _____ Ending date _____	Beginning date _____ Ending date _____
SLP Skills Ratings	SLP Skills Ratings	SLP Skills Ratings
1 5 4 3 2 1	1 5 4 3 2 1	1 5 4 3 2 1
2* 5 4 3 2 1	2* 5 4 3 2 1	2* 5 4 3 2 1
3* 5 4 3 2 1	3* 5 4 3 2 1	3* 5 4 3 2 1
4* 5 4 3 2 1	4* 5 4 3 2 1	4* 5 4 3 2 1
5* 5 4 3 2 1	5* 5 4 3 2 1	5* 5 4 3 2 1
6 5 4 3 2 1	6 5 4 3 2 1	6 5 4 3 2 1
7 5 4 3 2 1	7 5 4 3 2 1	7 5 4 3 2 1
8* 5 4 3 2 1	8* 5 4 3 2 1	8* 5 4 3 2 1
9* 5 4 3 2 1	9* 5 4 3 2 1	9* 5 4 3 2 1
10* 5 4 3 2 1	10* 5 4 3 2 1	10* 5 4 3 2 1
11* 5 4 3 2 1	11* 5 4 3 2 1	11* 5 4 3 2 1
12 5 4 3 2 1	12 5 4 3 2 1	12 5 4 3 2 1
13 5 4 3 2 1 N/A	13 5 4 3 2 1 N/A	13 5 4 3 2 1 N/A
14* 5 4 3 2 1	14* 5 4 3 2 1	14* 5 4 3 2 1
15* 5 4 3 2 1	15* 5 4 3 2 1	15* 5 4 3 2 1
16* 5 4 3 2 1	16* 5 4 3 2 1	16* 5 4 3 2 1
17* 5 4 3 2 1	17* 5 4 3 2 1	17* 5 4 3 2 1
18 5 4 3 2 1 N/A	18 5 4 3 2 1 N/A	18 5 4 3 2 1 N/A
SLPCF Mentor's Signature: _____ Clinical Fellow's Signature: _____ Date of Feedback Session: _____	SLPCF Mentor's Signature: _____ Clinical Fellow's Signature: _____ Date of Feedback Session: _____	SLPCF Mentor's Signature: _____ Clinical Fellow's Signature: _____ Date of Feedback Session: _____

Section 7. SLPCF Mentor's Recommendations and Verification of Information

☐ Yes ☐ No   I recommend that the SLPCF experience documented on this form be accepted by the CFCC as meeting the requirements for the CCC-SLP. (If No, attach a rationale and documentation for your answer.)

☐ Yes ☐ No   I affirm that there were at least 12 supervisory activities during each segment of the SLPCF, including 6 hours of on-site observations of direct client contact and 6 other mentoring activities. (If No, attach explanation)

☐ Yes ☐ No   I affirm that alternative methods of observation/mentoring activities were not used. (If alternative methods of observation/mentoring activities were used, prior approval was obtained from the CFCC before using those alternative methods.)

Section 8. Signatures of SLPCF Mentor and SLP Clinical Fellow
We, the SLPCF Mentor and the SLP Clinical Fellow, verify that we have discussed this report. We have verified that the mentor's certification was current throughout the CF experience. We verify that we have completed the required evaluations. We further verify that we are not related in any manner.

Signature of SLPCF Mentor _____   Date _____

Signature of SLP Clinical Fellow _____   Date _____

NOTE: This report must be signed/submitted AFTER the end date of the experience reported on this form. If it is signed prior to the end date, it will be returned and will delay the processing of your application for certification.

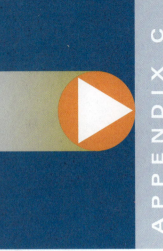

Code of Ethics

 ## Preamble

The preservation of the highest standards of integrity and ethical principles is vital to the responsible discharge of obligations by speech-language pathologists, audiologists, and speech, language, and hearing scientists. This Code of Ethics sets forth the fundamental principles and rules considered essential to this purpose.

Every individual who is (a) a member of the American Speech-Language-Hearing Association, whether certified or not, (b) a nonmember holding the Certificate of Clinical Competence from the Association, (c) an applicant for membership or certification, or (d) a Clinical Fellow seeking to fulfill standards for certification shall abide by this Code of Ethics.

Any violation of the spirit and purpose of this Code shall be considered unethical. Failure to specify any particular responsibility or practice in this Code of Ethics shall not be construed as denial of the existence of such responsibilities or practices.

The fundamentals of ethical conduct are described by Principles of Ethics and by Rules of Ethics as they relate to the responsibility to persons served, the public, speech-language pathologists, audiologists, and speech, language, and hearing scientists, and to the conduct of research and scholarly activities.

Principles of Ethics, aspirational and inspirational in nature, form the underlying moral basis for the Code of Ethics. Individuals shall observe these principles as affirmative obligations under all conditions of professional activity.

Rules of Ethics are specific statements of minimally acceptable professional conduct or of prohibitions and are applicable to all individuals.

 ## Principle of Ethics I

Individuals shall honor their responsibility to hold paramount the welfare of persons they serve professionally or who are participants in research and scholarly activities, and they shall treat animals involved in research in a humane manner.

© Copyright 2014 American Speech-Language-Hearing Association. All rights reserved.
Disclaimer: The American Speech-Language-Hearing Association disclaims any liability to any party for the accuracy, completeness, or availability of these documents, or for any damages arising out of the use of the documents and any information they contain.

Rules of Ethics

A. Individuals shall provide all services competently.
B. Individuals shall use every resource, including referral when appropriate, to ensure that high-quality service is provided.
C. Individuals shall not discriminate in the delivery of professional services or the conduct of research and scholarly activities on the basis of race or ethnicity, gender, gender identity/gender expression, age, religion, national origin, sexual orientation, or disability.
D. Individuals shall not misrepresent the credentials of assistants, technicians, support personnel, students, Clinical Fellows, or any others under their supervision, and they shall inform those they serve professionally of the name and professional credentials of persons providing services.
E. Individuals who hold the Certificate of Clinical Competence shall not delegate tasks that require the unique skills, knowledge, and judgment that are within the scope of their profession to assistants, technicians, support personnel, or any nonprofessionals over whom they have supervisory responsibility.
F. Individuals who hold the Certificate of Clinical Competence may delegate tasks related to provision of clinical services to assistants, technicians, support personnel, or any other persons only if those services are appropriately supervised, realizing that the responsibility for client welfare remains with the certified individual.
G. Individuals who hold the Certificate of Clinical Competence may delegate tasks related to provision of clinical services that require the unique skills, knowledge, and judgment that are within the scope of practice of their profession to students only if those services are appropriately supervised. The responsibility for client welfare remains with the certified individual.
H. Individuals shall fully inform the persons they serve of the nature and possible effects of services rendered and products dispensed, and they shall inform participants in research about the possible effects of their participation in research conducted.
I. Individuals shall evaluate the effectiveness of services rendered and of products dispensed, and they shall provide services or dispense products only when benefit can reasonably be expected.
J. Individuals shall not guarantee the results of any treatment or procedure, directly or by implication; however, they may make a reasonable statement of prognosis.
K. Individuals shall not provide clinical services solely by correspondence.
L. Individuals may practice by telecommunication (e.g., telehealth/e-health), where not prohibited by law.
M. Individuals shall adequately maintain and appropriately secure records of professional services rendered, research and scholarly activities conducted, and products dispensed, and they shall allow access to these records only when authorized or when required by law.
N. Individuals shall not reveal, without authorization, any professional or personal information about identified persons served professionally or identified participants involved in research and scholarly activities unless doing so is necessary to protect the welfare of the person or of the community or is otherwise required by law.
O. Individuals shall not charge for services not rendered, nor shall they misrepresent services rendered, products dispensed, or research and scholarly activities conducted.
P. Individuals shall enroll and include persons as participants in research or teaching demonstrations only if their participation is voluntary, without coercion, and with their informed consent.
Q. Individuals whose professional services are adversely affected by substance abuse or other health-related conditions shall seek professional assistance and, where appropriate, withdraw from the affected areas of practice.
R. Individuals shall not discontinue service to those they are serving without providing reasonable notice.

Principle of Ethics II

Individuals shall honor their responsibility to achieve and maintain the highest level of professional competence and performance.

Rules of Ethics

A. Individuals shall engage in only those aspects of the professions that are within the scope of their professional practice and competence, considering their level of education, training, and experience.
B. Individuals shall engage in lifelong learning to maintain and enhance professional competence and performance.
C. Individuals shall not require or permit their professional staff to provide services or conduct research activities that exceed the staff member's competence, level of education, training, and experience.
D. Individuals shall ensure that all equipment used to provide services or to conduct research and scholarly activities is in proper working order and is properly calibrated.

Principle of Ethics III

Individuals shall honor their responsibility to the public by promoting public understanding of the professions, by supporting the development of services designed to fulfill the unmet needs of the public, and by providing accurate information in all communications involving any aspect of the professions, including the dissemination of research findings and scholarly activities, and the promotion, marketing, and advertising of products and services.

Rules of Ethics

A. Individuals shall not misrepresent their credentials, competence, education, training, experience, or scholarly or research contributions.
B. Individuals shall not participate in professional activities that constitute a conflict of interest.
C. Individuals shall refer those served professionally solely on the basis of the interest of those being referred and not on any personal interest, financial or otherwise.
D. Individuals shall not misrepresent research, diagnostic information, services rendered, results of services rendered, products dispensed, or the effects of products dispensed.
E. Individuals shall not defraud or engage in any scheme to defraud in connection with obtaining payment, reimbursement, or grants for services rendered, research conducted, or products dispensed.
F. Individuals' statements to the public shall provide accurate information about the nature and management of communication disorders, about the professions, about professional services, about products for sale, and about research and scholarly activities.
G. Individuals' statements to the public when advertising, announcing, and marketing their professional services; reporting research results; and promoting products shall adhere to professional standards and shall not contain misrepresentations.

Principle of Ethics IV

Individuals shall honor their responsibilities to the professions and their relationships with colleagues, students, and members of other professions and disciplines.

Rules of Ethics

A. Individuals shall uphold the dignity and autonomy of the professions, maintain harmonious interprofessional and intraprofessional relationships, and accept the professions' self-imposed standards.

B. Individuals shall prohibit anyone under their supervision from engaging in any practice that violates the Code of Ethics.

C. Individuals shall not engage in dishonesty, fraud, deceit, or misrepresentation.

D. Individuals shall not engage in any form of unlawful harassment, including sexual harassment or power abuse.

E. Individuals shall not engage in any other form of conduct that adversely reflects on the professions or on the individual's fitness to serve persons professionally.

F. Individuals shall not engage in sexual activities with clients, students, or research participants over whom they exercise professional authority or power.

G. Individuals shall assign credit only to those who have contributed to a publication, presentation, or product. Credit shall be assigned in proportion to the contribution and only with the contributor's consent.

H. Individuals shall reference the source when using other persons' ideas, research, presentations, or products in written, oral, or any other media presentation or summary.

I. Individuals' statements to colleagues about professional services, research results, and products shall adhere to prevailing professional standards and shall contain no misrepresentations.

J. Individuals shall not provide professional services without exercising independent professional judgment, regardless of referral source or prescription.

K. Individuals shall not discriminate in their relationships with colleagues, students, and members of other professions and disciplines on the basis of race or ethnicity, gender, gender identity/gender expression, age, religion, national origin, sexual orientation, or disability.

L. Individuals shall not file or encourage others to file complaints that disregard or ignore facts that would disprove the allegation, nor should the Code of Ethics be used for personal reprisal, as a means of addressing personal animosity, or as a vehicle for retaliation.

M. Individuals who have reason to believe that the Code of Ethics has been violated shall inform the Board of Ethics.

N. Individuals shall comply fully with the policies of the Board of Ethics in its consideration and adjudication of complaints of violations of the Code of Ethics.

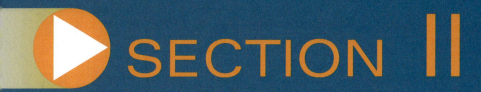

Developmental Communication Disorders

Section Outline

- **Chapter 6:** Speech Sound Disorders in Children, 139
- **Chapter 7:** Language Disorders in Young Children, 167
- **Chapter 8:** Spoken Language Disorders in School-Age Populations, 193
- **Chapter 9:** Written Language Disorders in the School-Age Population, 209
- **Chapter 10:** Autism Spectrum Disorders, 225
- **Chapter 11:** Stuttering and Other Fluency Disorders, 241

6
Speech Sound Disorders in Children

GREGORY L. LOF, PhD
AND MAGGIE WATSON, PhD

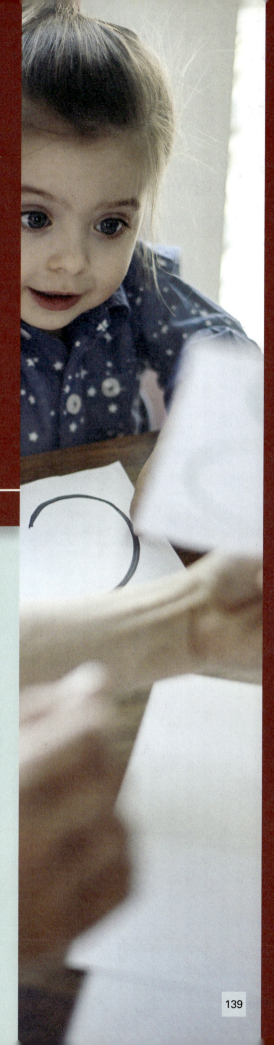

Chapter Outline
- Phonetics and Basic Terms, 140
- Models (Theories) of Acquisition and Disorders, 143
- Typical Development, 147
- Assessment of Speech Sound Disorders (SSD), 153
- Treatment of Speech Sound Disorders, 158
- References, 165

Phonetics and Basic Terms

Three Dimensions of English Consonants

1. Voicing: vibration of the vocal folds (Table 6-1).
   a. Voiced (+ voicing).
   b. Voiceless (− voicing).
2. Place of articulation: where the sound is formed in the oral cavity (Figure 6-1).
   a. Bilabial (bi = two; labial = lips): b, p, m, w, wh.
   b. Labiodental (labial = lips; dental = teeth): f, v.
   c. Interdental (inter = between; dental = teeth): θ, ð (*sometimes called dentals*).
   d. Alveolar (alveolar ridge): t, d, s, z, l, n.
   e. Palatal (hard palate): ʃ, ʒ, tʃ, dʒ, r, j.
   f. Velar (velum, or soft palate): k, g, ŋ.
   g. Glottal (vocal folds): h, ʔ.
3. Manner of articulation: how the sound is formed.
   a. Stops (Table 6-2).
      (1) Formed by a complete closure of the vocal tract in different locations in the oral cavity. The air is built up behind this closure and then released.
      (2) When the air is released, it may produce a short burst of noise called the "stop burst." This burst is why stops are sometimes called "stop plosives."
      (3) The six stop sounds are:
         (a) p (as in <u>p</u>it).
         (b) b (as in <u>b</u>it).
         (c) t (as in <u>t</u>ip).
         (d) d (as in <u>d</u>ip).
         (e) k (as in <u>k</u>ey).
         (f) g (as in <u>g</u>o).
   b. Nasals (Table 6-3).
      (1) Produced with a complete oral closure but with the velopharynx open so that the air travels through the nasal cavity.
      (2) The three nasal sounds are:
         (a) m (as in <u>m</u>om).
         (b) n (as in <u>n</u>ose).
         (c) ŋ (as in ri<u>ng</u>).
   c. Fricatives (Table 6-4).
      (1) A sound that is produced with a narrow constriction. The air escapes through this constriction and makes a continuous noise.

Table 6-1

Dimensions of Consonant Production		
VOICING	PLACE OF ARTICULATION	MANNER OF ARTICULATION
1. + Voice	1. Bilabial	1. Stop
2. − Voice	2. Labiodental	2. Nasal
	3. Interdental	3. Fricative
	4. Alveolar	4. Affricate
	5. Palatal	5. Liquid
	6. Palatal-Velar	a. Lateral
	7. Glottal	b. Rhotic
		6. Glide

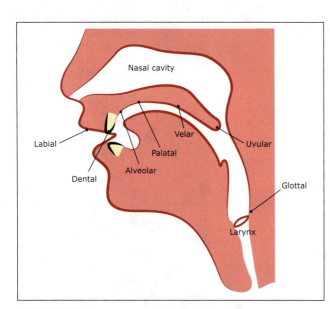

Figure 6-1 Anatomical Locations for Places of Articulation

Table 6-2

Manner: Stops			
	PLACE OF ARTICULATION		
	BILABIAL	ALVEOLAR	VELAR
− Voice	p	t	k
+ Voice	b	d	g

Table 6-3

Manner: Nasals			
	PLACE OF ARTICULATION		
	BILABIAL	ALVEOLAR	VELAR
+ Voice	m	n	ŋ

Table 6-4

Manner: Fricatives					
	PLACE OF ARTICULATION				
	INTERDENTAL	LABIODENTAL	ALVEOLAR	PALATAL	GLOTTAL
− Voice	θ	f	s	ʃ	h
+ Voice	ð	v	z	ʒ	

Table 6-5

Manner: Affricates	
	PLACE OF ARTICULATION
	PALATO-ALVEOLAR
− Voice	tʃ
+ Voice	dʒ

(2) The fricative sounds are:
    (a) θ (as in <u>th</u>umb).
    (b) ð (as in <u>th</u>ose).
    (c) f (as in <u>f</u>or).
    (d) v (as in <u>v</u>ote).
    (e) s (as in <u>s</u>oap).
    (f) z (as in <u>z</u>oo).
    (g) ʃ (as in <u>sh</u>oe).
    (h) ʒ (as in mea<u>s</u>ure).
    (i) h (as in <u>h</u>elp).
d. Affricates (Table 6-5).
   (1) A combination sound, with a stop closure followed by a fricative portion.
   (2) The two affricate sounds are:
    (a) dʒ (as in <u>j</u>eep).
    (b) tʃ (as in <u>ch</u>ip).
e. Liquids (also considered approximates).
   (1) A consonant that is vowel-like; the sound passes through the vocal tract that is constricted only somewhat more than for vowels.
   (2) Types of liquids.
    (a) Lateral: The sound is produced with the tongue tip against the alveolar ridge, with an opening along the sides of the tongue for the air to escape. The lateral liquid sound is:
      • l (as in <u>l</u>eg).
    (b) Rhotic: The sound is produced with the tongue tip curled back and not touching the alveolar ridge or by bunching the tongue in the palatal region. The rhotic liquid sound is:
      • r (as in <u>r</u>un).
f. Glides (also considered approximates) (Table 6-6).

   (1) Also known as a semivowel.
   (2) The production is a gliding motion of the articulators from being partially constricted to a more open state.
   (3) The three glide sounds are:
    (a) j (as in <u>y</u>ellow).
    (b) w (as in <u>w</u>e).
    (c) wh (as in <u>wh</u>ite).

Vowels

1. Vowels are voiced sounds that are produced with an unobstructed vocal tract.
2. Because they are necessary for a syllable, they are also called "syllabics."
3. Types of vowels (Table 6-7).
   a. Monophthongs: sometimes called "pure vowels," because they have a single, unchanging sound quality.

Table 6-6

Manner: Approximants			
	PLACE OF ARTICULATION		
	BILABIAL	ALVEOLAR	PALATAL
+ Voice	w	l	j, r
− Voice	wh		

Table 6-7

Vowel Phonetic Symbol and Exemplary Words			
MONOPHTHONGS		DIPHTHONGS	
i	he	aɪ	bye
ɪ	hid	ɔɪ	boy
e	ate	aʊ	how
ɛ	head	eɪ	bay
æ	had	oʊ	hoe
a	path		
ʌ	hub		
ə	<u>a</u>lone		
ɝ	her		
ɚ	fath<u>er</u>		
u	who		
ʊ	book		
o	hoe		
ɔ	law		
ɑ	hop		

b. Diphthongs: produced with a gradually changing articulation that produces a complex, dynamic sound quality.
  (1) The "onglide" is the position the articulators are in at the beginning of one vowel.
  (2) The "offglide" is the position at the end of the other vowel.
4. Monophthong vowel descriptions.
  a. Tongue height.
    (1) Refers to the relative vertical position of the tongue body.
    (2) High vowels have the tongue position near the roof of the mouth. Low vowels have the tongue in the most depressed portion of the mouth. Mid vowels are in between.
    (3) For example, in these words, the tongue movement for the vowel proceeds from high to low: meat → mitt → mate → met → mat.
  b. Tongue advancement.
    (1) Refers to the front-back, or anterior-posterior, positioning of the tongue in the mouth.
    (2) Descriptors for tongue advancement.
      (a) Front.
      (b) Central.
      (c) Back.
    (3) For example, in these words, the tongue movement for the vowel proceeds from front to back: heat → hurt → hoot.
  c. Tenseness/laxness.
    (1) Refers to the tenseness or laxness of the articulatory mechanisms during vowel production. Lax vowels are short, lower and slightly more centralized than are tense vowels.
    (2) Some prefer to use the word "length" rather than tenseness.
      (a) Tense vowels are longer in duration.
    (3) For example, /i/ is considered to be a tense vowel, while /ɪ/ is a lax vowel.
  d. Lip configuration.
    (1) Refers to the degree of lip rounding during vowel production. Rounded lips lengthen the vocal tract, which in turn produces acoustic changes.
    (2) Other terms for lip rounding include: protrusion, retraction, spreading, narrowing.
    (3) For example, /o/ is a rounded vowel, while /i/ is unrounded.
5. Vowel quadrangle (Figures 6-2 and 6-3).
  a. A schematic of how the different vowel sounds are displayed on the tongue.
  b. Front vowels: i, ɪ, e, ɛ, æ.
  c. Central vowels: ɝ, ɚ, ə, ʌ.
  d. Back vowels: u, ʊ, o, ɔ, ɑ.
6. Diphthong vowel descriptions.
  a. There are five diphthongs: aɪ, ɔɪ, aʊ, eɪ, oʊ.

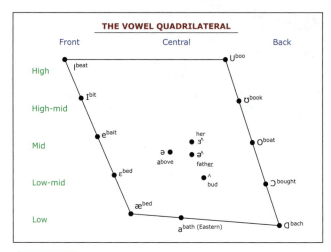

Figure 6-2 The Vowel Quadrilateral

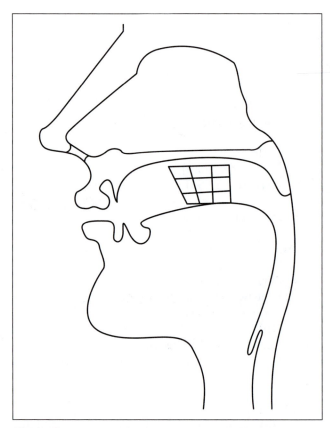

Figure 6-3 A Schematic of Possible Tongue Positions in the Mouth, with Regard to the Vowel Quadrilateral

  b. Phonemic diphthongs.
    (1) Cannot be reduced to a monophthong.
      (a) aɪ, ɔɪ, aʊ.
  c. Nonphonemic diphthongs.
    (1) Can be reduced to a monophthong.
      (a) eɪ, oʊ.

Other Phonetic Terms

1. Allophone: a nondistinctive phonetic variant for a phoneme.
   a. For example, the /k/ is produced differently for "ski," "key" and "caw," but it is still /k/.
2. Coarticulation: the influence of phonetic context on speech production.
   a. For example, the vowel in the word "man" is nasalized due to the surrounding nasal consonants.
3. Cognate: one of a pair of sounds that are different by just one phonetic feature.
   a. For example, /s/ and /z/ are voiced cognates.
   b. For English, the voicing aspect primarily distinguishes cognates.
4. Diacritics: a mark added to a phonetic character to indicate some form of a modification.
   a. Diacritics are used for narrow transcription.
   b. For example, there are diacritic marks for nasality or advanced tongue protrusion.
5. Dialect: different usage patterns in terms of pronunciation, vocabulary and/or grammar within the same language.
   a. For example, speakers in some parts of Louisiana speak the Cajun dialect.
6. Egressive sounds: formed from an outflowing stream.
7. Flap: a modified stop, in which a rapid flapping motion of the tongue tip contacts the alveolar ridge.
   a. The flap is used for the /t/ and /d/ in words like "city" or "ladder."
8. Homorganic: sounds that have the same place of articulation.
   a. For example, /m/ and /b/.
9. Ingressive sounds: formed from an inflowing airstream.
10. Morpheme: the minimal unit of meaning, the smallest unit of language that carries a semantic interpretation.
11. Obstruent: stops, fricatives and affricates because they have a complete, or narrow, constriction of the vocal tract.
12. Phoneme: the basic sound segment that has the linguistic function of distinguishing morphemes.
13. Phonology: the study of sound systems of language; the structure and function of sounds in languages.
14. Prevocalic: a sound that occurs before a vowel.
15. Prosody: involves the suprasegmental characteristics of intonation, stress patterns, loudness variations, pausing and rhythm.
16. Postvocalic: a sound that occurs after a vowel.
17. Rhotacization: a sound that has r coloring.
18. Sibilant: a speech sound with an intense, high-pitched noise.
    a. For example, /s/ and /ʃ/.
19. Strident: a speech sound with an intense frication noise like the sibilants but that also includes /f/ and /v/.
20. Suprasegmental: prosody characteristics that bridge across phonetic segments.
21. Syllable: unit of speech consisting of at least a vowel, which may be surrounded by one or more consonants.
    a. The syllable onset is at the beginning optional consonant.
    b. The nucleus is the vowel itself.
    c. The optional ending consonant sound is called the coda.

Models (Theories) of Acquisition and Disorders

Behavioral Theory

1. Aligns with traditional views of behavioral explanations of behavior, as discussed by individuals such as Skinner, Omsted and Mowrer.
2. Views verbal development as learned, using the processes of:
   a. Contingent reinforcement.
   b. Stimulus-response.
3. The development of speech sounds is shaped from infants' babbling by mature speakers in the environment.
4. During infancy, the vocalizations of caretakers' and infants' own vocalizations take on secondary reinforcement.
5. The consequences of the infants' vocalizations (i.e., reinforcement) is the impetus for learning.
6. Those sounds that best match those of the ambient language are selectively reinforced by the caregiver as well as the child noticing the similarity between their own productions and those produced by others.
7. Strengths of this theory.
   a. It is compatible with learning theories.
   b. It associates babbling with the development of meaningful speech.
   c. It acknowledges the role of input and speech sound perception.

8. Criticisms of this theory.
   a. There is a lack of data to support the role of caretakers' use of selective reinforcement of speech sounds for development.
   b. The child's role is seen as passive.
9. Clinical application of this theory.
   a. The use of reinforcement for correct production of speech sounds.
   b. Control of stimuli to elicit productions during intervention.
   c. Intervention can also be directed in helping children establish phonemic contrasts.

Distinctive Features Theory

1. Attributed to Roman Jakobson and colleagues, who defined a small set of "properties" or "features" to describe speech sounds.
2. Features represent acoustic and articulatory aspects of speech sounds.
3. Those features included were described as binary, since each feature was either present (+) or absent (–).
4. Groups of speech sounds that shared features were described as "natural phoneme classes."
5. In this theory, "marked" sounds are those that have additional features as compared to other sounds, e.g., /z/ is "marked" compared to /s/ because of its voiced feature.
6. Emphasizes the development of "feature contrasts," not individual speech sounds.
   a. Phonological development is realized as the development of feature contrasts, beginning with maximal contrasts (e.g., consonants vs. vowels, nasal consonants vs. oral consonants, etc.).
   b. Described a hierarchy of feature contrast development.
   c. Babbling is not related to the onset of meaningful speech.
7. Strengths of this theory.
   a. It acknowledges the rule-governed nature of phonological systems.
   b. Most children do acquire certain classes of sounds before others.
8. Criticisms of this theory.
   a. Universal order of development has not been proven.
   b. Most children do not acquire certain classes of sounds before others.
9. Clinical application of this theory.
   a. The analysis of speech sound substitutions according to distinctive feature properties that are/are not present.
   b. Intervention can be directed at training distinctive features with the potential of remediating a group of sounds that are affected by a particular missing feature such as stridency or voicing.

Generative Phonology

1. An expansion of Distinctive Features Theory by including concepts such as "underlying representations," "surface forms" and "phonological rules."
   a. Underlying representation: an abstract, mental representation or what is stored mentally about a word form.
   b. Surface form: the speaker's actual productions.
   c. Phonological rules: rules that explain the discrepancies between the underlying representation and surface form of a word.
2. Generative Phonology, similar to Generative Grammar Theory, proposes two levels of language, including the surface level (i.e., what is spoken) and a deep level (i.e., an abstract level of representation of language).
3. Generative Phonology also describes speech sounds as "natural" or "marked."
   a. Natural sounds: those that are relatively easy to produce and occur frequently in languages around the world.
   b. Marked sounds: those that are relatively more difficult to produce and occur less frequently in languages around the world.
4. The notion of underlying representations is used to account for what children know about speech sounds on a continuum of six knowledge types, ranging from "One," representing complete knowledge and always correct productions, to "Six," which encompasses sounds never produced correctly and not present in the phonetic inventory.
5. Phonological rules are expressed using a specific notation system that provides information about the sound change(s) and context (e.g., [s] → [t]/#___ means [s] becomes [t] in the initial positions of words).
6. Generative Phonological Theory focuses on describing phonological patterns that occur in language and identifying universal principles that apply to the phonological systems of languages.
7. Strengths of this theory.
   a. Compatible with other theories of language development.
   b. Attempts to account for differences in what children know about the phonological system and what they are able to produce.
8. Criticisms of this theory.
   a. The complex notation system associated with Generative Phonology is not widely used in clinical situations.

b. The concept of "phonological rules" has been questioned because of its abstract nature.
9. Clinical application of this theory.
   a. Children's speech sound errors are often described according to phonological rules.
   b. Intervention can be directed toward helping children acquire new and appropriate phonological rules.
   c. Levels of phonological knowledge have been used to account for generalization and choosing intervention targets.

Natural Phonology

1. Developed by Stampe (1969).
2. This theory attempts to explain children's phonological acquisition.
3. Children are born with a set of "natural phonological processes" that reflect their developing speech motor systems.
   a. Processes are innate and universal.
   b. These processes simplify the production of speech sounds and sound sequences, such as:
      (1) Replacing fricatives with stops.
      (2) Deleting one consonant from a consonant cluster.
      (3) Substituting glides for liquids.
   c. Application of these natural processes changes the child's productions to a more simplified version of the adult target.
   d. Processes are considered to be mental operations that are influenced by the limitations of human speech production and perception mechanisms.
4. Three broad categories of natural processes have been identified.
   a. Syllable structure processes change the complexity of how words are structured, for example:
      (1) Eliminating speech sound(s) from clusters (i.e., "blue" becomes "bwu").
      (2) Eliminating unstressed syllables from words (i.e., "umbrella" becomes "brella").
      (3) Deleting final consonants in words (i.e., "big" becomes "bi").
   b. Substitution processes change complexity of words by substituting relatively easier-to-produce sounds for more difficult ones, for example:
      (1) Substituting stops for fricatives (i.e., "fin" becomes "pin").
      (2) Substituting stops for affricates (i.e., "chip" becomes "tip").
      (3) Substituting alveolar stops for velar stops (i.e., "cap" becomes "tap").
   c. Assimilatory processes simplify the production of words by changing sounds in words to become more similar to each other, for example:
      (1) Producing "pip" for "lip" (labial assimilation).
      (2) Producing "nine" for "dime" (nasal assimilation).
5. Phonological development, according to the Natural Phonology Theory, is the result of changes in the system through:
   a. Limitation of processes by gradually reducing the instances in which certain processes are used.
   b. Process ordering, in which the application of certain processes reorganize and are no longer used in certain sequences.
   c. Process suppression, in which the process is no longer used.
6. In Natural Phonology Theory underlying representations are assumed to be adult-liked.
7. Strengths of this theory.
   a. Accounts for individual variations in acquiring a phonological system.
   b. Provides good descriptors for children's speech sound error patterns.
   c. Easily adaptable to account for phonological delays and disorders.
8. Criticisms of this theory.
   a. There is no evidence for the mental operations that govern the use and subsequent limitation of phonological processes.
   b. There is no evidence that children's underlying representations for words is adult-like.
   c. The child's role is relatively passive.
9. Clinical application of this theory.
   a. Analysis of children's speech sound errors using the three categories of phonological processes and other descriptors, such as:
      (1) Persistent use of processes used by typical children at younger ages.
      (2) Use of atypical or unusual processes.
      (3) Systematic sound preferences.
      (4) The inconsistent use of phonological processes.
   b. Treatment emphasizes the suppression of the use of inappropriate phonological processes.
   c. Treatment emphasizes the use of meaningful communication to assist with the progression of phonological process suppression.

Prosodic Theory

1. Emphasizes the perception of whole words as early word productions.
2. Early word productions are highly variable across children due to differences in input.
3. The salient features of words that children initially perceive and produce include prosodic information and syllable structure of words.

4. Children also perceive similarities across words that share certain features, such as nasality, and use that information to form patterns that influence their word productions.
5. Phonological development occurs as children's perception increases, allowing existing patterns to change and new ones to develop.
6. Strengths of this theory.
    a. Includes both perception and input.
    b. Accounts for individual learning due to variations in input.
    c. The child is viewed as an active learner by recognizing features shared by words.
7. Criticisms of this theory.
    a. Includes both perception and input.
    b. Does not consider the development of individual speech sounds or general patterns of development across children.
8. Clinical application of this theory.
    a. This theory does not have clinical application.

Interactionist-Discovery (Cognitive) Theory

1. This theory emphasizes the child's individual active learning processes as important for phonological development, primarily emphasizing the early phases of acquisition.
2. The child discovers the structure of language by forming and testing hypotheses about the language system.
3. Children create their own phonological rules as they attempt to bridge the gap between what is perceived and their own productions.
4. Phonological strategies and rules used by children are not viewed as innate.
5. Children apply their own strategies in an attempt to discover the rules and patterns of language.
6. Children's individual learning strategies account for the differences in phonological acquisition evident across children, especially in the early stages of development.
7. Strengths of this theory.
    a. Children are viewed as "active" learners and generate their own learning strategies.
    b. Accounts for individual variation in phonological development.
    c. Includes both perceptual and productive strategies.
8. Criticisms of this theory.
    a. The emphasis is on the earliest stages of development.
9. Clinical application of this theory.
    a. Useful for generating intervention plans for children at the earliest stages of development.

Nonlinear Theories

1. Nonlinear theories emphasize the hierarchical relationships that exist across production units, including speech segments, syllables and words.
2. A variety of nonlinear theories have been developed, with each emphasizing different aspects of the relationship across production units of segments and syllables.
    a. Metrical Phonology.
        (1) Focuses on the prosodic features within syllables, such as stress.
        (2) This theory examines the hierarchy of "syllables," "feet" and "segments."
        (3) Syllables are comprised of:
            (a) Onset: consonants that precede the vowel.
            (b) Vowel (also called the nucleus).
            (c) Rime: nucleus and consonants following the vowel.
            (d) In addition, the term "coda" refers to the consonants following the nucleus.
        (4) The foot consists of a stressed syllable and one or more unstressed syllables.
        (5) Variations in stress across syllables create the rhythm of speech.
    b. Feature Geometry.
        (1) This theory examines the relationship of features within segments.
        (2) Within a segment, some features dominate over other features.
        (3) Certain features tend to combine with each other more than others.
        (4) Differences in features are related to speech production capabilities, reflecting the individual or combined movements and functions of the articulators.
        (5) Each level is referred to as a tier, while the term "node" denotes those features that are dominant and thus higher in the hierarchy.
        (6) Feature spreading explains how some features affect the production of other features (referred to as "assimilation" in other theories).
    c. Optimality Theory.
        (1) Input representation: the mental representation for speech.
        (2) Output representation: the surface forms, or actual productions.
        (3) The term "output constraint" refers to the rules that limit production possibilities for words.
        (4) "Faithfulness constraints" strive to create the best match between the input and output representations.
        (5) Constraints are innate and universal.
        (6) Languages around the world vary in how constraints are ranked.

d. Gestural Phonology (also known as Articulatory Phonology).
   (1) The basic units of the phonological system are articulation gestures, which are abstract descriptions of articulation movements.
   (2) Utterances are produced that reflect a gestural score, or the articulation movements associated with an utterance.
   (3) Gestures are represented on different levels or tiers to denote independence, with some gestures grouped together to demonstrate production similarities.
   (4) Other tiers represent syllable structure and speech rhythm.
3. Clinical application of nonlinear theories.
   a. Clinical application of nonlinear theories for the analysis of speech sound disorders and choosing treatment targets has primarily involved case studies.

Typical Development

Development of Physical Structures for Speech

1. Changes in the size and shape of the vocal tract.
   a. When compared with adults, the infant has:
      (1) A shorter, flatter vocal tract.
      (2) A different shape for the vocal tract.
      (3) A shorter pharyngeal cavity.
      (4) Tongue mass that is placed more forward in the oral cavity.
      (5) More gradual bend in the oropharyngeal canal.
      (6) Higher laryngeal placement.
      (7) Close approximation of the velopharynx and the epiglottis.

Prelinguistic Development

1. Infant speech perception.
   a. Experimental methods to demonstrate perceptual skills include measuring sucking and visually reinforcing head turning.
   b. Abilities such as localization, discrimination of some phonemic differences and preference for human voice are present very early in development.
   c. Infants can be conditioned to discriminate speech sounds as young as four days old.
   d. Infants up to age 6–8 months have been shown to discriminate two similar nonnative speech sounds.
      (1) By age 10–12 months, this ability disappears.
2. Infant prelinguistic speech production.
   a. Phonation stage (birth–1 month).
      (1) Reflexive sounds.
      (2) Vegetative sounds, such as coughing, burping, sucking, grunting, and sighs.
         (a) Brief duration.
         (b) Consonantal (stops, fricatives and clicks).
         (c) Lack of voicing.
         (d) Ingressive airflow.
   b. Coo and goo stage (2–3 months).
      (1) Quasi-resonant nuclei, vowel-like sounds with limited resonance.
      (2) Sounds that are similar to back consonants (i.e., velars and glottals) and back vowels.
      (3) Vocal contagions and some self-imitations may occur.
   c. Exploration/expansion stage (4–6 months).
      (1) Vocal play.
      (2) Squeals, raspberries, trills, friction noises.
      (3) Fully resonated vowels.
      (4) Marginal babbling, consisting of consonant-vowel (CV) and vowel-consonant (VC) sequences.
      (5) Great variation in pitch and loudness.
   d. Canonical babbling (7–9 months).
      (1) Reduplicated babbling of strings of similar CV syllables.
      (2) Nonreduplicated, or variegated, babbling of adjacent CV syllables consisting of different consonants and vowels.
      (3) Stops, nasals and glides, vowels ɛ (bet), ɪ (bit) and ʌ (but).
   e. Jargon (10 months and older).
      (1) Production of variegated babbling with adult-like intonation.
      (2) Most frequent consonants include /h/, /d/, /b/, /m/, /t/, /w/, /j/.
      (3) Most common vowels include /ɑ/, /i/, /u/.
3. Transition to first words.
   a. Great deal of similarity between babbling and first words.
   b. Overlap between babbling and production of meaningful words.
   c. Use of protowords (also known as phonetically consistent forms [PCFs], vocables and invented words), whose characteristics include:
      (1) Not an adult-like word.

(2) Function as words for the infant.
(3) Produced with some phonetic consistency.
(4) Produced with some semantic consistency.

Phonological Characteristics of the First 50 Words

1. Single syllables and reduplicated syllables.
   a. Fewer closed syllables are used.
2. Stops, nasals and glides are the most frequently used sound classes.
3. The first vowels are typically /ɑ/, /i/, /u/.
4. May produce a few "progressive idioms," or words that are more advanced than the child's typical word productions.
5. May produce a few "regressive idioms," or words that are less advanced than the child's typical word productions.
6. Word productions at this stage are often called "pre-systematic," since application of systematic phonological rules and principles is often not evident.
7. Words that are attempted may evidence selectivity.
   a. Imitation may be limited to the child's production capacities.
8. A great deal of individual variability in production is evident.
   a. May produce some phones correctly in some words, but not others.
   b. May produce the same word in different ways.
9. Preference and avoidance of some speech sounds and words may be observed.

Two-Year-Olds: Beginning of Systematicity

1. Children between the ages of 15 and 24 months.
   a. More consonants in the initial position than the final position.
   b. Consonant inventories by age 24 months.
      (1) Word initial: [b, d, g, t, k, m, n, h, w, f, s].
      (2) Word final: [p, t, k, n, r, s].
   c. By age 24 months, the Percentage Consonants Correct (PCC) is 70%.

Speech Sound Development in Preschool-Age Children

1. Data is obtained from "large-*n*" studies or "cross-sectional" studies, since typically a large number of children serve as subjects and are not followed longitudinally.

2. These studies attempted to determine the following for each speech sound:
   a. Age of mastery, or the age at which 90% (some studies use 75%) of the subjects produced the speech sound correctly.
   b. Age of customary production, or the age at which 51% of the subjects produced the speech sound correctly.
3. Methodologies differed across these studies.
   a. Subject selection criteria.
   b. Elicitation methods.
   c. Training of examiners.
   d. Use of imitation.
   e. Criteria for determining age of mastery.
4. Generalization of results across studies by age (results accumulate with increased age).
   a. 3 years: [h, w, m, n, b, p, f].
   b. 4 years: [d, t, j, k, g].
   c. 6 years: [l, dʒ, r, s, z, θ, ð, ʒ].
5. Development of speech sounds can also be categorized according to early, middle and late developing.
   a. Early: [m, b, j, n, w, d, p, h].
   b. Mid: [t, ŋ, k, g, f, v, tʃ, dʒ].
   c. Late: [ʃ, ʒ, θ, ð, s, z, l, r].
6. Development of consonant clusters.
   a. Cluster development is complete by age 7;0.
   b. By age 4: [tw, kw, sp, st, sk, sm, sn].
   c. By age 4;6: [pl, bl, kl, gl, fl, pr, br, tr, dr, kr, gr, fr].
   d. By age 6: [skw, spr, str, skr].
   e. By age 7: [sw, sl, spl, θr].
7. Development of vowels.
   a. Limited information is available on vowel development.
   b. All vowels and diphthongs are produced with over 90% accuracy by age 3 years.
   c. The rhotic diphthongs reach mastery by age 5 or 6.

Early/Mid/Late 8 (In Continuous Speech)

1. Early: [m, b, j, n, w, d, p, h].
2. Mid: [t, ŋ, k, g, f, v, tʃ, dʒ].
3. Late: [ʃ, ʒ, θ, ð, s, z, l, r].

Use and Suppression of Phonological Error Patterns

1. Phonological patterns are systematic sound changes that affect sound classes and the syllabic structure of words.
2. See Table 6-8 for a listing of phonological patterns and their definitions.
3. Phonological pattern suppression.

Table 6-8

Phonological Patterns and Definitions

PROCESS	DEFINITION
Addition of a Syllable	• Addition of an entire syllable to a target word.
Addition of Consonants	• Addition of consonants that are not part of the adult production of the word.
Affrication	• Replacement of a fricative consonant with an affricate consonant. (1) • Addition of a stop component to a continuant phoneme. (2) • An affricate used for a fricative; may occur as a "half-way" step during therapy for elimination of Stopping of Fricatives: *sun*→/tsʌn/; *zoo*→/dzu/.
Alveolarization	• Replacement of consonants made with the lips or teeth with consonants made at the alveolar ridge. (1) • All fricatives move to the alveolar position: *four*→/sɔr/; *shoe*→/su/; *thick*→/sɔk/.
Assimilation, Alveolar	• Production of a phoneme that is more like an alveolar phoneme in the target word: *cat*→/tæt/; *bottle*→/dato/.
Assimilation, Labial	• Production of a phoneme that is more like a labial phoneme in the target word: *cup*→/pʌp/.
Assimilation, Nasal	• Production of a phoneme that is more like a nasal phoneme in the target word: *lunch*→/nʌnʃ/.
Assimilation, Progressive	• Replacement of the final consonant by a consonant that is the same as another consonant in the word or is similar in place, manner, or voicing.
Assimilation, Regressive	• Replacement of the initial consonant by a consonant that is the same as another consonant in the word or is similar in place, manner, or voicing.
Assimilation, Velar	• Production of a phoneme that is more like a velar phoneme in the target word: *kitty*→/kɪki/; *dog*→/gɔg/.
Backing	• Replacement of mid and front consonants with back consonants. • Substitution of a posterior consonant for an anterior consonant (posterior consonants include /k/, /g/, /ŋ/, /h/).
Backing of Alveolars	• Alveolars become velars: /t/→/k/, /d/→/g/.
Backing of Velars	• Alteration of the place of articulation from any consonant to a velar.
Cluster Deletion	• Omission of one or more consonants in a consonant cluster.
Cluster Reduction	• Deletion or replacement of one or more members of a cluster by another phoneme: *stop*→/dap/; *black*→/bæk/; *nest*→/nɛt/.
Cluster/Reduction Across Words	• In two-word phrases in which the first word ends with a consonant and the second begins with a consonant, the child omits one of the consonants: *wish to*→/wɪ tu/; *big boy*→/bɪ bɔɪ/; *is happy*→/ɪ hæpi/.
Cluster Simplification	• Simplification of a consonant cluster by deleting one of the consonants (one consonant may be replaced by another, the cluster may be omitted entirely, or the cluster may be replaced. • Simplification of a consonant sequence (cluster) by deleting one or more of the consonants or by inserting a schwa vowel between them.
Cluster Substitution	• Replacement of one or more consonants in a cluster with another consonant.
Coalescence	• Replacement of two phonemes by a new phoneme that has characteristics of both of the original phonemes. • Production of part of the beginning of a word with part of the end, so that the word is collapsed across syllables.
Consonant Deletion	• Omission of a consonant in the word-initial or word final position (does not include consonant sequences).
Consonant Harmony (Assimilation)	• Replacement of one sound in a word with a sound that is the same as or similar to a second sound occurring elsewhere in a word (the substituted sound assumes some or all of the characteristics of another sound in the word). • Influence of one consonant by another consonant in the same word, so that both are produced at a similar place of articulation.
Consonant Sequence Reduction	• Omission of any consonant in a sequence (consonants not separated by a vowel); (this includes all contiguous consonants as well as clusters that are within syllable boundaries).
Deaffrication	• Replacement of an affricate consonant with a fricative consonant. • Change of an affricate target phoneme to a continuant or a stop. • Replacement of an affricate with a fricative. • Deletion of the stop feature of an affricate, with retention of fricative or continuant feature. • The affricate loses either its stopping aspect or, usually, its fricative aspect /tʃ/→/ʃ/ or /t/; /dʒ/→/ʒ/ or /d/.

Table 6-8

Phonological Patterns and Definitions (*Continued*)

PROCESS	DEFINITION
Deletion of Final Consonants	• See Final Consonant Deletions.
Deletion of Initial Consonants	• Deletion of consonants or clusters in initial position.
Deletion of Medial Consonants	• Deletion of a consonant or cluster occurring between two vowels.
Deletion of Unstressed Syllables	• Unstressed syllables are deleted from multisyllabic words and/or unstressed single syllable words are deleted from phrases: telephone → /tɛfo/; I want to go → /a wa go/.
Denasalization	• Nasals become denasal: mom → /bab/; neck → /dɛk/.
Dentalized and Lateralized Production	• Distortion of consonants (particularly alveolar fricatives) by altering the place of articulation either dentally or laterally.
Devoicing, Initial and Medial	• Deletion of voicing from voiced consonants, not in word-final position.
Depalatalization	• Deletion of a palatal component from a palatal target phoneme. • Movement of the place of articulation of a palatal sound from the palate to a position forward in the mouth, typically the alveolar region.
Epenthesis	• Addition of consonants or vowels. • A schwa (/ə/) is inserted, usually between the two elements of a cluster: bread → /bərɛd/; elm → /ɛləm/; cat → /kætə/.
Final Consonant Deletions	• Deletion of the final consonant of a word. • Deletion of the final consonant or final cluster of a word. • Deletion of the final consonant, so that the production ends with a vowel.
Final Consonant Voicing	• A postvocalic voiceless consonant is replaced by a voiced sound (rare): leaf → /liv/.
Final Devoicing	• Deletion of voicing in word-final voiced consonants, leading to production as voiceless consonants.
Fronting	• Replacement of back consonants and palatal consonants with consonants produced at or in front of the alveolar ridge. • Substitution of an anterior consonant for a posterior consonant (this must be a major place of articulation shift). • Replacement of a velar sound with one produced further forward in the oral cavity (typically an alveolar sound replaces a velar sound). • A more "generalized fronting rule" to account for most sound errors at once: /ʃ/ → /s/; /ʒ/ → /z/; /s/ → /f/.
Fronting of Palatals	• Palatals become alveolars: /ʃ/ → /s/; /ʒ/ → /z/; /tʃ/ → /ts/.
Fronting of Velars	• Velars become alveolars: /k/ → /t/; /g/ → /d/.
Glide Deficiency	• Omission of /w/ or /j/ or substitution with another phoneme.
Gliding	• Replacement of a liquid sound with a glide /w/, /j/. • Substitution of a glide for a liquid sound before a vowel.
Gliding of Fricatives and Affricates	• Replacement of fricatives and affricates with glides. • Fricatives become glides, usually only in the initial position, with final fricatives becoming deleted or stopped: fish → /wɪt/; sun → /jʌn/; from → /wɔg/; soap → /jop/.
Gliding of Liquids	• Production of liquids /l/ and /r/ as glides /w/ and /j/.
Glottal Replacement	• Production of a glottal stop in place of another phoneme.
"H"ing of Stops	• Stops are replaced with the glottal fricative /h/, usually only for initial, voiceless stops: cow → /haʊ/; big → /hɪ/; tie → /haɪ/.
Initial Voicing	• See Voicing, Initial
Labialization	• Replacement of consonants made with the tongue tip with consonants made with the lips.
Liquid /l/ Deficiency	• Omission of /l/ or substitution with another phoneme.
Liquid /r/ Deficiency	• Omission of /r/ or /ɚ/ or substitution with another phoneme.

Table 6-8

Phonological Patterns and Definitions *(Continued)*

PROCESS	DEFINITION
Liquid Simplification	• Gliding or vocalization of liquids. • Replacement of the liquids /l/ or /r/ by /w/ or /j/.
Medial and Final Voicing	• Voicing of voiceless consonants that are not in the word-initial position.
Metathesis	• Transposition of phonemes or syllables (can occur across word boundaries and within words). • Transposition of the order of phonemes in a word or syllable. • The position of two sounds is reversed, although both sounds are produced correctly: ask→/æks/; animals→/æmɪnəlz/; spaghetti→/pɪsgɛti/.
Migration	• Transposition of a single phoneme in a word. • Movement of a sound to another position in the word.
Nasal Deficiency	• Omission of /m/, /n/, /ŋ/ or substitution with other nonnasal phonemes.
Palatal Fronting	• Fronting of a palatal consonant, usually to the alveolar ridge. • Replacement of /ʃ/, /ʒ/, /tʃ/, or /dʒ/ by a more anterior consonant.
Palatalization	• Addition of a palatal component to a nonpalatal target phoneme (manner remains the same). • Alveolar fricatives become palatals: sun→/ʃʌn/.
Postvocalic Singleton Consonant Omission	• Deletion of a singleton consonant that terminates a syllable; also referred to as CV preference, open syllable, or final consonant deletion.
Prevocalic Devoicing	• A voiceless sound replaces a prevocalic voice sound (rare): bee→/pi/.
Prevocalic Singleton Consonant Omission	• Deletion of a singleton consonant that initiates a syllable.
Prevocalic Voicing	• Voiceless sounds occurring before vowels or other voiced sounds become voiced: top→/dɑp/; cookie→/gʊgi/; pie→/baɪ/.
Reduplication	• Repetition of phonemes or syllables. • Production of an identical or nearly identical repetition of a syllable, usually to represent a multi-syllabic word. • Conversion of most multisyllabic utterances to two syllables, where the second syllable mirrors the first: rabbit→/wawa/; bottle→/baba/.
Sound Preference	• Use of one sound or type of sound significantly more often than others. • A favorite sound, particular to a child. Sometimes the Hing pattern is a sound preference.
Stopping	• Replacement of continuing consonants or affricates with stop consonants. • Substitution of a stop consonant for a continuant phoneme (does not include the affricates). • Substitution of a stop for a fricative or affricate (and occasionally for a liquid). • Replacement of a fricative or an affricate by a stop consonant (/h/ is not included as a fricative).
Stopping of Fricatives	• Fricatives become stops: zoo→/du/; fish→/pɪt/; five→/paɪb/.
Stopping of Fricatives and Affricates	• Stopping of a fricative, resulting in affricates or stops; or stopping of affricates, resulting in stop consonants (this does NOT include stopping of glides or nasals).
Stopping of Glides and Liquids	• Production of a stop consonant for continuants other than fricatives and affricates (liquids become stops).
Stridency Deletion	• Omission of strident consonants or replacement of them with non-strident consonants. • Lack of stridency in a normally strident consonant because of deletion or replacement by a non-strident sound.
Strident Deficiency	• Deletion of stridency either by means of total omission of a target strident phoneme or by substitution of a non-strident phoneme.
Syllable Deletion	• Omission of one syllable of a multi-syllable word, usually the weak or unstressed syllable.
Syllable Reduction	• Deletion of a syllable nucleus (vowel, diphthong, or vocalic consonant) in a stimulus word that has two or more syllables. • Reduction in the number of syllables in the target word.
Tetism	• Also called "consonant neutralization" where sounds move to the alveolar position (e.g., bee→/di/; cow /ta/; four →/sɔr/).
Unstressed Syllable Deletion	• Deletion of any syllable of a polysyllabic word.

Table 6-8

Phonological Patterns and Definitions (Continued)

PROCESS	DEFINITION
Velar Deficiency	• Omission of velar stops /k/ and /g/ or substitution with another phoneme.
Velar Fronting	• Production of an alveolar consonant for a target velar consonant in a syllable or word. • Replacement of /k/ or /g/ by /t/ or /d/.
Vocalization	• Use of a vowel in place of a syllabic or postvocalic liquid. • Final position vocalic /l/ and /ɚ/ becomes rounded vowels /u/ or /o/.
Vocalization of Liquids	• Production of a vowel for the syllabics /l/ and /r/.
Voicing, Initial	• Use of voiced consonants to begin words that should begin with voiceless consonants (place and manner of articulation may or may not be altered).
Vowel Change	• Substitution resulting in a change of voicing feature.
Vowelization	• Replacement of a liquid sound in word-final position with a vowel. • Substitution of a vowel for a consonant.
Weak Syllable Deletion	• Deletion of an unstressed syllable in a word.
Word Final Addition of Schwa	• Addition of a schwa to the final consonant of the production.

a. Phonological patterns expected to be suppressed by age 3 years.
   (1) Weak syllable deletion.
   (2) Final consonant deletion.
   (3) Doubling.
   (4) Diminutization.
   (5) Velar fronting.
   (6) Consonant assimilation.
   (7) Reduplication.
   (8) Prevocalic voicing.
b. Phonological error patterns occurring after age 3 years.
   (1) Cluster reduction.
   (2) Epenthesis.
   (3) Gliding.
   (4) Vocalization.
   (5) Stopping.
   (6) Depalatalization.
   (7) Final devoicing.

Development of Speech Intelligibility

1. Defined as how well a listener understands the speech of the speaker.
2. Intelligibility does not mean without speech errors.
3. Speech intelligibility is influenced by a number of variables.
   a. The speaker's articulation and phonological skills.
   b. Presence/absence of contextual cues.
   c. The speaker's language abilities.
   d. Listener familiarity with the speaker.
4. General guideline for levels of intelligibility of children to unfamiliar listeners.
   a. 25% to 50% intelligible in the age range of 19–24 months.
   b. 50% to 75% intelligible in the age range of 2–3 years.
   c. 75% to 90% intelligible in the age range of 4–5 years.
   d. 90% to 100% intelligible beyond the age of 5 years.

School-Age Children's Development of Phonemic Awareness Skills

1. Phonemic awareness (PA): the understanding that words are comprised of individual sounds.
2. PA skills.
   a. Identifying the first/last sounds in words.
   b. Segmenting words into component sounds.
   c. Deleting sounds from words.
3. PA abilities are correlated with the development of early reading skills.
4. Children with phonological disorders are at risk for the lack of development of PA skills.

Assessment of Speech Sound Disorders (SSD)

Purpose of Assessment

1. Screening: a concise appraisal of speech skills to determine if further assessment is necessary, typically rated as pass/fail.
2. Assessment: an in-depth analysis to determine if remediation is necessary.
   a. Strengths and weaknesses of speaking skills.
   b. Presence of other communication impairments besides speech sound disorder (SSD).
   c. Type of intervention.
   d. Frequency of intervention.
   e. Prognostic variables that support progress.

Assessment Procedures

1. Written case history.
   a. Designed to obtain pertinent background information to help determine assessment tasks.
   b. Typically completed by caregiver(s) before the assessment takes place.
2. Obtain information from other professionals who may have provided services to the client.
3. Oral interview with caregivers and other professionals.
   a. Provide information to the caregiver(s) about the assessment procedures.
   b. Attain additional information from the caregivers.
4. Hearing screening.
   a. To determine if the client has a hearing loss and is in need of further hearing testing.
   b. Typically screened at frequencies of 500, 1000, 2000 and 4000 Hertz (Hz) at 20 or 25 dB intensity level.
   c. Those failing the hearing screening should be referred for a full audiological evaluation.
5. Standardized measures of speech sound production abilities.
   a. Characteristics of standardized tests.
      (1) Most often elicit single-word productions using picture stimuli.
      (2) Most consonants elicited across word positions at least once.
      (3) Allow for recording of omissions, substitutions, distortions and additions.
      (4) Most generate a standard score and percentile ranking.
      (5) Some standardized tests also evaluate children's use of phonological error patterns.
   b. Scoring.
      (1) Correct productions and errors are noted.
      (2) Types of errors include omissions, substitutions, distortions and additions.
   c. Concerns.
      (1) Single-word responses are not representational of the child's speech sound system.
      (2) Tests do not provide enough information about the child's sound system.
      (3) Speech sounds are assessed in limited phonetic contexts.
      (4) Often vowels and consonant clusters are not adequately sampled.
6. Collect a connected speech sample of at least 80–100 different words.
   a. More representative of natural speaking abilities.
   b. The data can be analyzed using independent and relational analysis (see below for procedures).
   c. Can yield suprasegmental information.
   d. Concerns.
      (1) Transcription and analysis is often laborious and difficult.
      (2) Analysis results do not yield a standard score.
7. Examination of oral-motor structure and function.
   a. Structural integrity of the articulators.
      (1) Occlusion patterns of the teeth.
         (a) Class I: normal occlusion.
         (b) Class II: overbite.
         (c) Class III: underbite.
      (2) Ankyloglossia: restricted lingual frenum (tongue tied).
      (3) Macroglossia: too large a tongue.
      (4) Microglossia: too small a tongue.
   b. Movement of lips, mandible, tongue and velum using both speech (e.g., the production of syllables) and nonspeech (e.g., moving tongue back and forth) tasks.
   c. Measure diadochokinesis (DDK), or rate of repetition of syllables.
      (1) Also called alternating motion rates (AMRs) or sequential motion rates (SMRs).
      (2) Includes repetition of identical syllables (/pʌpʌ/) and different syllables (/pʌtʌkʌ/).
      (3) Limited data is available for comparison of DDK rates for children.
      (4) Movements are examined for rate, accuracy and ease or smoothness.
   d. Medical issues such as enlarged tonsils, health of teeth and gums, etc. may also be discerned.

8. Assess stimulability of sounds in error.
   a. Should be conducted once errored sounds are determined.
   b. Involves the use of a variety of cues to help the client achieve correct production.
   c. Can be used for prognostic information and determining treatment targets.
      (1) Generally, high stimulability is associated with a positive prognosis.
      (2) Sounds that are stimulable may be more easily remediated than sounds with little or no stimulability.
      (3) Targeting unstimulable sounds in intervention may lead to generalization to errored sounds not receiving treatment.
   d. Stimulability methods.
      (1) Providing auditory and visual cues related to production in isolation or syllable level.
      (2) Describing how to produce the speech sound(s).
      (3) Varying phonetic contexts to facilitate correct production.
      (4) Direct stimulation of the articulators.
9. Assess phonological and phonemic awareness skills.
   a. Assesses the awareness of the phonological structure of language.
   b. Phonemic awareness, a component of phonological awareness, is the ability to understand that words are comprised of individual sounds.
      (1) Phonemic awareness is critical for the development of early word decoding.
   c. Children with phonological impairment are at risk for the lack of development of phonemic awareness skills, especially if other language problems exist.
   d. Phonemic awareness skills may be assessed with a standardized test or informally.
      (1) Informal measures.
         (a) Identify the initial and/or final sounds in words.
         (b) Complete alliteration tasks.
         (c) Segment words into component speech sounds.
         (d) Blend isolated speech sounds to form words.
10. Informal measure of intelligibility.
    a. An overall impression or rating of how well the clinician understood the child.
    b. Most often uses a connected speech sample.
       (1) Can involve:
          (a) The clinician indicating how many words were understood out of a sample to determine the percentage of intelligible words.
          (b) Informally rating the client's intelligibility using a numbered rating scale.
          (c) Informally providing descriptive statements, such as "mildly unintelligible," "severely unintelligible," etc.
    c. Caregivers may also give their impression of how well the child is understood by themselves and others.
11. Assessing other language skills.
    a. See Chapters 3, 7, 8 and 9 in this book.
12. Assessing speech discrimination skills.
    a. Assess the client's ability to determine correct vs. incorrect productions of errored sounds.
    b. Locke's procedures (i.e., Locke's SPPT procedure) are often used for this discrimination task.
       (1) Components:
          (a) The target sound.
          (b) The sound the child uses as a substitute.
          (c) A control phoneme that shares similar characteristics to the target and substitute.
       (2) The clinician produces a variety of similar-sounding words to determine if the child can hear the differences.
    c. Auditory discrimination skills may also be assessed using formal testing procedures.
13. Contextual testing.
    a. Used to determine if facilitating phonetic contexts can evoke the errored sound.
    b. These phonetic contexts may be called "key words" or "key environments."
    c. May be assessed using informal procedures or a formal test.
    d. Examples of an informal procedure to assess the use of facilitating phonetic contexts to evoke /s/:
       (1) Use the alveolar place of production to facilitate correct production of /s/ by having the client imitate syllables such as "sty" and "eats."
       (2) Have the client produce multiple productions of the phoneme /t/ with increasing rate.
       (3) Note this aspect of assessment, contextual testing, is often within a stimulability protocol.

Analysis of Assessment Data

1. Relational analysis procedures compare the client's productions to the adult standard.
   a. Percentage Consonants Correct (PCC).
      (1) Compares the number of consonants produced correctly to the total number of consonants that should have been produced.
      (2) Procedures.
         (a) Selecting 80–100 different words from a connected speech sample is suggested.

(b) Child's production of consonants in each word is compared to the adult standard.
(c) Percentage of correct use is determined by comparing the number of correctly produced consonants to the number of consonants in the targets.
(d) Determines a severity level based on percentage of correctly produced consonants.
- 85%–100%: mild disorder.
- 65%–85%: mild-moderate disorder.
- 50%–65%: moderate-severe disorder.
- Less than 50%: severe disorder.

(3) Adaptations.
(a) Percentage Consonants Correct–Revised (PCC-R).
- All distortions are considered correct.
(b) Percentage Vowels & Diphthongs Correct–Revised (PVC-R).
(c) Percentage Phonemes Correct (PPC).

2. Error patterns.
   a. Place-Manner-Voicing (PVM) displays production abilities within the broad categories of place, manner and voicing characteristics of phonemes.
   b. Distinctive Feature Analysis categorizes children's productions and errors according to distinctive features that are present.
   c. Phonological Processes Analysis (also called Phonological Error Patterns Analysis) typically uses the error pattern categories of syllable structure, substitution and assimilation.
      (1) Useful for children with many errors.
      (2) Analysis determines the frequency of use for each pattern.

3. Phonological Mean Length of Utterance (PMLU) and Proportion of Whole-Word Proximity (PWP).
   a. Attempts to determine the length and complexity of words children attempt to say, and how well the child matches the target words.
   b. Procedures.
      (1) Minimum sample size of 25 different words is suggested.
      (2) The PMLU of the target words is determined by:
         (a) Assigning two points for every consonant and one point for every vowel in each word.
         (b) Dividing the total number of points by the total number of words.
      (3) The PMLU of the child's production attempts is determined by:
         (a) Assigning one point for every vowel and consonant produced by the child.
         (b) Assigning an additional point for every correct consonant.
      (4) The PWP is determined by comparing the PMLU of the target words with the child's PMLU.
      (5) Can be used to determine complexity of words attempted, to determine how well complexity was matched, to select intervention targets and to monitor progress.

4. Traditional analysis.
   a. Displays errors across word or syllable position.
   b. Records types of errors including omissions, substitutions, additions and distortions.
   c. May be most useful for those with few speech errors.

5. Independent analysis procedures examine the child's speech sound production skills without comparison to the adult model and include:
   a. Phonetic inventory (PI), which determines which consonants and vowels the client produced without considering correct vs. incorrect productions.
      (1) Sounds produced only once or twice are typically not included in the inventory or are considered "marginal."
      (2) Typically organized by manner and place of production, as well as word and/or syllable position.
      (3) Can be used to determine production strengths and weaknesses.

6. Analysis of use of words and syllable shapes.
   a. Provides a tally of the client's production of syllable types and how syllables are used to form words.
   b. Can be used to determine production strengths and weaknesses.

7. Standardized test(s) results can be used to determine:
   a. A standard score and percentile ranking.
      (1) Such scores are important for qualifying clients for intervention services across a number of settings.
   b. Independent analysis results, including a phonetic inventory, use of words and syllable shapes.
   c. Relational analysis results, including error patterns.
   d. Different tests will provide different kinds of information.

8. Determining a diagnosis of speech sound disorder.
   a. Interpretation of standardized scores and percentile ranks to determine if the client is eligible for speech intervention services.
   b. Comparing results to information provided by speech sound developmental charts to determine age-appropriateness of production skills.
   c. Determining if phonological error patterns are age-appropriate.
   d. Determining that errors are not related to use of a dialect or influence of other languages.

9. Nature of the disorder.
   a. Characteristics of articulation disorders.
      (1) Few errors and a pattern of error(s) cannot be discerned.

(2) Sound errors are related to some type of structural or functional problem.
(3) Client doesn't appear to have problems with using the phonological rules of language.
  b. Characteristics of phonological disorders.
    (1) Many errors and pattern(s) of errors can be discerned.
    (2) Highly unintelligible.
    (3) Limited production of word and syllable shapes.
    (4) Limited phonetic inventory.
    (5) Client appears to have difficulty using the phonological rules of language.
10. Analyzing and interpreting prognostic variables.
  a. A prognosis speculates clients' ability to benefit from treatment based on a variety of variables.
    (1) Severity: poorer prognosis associated with severity.
    (2) Chronological age: better prognosis associated with early intervention.
    (3) Motivation: better prognosis associated with higher motivation.
    (4) Inconsistent errors: speech sounds produced correctly some of the time may not need to be treated or may be remediated quickly.
    (5) Attention: inattention associated with poorer performance.
    (6) Family support: strong family support associated with better performance.
11. Considerations for assessing clients who are culturally and linguistically diverse.
  a. Essential information when assessing a nonnative English speaker.
    (1) Characteristics of the client's primary (or first) language.
    (2) Determining if and how the first language may be influencing acquisition of the second language.
    (3) Deciding if the client demonstrates a phonological disorder in both languages.
  b. Types of phonological errors often related to second language learning.
    (1) Underdifferentiation of phonemes (i.e., not differentiating phonemes in the second language if they are not differentiated in the first language).
    (2) Overdifferentiation of phonemes (i.e., producing allophonic variations of a phoneme in the second language as two separate phonemes if those variations are two separate phonemes in the first language).
    (3) Substitution of phonemes (i.e., substituting a phoneme from one language for one in the other language, especially if the phonemes share similar characteristics).
    (4) Omission of phonemes (i.e., a phoneme from the second language may be omitted if it is not a part of the first language).
  c. Theoretical positions on second language acquisition and phonology.
    (1) Two separate phonological systems (differentiated) or one phonological system (undifferentiated).
      (a) This debate is most applicable to speakers who acquire a second language simultaneously.
      (b) Speakers who acquire a second language after the establishment of a first language probably maintain differentiated phonological systems.
    (2) Critical age for second language acquisition and phonological development.
      (a) Critical age for second language acquisition and development of "native-like" phonological skills not established.
      (b) Generally, research shows that native-like phonological skills for second language acquisition is associated with age.
      (c) Propensity of native-like phonological skills for second language acquisition is influenced by numerous variables, including biological, environmental, instruction and motivation.
  d. Intervention considerations.
    (1) Culturally and linguistically diverse children do not require unique treatment approaches.
    (2) Treatment targets should consider characteristics of first and second language and what will improve intelligibility in the client's primary language the most.

Distinguishing Between Childhood Apraxia of Speech (CAS), Dysarthria and Speech Sound Disorders (Table 6-9)

Determining Goals and Objectives

1. Long-term goals target broad communication behaviors that may take a relatively long time to achieve and may include behaviors such as:
  a. Increased intelligibility to a specific level.
  b. Age-appropriate use of speech sounds.
2. Short-term goals that target specific phonological and articulation abilities, such as:
  a. Increased use of specific speech sounds.
  b. Reduced use of specific error patterns.

Table 6-9

Differentiating Between CAS, Dysarthria and SSD

VERBAL APRAXIA	DYSARTHRIA	SEVERE PHONOLOGICAL DISORDER
No weakness, incoordination or paralysis of speech musculature	Decreased strength and coordination or speech musculature that leads to imprecise speech production, slurring and distortions	No weakness, incoordination or paralysis of speech musculature
No difficulty with involuntary motor control for chewing, swallowing, etc. unless there is also oral apraxia	Difficulty with involuntary motor control for chewing, swallowing etc. due to muscle weakness and incoordination	No difficulty with involuntary control for chewing and swallowing
Inconsistencies in articulation performance—the same word may be produced several different ways	Articulation may be noticeably "different" due to imprecision, but errors generally consistent	Consistent errors that can usually be grouped into categories (fronting, stopping, etc.)
Errors include substitutions, omissions, additions, and repetitions, frequently includes simplification of word forms. Tendency for omissions in initial position. Tendency to centralize vowels to /ə/	Errors are generally distortions	Errors may include substitutions, omissions, distortions, etc. Omissions in final position more likely than initial position. Vowel distortions not as common
Number of errors increases as length of word/phrase increases	May be less precise in connected speech than in single words	Errors are generally consistent as length of words/phrases increases
Well-rehearsed, "automatic" speech is easiest to produce, "on demand" speech most difficult	No difference in how easily speech is produced based on situation	No difference in how easily speech is produced based on situation
Receptive language skills are usually significantly better than expressive skills	Typically no significant discrepancy between receptive and expressive language skills	Sometimes difference between receptive and expressive language skills
Rate, rhythm, and stress of speech are disrupted, some groping for placement may be noted	Rate, rhythm, and stress are disrupted in ways specifically related to the type of dysarthria (spastic, flaccid, etc.)	Typically no disruption of rate, rhythm or stress
Generally good control of pitch and loudness, may have limited inflectional range for speaking	Monotone voice, difficulty controlling pitch and loudness	Good control of pitch and loudness, not limited in inflectional range for speaking
Age-appropriate voice quality	Voice quality may be hoarse, harsh, hypernasal, etc. depending on type of dysarthria	Age-appropriate voice quality

Retrieved from: http://www.apraxia-kids.org/library/a-comparison-of-childhood-apraxia-of-speech-dysarthria-and-severe-phonological-disorder/.

3. General factors to consider when choosing treatment objectives.
   a. Targets that will make a significant impact on overall communication abilities.
   b. Targets that will be used and reinforced in the natural environment.
   c. Targets that will allow the client to further develop communication skills.
   d. Targets that are considered culturally and linguistically appropriate.
4. Specific factors that may be considered when choosing specific sounds and/or error patterns to target in intervention.
   a. Developmental norms.
      (1) Choosing speech sounds that are considered age-appropriate.
         (a) Belief that speech sounds develop in sequence.
         (b) Acquisition of speech sounds becomes more complex with age.
         (c) Earlier developing speech sounds considered easier to produce.
      (2) Choosing speech sounds that are considered developmentally complex.
         (a) Belief that by targeting more complex sounds, less complex sounds will generalize without intervention.
      (3) Problems with using developmental norms for choosing intervention targets.
         (a) Great deal of variability in development across children.
         (b) Conflicting evidence regarding the use of developmental norms for choosing treatment targets.
         (c) Not certain that children with SSD acquire articulation and phonological skills in the same way as typically developing children.
   b. Error patterns.
      (1) Choose error patterns that:
         (a) Interfere the most with intelligibility.
         (b) Reduce the use of homonymity.
         (c) Affect the greatest number of sounds.
         (d) Are demonstrated with the greatest frequency.

(e) Affect earlier-developing sounds.
c. Stimulability.
  (1) Choosing speech sounds for which the client is stimulable may indicate sounds the child will easily acquire and impact intelligibility quickly.
    (a) Early success in intervention is also associated with choosing these speech sounds.
  (2) Choosing speech sounds for which the client is not stimulable indicates sounds that are likely not to improve without intervention.
    (a) Some research has shown greater generalization than the remediation of stimulable sounds.
    (b) Stimulable sounds may improve without direct intervention as a result of targeting nonstimulable sounds.
d. Planning for generalization.
  (1) Sounds that represent maximal phoneme differences.
    (a) Implicates use of a word contrast intervention technique (i.e., sometimes the technique dictates or greatly influences treatment targets).
    (b) Associated with contrast intervention techniques.
    (c) Useful if the client has several errors.
    (d) Two phonemes that differ maximally in terms of distinctive features (e.g., /s/ and /g/) are targeted simultaneously in order to expose the child to more information about the speech sound system.
    (e) Intervention targets correct production of sounds in words (e.g., "sun" and "gun").
  (2) Sounds that represent multiple phoneme differences.
    (a) Implicates use of a word contrast intervention technique (i.e., sometimes the technique dictates or greatly influences treatment targets).
    (b) Associated with contrast intervention techniques.
    (c) Useful if the client has many errors.
    (d) Typically at least four different phonemes that differ across distinctive features are targeted simultaneously in order to expose the child to more information about the speech sound system.
    (e) Intervention targets correct production of sounds in words (e.g., "none" is contrasted with "sun," "gun," "run" and "fun").

Treatment of Speech Sound Disorders

Choosing Intervention Targets

1. Target selection follows a complete assessment.
2. Intervention targets should be chosen to achieve "in-class" and "across-class" generalization.
   a. "In-class" generalization involves skills generalizing to untreated sounds within the same sound class (e.g., working on /s/ generalizes to other fricatives).
   b. "Across-class" generalization involves skills generalizing to untreated sounds in different sound classes.
3. There are two broad methods for choosing targets.
   a. Developmental approach.
     (1) Uses the sequence of normal development of speech sounds for choosing targets that would be developmentally appropriate.
   b. Complexity approach.
     (1) Involves choosing intervention targets that are complex relative to the client's abilities, no matter where those speech sounds fall on the developmental chart.
4. Clinicians may choose to target individual phonemes, groups of phonemes, or to reduce the client's use of error patterns (i.e., phonological processes).
5. Variables to consider regarding target selection.
   a. Client's stimulability for errored sounds.
     (1) Clinicians may opt to target sounds that are highly stimulable in order to ensure early success.
     (2) Some research has shown that targeting sounds that are not stimulable produces more widespread generalization.
     (3) Other research has shown that targeting nonstimulable sounds does not produce widespread generalization.
   b. Client's developmental level.
     (1) Earlier developmentally acquired sounds are often recommended to be targeted early in treatment.
     (2) Targeting sounds that are acquired later in development has been shown to produce more system-wide generalization than targeting early sounds.
   c. Choosing targets that will make the biggest impact on intelligibility.

d. Choosing targets that will positively effect morpho-syntax skills, such as final "s" clusters that indicate plurality (i.e., "cups"), final clusters that indicate past tense, etc.
e. Target phonemes that are more "marked" than other phonemes.
   (1) Marked sounds are those that are less common in world languages.
   (2) Marked sounds tend to be acquired developmentally later.
   (3) Marked sounds are also described as more complex.
   (4) Unmarked sounds are more common in world languages and are acquired earlier.
   (5) The relationship between marked and unmarked sounds in a language can be defined in terms of implicational laws.
      (a) Implicational laws describe the relationship between marked and unmarked sounds.
      (b) Implicational laws are unidirectional, with more marked sounds implying the presence of less complex sounds (the reverse is not true).
      (c) Examples of implicational laws within phonological acquisition include:
         - Liquids imply nasals.
         - Fricatives imply stops.
         - Affricates imply fricatives.
f. Target phonemes of which the client has the least productive phonological knowledge (PPK).
   (1) Children's productions of phonemes are ranked on a 6-point continuum from "most knowledgeable" (i.e., always accurately produced) to "least knowledgeable" (i.e., sounds not in the client's inventory).
   (2) Some research has shown that targeting sounds with the least PPK results in more widespread generalization.
g. Target phonemes that will reduce homonymy and phoneme collapse.
h. Target phonemes that are considered easier to teach.
   (1) Visible sounds.
   (2) Stimulable sounds.
i. Consistency of the error(s).
   (1) Inconsistent errors may be targeted for early success.
   (2) Targeting consistent errors has been shown to produce more system-wide change, rather than targeting inconsistent errors.
j. The "distance metric."
   (1) Choose targets that are maximally distinct and characterize the sound classes that are represented by a single substitution (maximal classification).

6. Choosing targets that are not complex, inconsistently in error, and are highly stimulable may produce early success in intervention, but not widespread generalization.
7. Choosing targets that are complex, consistently in error, and are not stimulable may result in more widespread generalization.
8. Considerations for choosing targets for bilingual speakers.
   a. Target errors that are demonstrated with similar frequency in both languages.
      (1) Typically, these targets will make an impact on the client's speaking skills in both languages.
   b. After targeting errors that have equal frequency in both languages, target errors that are exhibited with unequal frequency in both languages.
   c. Next, target errors demonstrated in only one language.
9. Number of sounds or patterns to teach.
   a. "Goal attack" strategy is the term used to organize intervention to improve speech skills.
      (1) Horizontal goal attack strategy.
         (a) Several sounds or sound error patterns are taught in sequence.
      (2) Vertical goal attack strategy.
         (a) Each sound is targeted until a specific level of correct sound production is achieved.
   b. Some research has examined the efficacy of targeting a single error of multiple errors.
      (1) Targeting two errored sounds using a minimal pair format produced greater improvement than targeting one errored sound.
10. Learnability Theory.
    a. Providing children with complex input has been shown to assist language learning.
    b. Exposure to more complex language pushes children to learn and use more complex structures.
    c. Exposure to complexity gives children opportunity to detect and change their own phonological errors.
    d. Following Learnability Theory, targeting complex phonological targets predicts the greatest amount of change in the children's sound system.

Intervention Approaches

1. Variables to consider when choosing an intervention approach.
   a. Phonetic vs. phonemic errors.
      (1) Phonetic errors tend to be consistent errors and are attributed to faulty motor learning.
         (a) Intervention emphasizes helping the client learn how to produce speech sounds.

(2) Phonemic errors tend to involve groups of sounds or sound sequences.
  (a) Intervention emphasizes helping the client learn how speech sounds function in language to signal meaning.
(3) Clients with phonemic errors are often described as having reduced phonological contrasts.
  (a) This lack of contrast often results in the production of homonyms (e.g., saying "tu" for a number of words, such as "shoe," "sue" and "two").
b. Client variables to consider.
  (1) Stimulability skills.
  (2) Ability to self-monitor.
  (3) Attention, effort and motivation.
  (4) Cognitive skills.
  (5) Linguistic skills.
  (6) Oral motor skills.
  (7) Hearing acuity.
  (8) Age.

2. Intervention approaches for phonetic errors (articulatory-based approaches).
  a. These approaches tend to treat speech sounds individually, and a specific therapeutic sequence is often followed then gradually increased in complexity.
  b. Emphasis of intervention is placement and movement of the articulators.
  c. Typical phonetic techniques and strategies used in intervention.
    (1) Visual and auditory cues.
    (2) Description of articulator movements.
    (3) Providing a metaphor (i.e., "snake sound").
    (4) Shaping from other sounds.
    (5) Encouraging self-monitoring and evaluation.
    (6) Use of motor learning principles.
      (a) Repetition of the target in syllables, then gradually increasing phonetic complexity.
      (b) Early in treatment, using block practice and then later using random practice.
      (c) As accuracy improves, increasing specific feedback.
      (d) Over time, reducing extrinsic feedback.
  d. Phonetic approaches.
    (1) Van Riper (Traditional) Approach.
      (a) General therapy sequence of intervention.
        • Sensory-perceptual training (ear training): the client is trained to distinguish the "target" phoneme from other speech sounds.
        • The client isn't asked to produce the target yet, and this step may proceed in the following stages:
          – Identification of the clinician's production of the target vs. other sounds (this is done using isolation sound productions that may exaggerate certain aspects of the target).
          – Isolation involves having the client indicate every time the clinician produces the target in a variety of words and contexts.
          – In the stimulation stage, the clinician bombards the client with production of the target sound, and those productions will vary in loudness and rate and can include listening to audio productions by different speakers (the client will also identify when the target is produced).
          – In the discrimination stage, the clinician produces both the correct production of the target and the client's error in a variety of contexts (the client identifies the errored phoneme and may also tell the clinician how to correct the error).
      (b) Elicit and establish the sound in isolation or syllable level using a variety of sound establishment techniques.
        • Imitation of verbal models.
        • Visual cues.
        • Telling the client where to put the articulators.
        • Shaping the new sound from a sound the child can produce (e.g., using /s/ to shape /ʃ/).
        • Using phonetic context of known sounds to stimulate the new sound (e.g., having the client attempt /s/ in the context of /ts/ syllable endings).
      (c) Sound stabilization.
        • A gradual increase of the phonetic complexity in which the client can successfully produce the target (proceeds in the following stages):
          – Isolation.
          – Nonsense syllables.
          – Words that systematically vary where the target is located, including position (initial, intervocalic, final), number of syllables, clusters (initial, intervocalic, final).
          – Phrases, which may begin with carry phrases.
          – Sentences that gradually increase in length and complexity.
          – Conversation (structured and unstructured).
      (d) Transfer and carryover.
        • Also referred to as generalization.

- Emphasis on correct sound production outside the clinical setting with a variety of communication partners.
  (e) Maintenance.
  - The clinician may schedule follow-up sessions or interview others to ensure the child is maintaining the target.
(2) Sensory-Motor Approach.
  (a) Stresses the production of bisyllable units.
  (b) Key concepts.
    - Using facilitative phonetic contexts.
    - Gradual and systematic change of production units.
  (c) Begins with the production within a phonetic context in which the target is produced correctly (i.e., a facilitative phonetic context).
  (d) Intervention proceeds across various phases.
    - Production of bisyllables consisting of phonemes not in error.
      – Production varies in terms of loudness, rate and intonation patterns.
      – Production characteristics of different types of sounds are compared and contrasted.
    - Initially, production of the target sound in facilitating phonetic contexts is practiced (i.e., bisyllabic productions).
    - Gradual and systematic expansion of the phonetic contexts in which the client can produce the target successfully.
(3) Multiple Phoneme Approach.
  (a) Developed for children with multiple phoneme errors.
  (b) Simultaneous instruction on errored phonemes; a client may be at a different phase or step for each errored phoneme.
  (c) A highly structured approach with guidelines for number and type of stimuli to evoke correct productions, strict criteria for advancing to subsequent steps and phases of the program, type of stimuli and reinforcement schedule.
  (d) Consists of three phases, with substeps within each phase.
    - Establishment phase.
      – Correct production in isolation.
      – Productions are elicited by using graphemes.
      – Maximal cuing (auditory, visual and tactile) is provided initially.
      – Amount of cuing is gradually reduced.
      – Targets may be placed in a "holding" phase if accuracy at the isolation level is reached, but intervention cannot progress to the syllable level.
    - Transfer phase.
      – Intervention increases complexity, proceeding from syllables, to words, to phrases/sentences, to reading or storytelling, to conversation.
      – Once the child reaches the phrase/sentence level, whole-word accuracy is the goal (instead of individual phonemes in words) and self-monitoring is emphasized.
    - Maintenance phase.
      – The goal is 90% accurate production of whole words within conversations across different settings and with different listeners.
      – Accuracy rate must be achieved without direct intervention.
      – Authors recommend that the client be monitored for 3 months.
(4) Paired-Stimuli Approach.
  (a) Highly structured, sequenced approach.
  (b) Proceeds from single words, to sentences, to conversations.
  (c) Begins with the target being produced correctly in four "key words" (i.e., two with correct productions in the initial position and two with correct productions in the final position).
  (d) About 10 training words, or words in which the client produces the target in error, are then selected.
  (e) A picture board is created by placing a picture of the key word in the center, surrounded by pictures of the training word, keeping position of the target consistent across stimuli (e.g., all initial position).
  (f) The client alternates production of the key word with each training word until criterion is reached.
  (g) Next, the key word is changed to the final position and intervention continues until criterion is reached.
  (h) Intervention continues with the word pairings, but the client is encouraged to say the word pairs more quickly in succession.
    - The amount of reinforcement is reduced.
  (i) At the sentence level, the client is required to use the key word and each of the training words in sentences.
    - Complexity is increased by including words with the target in the initial and final position in each sentence.
  (j) At the conversation level, the clinician reinforces correct production of the target in any word.

(5) Integral Stimulation.
  (a) Emphasizes multiple input modes, mainly auditory and visual.
  (b) Cues are often provided simultaneously.
  (c) Cues are faded as client achieves more independent success with production.
(6) Enhancing Stimulability.
  (a) Designed to increase stimulability of unstimulable sounds and increased verbal communication attempts.
  (b) Associates the verbal production of sounds with a movement or gesture and a character (e.g., /f/ is paired with "fussy fish" and a hand motion).
  (c) Multiple sounds are targeted simultaneously, including both stimulable and non-stimulable sounds.
  (d) Games are played involving the characters, and the client can respond with the sound, word or gesture.
  (e) Intervention techniques also include modeling and requesting imitation.

3. Intervention approaches for phonemic errors (linguistic-based approaches).
  a. These approaches target groups of sounds or how sounds make up syllables (e.g., creating closed syllables, producing consonant clusters, etc.).
  b. Often most appropriate for children with multiple errors.
  c. Emphasis of intervention is helping the client develop and use appropriate phonological contrasts in natural communicative contexts.
  d. These approaches deemphasize phonetic training of sound productions.
  e. Intervention usually begins at the word level, and words are often presented in pairs to demonstrate phonemic contrasts (e.g., "tea" vs. "key").
  f. Typically more than one sound is targeted in intervention at a time.
  g. The goal is for the client to generalize new skills to errored sounds not targeted in therapy.
  h. Phonemic approaches.
    (1) Distinctive Features Approach.
      (a) Focus of intervention is on the distinctive feature(s) the client is missing from the phonological system.
      (b) Lack of distinctive features leads to reduced contrast in the client's repertoire.
      (c) The missing distinctive feature(s) are taught (e.g., continuant) in a few phonemes, and the client will generalize to other phonemes that share that feature.
      (d) Some distinct features programs include the use of nonsense syllables.
    (2) Phonological Contrast Intervention.
      (a) The goal of contrast therapy approaches is to create phonological contrasts in the client's speech.
      (b) In contrast intervention, the client's tendency to produce multiple word forms the same way (homonymy) is directly addressed.
      (c) Careful consideration is given to choosing treatment targets in order to maximize generalization.
      (d) Intervention is structured to show the client the need to produce different phonemes.
        • The listener will be confused unless the client produces a different word for each stimuli in the word pairs.
      (e) The sequence of intervention for contrast intervention is similar across the different types of contrasts used (although multiple oppositions uses multiple stimuli at one time).
        • Choose word pairs and familiarize the client with the pictures.
        • The clinician directs the client to point to the various pictures used in an activity.
        • The client produces the word pairs for the clinician in naturalistic activities.
        • Communication breakdowns will occur if the client fails to produce the appropriate contrasts.
        • The clinician provides appropriate feedback and opportunity for the child to produce the correct contrasts.
        • Some clients may need to be given articulatory instruction on correct sound production in order to succeed with the intervention tasks.
      (f) There are several variations of contrast therapy methods.
        • Minimal Pairs (Minimal Contrast Method).
          – The goal is to eliminate the client's creation of homonyms (e.g., saying "tea" for both "tea" and "key").
          – Minimal pairs are sets of words that differ by one phoneme, and that difference creates two different words.
          – The word pairs usually contrast the child's error with the target.
          – Typically, the focus of intervention is to present pairs of different words that the client typically produces as homonyms.
          – Intervention emphasizes the need to say the words in each pair differently (i.e., produce the phonological contrast).

- Minimal pair intervention follows the theoretical positions of Natural Phonology (i.e., targeting phonological error patterns) and the Principle of Informativeness (i.e., speakers using their listeners' feedback to improve speech).
- Generalization to other phonemes is expected.
• Maximal Oppositions (Maximal Contrasts).
- Word pairs in which the target is contrasted with another sound that is maximally distinct (differs across a variety of features) are the focus of intervention (e.g., contrasting "key" with "me").
- This approach exposes the child to more information about the sound system.
- The reduction of homonymy is indirectly addressed.
- Intervention emphasizes the need to say the words in each pair differently.
- Generalization to other phonemes is expected.
• Multiple Oppositions.
- This approach is useful for clients who have phoneme collapse or use one sound as a substitute for multiple sounds (e.g., /t/ is substituted for /k/, /s/, /ʃ/, /tʃ/, /f/, /ð/, /l/ and /st/).
- The target is contrasted with a number of different sounds based on the client's unique phoneme collapse(s), attempting to disrupt the client's unique deviant rule patterns.
- Targets used in this approach should also be maximally distinct from each other.
- The client is presented with a range of new sounds and exposed to different phonological patterns.
- A variety of errored sounds are treated simultaneously (e.g., the client is presented with pictures of "two/sue," "two/coo," "two/shoe" and "two/chew").
- A great deal of focused input during intervention is recommended, along with production opportunities and specific feedback about the semantic content of the child's productions.
- This approach attempts to reduce the client's tendency to use one phoneme to represent a variety of other sounds.
• Empty Set.
- Word pairs that contrast two errored sounds are used.
- Maximal contrast is recommended (i.e., "chip" vs. "rip").
(3) Cycles Remediation Approach.
(a) A main feature of this approach is the cyclical goal attack strategy.
• Different targets are addressed in succession without the need to reach criterion.
(b) Specific phonemes are targeted in an effort to reduce the client's use of error patterns.
• Generalization is expected.
(c) Each error pattern is addressed for approximately 2–6 hours, and once all significant error patterns are addressed, the first cycle is completed.
(d) Only one phoneme is targeted per session, with a different phoneme targeted each session.
(e) The authors provide suggestions for sequencing targets in intervention, generally following a developmental approach.
(f) Underlying tenets of this approach.
• Phonological development is gradual.
• Listening is a key component of phonological acquisition.
• Facilitating phonetic contexts are important for helping the client develop the movement and auditory awareness associated with phoneme production.
(g) Additional aspects of this approach.
• Auditory bombardment (at the onset and end of each intervention session) of words containing the targeted phoneme of the day.
• Targets such as s-clusters and liquids are addressed early.
• Addresses multisyllabic words and phonemic awareness skills in later cycles.
(4) Naturalistic Speech.
(a) A conversational based approach to treating phonological errors.
(b) Intervention takes place in natural place activities.
• Activities can be designed to contain a high frequency of words with the target.
(c) Frequent models and recasts of errors.
• Few direct elicitations of language and no direct reinforcement.
(5) Whole-Language Treatment Approach.
(a) Especially useful for children with phonological impairments and concomitant delays in other language skills.

(b) Based on the premise that phonological skills are influenced by a multitude of other variables.
(c) Improvements in one area of language can enhance changes in other areas of language.
(d) Multiple areas of language are often targeted simultaneously.
(e) Therapy is conducted in the context of meaningful and functional activities that reflect the client's development level, including:
- Play.
- Daily routines.
- Storytelling and retelling.
- Conversations.

(f) The therapist's role is to help the client verbally contribute to the conversation without correcting and evaluating communication performance.
(g) The therapist reacts to the client's utterances with a response that is more complex, anticipating the client will use the information to produce a more complex utterance.
(h) Typical techniques include modeling, recasting and visual information.
(i) Clients change their speech productions as they also advance the complexity of their language system.
(j) Changes in higher-level language processes (i.e., narration) are associated with changes in lower-level processes (i.e., phoneme production).

(6) Morphosyntax Approach.
(a) Designed for preschoolers who demonstrate SSD and syntactic and morphological (morphosyntactic) errors in their speech.
(b) Emphasis is on finite grammatical markers that mark tense and number.
- Also, complex morphemes that create final consonant clusters.

(c) Efficiency in intervention is accomplished by incorporating both grammar and phonology, thus capitalizing on a "cross-domain effect" for intervention.
(d) Generalization is expected to nonmorphological clusters (i.e., not just those involving bound morphemes).
(e) Generalization is also expected to nontargeted speech sounds.
(f) Therapy activities can be clinician-directed and naturalistic.
(g) Often targets are addressed in an alternate speech vs. morphosyntactic format.
(h) Focused stimulation is a primary intervention technique.
- Opportunities for natural productions are created (e.g., requesting) while elicited productions are also allowed.

(7) Metaphon.
(a) Metalinguistic approach to phonological disorders.
(b) Incorporates phonological awareness (PA) to change expressive phonological skills.
(c) Attributes phonological errors to the child not acquiring the rules of the sound system and not realizing the negative communication impact.
(d) Intervention is designed to help children change their deviant rules system by helping them realize they need to change their productions, and by giving them the skills to make the appropriate changes to assist in the change.
(e) Phase 1.
- Concept level: clinician and child "create" a common vocabulary to describe sound quality (e.g., noisy, short, long, etc.).
- Sound level: vocabulary created in the concept level is then used to describe speech and nonspeech sounds (e.g., balloons hissing, noisemakers, whispers, etc.).
- Phoneme level: common vocabulary is then used to describe speech sounds.
- Word level: child listens to word pairs and uses vocabulary to describe differences in the sounds between the word pairs.

(f) Phase 2.
- Child produces minimal word pairs.
- Child continues to use vocabulary to describe sounds.
- Clinician gives feedback regarding communication function.
- Later, the child can move on to sentences.

(8) Core Vocabulary Intervention.
(a) Designed for children who exhibit an inconsistent phonological disorder.
(b) Inconsistency may be associated with difficulty selecting and correctly arranging phonemes.
- Also described as difficulty with phonological planning.

(c) Typically targets whole words that are functional or important.
(d) Therapy sessions focus on 10–12 words to be produced for each specific target word.
(e) The goal is for the child to learn how to sequence phonemes for each specific target word.
(f) Ultimate goal is for the child to produce 70 words consistently.

(g) Once consistency for the 70 words is achieved, generalization of consistency is expected.
(h) Consistent errors (e.g., /w/ for /r/) are accepted.
   • These errors may be developmental or something to be targeted later.
(i) Cues include syllable segmentation, imitation, use of alphabet letters.

(9) Metaphonological Intervention.
   (a) Intervention integrates both phonological and phonemic awareness skill development, along with speech production skill development.
   (b) Many children with SSD also demonstrate difficulty with phonological and phonemic awareness skills, which can affect later literacy skills.
   (c) Research has shown that integrating PA instruction with therapy for SSD can positively affect literacy skills and speech production abilities.
   (d) PA activities in the context of SSD highlights the target(s) by having the client identify and manipulate sounds in words.
   (e) The client's awareness of sounds can be highlighted through such tasks as identifying specific phonemes in words, comparing words based on phonemic structure, etc.
   (f) Graphemes are often included to reinforce the client's awareness of the sound structure of words.
   (g) The client's awareness of sounds in words is used to help change errored productions.
   (h) This intervention is designed to increase both accurate speech productions and early literacy development.

(10) Nonlinear Phonological Intervention.
   (a) The emphasis is awareness and production of phonological forms in context.
   (b) This intervention is based on "nonlinear phonology" theories that describe the hierarchical relationship of phonological forms encompassing individual phonetic features through prosodic phrase.
   (c) Intervention should be preceded by nonlinear phonological analysis to determine appropriate targets.
   (d) Intervention typically addresses prosodic structures and/or speech segments and features.
   (e) Typical therapy techniques include the use of auditory, visual and tactile-kinesthetic cues to develop new word shapes, stress patterns and/or speech segments and features.

References

Baker, E., & McLeod, S., (2011). Evidence-based practice for children with speech sound disorders: Part 1 and Part 2. *Language, Speech and Hearing Services in the Schools, 42,* 102–152.

Bernthal, J.E., Bankson, N.W., & Flipsen, P. (2013). *Articulation and phonological disorders: Speech sound disorders in children* (7th ed). Boston: Pearson.

Bowen, C. (2015). *Children's speech sound disorders* (2nd ed.). New Jersey: Wiley-Blackwell

Shriberg, L.D., & Kent, R.D. (2013). *Clinical phonetics* (4th ed.). Boston: Allyn & Bacon.

Williams, A.L., McLeod, S., & McCauley, R.J. (2010). *Interventions for speech sound disorders in children.* Baltimore: Brooks Publishing.

7

Language Disorders in Young Children

AMY L. WEISS, PhD

Chapter Outline

- Terminology for Understanding Language Development and Disorders in Young Children, 168
- Models of Language Development and Disorders, 170
- Assessment of Language Disorders, 179
- Intervention for Children with Language Disorders, 184
- References, 191

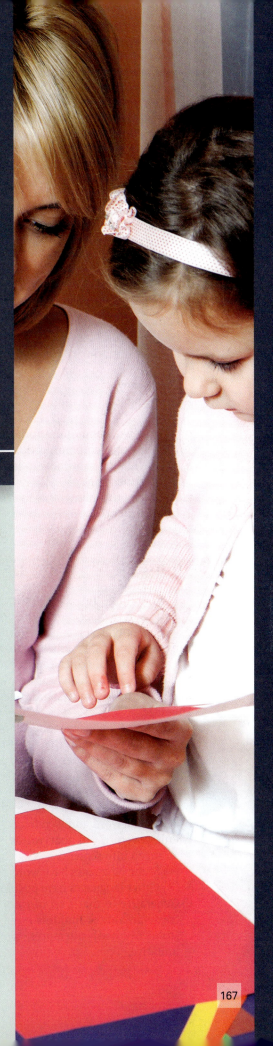

Terminology for Understanding Language Development and Disorders in Young Children

Communication Competence

1. Acquiring communication competence is the overall goal of language learning.
2. The successful exchange of information occurs between two or more participants.
   a. Assumed to be the primary motivation for language development.
   b. Speech-language pathologists (SLP) determine if there is a mismatch between a child's ability to communicate successfully and the demands placed on the child in his or her environment.
      (1) This is a primary consideration for assessment, intervention planning and for dismissal from therapy.
3. Developing understanding of the communication attempts of others and finessing the production of one's own communication attempts are keys to success within a communication context.
   a. Insufficient to know how to initiate with conversation partner only.
   b. Insufficient to know how to respond to conversation partner only.

Language Characteristics

1. Understanding the characteristics of languages is prerequisite to determining the presence of language disorders or typical language-learning patterns.
2. Languages can be verbal (spoken) or nonverbal (signed/gestured/written).
3. Majority of individuals learning language will eventually learn to understand and produce spoken language.
4. Regardless of language mode, all bona fide languages share a set of common characteristics.
   a. Socially-shared codes are rules governing language form, content and use and are common to a group of people, thus communicative.
   b. Arbitrary symbols: there is no inherent relationship between a word and its referent.
   c. Rule-governed, in that words are not randomly arranged into sentences.
      (1) Some languages have word-order constraints.
      (2) Other languages have position constraints.
   d. Generative in that a set of rules that can generate/create an almost limitless number of grammatical (rule-governed) utterances; productions are not imitative.
5. Dialectal differences must be distinguished from language disorders to prevent misdiagnosis, inappropriate labeling, as well as inappropriate referral for therapy.
   a. Standard dialect: arbitrary designation, typically given to the dialect spoken by the educated and/or wealthy classes in a society (e.g., Standard American English [SAE]).
   b. Non-standard dialect: arbitrary designation typically given to the dialect(s) or language variations spoken by those with less education or wealth (e.g., African American English [AAE]).
   c. SLP must know obligatory versus optional rules that differentiate standard versus non-standard dialects to accurately distinguish dialect differences from true disorders.
      (1) Specifying third-person singular verb forms or plural morphemes in SAE is (obligatory), but optional in AAE.
         (a) He run(s) to the corner.
         (b) Delia has two cookie(s).
      (2) Dialectal differences can be found in all components of language (e.g., semantics/vocabulary; syntax/morphology, pragmatics/language use in context and phonology/speech sound production).
         (a) Not all speakers of a dialect (standard or non-standard) use the exact same set of dialect features.
         (b) Not all speakers of a dialect who use specific dialect features use them in all contexts.
         (c) These factors make it both critical and difficult to assess dialect use on an individual basis.
         (d) Thus, expression of dialect use can differ from individual to individual and is not entirely predictable.
      (3) Typically, non-standard dialects are much more similar to the standard than they are different from one another.
         (a) This dialect feature often makes it possible for speakers of a standard dialect to understand the speakers of a non-standard dialect and vice versa.
         (b) This factor argues against the myth that non-standard dialects are less efficient for communication or are inaccurate/incorrect attempts to speak the standard version of a dialect.
         (c) There are exceptions to this generality (e.g., Mandarin and Cantonese are dialects of Chinese that are not mutually understandable).

(4) There is no inherent value in speaking one dialect of a language versus another; however, people who only speak a non-standard dialect variety may experience negative economic, academic and social ramifications.

(5) "Code switching" refers to the ability to speak more than one dialect and understand in what context it is appropriate/beneficial to speak one or the other.

6. Bilingualism.
   a. Simultaneous bilingualism.
      (1) Two or more languages are learned at the same time (i.e., child is exposed to . . .).
      (2) Typically, this means exposure begins shortly after birth and continues to be a feature of the caregiving environment.
      (3) Thus, the child's languages do not carry the traditional first versus second language distinction; both languages serve as first languages.
         (a) Sometimes children do demonstrate distinctive conceptual vocabularies depending on the context of language learning (e.g., foods in Spanish but clothing types in English).
         (b) Learning two languages simultaneously may slow down language development for a time to allow the child to sort out the rule systems in their languages.
         (c) The slowing of language learning is temporary and does not indicate the presence of a disorder.
   b. Successive bilingualism.
      (1) Second language (or additional languages) is learned after the acquisition of a first language.
      (2) The first, or dominant language, is known as L_1 and subsequent languages learned will be called L_2.
      (3) Determination of L_1 versus L_2 is critical because a language disorder can only be diagnosed if it is present in L_1.
         (a) SLP must be able to correctly determine the language that serves as a child's dominant language.
         (b) To prevent misdiagnosis of language differences versus language disorders, nonbiased evaluation in the dominant language is required.
         (c) Interference between the established L_1 and the learning of L_2 is not uncommon (e.g., child learning English as L_2 where L_1 is Spanish may place adjectives after nouns when speaking English).
         (d) Research has demonstrated that teaching in a child's L_1 facilitates learning of L_2 to a greater degree than teaching in L_2 only.

7. Components of languages must be evaluated during assessment and prioritized for therapy if needed.
   a. Consider both the receptive (comprehension) and expressive (production) aspects of these component parts of language in both typical language development and language disorders.
   b. Language comprehension tends to precede production although there are instances where children attempt to use words or syntactic forms before demonstrating their understanding.
      (1) Comprehension of language is often overestimated by caregivers.
         (a) Comprehension cannot be observed as directly as production but is inferred.
         (b) In the absence of full linguistic comprehension, children will respond to individual words or gestures to make guesses at linguistic messages.
         (c) Comprehension "guesses" or "strategies" demonstrate a child's recognition that a response is called for.
         (d) Comprehension "guesses" can also demonstrate a child's knowledge of routine contexts and object/action relationships.
      (2) Production is less likely to be overestimated because it can be directly observed (e.g., heard, seen, recorded and observed again).
   c. Teaching an aspect of language production will follow a distinctly different path if a child has no understanding of that expressive form/function.
      (1) If a child demonstrates understanding of a missing or inconsistently used language form or function, the SLP can capitalize on that understanding in teaching.
      (2) If not, teach understanding first or along with production.
   d. Bloom and Lahey (1978) divided language into form, content and use to make more evident how language components interface during typical language learning and are asynchronous when a language disorder is diagnosed.
      (1) Language form.
         (a) Syntax includes the rules for sentence construction (e.g., the production of grammatical declaratives, interrogatives and imperatives.
         (b) Morphology is the consistent use of the bound obligatory morphemes that specify verb tense (e.g., walks, walked), number (e.g., hats, gloves, boxes) or other affixes altering word meaning or word group classification (e.g., -ment, pre-, -ness); e.g., free morphemes are also acquired.
         (c) Phonology includes the development and use of a language's sound system, including phonemic inventory, phonotactic constraints and morphophonemic rules.

(2) Language content.
  (a) Development of vocabulary, both expressive and receptive.
  (b) Development of a system of semantic relations that describes roles and relationships of presyntactic word combinations (e.g., Agent + Action [daddy go], Action + Object [drive car]).
  (c) As more relationships are expressed per utterance, semantic relations are recombined (e.g., Agent + Action + Object).
(3) Language use.
  (a) Pragmatics is the use of language in context and can be divided into at least three different sets of competencies.
    - Communicative intentions/goals represent the functions of language use (e.g., requesting, demanding, negotiating).
    - Presupposition involves judging what the listener knows and making appropriate accommodations to facilitate successful communication (e.g., vocabulary choice, sophistication of syntactic structure).
    - Discourse management involves the rules for turn-taking, topic initiation, etc. that are understood by participants and necessary for successful communication (e.g., do not talk while another participant is talking).
(4) Examples of the interface among language components.
  (a) When a child's repertoire of syntactic structures increases (syntax), there is a greater likelihood that the child also has multiple ways to convey the same request (pragmatics).
  (b) When a child's consistency in the use of grammatical morphemes increases (morphology), there is a greater likelihood that the child can better specify the setting (i.e., time and place) of a narrative told to a naïve listener (pragmatics).
  (c) When a child's vocabulary grows (semantics), that child is better able to produce sentences with elaborated noun phrases (NPs) and verb phrases (VPs), an aspect of syntax.

Models of Language Development and Disorders

Models of Language Development

1. Most attempts to describe language development are variations on the relative contributions of nature (i.e., innate features of language learning) and nurture (i.e., environmental contributions).
2. Most investigators/theorists believe that there is some balance between the two types of input to the language-learning process; both are needed and interface to foster language learning.
   a. The child is specially designed to make use of the language input provided by the environment (e.g., cognitive/perceptual mechanisms are attuned to the human voice, human faces).
      (1) The input, called child-directed speech or motherese, provided in language-learning contexts (e.g., caregiver-child interactions) tends demonstrate a set of characteristics.
         (a) It tends to be repetitive.
         (b) It has prosodic emphasis placed on new information.
         (c) It is constructed to maintain the attention of young children through prosodic variations and exaggerated gestures.
      (2) The features are used to highlight the connection between the context and language used.
3. Connectionist and information processing models have also been promoted as explanations for children's language learning.
   a. Connectionist modeling focuses on the strengthening of relationships between frequently co-occurring events and language forms.
   b. Information processing models of learning focus on the role played by memory stores, both short-term and long-term, in language learning.
4. Language learning is a lifelong process, although a significant portion of language learning typically is mastered by the time a child enters elementary school (i.e., 5–6 years of age).
   a. Amount of language learning (e.g., vocabulary) and trajectory of language learning is unparalleled during the preschool years.
   b. All language aspects (e.g., pragmatics, vocabulary) continue to develop throughout an individual's lifetime, barring extraordinary illness, sensory deprivation without compensation, etc.
5. Cultures differ regarding who is the primary caregiver (i.e., typically mother or sibling), who is an appropriate conversation partner for a young child (i.e., adults, peers, both), the role the caregiver assumes in terms of teaching language to children and whether a child can initiate a conversation with an adult.

a. Cross-cultural competence is needed by the SLP to understand the framework of typicality for an individual learning language.
b. Cross-cultural competence is essential for the development of intervention programs that make sense for individual families.
c. Differences may affect both quantitative and qualitative aspects of language acquisition.
6. Differences may affect opportunities for exposure and the quality of language data to which the child is exposed and context for practicing language learning. Language learning presupposes some prerequisite skills and contextual supports.
   a. Cognitive or intellectual capacities sufficient for language learning.
      (1) Most children will learn some language despite significant cognitive deficits although normalization may not be an appropriate expectation or goal in this case.
      (2) Functional language goals may be more appropriate in some cases, including teaching a limited language repertoire that targets specific vocational and/or recreational needs.
         (a) Teach production of useful vocabulary and syntactic structures that reflect communicative needs in the child's activities of daily living (i.e., expressive language).
         (b) Teach understanding of useful vocabulary and syntactic structures that reflect communicative needs in the child's activities of daily living (i.e., language comprehension).
      (3) Cognitive competencies underlying language learning allow a child to observe and learn how the world works in terms of people, things and events (e.g., people can embody an "agent" role in semantic relationships because they can get things done, things out of sight do not cease to exist, etc.).
         (a) Consider how terms like "on top of" or "next to" require some understanding of the relationships that people and objects can have to one another in space before one can map language onto them.
         (b) Consider that it is necessary to compare two words or two situations to determine relative similarities and differences for generalization to occur (i.e., can the same rule be applied in both instances?).
         (c) Cognitive competencies also relate to organizing experiences then storing them in a logical way in memory to facilitate ease of retrieval.
   b. Perceptual abilities sufficient to make use of visual, auditory, tactile (less typically taste and smell) cues from the environment.
   c. Sufficient environmental input, both direct and indirect, to foster the learning of the connections between language symbols (e.g., oral, gestural or written) and the context in which they are used, is sometimes referred to as "mapping language onto context."
   d. General health and well-being of the child and family unit as well as the availability of ongoing, adequate medical care, nutrition and shelter for them.
      (1) A child's fragile health early on can negatively affect maternal bonding with the child with or without hospitalization.
         (a) Inconsistent cuing by the infant makes scaffolding difficult or impossible; input for the child may not be accessible.
         (b) Increased stress in the family unit (i.e., will my child survive?) negatively affects bonding.
      (2) History of pre-, peri- and/or postnatal medical problems (e.g., anoxia, presence of drugs/alcohol in utero) can lead to language-learning difficulties for a child.
      (3) Premature infants or those who are small for gestational age are at higher risk for several developmental disorders, including language development.
      (4) Diagnosis of a syndrome with a high probability of concomitant speech and language development concerns (e.g., Down syndrome, fragile X, fetal alcohol syndrome).
      (5) Instability in the family unit due to financial, maturational (i.e., immature parents) and health issues can place a child at risk for atypical development, including speech and language acquisition.
7. Elements of language learning interact with one another so that advances in the sophistication of one area of language learning will enhance a child's ability to express himself/herself in another.
   a. With increases in vocabulary and syntax development, children learn different forms for conveying the same meaning (e.g., asking for another cookie or more milk) that vary in formality and politeness.
      (1) "It would be nice to have another cookie."
      (2) "Maybe you will bring me some more milk later."
      (3) "Please may I have some more milk?"
      (4) "Give me another cookie!"
   b. Finessing vocabulary and syntax can facilitate the development of a richer repertoire of alternatives for the requesting communicative function/intention, a part of pragmatic development.
   c. Remember that observing or analyzing language on a component-by-component basis is artificial,

Basic Language Development Milestones Component

1. Pragmatic development.
   a. Consider both the quantity and quality of what is developing and the trajectory of that development over time.
   b. Before the development of words, children recognize that gestures (e.g., eye gaze, pointing) can be useful for getting what they want (see protoimperatives and protodeclaratives in semantic development below).
   c. Children learn by using nonverbal communication early on. Communication is a two-process system, involving both receiving information from others and conveying information to others.
   d. Communicative intentions develop as intentionality becomes evident (e.g., requests for action, requests for objects, statements and comments).
      (1) The child's repertoire of different communicative intentions expands.
         (a) The ability of the child to add vocalization or words to gestures.
         (b) The flexibility of different words that can be used to convey specific communicative intentions.
   e. Presupposition has begun to develop when a child takes the perspective of the conversation partner and makes accommodations to communication attempts, verbal or nonverbal, to facilitate successful communication.
      (1) Early evidence of presupposition is seen in toddlers' use of motherese, a language register typically used by caregivers to maintain the attention of babies.
      (2) Toddlers assume that their smaller conversation partners are less sophisticated conversation partners.
      (3) Eventually they learn that this parameter (i.e., size of the partner) is insufficient for gauging partner sophistication.
      (4) Any accommodations (i.e., changes) of vocabulary, syntax or increased precision of phonetic productions by a child can be interpreted as attempts to meet the communication needs of the listener and avoid the need for clarification (e.g., "What? Can you tell me that again? I'm confused.").
      (5) Responding to requests for clarification (e.g., repetition of the message, altering semantic choice, altering syntactic choice, providing additional information of an explanatory nature) demonstrates concern for the listeners' understanding as a prerequisite for successful communication.
      (6) Increase in language sophistication of a young speaker can be reflected in the manner of responding to clarification requests and success in keeping conversation relatively free from communication breakdowns.
      (7) Theory of Mind is a complex type of presupposition wherein a child demonstrates he/she can understand what another believes to be true (e.g., "Where does Betty believe the cookies are?").
         (a) Children diagnosed on the autism spectrum typically have difficulty with Theory of Mind tasks.
         (b) These children will demonstrate they know where the cookies are but cannot separate that knowledge from consideration of what Betty's different perspective is regarding the location of the cookies.
   f. Discourse management begins to develop when children engage in conversation frameworks often fostered by their caregiver's turn-taking behavior.
      (1) Depending on cultural influence, children will learn that conversations are comprised by nonoverlapping turns among participants fairly early on.
         (a) In mainstream culture, caregivers accept gurgles and random movements as children's turns.
         (b) Caregivers wait for the child to take a turn and then take their own.
         (c) Caregivers' goal is to frame a conversation around the child participant regardless of the child's communication immaturity or lack of intentionality.
         (d) This behavior pattern is very different from that observed in adult-adult conversations where there is typically less waiting for others' turns and more competition for conversation control.
         (e) This pattern of interaction may not be typical in a child's home if young children are not seen as appropriate conversation partners for adults except when the caregiver initiates conversation with the child.
      (2) Successful development of conversation or any discourse type rests on the child's knowledge of and ability to demonstrate:
         (a) Joint attention, or focusing on what the caregiver is focused on, as a prerequisite to establishing a topic.

(b) Following the caregiver's line of regard, or recognizing that the caregiver is attending to someone or something, and seeking out the point of attention.
(c) Joint action routines (JARs), or repetitive, predictable patterns of interaction (e.g., "peek-a-boo," rolling a ball back and forth between participants), that include specified roles and responsibilities for each participant.
- JARs provide predictable contexts for the overlay of relevant words, actions, semantic relations and/or sentences (e.g., "I'm rolling the ball. Now you roll the ball").

(3) There is very little about a conversation that is predictable, including topic choices, length of turns, number of turns per topic, whose turn it is in multiple-participant conversations, etc.
(4) Conversation management is generally negotiated among the participants with a combination of verbal and nonverbal information (e.g., I can look at my partner to indicate it is his turn and I can also say, "Fred, what do you think?").
(5) Discourse can refer to any text comprised of multiple sentences, not just in a conversation context. However, all discourse needs to be constructed logically to enable comprehension and facilitate participation with others.
    (a) Narratives are stories that follow a prescribed story grammar to be understood and can be original stories or story retelling; they can be fictional/fantasy or based on personal experiences.
    (b) Expository text is a description of how to do something; it is a set of instructions provided to an audience in need of the information (e.g., How do you make the best peanut butter and jelly sandwich?).
(6) Forms of discourse begin their development during the preschool years facilitated by experience as a participant, being a recipient of helpful feedback indicating when a child's contribution has been constructive to conveying the communication type.
    (a) Discourse success is also aided by development of perspective-taking skills.
    (b) Discourse success is also aided by ongoing developments in vocabulary learning, increasing sophistication of syntax, reading, etc.

g. Closely related to pragmatics of language learning is the development of metalinguistics.
   (1) Using language to talk about language is a simple definition for metalinguistics.
   (2) A key to metalinguistics is that to evaluate language (e.g., "That's a good sentence." or "What does that word mean?") the child has to first objectify language, study it and then judge it based on internalized criteria for acceptability.
   (3) Metalinguistic competencies are critical to learning how to divide words up into their component syllables and sounds.
       (a) This skill is known as demonstrating phonological awareness and it is a prerequisite to learning to decode written symbols for reading.
       (b) Phonological awareness is an important part of literacy learning and preschool-age children typically demonstrate the ability to rhyme words and recognize that compound words like "lakehouse" can be divided into two separate words.
       (c) Phonological awareness includes the manipulation, blending and segmenting of syllables and phonemes within words (e.g., "House. Drop the last sound and what do you have?").

2. Early sound production.
   a. Consider the quantity and quality of what is developing as well as the trajectory of that development.
   b. Generally, infants → toddlers → preschoolers are gaining motor control over their sound systems, resulting in reduction in variability over time for both consonants and vowel productions.
   c. Reflexive vocalization in response to pleasure or pain is not intentional but may be interpreted as such (e.g., crying and fussing).
   d. "Cooing" and "gooing": Infant produces approximations of consonants (i.e., there is some obstruction of the airstream in the vocal tract) and vowels (i.e., relatively unobstructed airstream through the vocal tract) in sequence sounding like /k/ or /g/ + vowel, usually a low back vowel.
   e. Babbling (e.g., marginal, reduplicated, nonreduplicated) is comprised of consonants and vowels more closely approximating the acoustic properties of adult vowels and consonants that are produced in sequence.
      (1) Reduplicated babbling is constituted by repeated CV sequences (e.g., /bababab/).
      (2) Nonreduplicated babbling represents a more complex pattern of CV syllables that are not identical (e.g., /pabadito/).
      (3) When accompanied by prosodic intonation contours (e.g., rising or falling intonation), toddlers may sound like they are actually speaking.

(4) Caregivers often mistake nonreduplicated babbling/jargon as real speech because of the addition of prosodic contours.
f. For many children, the first real words appear around 12 months of age but there is a great deal of variability and they must meet three criteria.
(1) They are produced with consistent phonetic forms.
(2) They approximate an adult word.
(3) They are used in consistent contexts.
g. First words are typically consonant (C) + vowel (V) in shape and often include nasal, glide and/or stop consonants.
h. Use of first words and babbling overlap in most children; do not expect a clear demarcation between pre- and postverbal productions.

3. Development of meaning or language content.
a. Consider the quantity and quality of what is developing as well as the trajectory of that development.
b. Appearance of intentionality occurs when there are persistent attempts to reach a goal.
c. Gestures are used in triadic interactions with caregivers and objects.
(1) The child uses objects to get the attention of a caregiver (i.e., protodeclaratives); child uses gestures and/or vocalizations and eye gaze to convey intended meaning.
(2) The child signals the caregiver to get objects for him or her (i.e., protoimperatives); child uses gestures and/or vocalizations and eye gaze to convey intended meaning.
d. Children's first words almost always develop in their receptive vocabulary before they appear in their expressive vocabulary.
(1) Lag between receptive and expressive vocabulary in terms of numbers of vocabulary items and rate of acquisition continues for the first few years of development.
(2) Research findings indicate that when the first 10 words in the expressive vocabulary have appeared, it is typical to have approximately 50 words in the receptive vocabulary.
e. Children's definitions of words develop over time with experience, including direct and indirect feedback, so their concepts of words are much less comprehensive when they first begin to use them.
f. Demands to participate in communication may be hampered by limited vocabulary choices.
(1) Early word use may be characterized by underextensions (e.g., "Annie," the name of the child's sister is used for all little girls).
(2) Overextensions (e.g., *cow* for *horse*, *car* for *truck*) may also occur because of limited breadth of vocabulary choices.
(a) Overextensions that appear in production may not appear in comprehension (e.g., child recognizes that horses and cows are not the same but does not have two different words for them).
g. Vocabulary development should reach at least 50 different words in the expressive vocabulary by age 2.
(1) For many children, reaching the milestone of an expressive vocabulary of 50 different words serves as a precursor for the appearance of word combinations.
(2) If 50 different words and two-word combinations do not appear by 2 years of age, the diagnosis of "Late Talker" is appropriate and child has an increased chance of continuing to have difficulty learning language.
h. Semantic relations develop as children begin to combine words.
(1) Before word combinations, children are learning words with meanings that will be helpful in constructing multi-word utterances (e.g., more = recurrence; no = negation, denial).
(2) Children are learning the roles that words can play in combinations with other words as well as meanings.
(a) "Mommy" can serve as a doer of actions or agent, as in "Mommy fall."
(b) "Mommy" can also be a recipient of actions or object, as in "hug Mommy."
(3) Taxonomies of semantic relations reveal that children are learning similar categories of meanings expressed in their pre-sentential utterances regardless of the language learned.
(4) Development of semantic relations follows two parameters.
(a) Acquisition of a comprehensive set of different semantic relationships that can be expressed.
(b) Flexibility to use a variety of words to convey the meaning represented by the semantic relationship.
(5) True semantic relationships (i.e., nonimitative, productive utterances).
(a) Are not relegated to one position only (not no + X or X + no only, but both).
(b) Are not relegated to one word combination (not no + doggie only, but no + X, no + Y, no + Z).
(c) Demonstrate some creativity so it is unlikely the child has imitated the two-word combination (e.g., "open shoe" produced to request that the child's shoe be removed or untied).

(6) After children have acquired several different two-role semantic relationships, they begin to combine them into longer strings of meaning.
   (a) Agent + Action and Action + Object = Agent + Action + Object.
   (b) "Bob walk" and "Walk dog" = "Bob walk dog," for example.
   (c) Note that the redundant term, in this case the action, is not repeated but expressed once.
   (d) With development as noted above, a child's repertoire of semantic relations increases; the number of examples within categories of semantic relations increases.
(7) When children begin producing longer and more complex sentences, syntax, rather than semantics, is typically the focus of assessment, although underlying the syntax, semantic relations are present.
(8) Children adopt strategies for word learning, including utilizing spoken context and requesting information from more knowledgeable peers or adults (e.g., "What that?").
   (a) "Fast mapping" refers to a child's ability to correctly use a new word after one exposure to it by relying on context cues.
   (b) "Rote learning" accounts for many instances of word learning; adults draw a child's attention to a new word and provide a definition and an example of how to use the word, often without the benefit of supporting context.
i. Concept development continues to grow and change with language experience, including direct and indirect verbal input/teaching and later from exposure to text.
j. By the time a typical child enters kindergarten, he or she will have approximately 1100 different words in his or her expressive and receptive vocabularies, respectively, and there is less distinction between the size of the receptive and expressive vocabularies than there was earlier in the preschool period.

4. Syntactic development.
   a. Consider what develops as the trajectory and quality, as well as quantity, of development.
   b. Syntax is a part of language form and can be considered part of the code of the linguistic message.
   c. Syntax is made up of the rules and regulations that govern the construction of grammatical sentences, those sentences that abide by all of the grammatical constraints of a language.
      (1) Children learn to produce different sentence types to convey their intended meanings (e.g., declaratives, interrogatives, imperatives).
      (2) Languages differ in terms of syntax complexity; not all languages have word-order constraints that are as restrictive as English, for example.
      (3) When children are acquiring syntactic structures that enable them to create longer and more complex sentences during the preschool years, they are typically utilizing coordination and embedding to do so.
         (a) Coordination links clauses or other sentence parts through the use of conjunctions (e.g., and, but, if . . . then) as in, "An enormous vehicle lumbered down the road and then it veered sharply to the right."
         (b) Embedding refers to the use of main and subordinate clauses in the same sentence as in "Fred, the guy who lives in the apartment next to mine, owns a sheepdog."
      (4) Use of more sophisticated and elaborate noun phrases (NPs) and verb phrases (VPs) not only yields longer and more complex sentences but also permits the production (and understanding) of more descriptive and precise conversations, narratives and expository text.
         (a) NPs can be single words (e.g., bat) or multi-word (e.g., the brown, hairy, scary-looking bat).
         (b) VPs can also be simple (e.g., ran fast) or multi-word (e.g., ran quickly down the road and into the village).

5. Morphology development.
   a. Consider what is developing as well as the trajectory and quality and quantity of that development.
   b. Morphological development refers to the acquisition and consistent use of obligatory morphemes that are required for grammatical sentence production.
      (1) Free morphemes refer to any morphemes that can stand alone, thus any word is also a free-standing morpheme (e.g., car, recognizes, after).
      (2) Bound morphemes cannot appear alone, but instead are attached to a word stem (e.g., walk**s**, walk**ed**, **pre**nuptial).
      (3) Counting morphemes produced in language samples, averaged across utterances, yields a Mean Length of Utterance measure (Brown, 1973; Miller & Chapman, 1981).
   c. Language dialects differ in terms of the categorization of morphemes as obligatory or optional.
      (1) An example of an obligatory context for a third-person singular verb morpheme in SAE is walks.
      (2) In AAE, the third-person singular verb morpheme is optional in many instances so that walk or walks would be grammatical and acceptable.

d. Consistency of usage in obligatory contexts is key in the assessment of morphological development.
      (1) Children who are diagnosed with Specific Language Impairment and other language-learning disorders typically present with a lag in acquisition of consistent bound morpheme use.
      (2) Consistency of morpheme use in obligatory contexts can be calculated as a percentage.
         (a) It is the number of times the child correctly produced a specific morpheme (in obligatory context) divided by the total number of opportunities for that specific morpheme to have been produced in a spoken or written passage.
         (b) Traditionally, 90% of use in obligatory contexts has been used as the standard for establishing the acquisition of a morpheme.
      (3) Most morphemes emerge in a child's repertoire long before acquisition has occurred and thus morpheme development is a process.
   e. Morphological development is essential to finessing meaning in sentences and text forms by providing children with the tools for specifying time, number, possession and other conceptual pieces of information.
   f. In language sample analysis, SLPs can use Brown's 14 Grammatical Morphemes as a standard list to measure preschool-age children's appropriateness of morphological development.
      (1) Not all grammatical morphemes are included in this list (not exhaustive).
      (2) Brown believed that these 14 morphemes showed the most dramatic acquisition trajectory in the first few years of language development.
      (3) SLPs calculate percentage of usage of each morpheme in obligatory contexts.

Models of Language Disorders

1. Language disorders can be viewed from a normative perspective. When compared with data available from typically developing children of the same chronological age, does the child demonstrate a comparable skill set?
   a. Clinicians should be careful to note that this perspective yields a deficit model, where the child's needs are highlighted but their abilities are not.
   b. Mental age is not an appropriate comparison point.
   c. It is useful to have standardized/objective data to help define a language disorder but clinicians should note their limits.
      (1) Many test instruments we use take a decontextualized view of language and neglect how language is actually used by the child; this must be inferred from test results.
      (2) Not all standardized tests are equal in validity and reliability and may not be appropriate for particular clients.
2. Language disorders can be viewed from a communication perspective. When the communication demands of the child's environment are considered, does this child have sufficient language competencies to meet those age-appropriate language demands?
   a. A mismatch between language demands in the child's activities of daily living and the language skill set yields communication breakdowns and frustration.
   b. This model represents a functional approach to describing language disorders.
3. Language disorders can be viewed from the perspective of a child's apparent understanding of the use of language as a tool for conveying information to a conversation partner as well as responding to the conversation bids of a partner.
   a. Is the child an assertive language user?
      (1) Is the child able and willing to initiate language in a conversation (e.g., request for information, comment)?
      (2) If assertiveness is demonstrated, the child is assumed to understand that language can be used to engage others.
   b. Is the child a responsive language user?
      (1) Is the child able and willing to respond to the conversation bids of conversation partners (e.g., responses to requests for information, responses to requests for action)?
      (2) If responsiveness is demonstrated, it is assumed the child understands that language can be used to respond to the requests of conversation partners.
   c. Does the child understand the reciprocal nature of conversation and use language to respond to the communication bids of a conversation partner?
   d. Intervention for children with different profiles of +/− assertiveness and +/− responsiveness competencies is not uniform but planned to establish a foundation of these two prerequisite conversation abilities.
4. Definitions of language disorders.
   a. There is not total agreement about how to best describe children with language disorders and there is overlap in definitions used.
   b. ASHA defines a language disorder as "impaired comprehension and/or use of spoken, written and/or other symbol systems. The disorder may involve
      (1) the form of language (phonology, morphology,

syntax), (2) the content of language (semantics), and/or (3) the function of language in communication (pragmatics) in any combination."
c. Multiple terms are used; in all cases terminology should be person-first: "Children who are diagnosed as/with . . . (e.g., Late Talkers, Specific Language Impairment, Language-Learning Disabilities, Language Disorders, Pragmatic Language Impairment).
  (1) Different terms may relate to different points along the age span (e.g., "Late Talkers" versus "Specific Language Impairment").
  (2) Different terms may relate to different areas of language learning most likely to be affected (e.g., "Pragmatic Language Impairment" versus "Pervasive Developmental Disorder").
  (3) Different terms may relate to a generality of the group of children described (e.g., "Learning Disabilities" versus "Language-Learning Disabilities").
  (4) Different terms may relate to the popularity of term use by different researchers or preferences in different countries (e.g., "Pragmatic Language Impairment" versus "Autism Spectrum Disorder").
d. What is to be gained by the use of an appropriate diagnostic term?
  (1) Does the diagnosis provide a better description of the language disorder?
  (2) Is the diagnosis more likely to provide eligibility for services?
  (3) Does the diagnosis provide direction to the SLP for the planning of services?
e. Language disorders may represent an underlying deficit in language symbol processing that may continue to be exhibited across the age span (e.g., reading, speaking, writing, mathematics).
f. Continuity of language-learning difficulties across the lifespan is commonly observed in this population.
g. Quality of life for adults with life-long language-learning disorders may be diminished in terms of education achievement and income.
h. Heterogeneity is more the rule than the exception within groups of children with language disorders.
  (1) Differences evident in areas of language affected or scope of the language disorder as well as severity.
  (2) One commonality observed for young children diagnosed with Specific Language Impairment is difficulty with grammatical morphemes.
i. The traditional definition of children classified as "Late Talkers" is children who reach the age of 24 months and do *not* demonstrate the use of 50 different words in their expressive vocabularies and do not yet combine words.
j. The traditional definition of children classified with "Specific Language Impairment" is that these children do not demonstrate deficits in cognitive, socio-emotional, or motor development; there is no evidence of hearing impairment, but a deficit in language learning is evident.
  (1) Thus, a disorder of exclusion.
  (2) Heterogeneity is a key characteristic but most have significant difficulties acquiring the grammatical morphemes of their language.
k. Children with Non-specific Language Impairment (NLI) have cognitive test scores less than 1 standard deviation below the mean and meet other criteria for SLI.
l. Learning Disability (LD).
  (1) "An unexpected difficulty" in learning relative to age.
  (2) "A disorder in one or more of the basic psychological processes involved in understanding or in using language spoken or written that may manifest itself in an imperfect ability to listen, think, speak, read, write, spell, or do mathematical calculations . . . ." (IDEA, 2004).
    (a) Note that problems associated with mental retardation, perceptual deficits, emotional disturbance, etc. are excluded from this definition.
m. Language-Learning Disability (LLD).
  (1) The most common type of LLD, typically with a history of both oral language disorder and reading disorder.
  (2) Reading, writing and spelling are most commonly deficient; the nature of these specific disorders is heterogeneous within the group of individuals defined with LLD.
  (3) Because the preschool child has not typically begun to read, these topics are beyond the scope of this chapter.
    (a) Note that phonological awareness, an important foundational skill for reading success, does emerge during the late preschool years.
    (b) SLPs and caregivers can foster recognition and practice of rhymes as well as phoneme manipulation, blending and segmenting through book-reading activities.
    (c) Encouraging the presence of text in households is important to increase the likelihood a child will become curious about and motivated to learn the code of reading.
n. Autism Spectrum Disorders (ASD).
  (1) DSM-V (2013) updated the definition of ASD to create a more general umbrella term.
    (a) Core challenges to social communication/social interaction with specific deficits in

social reciprocity, nonverbal communication and developing/maintaining relationships.
- (b) Repetitive, stereotypical behaviors, activities or interests (e.g., routinized or restricted behaviors, excessive reactivity to stimuli).
- (c) Symptoms first emerge in early childhood and may exacerbate as context demands increase.
- (d) The child's activities of daily living (ADLs) are subsequently restricted.
- (e) Children with ASD present with a range of verbal competencies; all have difficulties using the language they have in social contexts. ASD is probably "the most variable in terms of cognitive profile, language ability, co-morbid diagnoses, and eventual outcomes" (Paul and Norbury, 2012, p. 119).
- (f) The focus of research and SLP practice is to identify children with symptoms of ASD as early as possible and provide treatment to teach prerequisite, nonverbal communicative behaviors (e.g., joint attention, gesture).

Potential Causal Factors for Language Disorders

1. Cognitive differences/limitations.
   a. Limited processing capacity.
      (1) Difficulties utilizing working memory and phonological memory, paired with perceptual deficits, can negatively affect language-learning ability in young children.
      (2) When processing demand increases as tasks become more complex, a child's limited processing capacity is further minimized.
   b. Auditory processing deficits.
      (1) Children with language disorders have an extraordinarily difficult time accurately processing rapid auditory information (e.g., grammatical markers, phonemes).
      (2) Auditory processing deficits frequently occur in the population of children with language disorders, but not all.
2. Environmental features of the language-learning environment.
   a. Differences across language-learning environments alone probably do not explain the presence of language disorders.
   b. Paul and Norbury (2012) noted that language learning is a robust phenomenon, not likely to be negatively affected by environmental factors alone.
3. Biological feature differences.
   a. Anatomical and/or physiological differences in the brain.
      (1) New technologies have allowed studies of brain structure and function to begin amassing comparative data.
         (a) Magnetic Resonance Imaging (MRI) studies have shown asymmetry in the brains of children with language disorders not observed in children with typical language development.
         (b) Recent work has identified different clusters of anatomical features in children with language comprehension difficulties versus children with phonological impairments.
   b. Brain function as assessed with Functional Magnetic Resonance Imaging (fMRI) has also demonstrated differences in activation levels and areas of activation when individuals with language disorders are compared with typical language learners in adolescence.
   c. Genetic features of language disorders.
      (1) Language disorders have a tendency to be inherited.
         (a) Specific genes on chromosomes 7, 16 and 19 have been shown to be associated with language disorders as well as other neurodevelopmental disorders.
         (b) The relationship between genes and specific language behavior is complex; prediction of language behaviors by specific gene is not a reality.
      (2) Twin studies have been useful in studying heritability of language disorders; monozygotic twins (identical) are more likely to both have language disorders than dizygotic (fraternal) twins.
4. Often families are told that it is uncertain what the causal factor or factors were in language disorders.
   a. It is likely that the more risk factors present, the more likely the presence of a disorder.
   b. The relationships among the potential factors of language disorder are not fully known.

Assessment of Language Disorders

Assessment Focus and Other Pre-assessment Data

1. The referral source may suggest a focus for the assessment (e.g., child is unintelligible, produces immature sentences, says few words), although it is a good idea when a language disorder is suspected to evaluate all areas of language, both in comprehension and expression, where possible.
   a. The family is included as a full partner in assessment planning, as per family-centered practice required by law (IDEA, 2004).
   b. Family members should be consulted regarding who should be present at the time of the assessment, who is the most appropriate informant for history gathering and the timing of the evaluation.
   c. Find out what the family hopes to gain as an outcome of the assessment (e.g., Is my child retarded? Does my child qualify for special services? What is the best way to help my child?).
2. The SLP can highlight the specific concern the referral source conveyed in the formal report of the assessment outcome by reporting this information first.
3. Determine whether information from other professionals or agencies will add to the validity of the findings and, if so, arrange with the family ahead of time for legal permission to gather outside information.
   a. Audiological evaluations completed within the last few months will be essential to access; many young children with and without language disorders present with histories of conductive hearing losses with episodes of concomitant hearing loss.
   b. It is critical to establish the hearing status of any child suspected of a language disorder prior to assessment.
   c. If recent audiological evaluation data are not available and if a hearing loss is suspected, either refer elsewhere for an audiological evaluation or plan to provide one prior to testing.
   d. May delay evaluation if hearing assessment outcome data are not available.
   e. If the child has been previously assessed by other agencies, request access to those reports; recognize that a family may be using your assessment as a second opinion and may not want you to have access to reports from other agencies.
   f. As part of preassessment data gathering, determine if the child has been previously evaluated for developmental concerns and/or received services from physicians, psychologists, physical therapists, occupational therapists, early intervention (EI) teams, etc.
   g. In lieu of access to official reports from other professionals, ask the informant for the family's impression of previous findings.
4. Be sure to explain to the caregiver/informant what to expect from the assessment process; unfortunately, these questions from the caregiver are not often addressed until the day of the assessment.
   a. How long will the assessment take?
      (1) Will the assessment take place all in one day?
      (2) Will there be opportunities for breaks for the child?
   b. Who will be involved with the assessment?
      (1) Be prepared to explain the expertise represented by all assessment team members.
      (2) How will the team ensure that the family understands the team members (i.e., What will be the language of the assessment? Will a translator be present?)
   c. What should the family expect in terms of their direct involvement in the assessment process?
      (1) Who would the family like to have present at the evaluation (e.g., extended family members, trusted individuals in the community)?
      (2) Has the caregivers' role in the assessment been explained in terms of serving as informants, completing documentation, facilitating the child's cooperation but not answering for the child?
   d. Should the family bring anything with them from home (e.g., favorite toy or book, where appropriate; a snack)?
      (1) A familiar toy, book or game may be comforting to a child because it is reminiscent of home when a child is assessed elsewhere.
      (2) A familiar toy, book or game may give a child something to talk about to the SLP; it creates a mismatch in background knowledge.
   e. Will I get answers to my questions today or will I have to wait for my answers?
      (1) Facilities differ in terms of how they handle debriefing following an assessment.
      (2) Some facilities prefer to conduct debriefing with families on a separate date following the assessment.
         (a) This can be helpful for the assessment team in providing sufficient time for analysis of data collected and/or received from other agencies.

(b) This can be helpful for families who may be fatigued following the assessment and not prepared to attend carefully to diagnostic information and recommendations.

(c) This can be difficult for families when they are worried about their children and want results as soon as possible.

Resources for Assessment Data

1. Selecting tasks for assessment of language.
   a. For young children or those who are noncompliant.
      (1) Data gathering may be accomplished through observation.
      (2) Data gathering may be accomplished through interviewing a caregiver/informant who is knowledgeable about the child's development.
   b. Data gathering for all young children may be accomplished through a combination of observation, informant information and elicitation of the language features to be assessed.
2. Tasks for assessment of language comprehension.
   a. Identification (by pointing) as in "show me *turkey*" when the child is shown a display of two- or three-dimensional stimuli.
   b. Identification tasks can be used for assessing aspects of vocabulary, morphology, syntax, phonology or pragmatics development.
   c. Identification tasks vary in stimuli length from a word, as in the case of The Peabody Picture Vocabulary Test-4, or several words or a sentence in length, as in the Test of Auditory Comprehension for Language-3. Acting-out tasks, as in "show me the cow is chased by the elephant," may be assessed when the child is provided with a toy cow and elephant.
   d. Responses to questions to demonstrate comprehension of the constraints inherent in different question types, as in Yes-No questions versus Wh-question types.
      (1) Yes/No questions require a verbal or nonverbal indication of affirmation or negation.
      (2) Appropriate answers to questions follow the linguistic constraint of the Wh-word.
         (a) "Where questions" must include a location.
         (b) "When questions" must include some indication of time.
   e. Correctness and appropriateness are two different considerations when evaluating responses to questions.
      (1) A correct answer to "when is your soccer game this afternoon?" could be "4 o'clock."
      (2) An appropriate answer to the same question could be any response that includes a time response (e.g., "2:30" or "7 p.m.") although the answer may not be correct.
3. Tasks for assessment of language production.
   a. Imitation tasks differ in terms of the amount of time that elapses between the presentation of the model and the expectation of an imitated response by the child.
      (1) The longer the interval and if there is inclusion of intervening language to process, the more difficult the imitation task becomes.
      (2) Immediate Imitation versus Delayed Imitation reflects this difference.
      (3) Care should be taken to not assume that language forms imitated reflect true productive use by a child; if not, what a child can easily produce without prompting may be overestimated.
      (4) Imitation tasks may be used when working with reticent children who are not providing much language production data.
      (5) Using "choice" questions can also serve this purpose of providing an example of an acceptable answer embedded in a question such as, "do you like parades or Ferris wheels better?"
      (6) Imitation tasks can also serve as a validation check of language produced in a spontaneous language sample or to augment language structures expected but missing from a sample.
   b. Fill-in or cloze procedure can be used to have a child "fill in the blank" to demonstrate ability to produce vocabulary that fits a context or grammatical morpheme obligated by the context.
      (1) "This is a bear. Here are two _____."
      (2) "Sally runs a race every day. Tomorrow she will _____ it again."
   c. Collection and analysis of a spontaneous language sample provide an opportunity to infer the grammatical rule system the child has acquired by collecting a representative corpus of utterances.
      (1) The representative sample is a subset of all the utterances a child is capable of producing.
      (2) The representative sample is assumed to be prototypical of a child's entire repertoire of utterances.
      (3) Thus, the SLP can infer the set of language structures and forms in a child's repertoire by collection and analysis of a much smaller set of utterances.
      (4) Collection of a representative language sample takes planning and cannot be accomplished without consideration of the materials, the topics of conversation partners made available for the collection period.
         (a) Consider observing a child with a caregiver as well as the SLP where possible.

(b) Interactions with siblings or peers provide for a variety of conversation partners and insight into consistency of language form and function.
(c) Language sampling does not have to occur during a discrete segment of the assessment period; incidental conversations during testing may yield useful utterances.
(5) Multiple methods of language sample analysis are available via computer or by hand calculation.
(6) Language samples can contain conversation, narratives or expository text; any combination of these can be revealing.
(7) Language sample analysis can focus on the child's production of utterances as well as the way those utterances constitute a coherent text.
d. Story-retelling tasks provide children with a model story with visual and/or auditory stimuli to support memory load.
(1) The child is asked to listen to and/or watch a story (i.e., video presentation) being told and then repeat it to the SLP (or caregiver, peer, etc.).
(2) It is helpful if the listener/recipient is naïve to the story to create a genuine context for communication.
(3) Retelling of the story can be prompted with use of supportive stimuli as well as questions from the SLP.
(4) Syntactic structures included in the retelling are probably part of the child's productive repertoire.
4. When selecting assessment tools, consider not only the area(s) of language addressed but also the task type used to elicit that information.
a. Failure on particular tests or subtests could be related to the task type selected.
b. Not all task types are familiar to children across cultures (e.g., sharing information the child knows that the SLP already knows, creating fantasy narratives that are not "true").
c. If failure is related to a task type, select another standardized test or create a nonstandardized probe that incorporates a different task type.
5. Standardized versus nonstandardized assessment.
a. Standardized testing includes prescribed stimuli, tasks, administration and interpretation procedures as well as normative data for comparison of client performance.
b. SLPs look for "converging data," evidence from several sources pointing to a disorder (or typical development) before reaching a diagnostic conclusion.
c. Although standardized testing is generally preferable for decision-making purposes, there are gaps in the availability of reliable and valid standardized tests to assess all areas of language (both receptive and expressive aspects).
(1) Where gaps in the availability of a standardized test exist, nonstandardized testing or probing will be necessary (see "7. Nonstandardized testing," below).
(2) There may not be a standardized test available that can be administered to a given child without introducing testing bias, and thus nonstandardized testing will be needed.
(3) Sometimes few examples of a language form or function are included in a test when more in-depth information is needed, thus nonstandardized testing will be necessary.
6. When selecting tests to include in a test battery, determine whether the test publishers can claim their test is both valid and reliable.
a. Understand the concepts of validity: Does a test actually test what it advertises it will test; and reliability: Does the test yield consistent outcomes across examiners, within examiners?
b. SLPs must be familiar with information available in a standardized test's manual to determine whether sufficient evidence of validity and reliability is present to support the inclusion of a test in an assessment.
(1) Test manuals are also essential resources for administration, scoring and interpretation guidelines.
(2) SLPs cannot administer, score or interpret the results of a test without thoroughly reading the test manual and practicing a test prior to its official use even if tests appear deceptively simple.
7. Nonstandardized testing.
a. Nonstandardized testing is often an ad hoc response by an SLP to gather information about a child's ability in an area of language learning that is not sufficiently covered by standardized test(s).
(1) Do available tests demonstrate adequate validity and reliability?
(2) Are available tests biased in terms of the stimuli, tasks or scoring criteria established?
(3) Have available tests used a standardization sample that is not inclusive to the client?
(4) Do available tests have too few items included to sufficiently assess the scope of the language problem?
b. Nonstandardized testing is sometimes referred to as the use of nonstandardized probes.
(1) Can it be used during diagnostic therapy (post-diagnosis) to investigate those language areas on a standardized test that may have been

difficult for a child? Sometimes this is called deep testing and it provides verification of where to begin therapy.
  (2) Can it be used prior to a diagnosis to evaluate any area of language not covered at all or adequately by a standardized measure or elicited through language sample collection (e.g., production of Wh-questions, production or understanding of passive sentences, use of presupposition in conversation)?
 c. Because of their specific nature, nonstandardized probes may have to be developed individually to serve the needs of the SLP and the child/family.
  (1) Determine the feature of language that needs to be deep tested and select 10–20 examples that were not utilized on the test.
  (2) Does this language form or function need to be assessed in comprehension, production or both?
  (3) What is known about the typical acquisition of this language form or function in terms of its common developmental pattern, and how can this information be incorporated so that more challenging items are placed later than developmentally less challenging items?
  (4) Given what we know about this child, what type of task is likely to elicit the information needed (i.e., avoid tasks that may include inherent cultural biases)?
  (5) What task types have already been attempted and is there any concern that the child cannot reasonably adapt to this task?
  (6) Following administration of the nonstandardized test, determine the pattern of performance, percentage correct, and determine the developmental level of correct responses.
 d. Nonstandardized probes also have utility in intervention to determine progress in therapy. (See "Measuring Progress in Therapy" in Intervention for Children with Language Disorders, later in this chapter.)

Selecting Assessment Materials

1. Know and evaluate the psychometric parameters of the standardized test reported in the test's manual.
 a. Adequate validity (e.g., content, construct): Does the test assess what it says it will test?
 b. Adequate reliability (e.g., test-retest, interrater reliability): Are test scores consistent?
 c. Adequate standardization sample for use of the normative data provided (e.g., size of sample, stratification re current census data)?
 d. Appropriate standardization sample for comparison, given the child being tested (e.g., SES, race, ethnicity, geographic region)?
 e. Availability of normative data adequate for diagnosis and/or screening?
 f. Are the stimuli engaging? Good representations of the concepts to be tested? Age appropriate?
2. Does the test provide the SLP with information relevant to the diagnostic question being asked (e.g., comprehension versus production)?
3. Is the SLP sufficiently familiar with the administration, scoring and interpretation of the test?
 a. Does the test manual provide explicit instructions so that SLPs unfamiliar with the test can become appropriate administrators, scorers and interpreters?
 b. Are ancillary materials available for teaching these procedures (e.g., practice videos, courses to teach administration)?
 c. Practicing administration, scoring and interpretation is a good professional procedure.
4. Is the version of the test used the most current available?
5. Has the SLP determined that the test represents a nonbiased assessment tool for the client in question?
 a. This information may be explicitly provided in the test manual.
 b. SLPs should be able to examine test stimuli, administration procedures, scoring and interpretation guidelines to determine whether and, if so, where potential sources of biased assessment may lie.

Creating a Test Battery and Assessment Appointment

1. Consider context available for assessment.
 a. Will the child be evaluated in the home environment and, if so, are there any inherent constraints imposed?
  (1) Agencies may require specific sets of tests to be used.
  (2) Agencies may also require time limits on the amount of time for each visit.
  (3) Timing of visit may be critical (e.g., before nap, after nap, before or after mealtime, availability of caregivers).
  (4) Will the home environment be (relatively) free from distractions?
 b. Will the child and family be evaluated in a location outside of their home?
  (1) Transport to and from the location must be feasible.
  (2) Child care may be needed for accompanying siblings.

(3) The test environment may be too clinical for the comfort of the child and/or family members (e.g., lab coats, formality, unfamiliarity).
(4) Child may be more anxious in an unfamiliar context.
c. Regardless of setting, what are the time and space constraints imposed?
2. Consider the question(s) the SLP wants to answer through assessment.
a. Is there a bona fide language disorder?
(1) Diagnostic tests and not screening tests are needed to answer this question (make this diagnosis).
(2) Screening tests answer the question: Should we evaluate further for a language disorder?
(3) Converging data from several sources are needed to confirm a diagnosis; no one test is sufficient to establish a diagnosis.
(4) When standardized sources are selected, they must be suitable and unbiased regarding the child and the child's family.
b. If there is a bona fide language disorder, what is the scope of the language disorder?
(1) Information about scope relates to the prognosis for the disorder.
(2) Does the language disorder encompass both receptive and expressive language modalities?
(a) When only an expressive language disorder is diagnosed, this typically indicates more rapid recovery than a language disorder characterized by both receptive and expressive deficiencies.
(b) Diagnosis of both receptive and expressive deficiencies will indicate a different approach to therapy than expressive language deficiency only.
(3) Scope of the language disorder also refers to the components of language that are affected.
(a) Language disorders may be characterized with deficiencies in one or more component parts of language.
(b) Typically, the greater the number of language components affected, the more difficult it will be for the child to communicate within activities of daily living.
(4) As the scope of the language disorder increases, a child's eligibility for therapy may also increase; a child is then at greater risk for negative social and academic outcomes.
c. What is the child's prognosis for catching up or otherwise benefiting from therapy?
(1) Did the child demonstrate knowledge of the underlying foundations of communication, including assertiveness and responsiveness in conversation, either verbal or nonverbal?
(2) Does the child demonstrate attention and discrimination skills necessary for benefiting from focused stimulation?
(3) Is there a supportive environment for the transfer of learning into activities of daily living?
(4) Has the child demonstrated inconsistent usage of some of the age-appropriate forms and functions of language?
(5) Does the child demonstrate awareness of or frustration with communication failures?
(6) Has the child demonstrated self-correction behaviors or other evidence of monitoring speech and language output?
d. Does periodic assessment reveal successful therapy outcomes?
(1) Assessment is also a critical part of the treatment phase of service delivery.
(a) Administration of untrained probe items will reveal the extent of the child's learning of the targets.
(b) Information gleaned from administration of probes will yield clues to ways of increasing the efficacy of the treatment (e.g., changes to stimuli, feedback provided, modeling used).
(2) SLPs should assess for timely progress toward stated goals.
(3) SLPs should consider progress toward stated goals as rationales for dismissal.

Interpreting Test Data

1. The initial decision is to determine if a language disorder exists.
2. Although beneficial to answering questions about scope and prognosis following the initial meeting, these questions may require diagnostic therapy (postenrollment service delivery) for comprehensive answers.
3. If a language disorder is diagnosed, prioritize targets for therapy.
a. Use normative data to determine the aspects of communication that are most significantly deficient.
b. Use information from the family and observations as well as observations of others to determine what the communication demands are on the child and how they are met.
c. Choose functional goals.
(1) Can the child compensate for lack of speech and language competencies?

(2) Activities of daily living (ADL): Will the child have opportunities to immediately incorporate the forms and functions targeted in therapy?
(3) What types of activity participation would help the child practice and normalize?
(4) How does the family support the child's use of new language forms and functions?
4. Check for language forms and functions that are used inconsistently versus not at all.
   a. If used inconsistently, the child has more knowledge of the form or function than if not used at all.
      (1) Similar to the "stimulability" concept in speech sound disorders.
      (2) Child is likely to make more progress more quickly on forms and functions used inconsistently.
   b. Recognize that sampling error can lead to false expectations of performance in therapy.
      (1) Inconsistent use may represent insufficient opportunity to perform in the evaluation session.
      (2) Troubleshoot data gleaned from diagnostic testing to be certain.
      (3) Consider use of probes to provide additional opportunities for elicitation of specific forms or functions.
   c. Check for forms and functions that may be part of the child's repertoire in comprehension but not in expression.
      (1) It is not typical for forms and functions to appear in expression; however, it is typical in comprehension.
      (2) Forms and functions understood but not expressed also signal that the child has more foundational knowledge and may be easier to teach/be taught more quickly.

Dynamic Assessment

1. A type of assessment used to determine if the child can be a successful learner when sufficient supports are in place.
   a. Intensive, individualized instruction.
      (1) May involve additional examples.
      (2) More explicit instruction or observational learning opportunities.
2. Used to distinguish between a child with severe developmental disability and a child who may not have received adequate instruction.
   a. Can eliminate or greatly reduce overdiagnosis of children from cultural and linguistic minorities as needing special services.
   b. Can reduce the number of children needlessly assessed, incorrectly diagnosed and eventually provided with special education.
3. In SLP practice, dynamic assessment is closely related to "response to intervention" (RTI).
   a. Attempt by school district personnel to reduce numbers of children not educated in general education classrooms.
   b. Attempt by school district personnel to avoid labeling children as having special needs.
   c. Attempt by school district personnel to provide intensive, appropriate services to children who may not have received best practices instruction.
4. In SLP practice, dynamic assessment is closely related to "diagnostic therapy."
   a. Attempt by SLP to bridge the gap between assessment and therapy planning.
   b. As noted above, delineates the scope of the language problem.
   c. As noted above, eliminates sampling error from data gleaned at the time of the assessment.

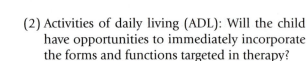

Intervention for Children with Language Disorders

Techniques to Modify Language Understanding and Use

1. Language therapy, language treatment, language intervention all refer to a set of techniques that serve to modify a child's understanding and use of language in ADL.
2. The overall goal is to increase a child's ability to be a successful communicator to a level expected, given the child's chronological age.
3. Intervention goals for a child are closely related to the deficits gleaned from assessment and subsequent monitoring of the child in a variety of communication contexts.
4. The purpose of language-based intervention is to make clear to the child the connection between language symbols (spoken or written or signed) and the contexts where used for communication.
   a. This can be referred to as "mapping language onto context."
   b. These contexts are in the here and now, early on when children are less cognitively and linguistically sophisticated.
   c. With development, contexts for using language will be in past time, future time, real or imagined.

5. The techniques used in intervention will provide the child with support for success during the learning process.
   a. Supports include supplementary visual/auditory/tactile information.
   b. Supports include frequent opportunities for practice.
   c. Supports include frequent opportunities for feedback, either direct or indirect.
6. Generalization, both response and stimulus generalization, indicates that the child has learned the targeted form(s) or function(s).
   a. Response generalization refers to a child's production of untrained targets at the same or at a different linguistic level.
      (1) "Is + verb + ing" taught in "catching," "sleeping" and "drawing" as individual words. Child produces "laughing."
      (2) "Is + verb + ing" taught in "catching," "sleeping" and "drawing" at the word level. Child produces "catching Noah cold."
   b. Stimulus generalization refers to a child's production of the same level of accuracy in an untrained setting, with new stimuli, with a new clinician.
      (1) "Is + verb + ing" taught as responses elicited following SLP A's modeling; same percentage of successful production following SLP B's modeling.
      (2) "Is + verb + ing" taught in a preschool classroom; same percentage of successful production when child is at home.
   c. If generalization is not achieved, therapy was not truly successful because the child continues to rely on the support provided by the SLP.
   d. Generalization is not just hoped for but has to be planned for through creation of periodic changes in the degree of stimulus support provided or therapy context.
7. Facilitation or induction techniques?
   a. Facilitation refers to increasing the rate at which a targeted form or function is learned.
      (1) It is assumed that this target would be learned without therapy.
      (2) Increasing the rate of learning makes the targeted form or function available sooner to the child for subsequent academic and/or social benefits.
      (3) Frequent and exaggerated modeling of a targeted form or function, when presented in a meaningful context, may facilitate its appearance in a child's repertoire.
   b. Induction teaching refers to using a more explicit and systematic set of teaching steps beyond modeling.
      (1) It is not assumed that this target would have been learned without intervention or learned to the same degree.
      (2) Because of the usefulness of the targeted form or function, induction teaching leads to concomitant achievements in academic and/or social contexts.
8. Focused or general stimulation techniques?
   a. Focused stimulation refers to the targeting of specific forms and functions by the SLP through repetition, modeling, exaggerated productions, etc.
      (1) Wh- question production is targeted and through focused stimulation, child is exposed to many meaningful examples and begins to incorporate this form.
      (2) Requests are targeted because they are infrequently used by the child and thus the child is exposed to many meaningful examples of the request function.
      (3) Appropriate outcome would be greater number/proportion of correct examples of production or comprehension of targets.
   b. General stimulation refers to provision of an enriched language-learning environment but there are no specific forms or functions targeted for learning.
      (1) Child is encouraged to "tell me more."
      (2) SLP models several ways of expressing the same idea.
      (3) Appropriate outcome would be child increases the length and complexity of utterances, understands more complex utterances.

Factors for Language Intervention Success

1. The SLP attempts to find meaningful form and function targets for the child.
   a. The child will be more motivated to learn a target that can be immediately useful for better communication.
   b. The child will have more opportunities for feedback provided indirectly from the environment (was communication successful?) or directly from an SLP, teacher, peer, caregiver regarding accuracy or appropriateness of the language used.
   c. The SLP varies the naturalness of the therapy context.
2. Level of awareness by the child that he/she has a language deficit.
   a. Frustration because of failure to communicate initially may lead to "acting out" behaviors or avoidance of communication attempts.
   b. When usefulness of language targets is demonstrated, child may become more invested in therapy.

3. Intensity of therapy provided.
   a. Language intervention may be more effective if provided more frequently, especially when teaching something that is not part of a child's repertoire.
   b. Once the basic foundations of a form or function are learned, less frequent therapy sessions may be useful to determine if the child can generalize the skill to untrained examples of the targeted form or function.
4. Explicitness of therapy provided/needed for learning.
   a. Children differ in terms of the number of examples they need to learn a new language form or function.
   b. Some children will need exposure to a specific rule, led through overgeneralization, and specifically taught exceptions to the rule.
5. Support for new language forms and functions outside of the therapy setting (e.g., classroom, home).
   a. Are caregivers in the home environment (if the child receives language intervention outside the home) able and willing to provide the child with opportunities for practice?
   b. Are caregivers in the home environment (if the child receives language intervention outside the home) able and willing to provide models of the form or function taught?
   c. Is support provided in the classroom to prompt the child to use the information worked on in therapy where appropriate (opportunities) and receive feedback?
   d. If therapy is provided in the home, do the caregivers model the targeted forms and functions as well as provide opportunities for use that are part of the child's ADLs?
   e. Does the therapy plan include a systematic plan for incorporating caregiver input?
      (1) Language therapy plans can be designed to include home programs, where caregivers are asked to *monitor* the child's use of therapy targets in the home environment beyond the presence of the SLP and provide this information to the SLP.
      (2) Language therapy programs can also be designed to include a caregiver training component so that the caregiver is *coached* to become the SLP in absentia.
         (a) When caregivers serve as coaches, generalization is facilitated.
         (b) When caregivers serve as coaches, primary responsibility for the child's success is shifted from the SLP to the caregiver.
         (c) Response to coaching methods may be more or less successful with some caregivers, given their degree of self-esteem, buy-in to family-centered approaches to therapy, etc.
         (d) For older preschool-age children receiving therapy outside the home, consider some at-home activity to enhance stimulus generalization.
         (e) Recognize time constraints on families but balance this acknowledgment with the importance of eventually transitioning out of therapy.
6. Does the child have prerequisite attention competencies for learning the language targets selected?
   a. Is the child able to focus simultaneously on the targeted language and the relevant context?
   b. Are cues provided by the SLP salient to the child?
   c. Does the child have the ability to discern similarities and differences between examples provided?
7. Does the child have the cognitive/linguistic prerequisites necessary to incorporate the information presented?
   a. SLPs must determine the cognitive and linguistic prerequisites for the targets selected.
   b. SLPs must also ascertain the child's level of competence relative to the prerequisite skills delineated prior to therapy planning.
   c. For example, teaching the client comprehension or production of "why?" questions would probably be unsuccessful if the child did not understand the concept of causality or did not already use "do" as an auxiliary form in question structures.

Early Intervention

1. Adoption of a prevention model.
   a. Intervention is provided when a child meets the eligibility requirement of being at significant risk for developing a language disorder although a bona fide diagnosis has not been made.
   b. Principles of early intervention.
      (1) Services are family-centered, culturally and linguistically responsive.
      (2) Services are developmentally supportive and promote children's participation in their natural environments.
      (3) Services are comprehensive, coordinated and team-based.
      (4) Services are based on the highest-quality evidence that is available.
2. SLPs are responsible for transition planning for children who continue to need therapy beyond age 3.
3. Individual Family Service Plans (IFSPs) are developed (analogous to Individual Educational Plans (IEPs)) to monitor presenting performance characteristics, describe the programming to be provided and

periodically document behavior changes as well as monitor viability of the service delivery plan.
   a. Most often, families receive services in their homes, as the least restricted environment.
   b. Multiple service providers may assess and provide therapeutic services to the child and caregivers; multidisciplinary, interdisciplinary or transdisciplinary team models may be used.
      (1) Transdisciplinary teams include the concept of "role release" so that professional role boundaries are less clear.
      (2) Transdisciplinary teams are family-centered; the whole child within the family unit is the recipient of intervention.
4. A coaching model should be used by the SLP to help caregivers assume the responsibility of facilitating the child's language learning.
   a. This is preferable to providing child-directed services only.
   b. Increasing the caregivers' empowerment and self-esteem will be enhanced through coaching.
   c. SLPs teach the caregiver how to facilitate the child's age-appropriate language competencies.
      (1) Provide modeling.
      (2) Provide opportunities for practice.
      (3) Provide feedback.

Techniques Used in Language Therapy

1. The goal of therapy techniques is to provide examples of the targeted forms and functions in meaningful contexts.
   a. Many exaggerated or otherwise highlighted productions (e.g., use of increased prosodic cueing) create an environment where the targets are more salient than in incidental conversation.
   b. Design of meaningful, if sometimes contrived, contexts will create an environment where the usefulness of the targeted forms and functions is more evident than in incidental conversation.
2. Therapy approaches differ in terms of their naturalness or how close the therapy setting resembles nontherapeutic interactions.
   a. The more natural the therapy setting, the less dramatic the bridge to generalization or carryover to ADLs.
   b. Therapy provided in the home environment is inherently more natural than that provided in an SLP's office or clinic.
   c. Therapy provided by a caregiver or any more knowledgeable, familiar language user is inherently more natural than therapy provided by an unfamiliar adult (typically portrayed by an SLP).
3. Approaches to language therapy vary along a clinician-centered to client-centered continuum.
   a. Clinician-centered approaches to language therapy.
      (1) The clinician chooses the targets.
      (2) The clinician sets the agenda for the therapy session, including the time allotted for working on specific targets.
      (3) Often regarded as being more structured and less conversation friendly.
      (4) May appear less natural than client-centered approaches.
   b. Client-centered approaches to language therapy.
      (1) The client interacts with the clinician and the clinician uses the interests of the client to direct the order and substance of the language intervention session.
      (2) The clinician "follows the child's lead," so it is critical that the clinician understands the child's language goals.
      (3) Often regarded as less structured and more conversation friendly.
      (4) May appear more natural than clinician-centered approaches.
      (5) May enhance generalization because learning occurs in an appropriate context.
   c. Hybrid approaches to language therapy.
      (1) Borrow characteristics of both clinician- and client-centered language intervention approaches.
      (2) "Incidental language teaching" is a hybrid approach; the clinician has a specific set of targets and uses a conversation framework developed from materials in which the child is already engaged.
4. Experiential language intervention techniques, based on conversation contexts, have their genesis in the interaction patterns commonly observed between caregivers and young children in middle-class, Western households.
   a. Taken together, these techniques foster a conversation framework.
      (1) Turn-taking patterns are evident.
         (a) Children are viewed as full-fledged members of the conversation and thus must take turns.
         (b) Through this experience children learn about the back-and-forth nature of conversation, that two participants do not talk at the same time.
      (2) When caregivers expect to share the "conversational floor" with the children, they make accommodations they would likely not make with other adults.
         (a) Wait longer for child's turns (i.e., increased turn latency).

(b) Accept verbal or nonverbal, intentional or random vocalizations or movements as child's turn.
(3) Caregivers will ask internal state questions although they do not really expect the child to answer (e.g., "Are you hungry?" "You look sleepy.").
b. Each technique provides a caregiver/SLP with an opportunity to acknowledge a child's participation.
(1) Provides alternatives that will enhance the child's communication success.
(2) Can provide direct feedback (e.g., "Yes, you said . . .") or indirect feedback (e.g., SLP follows the child's utterance with one of her/his own).
c. The caregiver behaviors observed during typical caregiver–child routines build a back-and-forth conversational framework long before the child can be making purposeful attempts at conversation.
(1) Caregivers in the cultural mainstream gauge their expectations to the child's abilities so that expectations for quality of turns increases as the child's abilities become more sophisticated.
(2) This happenstance has been called a "dance of conversation."
(3) There is synchrony in the turn-taking efforts, controlled by the caregiver who is more skillful.
d. Experiential language intervention types: All are techniques to provide modeling of accurate/appropriate language within specific language-learning contexts.
(1) Self-talk: Caregiver/SLP talks about what she or he is doing, matching language to context; child is not required to say or do anything.
(2) Parallel talk: Caregiver/SLP talks about what the child is doing, matching language to context; child is not required to say or do anything.
(3) Imitation: Providing a model and expecting the child to replicate what the caregiver/SLP said or wrote or signed.
 (a) Direct imitation: There is little time lapse and no language between the clinician's model and the child's production. SLP says, "Say 'apple.'"
 (b) Delayed imitation: There is some intervening language between the SLP's model and the child's production. SLP says, "Apple. What is this?"
(4) Expansion or recast: SLP provides a corrected version of a child's word or utterance. Child says, "Daddy go play" and the SLP says, "Daddy's going to play."
 (a) Note that expansions/recasts attempt to stay true to the child's intended meaning and do not introduce additional information to the utterance.
 (b) Note that expansions/recasts can address one or many parts of the child's utterance at the same time (e.g., phonetic accuracy, syntax, lexical choice).
 (c) Note that the child initiates an expansion/recast with the SLP.
 (d) SLP acknowledges the child's participation in a conversation although there are one or more errors in that turn.
(5) Expatiation: SLP provides a corrected version of a child's word or utterance and goes beyond child's original meaning. Child says, "I like cookie" and the SLP says, "I like cookies, too, especially chocolate chip cookies."
 (a) This technique must also be initiated by the child.
 (b) This technique is useful for teaching topic maintenance options (i.e., What else can we say about this topic?).
e. Deciding on the language therapy mode to be employed.
f. Therapy modes express different points along a continuum from most structured to least structured.
(1) Drill is most structured.
(2) Play is least structured.
(3) Position on the continuum of structure depends on the presence or absence of four critical components.
g. Each therapy mode or teaching type can be described in terms of major components.
(1) Antecedent instructional events (AIE): Whatever method(s) the SLP employs before the child's attempt to use the language target (e.g., modeling, sequence pictures, explicit rule description).
(2) Subsequent instructional events (SIE): The feedback the SLP provides the child following the attempt to use the language target (e.g., "right," "no, not quite" and "try it again").
(3) Antecedent motivational events (AME): Any activity not directly related to the learning of the language target that fosters the child's attention and encourages work on the language target(s) (e.g., blocks for building, board game) and occurs prior to the child's attempt at the target(s).
(4) Subsequent motivational events (SME): Reinforcement is anything that occurs following a child's attempt at the language target(s) that is likely to foster continued success and attention (e.g., "Good job," "You can take a sticker").
h. Drill is the most structured of the therapy modes.
(1) The only component *not* found is an antecedent motivational event.

(a) AMEs take time away from learning.
(b) If not needed (i.e., the child is sufficiently motivated), they hinder progress.
(2) SMEs are provided only if the child produces an accurate/appropriate attempt at a language target.
(3) SIEs (feedback) are always provided by the SLP clearly and immediately so that the child can begin to determine where the boundaries are between correct and incorrect language targets.
(4) Drill is an appropriate therapy mode when the client is motivated, when a new language target (either rarely observed or absent from the child's repertoire) is a goal.

i. Drill Play is considered to be a therapy mode slightly less structured than Drill.
(1) All of the components are present.
(2) AMEs are added to the Drill template.
(3) Addition of the AME indicates the child either needs some motivation to complete the task or some naturalness to increase the task's difficulty.
(4) Drill Play is an appropriate therapy mode when the client is generally motivated, is being taught a new language target (rarely observed or absent from the child's repertoire) and can tolerate some extraneous activity to promote naturalness.

j. Structured Play is considered to be somewhat less structured than Drill Play but more structured than Play.
(1) All of the components are present.
(2) SME is provided whether or not the client's attempt at the targeted language form or function is correct.
(3) SIE is also provided but done so differentially to provide feedback distinguishing between correct and incorrect attempts.
(4) Structured Play is appropriate for children who are becoming acclimated to therapy and cannot tolerate too much structure or who have been working on a language target for a while and are trying to demonstrate independent learning in a more natural setting.

k. Play is the most natural and least structured of the therapy modes.
(1) AMEs and SMEs are always provided.
(2) AIEs and SIEs are provided only if they do not interfere with the play activity.
(3) Play is an appropriate therapy mode for assessing generalization to a more natural setting because feedback is only intermittently present, if at all.

l. Selection of a therapy mode.
(1) Appropriateness of the therapy mode selected will change over time as a function of how much learning by the client has occurred (e.g., no usage, inconsistent, consistent).
(2) Appropriateness of the therapy mode selected will change over time as a function of what the SLP wants to assess (e.g., generalization, correct responses to modeling).
(3) SLPs should expect to alter the therapy modes used with individual clients based on the client's skill level.
(4) No one therapy mode is inherently better than another.
(5) Therapy mode provides the framework for the actual learning to take place.

Measuring Progress in Therapy

1. Periodic measurement of client performance is critical.
   a. Must determine if client is making progress that is connected to provision of therapy.
   b. Changes in client performance could be related to maturity and not therapy.
   c. Important to determine progress matched against longer-term goals and shorter-term objectives.
2. Utilize untrained exemplars to evaluate progress when eliciting language.
   a. Target is third-person singular verb forms with specific teaching for "comes" and "walks."
      (1) "Jane was walking and now she walks."
      (2) Can client transform "talking" into a third-person singular verb form?
      (3) "Phil was talking and now he _____."
   b. Look for untrained exemplars in language sample data when collecting spontaneous language production.
      (1) Collect a language sample where client is given some cuing to assume present tense.
      (2) "Have you ever listened to a sports broadcast? Well, most broadcasters talk in the present tense (e.g., 'He shoots, he scores'). Now you try that . . . ."
3. Measuring a client's progress via language change is not the same as data collection within a session (to determine if the client is responding correctly to trained exemplars).
   a. Important to collect both types of data.
   b. Determine whether teaching strategy is working.
   c. If the teaching strategy is not working, how/what can be changed to facilitate improvement in a child's performance?
      (1) Change the examples provided so they are more similar to one another (i.e., training deeply).
         (a) When examples are too different from one another they require some generalization to detect similarities.
         (b) Use of highly similar examples allows the client to focus on essential features of the stimuli.

(2) Use fewer examples (i.e., training deeply).
   (a) Use of too many examples may be distracting.
   (b) Use of too many examples may make less obvious the essential features of the stimuli.
(3) Provide more explicit feedback.
   (a) Children who need language therapy have typically been unable to infer language rules and regulations without explicit feedback.
   (b) Explicit feedback provides children with a focus on what is most essential in the language-learning task.
(4) Provide feedback in a manner conducive to the client's understanding.
   (a) Decrease rate of teaching overall (including response latency) and particularly provision of feedback.
   (b) Recheck accuracy and consistency of feedback.
(5) Look for an intermediate step in the teaching process.
   (a) Child should have some success with each task.
   (b) If not, the specific objective selected is too much of a cognitive "leap" from a prior level of learning.
   (c) Analyze the task to determine how to revise the objective to a challenging but not frustrating level.
   (d) Task analysis and change may involve one or more of the suggestions listed here.
(6) Make clearer the benefits of using this language form or function.
   (a) The usefulness of language is a child's prime motivator for learning how to use it.
   (b) Sometimes the utility of language use can be lost in its teaching (i.e., decontextualized).
(7) A change in the therapy management mode may be indicated.
   (a) Configuration of the therapy task in terms of feedback and reinforcement may have a direct impact on a child's success.
   (b) As noted, therapy modes are well or less well suited to particular therapy goals.
   (c) An adjustment in therapy intensity (i.e., number of sessions per week, number of minutes per session) could be warranted.
   (d) A change in the degree that family is included in programming could be warranted.
(8) As a final consideration, is the client still an appropriate candidate for therapy?
   (a) This factor may be related to the child (and family/caregiver's) motivation to support the child's language change.
   (b) When dismissal is considered, it is not as a final decision but appropriate at this time and temporary in nature.

Dismissal from Therapy for Child Language Disorders

1. Has the child met the goals and objectives delineated based on the original and subsequent assessments?
   a. It is critical to have some objective measures (as well as functional ones) to determine progress over time.
   b. Recognize that assessments of progress should be made periodically.
      (1) Make a judgment about the trajectory of rate/change over time.
      (2) Has sufficient time elapsed to accurately gauge progress?
2. Is the child currently able to meet the communication demands imposed through activities of daily living?
   a. This will require a careful investigation of all language-use contexts.
   b. This will involve input from the child's family and others who are familiar with both the child's language competencies and daily language milieu.
   c. Family members or caregiver may be satisfied that the child's progress warrants dismissal.
3. Are the child and family motivated to facilitate the child's language learning in the current therapy context?
   a. Sometimes clients and families are tired of therapy; if other configurations for service delivery have been exhausted, maybe all parties need a break.
      (1) This recommendation must be carefully documented if an IEP is in place.
      (2) Other service delivery types and contexts should be considered.
      (3) SLP can informally and periodically monitor a child's progress with input from caregivers and school personnel, if relevant.
   b. Breaks from therapy provide an opportunity to evaluate generalization (both stimulus and response generalization) to determine if treatment is no longer needed.
   c. Breaks from therapy may make more evident that the child continues to be in need of therapy.
   d. If a child and family are not currently motivated to support change, should they have a spot on the clinician's caseload?
4. Decisions for therapy dismissal are not irrevocable but must be deemed appropriate at the time they were made.

References

American Speech-Language-Hearing Association. (1988). *Prevention of Communication Disorders* [Position Statement]. Available from www.asha.org/policy.

American Speech-Language-Hearing Association. (1993). *Definitions of Communication Disorders and Variations* [Relevant Paper]. Available from www.asha.org/policy.

American Speech-Language-Hearing Association. (1998). *Provision of Instruction in English as a Second Language by Speech-Language Pathologists in School Settings* [Technical Report]. Available from www.asha.org/policy.

American Speech-Language-Hearing Association. (2003). *American English Dialects* [Technical Report]. Available from www.asha.org/policy.

American Speech-Language-Hearing Association. (2004). *Knowledge and Skills Needed by Speech-Language Pathologists Providing Services to Infants and Families in the NICU Environment* [Knowledge and Skills]. Available from www.asha.org/policy.

American Speech-Language-Hearing Association. (2005). *Evidence-Based Practice in Communication Disorders* [Position Statement]. Available from www.asha.org/policy.

American Speech-Language-Hearing Association. (2006). *Roles and Responsibilities of Speech-Language Pathologists in Diagnosis, Assessment, and Treatment of Autism Spectrum Disorders Across the Life Span* [Position Statement]. Available from www.asha.org/policy.

American Speech-Language-Hearing Association. (2008a). *Roles and Responsibilities of Speech-Language Pathologists in Early Intervention: Position Statement* [Position statement]. Available from www.asha.org/policy.

American Speech-Language-Hearing Association. (2008b). *Core Knowledge and Skills in Early Intervention Speech-Language Pathology Practice* [Knowledge and Skills]. Available from www.asha.org/policy.

Bloom, L., & Lahey, M. (1978). *Language Development and Language Disorders*. New York: Wiley.

Brown, R. (1973). *A First Language: The Early Stages*. Cambridge: Harvard University Press.

Carrow-Woolfolk, E. (1999). *Test for Auditory Comprehension of Language—3*. Austin, TX: Pro-Ed.

Chapman, R. (1978). "Comprehension Strategies in Children." In J. Kavanaugh & W. Strange (Eds.), *Speech and Language in the Laboratory, School, and Clinic*. Cambridge: MIT Press.

Dale, P., Price, T., Bishop, D., & Plomin, R. (2003). Outcomes of early language delay: I. Predicting persistent and transient language difficulties at age 3 and 4 years. *Journal of Speech, Language, and Hearing Research, 46*, 544–560.

Diagnostic and Statistical Manual of Mental Disorders—V (DSM V). (2013). American Psychiatric Association.

Dollaghan, C. (2004, April 13). Evidence-based practice: Myths and realities. *The ASHA Leader, 12*, 4–5.

Dunn, L., & Dunn, L. (2007). *Peabody Picture Vocabulary Test—IV*. San Antonio, TX: Pearson Assessments.

Fenson, L., Marchman, V., Thal, D., Dale, P., Reznick, S., & Bates, E. (2007). *MacArthur-Bates Communicative Development Inventories—III*. Baltimore: Paul H. Brookes.

Fey, M. (1986). *Language Intervention in Young Children*. Needham Heights, MA: Allyn & Bacon.

Hoff, E. (2006). How social contexts support and shape language development. *Developmental Review, 26*, 55–88.

Individuals with Disabilities Improvement Education Act of 2004, PL 108-446 (2004).

Leonard, L. (1998). *Children with Specific Language Impairment*. Cambridge, MA: MIT Press.

Miller, J., & Chapman, R. (1981). The relation between age and mean length of utterance in morphemes. *Journal of Speech and Hearing Research, 24*, 154–161.

Paul, R., & Norbury, C. (2012). *Language Disorders from Infancy Through Adolescence: Listening, Speaking, Reading, Writing, and Communicating*, 4th ed. St. Louis: Elsevier/Mosby.

Rescorla, L. (1989). The language development survey: A screening tool for delayed language in toddlers. *Journal of Speech and Hearing Disorders, 54*, 587–599.

Roth, F., & Spekman, N. (1984). Assessing the pragmatic abilities of children: Part 1. Organizational framework and assessment parameters. *Journal of Speech and Hearing Disorders, 49*, 2–11.

Shriberg, L., & Kwiatkowski, J. (1982). Phonological disorders II: A conceptual framework for management. *Journal of Speech and Hearing Disorders, 47*, 242–255.

Stein, N., & Glenn, C. (1979). "An Analysis of Story Comprehension in Elementary School Children. In R. Freedle (Ed.), *New Directions in Discourse Processing: Vol. 2*. Norwood, NJ: Ablex, pp. 53–120.

Van Kleeck, A. (1994). Potential cultural bias in training parents as conversational partners with their children who have delays in language development. *American Journal of Speech-Language Pathology, 3*, 67–78.

Weismer, S. E., Plante, E., Jones, M., & Tomblin, J. B. (2005). A functional magnetic resonance imaging investigation of verbal working memory in adolescents with Specific Language Impairment. *Journal of Speech, Language, and Hearing Research, 48*, 405–425.

8

Spoken Language Disorders in School-Age Populations

SANDRA LAING GILLAM, PhD
AND VICKI SIMONSMEIER, MS

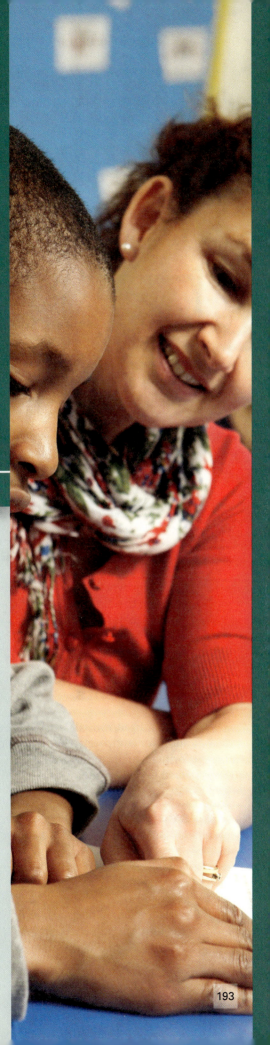

Chapter Outline

- Definitions/Terminology, 194
- Prevalence, 194
- Assessment of School-Age Language Disorders, 194
- Considerations for Culturally and Linguistically Diverse Populations, 198
- Intervention, 199
- Response to Intervention (RTI), 200
- Evidence-Based Practices, 201
- Causal Categories, 202
- Congenital Syndromes, 202
- Cognitive/Intellectual Disability, 202
- Down Syndrome, 203
- X-Linked Syndromes, 203
- Attention Deficit/Hyperactivity Disorder (ADHD), 204
- Specific Learning Disabilities (SLD), 204
- Neural Tube Defects (NTD), 204
- Cerebral Palsy, 204
- Traumatic Brain Injury, 205
- Autism Spectrum Disorders (ASD), 205
- References, 206

Definitions/Terminology

Population and Language Disorder

1. School-age population—children in kindergarten through high school, generally between the ages of 5 and 21.
2. A language disorder involves impairment in comprehension and/or use of spoken, written or other symbolic language system.
   a. May manifest in difficulties in *form* (phonology, morphology and syntax), *content* (semantics) and/or *use* (pragmatics) or any combination of the three.

Prevalence

Number and Percentages

1. Six million children under the age of 18 present with a speech or language disorder, two-thirds of whom are male.
2. Approximately 85% of all school-age children with communication disorders are educated in regular classroom settings.
3. Approximately 6% of school-age children present with language impairment.

Assessment of School-Age Language Disorders

Purpose of Assessment

1. Determine whether a disorder exists.
2. Establish baseline functioning.
3. Identify goals for instruction.
4. Measure response to instruction.

Standardized/Formal Assessments

1. Standardized/formal assessments are designed to allow for comparison among children at various ages for performance on specific skills; typically administered to large groups.

Psychometric Properties of Standardized Assessments

1. Reliability—the extent to which a test yields consistent scores.
   a. Inter-rater reliability—the consistency of scores obtained on a measure administered under similar conditions across examiners.
   b. Test-retest reliability—the consistency of scores obtained on a measure across time under similar conditions.
   c. Internal consistency reliability—the consistency of scores or results across items within a measure.
2. Validity—the extent to which a test measures what it is designed to measure.
   a. Face validity—property of a test in which observers agree superficially that it appears to measure what it is designed to measure.
   b. Content validity—property of a test in which statistical tests confirm that it measures all facets of a given construct or topic area.
   c. Construct validity—property of a test in which statistical tests confirm that the measure correlates with the underlying theoretical construct that it is designed to measure.
   d. Criterion-related validity (also termed instrumental or concurrent validity)—property of a test in which statistical tests confirm that a measure is accurate because it correlates with a valid measure of the same construct type.
   e. Predictive validity—a type of criterion-related validity used to determine the extent to which a measure "predicts" later performance on a related measure.

3. Sensitivity—the extent to which a test accurately identifies children who have a language impairment.
4. Specificity—the extent to which a test accurately identifies children who have not been diagnosed as language impaired.
5. Positive predictive value—proportion of true positives.
   a. 0.80 or higher is very good.
   b. 0.90 or higher is excellent.

Criterion-Referenced/Curriculum-Based Assessments

1. Assessments designed to measure a specific linguistic skill.
2. No comparison is made of performance between children.
3. Performance is used to identify current level of performance so that linguistic targets may be selected for instruction and monitored over time.

Dynamic Assessments

1. Assessment designed to measure the extent to which a child's performance on a specific task may be modified or extended with contextual support.
2. Performance is used to identify learning processes and response to differential instruction.

Functional/Ecological Assessments

1. Assessments measure the extent to which a child's communication disorder impacts daily living.
2. The assessments select linguistic targets that may improve daily living.
3. The assessments also monitor progress on these skills over the course of instruction.

Curriculum-Based Assessments

1. Assessments designed to measure the extent to which a child's communication disorder impacts academic functioning, to select linguistic targets that may improve daily living and to monitor progress on these skills over the course of instruction.
2. Discourse.
   a. Narrative comprehension and production—narratives are orderly, continuous accounts of events or series of events.
      (1) Advantages of narrative skill.
         (a) Provides cognitive linguistic, academic and social benefits.
         (b) Allows students to express complex ideas, engage in complex cognitive processing, interact with peers and engage in classroom discussion.
         (c) Experience with narrative comprehension and production supports reading comprehension.
      (2) Difficulties in comprehending and producing narratives.
         (a) Children with language impairments have difficulty understanding critical elements and "gist information" and in drawing inferences.
         (b) Children with language impairment demonstrate greater variability across stories, make incomplete references to character and story contexts, include fewer story grammar propositions and receive lower holistic scores.
         (c) Children with language impairment have difficulty answering questions related to information contained in discourse, both factual and inferential, and in recall of stories.
      (3) Types of narratives.
         (a) Recounts—prompted narratives that relate unique, shared experiences using past tense.
         (b) Personal narratives (accounts)—spontaneous narratives relating specific experiences or events.
         (c) Event casts—narratives produced as descriptions of ongoing activities, often during play, may resemble "broadcasting" or "directing."
         (d) Scripts—narratives that relate routine events or activities that occur with some degree of frequency (e.g., going to McDonald's).
         (e) Fictional narratives—recountings or novel generation of fictional stories about characters motivated by goals and that respond to events or problems.
      (4) Macrostructure—story grammar or story elements.
         (a) Characters—agents who perform actions in stories.
         (b) Setting—the time and/or place that the story took place.
         (c) Initiating event—an event or problem that requires the character to take action to resolve.
         (d) Internal response—indicates how a character felt in response to an initiating event.
         (e) Plan—information in the story that indicates characters intend to solve a problem, or a comment regarding their thoughts or decisions in relation to the problem. The presence of a plan is often marked by words such as *thought*, *decided* or *wanted*.

(f) Attempt—an action taken by the character in response to the initiating event.
(g) Consequences—statements in the story that relate to successful or unsuccessful ramifications of actions taken by characters in direct relation to the initiating event.
(h) Reaction—often a "metacognitive" comment made by a character that relates to the story as a whole.

(5) Development of macrostructure.
(a) Basic episode = initiating event, attempt, consequence (ages 3–4).
(b) Complete episode = initiating event, internal response, plan, consequence/resolution, reaction (ages 4–5).
(c) Complex episode = multiple embedded or associated episodes (ages 6–7).

(6) Narrative episode levels.
(a) Descriptive sequence (1) = description of a character and/or his or her surroundings. Includes actions that are not causally related to an initiating event.
(b) Action sequence (2) = coded when a narrative contains a series of actions that follow a chronological order but are not causally linked.
(c) Reactive sequence (3) = coded when a narrative contains a series of actions that follow a chronological order and which are causally linked.
(d) Abbreviated episode (4) = contains causally related actions that are not associated with an initiating event or specific, goal-directed behavior.
(e) Incomplete episode (5) = contains two of the following, but not all three: initiating event, action or consequence.
(f) Compete episode (6) = coded when a child's narrative includes an initiating event and at least one action and consequence related to the initiating event.

(7) "High-point" analysis.
(a) Identifying an introducer (story opening).
(b) Identifying an orientation (background, setting).
(c) Identifying a complicating action (action leading to a high point or climax).
(d) Identifying evaluation (emotional content).
(e) Identifying a resolution (resolution of conflicts, event ends) and coda (story closing).

(8) Microstructure.
(a) Literate language.
- Elaborated noun phrases—noun phrases are elaborated when determiners (a, the) or modifiers precede a noun and/or when qualifiers (prepositional phrases, relative clauses) follow a noun. Serve to make the story more detailed.
- Conjunctions.
- Coordinated (for, and, nor, but, or, yet, so).
- Subordination (after, although).
- Sentence complexity (dependent clauses).
- Infinitives (I stopped to look at the giant elephant).
- Clausal complements (I knew you couldn't stay angry with him for long).
- Relative clauses.
  - Subjective (The boy who told on you got in trouble at recess).
  - Objective (I saw the boy who told on you).
- Mental and linguistic verbs (knew, felt like, thought, decided to, said).
- Adverbs (when, after, because, if, since).

(b) Cohesion.
- Microstructure encompasses the notion of cohesive adequacy. Cohesive markers may be identified and judged as clear (unambiguous) or unclear (ambiguous).
  - Unambiguous cohesive markers: coded when no further information is necessary to determine the cross-C-unit referent.
    ○ Example:/One day *John* saw the aliens//and *he* was scared/.
  - Ambiguous cohesive markers: coded when the cross-C-unit referent is unclear.
    ○ Example:/One day *he* saw the aliens// and *he* was scared/.
- Five categories of cohesive markers include reference, conjunctive, lexical and substitution or ellipses.
  - Reference cohesive marker—a word that marks personal reference or demonstrative reference.
    ○ Example: I, you, us, he, him, she, her, they, them, their, our, mine, its, the, this, that, these, those, here, now, then.
  - Conjunctive reference—a word or words that specify cross-C-unit semantic relationships.
    ○ May be additive (e.g., and, also, nor, or, furthermore, besides).
    ○ May be adversative (e.g., but, however, yet, though, only, except).
    ○ May be causal (e.g., so, because, as a result).

- May be temporal (e.g., then, next, after that, finally).
- May be continuative (e.g., well, surely, now, of course).
   - Lexical ties—include words that are related through specific selection of vocabulary.
      - Repetition (e.g., /A *bird* was in the tree//The *bird* was red/).
      - Synonymy (e.g., /A *rat* saw some cheese//The *rodent* was happy/).
      - Antonymy (e.g., /The birds looked *different*//One was *fat*, one was *skinny*/).
      - Part-whole (e.g., /The *car* was broken//The *wheel* fell off/).
      - Superordinate–subordinate relationships (e.g., /He wanted a *bike*//The store didn't carry *cycling* equipment/).
      - Substitution-ellipses (e.g., /She is having *cake*//I want *that* too/).
3. Expository.
   a. Sequence—topic is described through lists of items or events in some logical order (e.g., numerical, chronological, sequence).
   b. Comparison—topic is described by outlining how two or more events, topics, concepts, theories, problems or objects are similar or dissimilar.
   c. Cause and effect—topic is described by presenting facts, ideas, concepts, events or problems as causes or catalysts for resulting events, etc.
   d. Problem and solution—topic is described by presenting a problem with one or more potential solutions.
4. Conversational areas.
   a. Conversational language may be used to convey various cognitive functions or "intents" as children use language to explain, describe, direct, interpret, relate, reason and hypothesize about topics or concepts they encounter. As children mature, they begin to understand that language used in social contexts must be "appropriate" to the audience or listener, situation and/or contexts in the immediate surroundings.
      (1) Types of perspective taking that affect children's communicative behaviors include perceptual, cognitive and linguistic.
         (a) Perceptual perspective taking—develops during preschool and involves the ability to determine what another sees and how it is seen when the other person is in a different location.
         (b) Linguistic perspective taking—develops during preschool and involves the ability to modify the form, content and/or use of language in relation to the listeners' needs.
         (c) Cognitive perspective taking—develops during the school-age years and involves a child's ability to infer other people's thoughts, feelings, beliefs and/or intentions and involves making judgments about the internal psychological states of another person.
   b. Contextual variation strategies and linguistic devices that are used to mediate social use of language in school-age children.
      (1) Register variation (e.g., altering tone, pitch, choice of words).
      (2) Presupposition (articles, demonstratives, pronouns, proper nouns, some verbs such as "know" and "remember", wh- questions "that + clause", forms of address "dear" and "honey").
      (3) Ellipses (deletion of redundant information).
      (4) Indirect requests (do not refer directly to what the speaker wants).
   c. Discourse management.
      (1) Mediation of turn, topic initiation, maintenance and termination and repair of conversational breakdowns and requests for clarification.
      (2) Children with language impairments often demonstrate disrupted speech (e.g., mazing) and difficulties with persuasion and negation.
5. Vocabulary.
   a. Instructional vocabulary—words used in daily classroom instruction that students need to know to follow directions and complete assignments (e.g., spatial, temporal, connective, logical, directive, words unique to the classroom environment).
   b. Content vocabulary—words that are specific to the information contained in instructional or curricular materials.
6. Syntax.
   a. Simple (appropriate for children ages 3 and 4; MLU = 4).
      (1) Simple infinitive.
      (2) Full propositional complements.
      (3) Simple wh- questions.
      (4) Simple conjoining.
   b. Complex (appropriate for children over age 4; MLU > 4).
      (1) Multiple embedding.
      (2) Embedded and conjoined.
      (3) Infinitive clauses with different subjects.
      (4) Relative clauses.
      (5) Gerunds.
      (6) Wh- infinitives.
      (7) Unmarked infinitives.

Table 8-1

Brown's Stages of Morphological Development

BROWN'S STAGE	AGE	MORPHOLOGICAL STRUCTURE(S)	FUNCTION	EXAMPLES
Stage II	2.0–2.5	Copula be (is)	Used with adjectives, nouns or prepositional phrases	She **is** happy.
		Auxiliary be (is)	Used with progressive -ing to form progressive aspect	He **is** running.
		Modals (gonna, wanna, gotta, hafta)	Indicate attitude, add meaning to sentences	I **wanna** go.
		Irregular past tense		He **went** to the airport.
Stage III	2.5–2.9	Copula be (is, am, are)	Used with adjectives, nouns or prepositional phrases	I **am** happy.
		Auxiliary be (is, am, are)	Used with progressive -ing to form progressive aspect	I **am** talking.
		Possessive -s		Doggie**'s** bone.
		3rd-person present		She like**s** tea.
		Regular past tense		He **finished** the painting.
Stage IV	3.0–3.5	Auxiliary do (do, does, did)	Used to form negatives, questions, elliptical responses and to provide emphasis	I **do**n't eat dairy. **Did** he eat?
		Modals (can, may, will, shall, could, might, would, should)	Indicate attitude, add meaning to sentences	He **can** do it.
Stage V+	4.5–5.0	Auxiliary have (have, has, had)	Used with past participle to form perfective aspect	I**'ve** already seen it. **Has** he seen it?

7. Morphology (Table 8-1).
8. Phonological awareness and literacy.
   a. Sound categorization, blending, segmentation, elision/deletion—students with poor phonological awareness skills often go on to experience difficulties in learning to read.
   b. Complex phonological production—students with a language disorder often have difficulty producing words containing complex syllable structures.
   c. Nonword repetition—students who demonstrate difficulty repeating nonwords often have unstable underlying phonological representations. This is suggestive of a language disorder.

Considerations for Culturally and Linguistically Diverse Populations

Preventing Over- or Underdiagnosis of Disabilities in CLD Populations

1. Content bias.
   a. Test stimuli, methods or procedures reflect the assumption that all populations have the same life experiences and have learned similar concepts and vocabulary.
2. Linguistic bias.
   a. Disparity between the language or dialect used by the examiner, the child and/or the language or dialect expected in the child's response.
3. Disproportionate representation in normative samples—many tests do not include CLD populations in their samples.

Alternative Assessment Procedures

1. Criterion-referenced measures—compares a child's performance to predetermined criteria.
2. Processing-dependent measures—minimally dependent on prior knowledge or experience.
   a. Digit span, working memory, nonword repetition.

3. Dynamic assessment—diagnostic teaching.
   a. Test-teach-retest—test a skill, provide instruction, retest the skill.
   b. Task/stimulus variability—modify the way the test is presented.
   c. Graduated prompting—assessment and intervention occur simultaneously.

Intervention

Purpose

1. To remediate or modify underlying problems contributing to the language impairment or to assist in the development and use of compensatory strategies to lessen the functional impact of the language impairment in academic, social and vocational settings.

Legislation

1. Rehabilitation Act of 1973—prohibited discrimination on the basis of disability by programs and agencies receiving federal funding.
2. Education for All Handicapped Children Act (PL 94-142)—mandated that all children with disabilities be afforded a free and appropriate public education.
   a. Individuals with Disabilities Education Act (IDEA 2004); Reauthorization of PL 94-142—law ensuring services to children with disabilities. Governs how states and public agencies provide early intervention, special education and related services. Emphasized least restrictive environment and extended services to those with autism and traumatic brain injury; added transition services from school to postschool contexts.
3. Individual Educational Plans (IEPs)—legal document written by health care professionals and caregivers that outlines long-term and short-term educational goals for children with disabilities. Includes information about how students learn and what teachers, clinicians and service providers plan to do to assist the student in learning effectively.
   a. Must include:
      (1) Present level of performance.
      (2) Special education services.
      (3) Requirements, aids, modifications, long- and short-term goals, benchmarks and information regarding additional services and least restrictive environment.

Service Delivery Models

1. Direct services—one-to-one or small group intervention is provided by the SLP in a self-contained setting or within a classroom setting.
2. Indirect services—SLP provides services to children with speech and language disorders or delays in consultative or collaborative contexts.
   a. Consultant—SLP provides professional or expert advice to teachers, parents and paraprofessionals working with a child with speech or language needs.
   b. Collaborative—SLPs, teachers, parents and paraprofessionals work together to assess, provide intervention and/or curricular support to a student with speech or language needs. The SLP may provide instruction in the regular classroom context or even co-teach lessons with the classroom teacher.

Approaches

1. Clinician-directed or discrete trial intervention—instruction implemented in a way that allows clinicians to specify the materials that are used in intervention, how the materials are used, the type and frequency of reinforcement, the form of responses expected from the client and the order in which activities will be conducted.
   a. Advantages.
      (1) Provides clinician with ways to make target linguistic stimuli highly salient by reducing irrelevant or distracting stimuli.
      (2) Allows clinician to maximize the opportunities provided for a child to produce a target response.
   b. Disadvantages.
      (1) Less naturalistic.
      (2) Skills learned may not generalize into new contexts readily.
   c. Clinician-directed instructional approaches.
      (1) Drill—highly structured context in which a stimulus is introduced, a response is elicited and a consequence is imposed; designed to increase the likelihood that a certain behavior will occur.
      (2) Drill play—less structured context in which a stimulus is introduced in a highly motivating context such as play; as in drill contexts, a response is elicited and a consequence is imposed.
      (3) Modeling—highly structured procedure in which numerous examples of a target structure are provided during an interactive activity; child is not required to produce the target during the session.

2. Child-directed instruction.
    a. Provided to improve overall communication skills.
    b. Indirect language stimulation, whole-language techniques (recasting, modeling, use of themes, naturalistic consequences) and naturalistic contexts are used to expose children to language form, use and content.
        (1) Indirect language facilitation techniques.
            (a) Demonstration—repeated but variable use of a sentence or text pattern.
                - Sentence pattern: The girl walked home. The cat walked home. Everyone walked home (emphasizing the past tense –ed).
                - Text pattern: The girl saw the spaceship (take off). She went to meet the aliens (action). They became friends (consequence). The boy found a boat on the lake (take off). He went to get in the boat (action). He rode around on the lake all day (consequence).
            (b) Expansions—contingent verbal responses that increase the length or complexity of the child's utterance.
                - Example: Child: Doggy. Teacher: That is a doggy. (The utterance is contingent because it incorporates the word the child used—doggy. It is an expansion because it increased the length of the utterance.)
            (c) Expatiations—contingent verbal responses that add new but relevant information to the child's utterance.
                - Example: Child: Doggy. Teacher: That is a friendly doggy. (The utterance is contingent because it incorporates the word the child used—doggy. It is an expatiation because it added new information to the child's utterance.)
            (d) Vertical structures—clinician/teacher asks questions to construct a syntactically complete sentence.
                - Example: Child: Doggy. Teacher: What is the doggy's name? Child: Bubba. Teacher: The doggy's name is Bubba.
            (e) Prompts/Questions—comments and questions that serve to extend what the student has said or written.
                - Example: Child: Doggy. Teacher: What does the doggy like to do?
3. Hybrid.
    a. Instruction contains elements of structure provided by the clinician and of child-directed, naturalistic instruction.

Response to Intervention (RTI)

Approach and Use

1. RTI is a multitiered approach to providing academic instruction.
    a. The RTI initiative, as supported by federal IDEA laws, provides the possibility for SLPs to work within general education settings in prevention-based activities.
    b. School-based models of RTI are implemented early to prevent academic failure, to differentiate children whose academic challenges result from environmental etiologies (e.g., poor or inadequate instruction, limited home support for literacy) from those who exhibit neurologically based learning problems that may require ongoing support. RTI typically involves a three-tiered instructional process in which students move into and out of tiers based on an established set of procedures designed to ensure that optimal learning is taking place.
    c. At Tier 1, students receive evidence-based, high-quality core curriculum instruction in the general education environment.
    d. Students who do not respond to Tier 1 instruction receive more supportive and/or different instruction in Tier 2.
    e. Students who respond well in Tier 2 go back to the regular classroom for further instruction. Students who do not respond sufficiently in Tier 2 may move into Tier 3.
    f. Tier 3 may involve more intensive instruction, specialized supports or in some cases, referral for special education services.
2. The use of criterion-referenced progress-monitoring measures that can reliably capture a student's growth over time is critical within an RTI framework.
    a. Progress-monitoring tools should be easy to administer, score and analyze, because they are designed for frequent implementation (sometimes biweekly) to permit rapid analysis of students' progress.
    b. These tools must be psychometrically sound with respect to internal consistency, inter-rater reliability and construct/concurrent validity.
    c. Progress-monitoring tools are used to make informed decisions about intervention approaches or to compare a student's performance to that of students with similar abilities receiving the same or different instruction.

Evidence-Based Practices

Integration and Evaluation

1. The process by which clinicians integrate external and internal research evidence, as well as their own expertise, to make decisions about best practices for clients.
2. Critical appraisal of external evidence—the process by which published research findings are evaluated for quality.
3. Types of evidence.
   a. Systematic meta-analyses of multiple well-designed randomized controlled studies and single randomized controlled trials constitute the highest level of external evidence for a particular approach or instructional technique.
      (1) Randomized controlled trials—experiments in which participants are randomly assigned to treatment and control groups.
      (2) Systematic review—analysis of a number of studies related to a specific approach or technique that allows for summarization of findings across multiple experiments.
      (3) Nonrandomized, quasi-experimental trials, and multiple-baseline designs.
      (4) Nonrandomized quasi-experimental clinical trial—an experiment in which participants are not assigned randomly to treatment and/or control groups, but are assigned on the basis of a theoretical or matching variable.
      (5) Multiple-baseline designs—an experiment in which participant traits, behaviors and/or outcomes of instruction are measured across multiple individuals in a systematic, controlled fashion.
      (6) Expert opinion—opinions of respected professionals.
4. Evaluation criteria for external evidence.
   a. Comparisons—studies that compare experimental and control groups are viewed as higher levels of evidence than those that do not.
   b. Random assignment—studies in which participants were randomly assigned to treatment and control groups are viewed as higher levels of evidence than those that do not.
   c. Participants—studies in which participants are clearly described in terms of age, gender, race, ethnicity, socioeconomic status, speech, language and cognitive abilities are ranked more highly in terms of the level of evidence provided than those that do not include this information.
   d. Initial group similarity—studies in which comparison groups are well matched at the outset of the experiment are ranked more highly in terms of the level of evidence provided.
   e. Blinding—studies in which evaluators are blind to the purpose of the experiment and/or the groups to which participants have been assigned are ranked more highly in terms of the level of evidence provided.
   f. Measures—studies using valid and reliable outcome measures are ranked more highly in terms of the level of evidence provided.
   g. Statistical significance—studies reporting p-values of less than 0.05 with appropriate statistical controls and considerations are ranked more highly in terms of the level of evidence provided.
   h. Practical significance—studies reporting medium to large eta-squared and/or standardized d-values are ranked more highly in terms of the level of evidence provided.
   i. Critical appraisal of internal evidence—the process by which clinical expertise, client and institutional factors are combined to make decisions about instruction.
5. Evaluation criteria for internal evidence.
   a. Student/parent factors.
      (1) Cultural values—consideration of familial cultural values and beliefs in the selection of approaches or techniques.
      (2) Student/parent activities and participation—consideration of child interest, ability and motivation in the selection of approaches or techniques.
      (3) Financial resources—consideration of familial resources in the selection of approaches or techniques.
      (4) Interest and engagement—consideration of the level of active participation required of families and children in the selection of approaches or techniques.
      (5) Opinion—consideration of parent/family wishes and opinions in the selection of approaches or techniques.
   b. Clinician/agency factors.
      (1) Education—consideration of clinician knowledge, education and training in the selection of approaches or techniques.
      (2) Agency policies—consideration of setting/district policies and resources in the selection of approaches or techniques.
      (3) Clinician data—application of clinical-generated outcome data in the selection of approaches or techniques.
      (4) Theoretical orientation—consideration of clinician philosophical and theoretical convictions in the selection of approaches or techniques.

Causal Categories

Syndromic and Nonsyndromic

1. Syndromic—a collection of symptoms, anomalies and signs all having a common cause.
2. Nonsyndromic—many causes that can result in similar effects.
   a. Birth trauma.
   b. Family history.
   c. Iatrogenic effects of medications.

Congenital Syndromes

Genetic

1. Runs in families and is presumed to be transmitted in genetic makeup.
2. The majority of genetic syndromes cause language disorders because of the effects on the auditory system (e.g., congenital deafness).
3. Speech-language impairments, stuttering and dyslexia have a genetic contribution.
   a. Concordance higher in monozygotic than in dizygotic twins.

Chromosomal

1. Arise from a difference in the structure or complement of chromosomes.
2. Can be isolated cases and do not necessarily run in families.
3. Two types.
   a. Autosomal disorders.
      (1) Trisomy 21 or Down syndrome.
      (2) Cri du chat syndrome.
   b. Sex-linked chromosomal disorders.
      (1) Turner syndrome.
      (2) Klinefelter syndrome.
      (3) Fragile X syndrome.
      (4) Cornelia de Lange.
      (5) Neurofibromatosis.
      (6) Prader–Willi.
      (7) Williams.
4. Metabolic disorders.
   a. Phenylketonuria.
   b. Mucopolysaccharidoses.
   c. Hurler syndrome.
   d. Enzyme deficiency.
5. Degenerative.
6. Diseases acquired postnatally.
   a. Respiratory disorders.
7. Infections and toxins.
8. Trauma.

Cognitive/Intellectual Disability

Prevalence

1. The 2010 U.S. Census indicates that the population of school-age children with special needs or disabilities is approximately 5% in metropolitan areas and >6% outside of metro areas.
   a. Of these children identified in the census, the greatest majority were identified as having a cognitive or intellectual disability (approximately 4% in metro areas and 5% outside of the metro areas).
   b. The degree of a child's cognitive disability (mild, moderate, severe, profound) is important for aligning services within the educational setting.
      (1) The American Association on Intellectual and Developmental Disabilities indicates that there must be limitations in two or more areas:
         (a) Communication.
         (b) Self-care.
         (c) Home living.
         (d) Social skills.
         (e) Community use.
         (f) Self-direction.
         (g) Health and safety.
         (h) Functional academics.
         (i) Leisure.
         (j) Work.

c. Diagnosis is a combination of standardized cognitive testing and adaptive measures.
d. The Vineland-II is commonly used to determine adaptive function. This is a semistructured interview completed with caregivers that identifies skills in communication, socialization, daily living and motor skills.
e. Adaptive skills are sometimes more amenable to intervention than are overall cognitive skills.

Cognitive Disability

1. Cognitive disability can co-occur with a wide variety of low-incidence disabilities and special health care needs.
    a. There tends to be a higher incidence of behavioral disorders among children with cognitive disability.
    b. Behavior management programs can be helpful, and sometimes children require pharmacological intervention.

Associated Language Difficulties

1. Delayed morphological development as students with cognitive impairment tend to use less complex sentences and fewer relative clauses.
    a. There are additional difficulties in semantics as the children may be more concrete in their understanding and use of certain vocabulary. They may tend to use fewer adjectives and adverbs.
    b. Pragmatics may be commensurate with mental age. Students with cognitive impairment may not understand the proxemics, or how far to distance themselves from a communication partner, in specific communication situations.

Down Syndrome

Chromosomal Abnormality

1. Sometimes referred to as trisomy 21.
2. There are several different types of Down syndrome; however, the manifestations of cognitive and language skills are not significantly different.
3. Current prevalence is 1/800 births, and Down syndrome is highly correlated with cognitive impairment.
4. The hierarchy of development is the same as in neurotypical children, except more slowly in some areas.
5. Hearing deficits are common and may additionally affect language comprehension and expression.

Associated Language Difficulties

1. Language production is often more affected than language comprehension.
2. Syntax is more affected than semantics.
3. Vocabulary and syntax growth is asynchronous, causing an uneven pattern of language development.

X-Linked Syndromes

Fragile-X

1. Fragile-X is the most common inherited form of intellectual handicap. It can vary in degree and manifestation of symptoms.
2. Prevalence is 1:750–1000 male births; 1:500–750 female births.
3. Symptoms include moderate intellectual handicap, language-learning difficulties beyond what would be predicted by cognitive levels.
    a. Symptoms are less severe in females.
4. Some students with fragile-X have characteristics of autism.
5. Language disorders are primarily expressive, often with associated articulation problems.
    a. Delayed onset and development of expressive syntax.
    b. Difficulties in organization.
    c. Difficulties in auditory memory.
    d. Pragmatic deficits including fluency and prosody. Receptive language and vocabulary skills and visual skills are relative strengths.
6. Hyperactivity and impulsivity are common, as is short attention span, which can prove to be barriers to learning language.
7. Speech-language therapy that focuses on auditory skills and listening for following directions is helpful.
    a. Direct therapy on pragmatic skills is also warranted.

Attention Deficit/Hyperactivity Disorder (ADHD)

Characteristics

1. This is the most prevalent mental health diagnosis made in childhood.
2. ADHD can be comorbid with a number of other disorders.
    a. Interventions include psychological and language therapies along with educational supports.
    b. Pharmacological management is often used.
3. Difficulties in concentration, organization, impulse control, planning and distractibility.
4. Those students with the hyperactivity component may also be restless, fidgety, and this may manifest as excessive talking as well.
5. They may exhibit short-term memory problems secondary to their attention problems.
6. Problems in self-monitoring also exist.
7. Difficulties in social language are best mediated with social skills training in naturalistic settings that include a parent training component as well.

Specific Learning Disabilities (SLD)

Characteristics

1. Includes Specific Reading Disability, which is the most common SLD.
2. Symptoms related to language, in addition to reading difficulties, include difficulties with executive functions, including planning, organizing and problem solving.
    a. May also exhibit written language difficulties, or dysgraphia.
        (1) May result from specific difficulties in coordinating pen/paper activities, in addition to the metalinguistic needs involved in writing.
3. Difficulties in short-term memory affect spoken language and reading skill development.
4. Difficulties in social skills are also evident.
    a. Other difficulties include emotional/behavioral problems.

Neural Tube Defects (NTD)

Characteristics

1. The most common neural tube defect is spina bifida.
2. NTDs can affect the spinal cord, brain and associated vertebrae.
3. Because of the specific areas affected, approximately 25% of children with NTD have intellectual disability or learning disability and may have subsequent seizure disorder as well.
    a. Comorbidity of ADHD is also noted.
4. Despite average intellectual abilities, children with NTD have perceptual deficits and difficulties in organizational skills, attention and academic fluency.

Cerebral Palsy

Characteristics

1. Developmental, nonprogressive disability caused by a disturbance in the brain.
2. There are many causes of cerebral palsy, but it is often a consequence of brain injury.
    a. Associated disabilities include visual, hearing, cognitive, speech-language, feeding and emotional/behavioral.

(1) Approximately half of all individuals with cerebral palsy have intellectual disability as well.

(2) Difficulties in both receptive and expressive language.

Traumatic Brain Injury

Characteristics

1. Varies from mild to severe.
   a. Severe brain injury is the most common cause of disability in childhood.
2. 1:25 children receive treatment for a head injury, but 1:500 is severe enough to cause anatomical changes in the brain.
3. Difficulties in language are specific to the area of the brain injured.
   a. Generally, if the TBI is on the left, there will be auditory perceptual problems.
4. Comprehension difficulties.
5. Speech is often telegraphic.
6. Problems in semantics and specifically word finding are often evident.
7. Disorganized language secondary to decreased executive functioning is also evident.
8. Pragmatic difficulties may be present based on the severity of the TBI.

Autism Spectrum Disorders (ASD)

Deficits

1. Impairment in social interaction.
2. Impairment in communication.
3. Restricted repertoire of activity and interests.

DSM-V Category

1. Currently in the DSM-V (publication date May 18, 2013) the category is listed as Autism Spectrum Disorders.
   a. Two broad areas of concern.
      (1) Social communication.
      (2) Restricted behaviors and activities.
   b. All diagnoses (ASD, Asperger's, PDD-NOS) are encompassed under one diagnostic category of Autism Spectrum Disorder.

Comorbidity and Treatments

1. Can be comorbid with intellectual difficulties.
2. Treatments should address the core symptoms of problems in communication and decreased social reciprocity.
   a. Behavioral interventions.
      (1) Teach compliance, attending and imitating.
      (2) Use 1:1, trial-by-trial training.
      (3) Reinforce correct responding.
      (4) Use prompting techniques.
      (5) Provide intensive, teacher-directed instruction.
      (6) Train functional skills.
      (7) Train to generalize.
      (8) Data-based instruction.
   b. Developmental–Individual Relationship (DIR model).
      (1) Floor time.
      (2) A systematic way of working with children to help them move forward developmentally.
      (3) Efficacy at single-subject level and chart review info; however, it is promising.
      (4) Respond to all communication as purposeful.
      (5) Helps child establish affective contact with primary caregivers.
      (6) Increased gestural and verbal interactions lead to decrease in odd or stereotypic behaviors.
      (7) Interactions capitalize on children's emotions by following their interests and motivations.
      (8) As communication circles (turn taking) increase in length, child achieves relating to parent and higher levels of emotional development.
   c. Relationship development interventions.
      (1) Pivotal Response Training (PRT).
      (2) Well established.
      (3) Focus is on increasing motivation through choices, reinforcing, modeling and natural consequences.
      (4) Pivotal behaviors are behaviors central to a child's day-to-day functioning.

(5) Train behaviors for generalization across environments.
   (a) Motivation.
   (b) Responsivity to multiple cues.
   (c) Self-initiation.
   (d) Empathy.
   (e) Self-regulation.
   (f) Social interaction.
(6) Intermix tasks that are novel with one the child does automatically.
(7) Give child some choice or shared control.
(8) Respond to child's behaviors and provide scaffolds and structure.
(9) Reinforce behavior.

3. Social Stories Guidelines gather information about the child and the social situations that present challenges.
   a. Determine where the social situations occurs, who is involved, how long the event is, how it begins and ends, what happens and why.
   b. Interview those working with the child and familiar with the situation.
   c. Observe and record the information observed objectively.
   d. Assume the perspective of the student with ASD.
   e. Facilitate perspective taking by asking the student questions about the relevant cue.
   f. Avoid words like *always* and instead substitute words such as *usually* or *sometimes* to ensure flexibility in events/reactions.
   g. Consider reading and comprehension level of the student.
   h. Photographs, illustrations or drawings can be useful to some students.

References

American Speech-Language-Hearing Association. (2006). *Guidelines for Speech-Language Pathologists in Diagnosis, Assessment, and Treatment of Autism Spectrum Disorders Across the Life Span* [Guidelines]. Available from www.asha.org/policy.

Armstrong, J. (2011, August 30). Serving children with emotional-behavioral and language disorders: A collaborative approach. *The ASHA Leader.*

Bates, E., & Roe, K. (2001). "Language Development in Children with Unilateral Brain Injury," in C.A. Nelson & M. Luciana (Eds.), *Handbook of Developmental Cognitive Neuroscience.* Cambridge, MA: MIT Press, 281–307.

Batshaw, M. L., Pellegrino, L., & Roizen, N. J. (2007). *Children with Disabilities,* 6th ed. Baltimore, MD: Paul H. Brookes Publishing, Co.

Boudreau, D. M., & Chapman, R. S. (2000). The relationship between event representation and linguistic skill in narratives of children and adolescents with Down syndrome. *Journal of Speech, Language, and Hearing Research, 43,* 1146–1159.

Cleland, J., Wood, S., Hardcastle, W., Wishart, J., & Timmins, C. (2010). Relationship between speech, oromotor, language and cognitive abilities in children with Down syndrome. *International Journal of Language and Communication Disorders, 45,* 83–95.

Cone-Wesson, B. (2005). Prenatal alcohol and cocaine exposure: Influences on cognition, speech, language, and hearing. *Journal of Communication Disorders, 38,* 279–302.

Fidler, D. J., Hodapp, R. M., & Dykens, E. M. (2002). Behavioral phenotypes and Special Education: Parent report of educational issues for children with Down yndrome, Prader-Willi Syndrome, and Williams Syndrome. *The Journal of Special Education, 36*(2), 80–88.

Fidler, D. J., Philofsky, A., & Hepburn, S. L. (2007). Language phenotypes and intervention planning: Bridging research and practice. *Mental Retardation and Developmental Disabilities Research Reviews, 13,* 47–57.

Giangreco, M. F. (2000). Related services research for students with low-incidence disabilities: Implications for speech-language pathologists in inclusive classrooms. *Language, Speech, and Hearing Services in Schools, 31,* 230–239.

Gray, C. A. (1995). Teaching children with autism to "read" social situations. In K. Quill (Ed.), *Teaching Children with Autism: Strategies to Enhance Communication and Socialization.* New York: Delmar, 219–242.

Greenspan, S. I., Wieder, S., & Simons, R. (1998). *The Child with Special Needs: Encouraging Intellectual and Emotional Growth.* Cambridge, MA: DeCapo Press.

Hurvitz, E. A., Beale, L., Ried, S., & Nelson, V. S. (1999). Functional outcome of paediatric stroke survivors. *Pediatric Rehabilitation, 3*(2), 43–51.

Kaderavek, J. N., & Rabidoux, P. (2004). Interactive to independent literacy: A model for designing literacy goals for children with atypical communication. *Reading & Writing Quarterly, 20*(3), 237–260.

Kumin, L. (1996). Speech and language skills in children with Down Syndrome. *Mental Retardation and Developmental Disabilities Research Reviews, 2,* 109–115.

Lund, N., & Duchan, J. F. (1993). *Assessing Children's Language in Naturalistic Contexts,* 3rd ed. Englewood Cliffs, NJ: Prentice-Hall.

McDuffie, A. S., Sindberg, H. A., Hesketh, L. J., & Chapman, R. S. (2007). Use of speaker intent and grammatical cues in fast-mapping by adolescents with Down syndrome. *Journal of Speech, Language, and Hearing Research, 50,* 1545–61.

McLean, L. K., Brady, N. C., McLean, J. E., & Behrens, G. A. (1999). Communication forms and functions of children and adults with severe mental retardation in community and institutional settings. *Journal of Speech, Language, and Hearing Research, 42,* 231–240.

Mervis, C. B., & John, A. E. (2008). Vocabulary abilities of children with Williams Syndrome: Strengths, weaknesses, and relation to visuospatial construction ability. *Journal of Speech, Language, and Hearing Research, 51*, 967–982.

Nichols, S., Jones, W., Roman, M. J., Wulfeck, B., Delis, D. C., Reilly, J., & Bellugi, U. (2004). Mechanisms of verbal memory impairment in four neurodevelopmental disorders. *Brain and Language, 88*, 180–189.

Paul, R. (2007). *Language Disorders from Infancy through Adolescence: Assessment & Intervention*, 3rd ed. St. Louis, Missouri: Mosby Elsevier.

Philofsky, A., Fidler, D. J., & Hepburn, S. (2007). Pragmatic language profiles of school-age children with Autism Spectrum Disorders and Williams Syndrome. *American Journal of Speech-Language Pathology, 16*, 368–380.

Prelock, P. A. (2006). *Autism Spectrum Disorders: Issues in Assessment and Intervention*. Austin, TX: PRO-ED, Inc.

Retherford, K. (1993). *Guide to Analysis of Language Transcripts*, 2nd ed. Eau Claire, WI: Thinking Publications.

Richard, G. J. (2008, September 23). Autism spectrum disorders in the schools: Assessment, diagnosis, and intervention pose challenges for SLPs. *The ASHA Leader*.

Roberts, J., Martin, G. E., Moskowitz, L., Harris, A. A., Foreman, J., & Nelson, L. (2007). Discourse skills of boys with Fragile X Syndrome in comparison to boys with Down Syndrome. *Journal of Speech, Language and Hearing Research, 50*, 475–492.

Vanderett, J., Maes, B., Lembrechts, D., & Zink, I. (2010). Predicting expressive vocabulary acquisition in children with intellectual disabilities: A 2-year longitudinal study. *Journal of Speech, Language, and Hearing Research, 53*, 1673–86.

Vigil, V. T., Eyer, J. A., & Hardee, W. P. (2005). Relevant responding in pragmatic language impairment: The role of language variation in the formation-soliciting utterance. *Child Language Teaching and Therapy, 21*(1), 1–21.

Wodrich, D. L. (2006). Children with epilepsy in school: Special services usage and assessment practices. *Psychology in the Schools, 43*(2), 169–181.

9
Written Language Disorders in the School-Age Population

CHARLES W. HAYNES, EdD
AND PAMELA HOOK, PhD

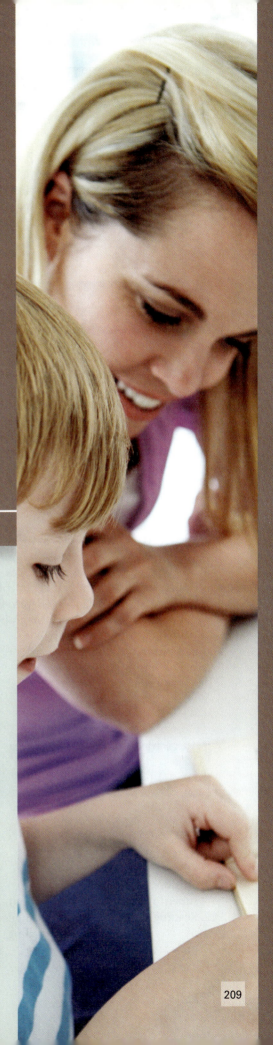

Chapter Outline

- Introduction, 210
- Roles, Responsibilities, Knowledge and Skills Required for Addressing Literacy, 210
- Nature of Literacy: Spoken-Written Language Relationships, Reading and Writing, 210
- Assessment of Literacy Skills, 215
- Reading- and Writing-Related Disorders, 218
- General Considerations for Reading and Writing Instruction, 218
- The Individuals with Disabilities Education Act (IDEA), 220
- References, 221

Introduction

What Is "Literacy"?

1. According to the United Nations Educational, Scientific and Cultural Organization (UNESCO), literacy refers to the "ability to identify, understand, interpret, create, communicate and compute, using printed and written materials."
2. This chapter outlines key knowledge for understanding, preventing, assessing and intervening for literacy disorders related to reading and writing.

Roles, Responsibilities, Knowledge and Skills Required for Addressing Literacy

General Role of SLP

1. According to the American Speech-Language-Hearing Association policy (ASHA, 2001), SLPs can play direct and/or collaborative roles in supporting literacy skills in children, adolescents and adults with developmental and/or acquired literacy communication disorders, including persons with severe or multiple disabilities.

Specific Roles of SLP

1. Specific roles and responsibilities of the SLP with respect to reading and writing in children and adolescents in the area of literacy (adapted from ASHA, 2001).
   a. Preventing written language problems.
   b. Identifying children at risk.
   c. Assessing reading and writing.
   d. Providing intervention and documenting outcomes.
   e. Other roles.
      (1) Assisting general education teachers, parents and students.
      (2) Adding to the knowledge base.
2. Specific knowledge and skills expected of the SLP working with literacy (adapted from ASHA Ad Hoc Committee on Reading and Writing, 2002).
   a. Knowledge areas.
      (1) Nature of literacy.
      (2) Normal (typical) development of reading and writing.
      (3) Disorders of language and literacy.
      (4) Clinical tools and methods.
      (5) Collaboration, leadership and research principles.
   b. Skill areas.
      (1) Prevention of written language problems.
      (2) Identification of at-risk children.
      (3) Assessment of reading and writing skills.
      (4) Providing intervention.
      (5) Other roles.

Nature of Literacy: Spoken-Written Language Relationships, Reading and Writing

Characteristics of Written Language

1. Orthography is a secondary symbolic system superimposed on the primary oral language system.
2. Reading and writing (written language) are comprised of receptive processes (reading) and expressive processes (writing).
3. Written language performance is supported by cognitive factors such as attention, executive functions and memory.
4. Written language is influenced critically by cultural and linguistic differences, such as bilingualism, richness of home language and literacy, socioeconomic status, and quality and characteristics of school curriculum.

Component Processes That Influence Reading and Writing

1. Reading and writing are comprised of two major elements: word identification/spelling and comprehension/written formulation.
2. Components of word identification/spelling include phonic word attack and encoding strategies based on phonological structure, structural analysis based on morphological structure and sight-word recognition, which relies heavily on orthographic memory.
   a. Phonic word attack and encoding involve phonological awareness, grapheme-phoneme correspondence and syllable recognition skills.
      (1) Phonological awareness refers to the capacity to reflect on, analyze and manipulate speech information; general phonological awareness skills predict later word-recognition skills.
      (2) There is a developmental progression for phonological awareness in English, from earlier to later developing.
         (a) Rhyme awareness refers to the ability to recognize or produce words that rhyme: "I saw a frog. It sat on a (log)."
         (b) Word awareness pertains to the ability to recognize words as units in phrases or sentences (i.e., clap the words in "I feel happy today").
         (c) Onset-rime awareness refers to the ability to detect and identify initial sounds in onset-rime words (e.g., which words start with the same sound as "bed": "bug, truck, or boy"?).
            - *Onset* refers to any consonant sounds preceding vowel sounds in a syllable.
            - *Rime* refers to the vowel sounds and any other consonants that occur after the initial consonant sound.
            - Onset-rime awareness is a prerequisite for phonemic awareness.
         (d) Phonemic awareness is the capacity to reflect on, analyze and manipulate speech at the phoneme level.
            - Classic phonemic awareness tasks include blending: /h/ + /æ/ + /p/ + /i/ = "happy"; segmentation: "trip" = /t/ + /r/ + /ɪ/ + /p/; elision (or manipulation): "trim" without /t/ = "rim."
            - Phonemic awareness skill correlates significantly with word recognition and spelling performance for regular words.
            - Development of phonemic awareness occurs synergistically with the development of phonic reading and spelling skills.
      (3) Grapheme-phoneme (symbol-sound) correspondence (GPC) refers to the ability to connect letters with corresponding phonemes.
         (a) Examples of GPC include b = /b/; c = /s/ or /k/; i = /ɪ/ or /aɪ/; ch = /tʃ/, /ʃ/, or /k/; ee = /i/.
         (b) Grapheme-phoneme correspondence knowledge and skills (regular spelling) are predicted by letter-naming performance; together these skills predict and correlate with acquisition of word-recognition skills.
      (4) Syllable-type recognition skills are needed for decoding one- and two-syllable words once GPC has been acquired.
         (a) The following six syllable types provide orthographic cues to vowel pronunciation (C = consonant, V = vowel); knowledge of how to recognize them is critical for struggling readers learning to identify words.
            - Closed = (C)VC (fit, pan, bed).
            - Open = CV (fi- in final, mu- in music, se- in sequin).
            - Silent e = CVCe (fine, late, cede).
            - Vowel team or vowel combination = (C)VV(C) (main, seam, coin).
            - R-controlled = -Vr in stressed syllables (-ar in car, -or in fort; -er in fern, -ir in bird, -ur in burn).
            - Consonant + le = Cle (-fle in rifle, -gle in bugle, -dle in riddle).
      (5) Syllabication rules for two- and some three-syllable words are as follows.
         (a) Splitting the word between medial consonants in (C)VC/CV(C) words (rab/bit, el/bow, pic/nic) and the "flex" rule.
         (b) Splitting the word before or the medial consonant in CV/C/VC words (pa/per, fi/nal; lem/on, cab/in).
   b. Structural analysis, based on morphological structure, involves breaking words down according to base words and affixes.
      (1) Examples of application of structural analysis.
         (a) bio (life) + logy (study of) = biology (study of life).
         (b) re- (back) + tract (pull) + -able (capable of) = retractable (able to be pulled back).
      (2) Highest-frequency morpheme groups targeted for instruction of English are Anglo-Saxon, Latin and Greek.
   c. Sight-word reading involves gestalt, or whole-word, recognition of regular (dog, sprint, magnet) or irregular words (one, friend, yacht).
      (1) The ultimate goal of sight-word reading is automatic word identification.

(2) Sight-word reading places heavy demands on orthographic memory for visual word forms.
d. Automaticity and fluency pertain to reading efficiency (speed and accuracy).
(1) Automaticity refers primarily to word-recognition skills. When word-recognition skills are "automatic," they require minimal cognitive resources. Automaticity contributes to development of fluent reading.
(2) Fluency refers to reading at the phrase, sentence and discourse levels.
(a) Fluent oral reading is prosodic—reflecting appropriate rhythm, intonation and syntactic chunking in combination with automatic word-recognition skills.
- Fluent readers leverage syntactic and discourse contexts to anticipate upcoming words and phrases.
(3) Automaticity and fluency contribute to and interact with reading comprehension.
3. Reading comprehension refers to the complex cognitive process involving the intentional interaction between reader and text to extract meaning.
a. Spoken and written linguistic factors that influence reading comprehension include, but are not limited to:
(1) The reader's knowledge and skills of word recognition.
(2) Reading automaticity and fluency.
(a) Automaticity of word recognition and text-level fluency are important for efficient extraction of meaning from text.
(3) The reader's knowledge and skills of morphology and syntax.
(4) The reader's concept knowledge.
(5) The reader's vocabulary-related semantics.
(a) In persons with adequate word-recognition skills, vocabulary is the individual component of language ability that best predicts reading comprehension.
(6) The reader's knowledge and skills of discourse processing and higher-order thinking.
(a) After vocabulary knowledge and skills, sentence processing and production (the capacity to hold in memory, make sense of and produce word-order patterns in sentences of varying length and complexity) is the second most powerful linguistic predictor component of reading comprehension performance.
(b) Processing and production of discourse (multi-sentence language) comprises the aggregate operations of semantic, syntactic and text structure knowledge and skills.
b. Discourse structures vary on a continuum from narrative to expository.
(1) Narrative, or story structure, is typically more familiar and easier for early grade schoolchildren to understand and produce than is expository, or informational, text.
(2) Mainstream middle-class narrative structure typically requires the reader to understand the following sequence of story elements:
(a) Characters and setting → initiating event → emotional response → internal plan → attempt → consequence → ending.
(3) African American English as well as working-class narrative structure may contain the above elements elaborated with anecdotal, topical associations.
(4) Expository structure is informational in nature and is typically found in newspaper reports, content-area texts such as geography, science and biology and essays.
(a) Standard expository structures include, but are not limited to, descriptive, sequential/enumerative, comparison/contrast and persuasive.
c. Higher-order thinking skills (HOTS) support and direct the reader's interaction with and derivation of meaning from the text. Examples of key HOTS include, but are not limited to, getting facts, identifying the main idea drawing inferences and drawing conclusions.
(1) Fact-oriented comprehension tasks require the reader to identify or produce key information that is directly represented in the text.
(2) In order to identify the main idea, the reader must differentiate between relevant versus irrelevant details.
(3) Drawing inferences requires the reader to extrapolate information that is implied but not explicitly stated in the text.
(4) In order to identify a main idea or draw an inference, the individual must create a mental model that combines information from the text with prior knowledge. The reader then tests this model to determine viable main ideas and/or draw inferences.
d. Components of writing largely parallel those involved in word recognition and reading comprehension; they include spelling and language formulation, as well as cognitive processes of attention, executive function and memory.
e. Planning.
(1) Evaluate the writing assignment, including the topic, audience and any motivating cues.
(2) Retrieve from long-term memory (LTM) stored knowledge of topic (schema, vocabulary,

concepts) and audience (preferences) as well as previously learned strategies and plans for writing.
  (a) Set goals for the writing product.
  (b) Organize the plan.
  (c) Monitor plans being formulated.
    - Monitoring draws heavily on attention, executive functioning and verbal working memory.
f. Translation comprises formulating underlying language based on plans and converting this language into print.
  (1) Generation of internal oral language including word choice and sentence formulation, as well as text formulation of discourse structures such as narrative or expository forms.
  (2) Transcription to print, which involves application of spelling knowledge and skills.
    (a) Regular word spelling (/b/ + /æ/ + /t/ = bat; /ʧ/ + /ɪ/ + /n/ = chin), which draws heavily on mastery of phoneme-grapheme associations.
    (b) Rule-based spelling ("doubling rule": chip + -ing = chipping; "drop y change rule": party + s = parties), which relies on systematic instruction of such rules.
    (c) Irregular word (yacht, buoy, any) and homophone (/meɪn/ = mane, main, Maine; /saɪn/ = sine, sign) spellings, which draw heavily on learning semantic-orthographic associations.
    (d) Transcription of language to print draws heavily on automaticity.
      - Fine motor skills of handwriting and/or digital keyboarding.
      - Punctuation (commas, colons, end punctuation) and capitalization, both of which rely in part on awareness of sentence prosody and intonation.
    (e) Transcription processes require ongoing monitoring of execution and draw heavily on cognitive functions of attention, executive functioning and verbal working memory.
  (3) Reviewing pertains to reading and editing what has been translated.
    (a) Reading relies heavily on decoding skills as well as monitoring for match versus mismatch between the product, the plan and the assignment.
    (b) Editing involves changing the text to make it approximate the plans and goals.
    (c) The process of editing and revising re-invokes transcription processes.
    (d) Reviewing, like planning and editing, draws heavily on attention, executive functioning and verbal working memory.

4. Writing skill development has been most extensively researched in the areas of spelling as well as language formulation.
  a. Spelling develops in a sequence of five general stages: preliterate, semiphonetic, later phonetic, syllable juncture and derivational, as outlined by Louisa Moats, Ed.D.
    (1) During the preliterate, or emergent, stage, children show the awareness that spelling involves making markings on a page that are intended to communicate language. During this period, children make nonalphabetic squiggles or other marks to record what they have to say.
    (2) In the semiphonetic, or letter-name, stage, children use letter names to convey spellings of words; for example: R U DF = "Are you deaf?" I M SLE = "I am silly." KNOPNR = "can opener."
    (3) In the later phonetic stage, children represent most sounds accurately, with the exception of simplifications of some blends; for example: JUP = "jump"; LITL = "little"; POWLEOW = "polio."
    (4) During the syllable juncture stage, children graduate to using spellings that reflect emergent knowledge about orthographic patterns within words: for example: YOUNITED = "united"; EIGHTEY = "eighty"; TAOD = "toad."
    (5) During the derivational stage, the child shows knowledge of morphological roots and affixes; for example: BIGGER, REHEAT, BIOLOGY.
  b. Development of composition/formulation skills can be broken down into two broad phases—emergent and school age.
    (1) The emergent writing phase typically occurs between ages 4–6. This period is characterized first by drawing of pictures, then by drawing mixed with some alphabetic spelling. Writing serves a social and communicative function—children are telling others their thoughts or are seeking understanding of what others have written.
    (2) The school-age (or conventional) writing phase typically occurs from the end of first grade onwards. This phase has numerous distinguishing characteristics:
      (a) Sentence or multi-sentence writing follows at least rudimentary writing conventions (at least alphabetic, with beginnings and endings of sentences, often with narrative elements).
      (b) Drawing may serve an illustrative function but is distinct from text formulation.
      (c) Early conventional writing is characterized by knowledge telling, with limited planning and monitoring.

(d) In grades 1-2, children primarily learn and develop narrative genre and some object description skills.

(e) Students first learn to relate egocentric personal sequence narratives; for example: "Yesterday, I went skiing with my mom. We rented skis. I went down the easy slope. It was fun."

(f) Personal sequence narratives are often followed by third-person story retell structures; for example: "Mr. Toad had a party. All his friends came. They ate tons of cake and ice cream. Then they all went home. They were stuffed!"

(g) Proto-expository object descriptions may be taught. These structures are rudimentary, typically involving listing of basic adjectival attributes and functions; for example: "An apple is red. It is sweet. You cook apples in a pie."

(3) In the school-age writing phase, from grades 2 or 3 on, children begin to learn and develop classic expository text structures, first at the paragraph level and then in multi-paragraph texts. Examples of expository text forms learned include, but are not limited to, process, descriptive, persuasive and comparison. Multi-paragraph essays often contain combinations of these expository paragraph forms.

(a) Development of writing skills parallels and interacts with development of executive functioning and higher-order thinking skills.

(b) As students progress from grade school through high school, they exhibit increased use of key strategies for enhancing the coherence and quality of their writing, employing intra- and intersentence cohesive ties and discourse structure cohesive devices to promote textual coherence and integrity.

- Examples of sentence and intersentence cohesive ties include, but are not limited to, pronominal referencing, use of conjunctions and use of synonyms.
- Examples of discourse-level cohesive devices include use of introductory and concluding sentences within paragraphs and employing introductory and concluding paragraphs within essays. Students also learn planning and revising strategies for composing and elaborating different types of narrative and expository structures and employ and monitor for rationales to support points of view as well as analyze and discuss competing points of view.

5. The cognitive factors of attention, processing speed, executive functions and memory are integrally involved in supporting reading.

a. Attention refers to the capacity to attend selectively to stimuli as well as adaptively shift focus when necessary.
   (1) Approximately one-third of students with Attention Deficit Disorders (ADD) exhibit concomitant reading disabilities.

b. Processing speed reflects the individual's general rate of processing cognitive information in different modalities.
   (1) Slow retrieval speed has a negative effect on automaticity and fluency of reading, which in turn detracts from performance on timed reading comprehension tasks.

c. Executive functioning refers to the mental capacities for planning (strategizing), self-monitoring and adaptively changing plans when the situation demands it.
   (1) Executive functioning reading requirements:
      (a) Form and enact plans for reading text as well as for understanding meaning in the text.
      (b) Self-monitor for accuracy of reading as well as accuracy of understanding.
      (c) Change strategies when self-monitoring, which indicates that the current approach or understanding is inaccurate.

d. Memory functions are vast in scope. A simple model would include long-term memory, short-term memory and verbal working memory.
   (1) With respect to memory functions, long-term memory (LTM) refers to the mind's permanent store of knowledge and associations.
      (a) LTM knowledge and associations for sound-symbol rules, procedures for word recognition, vocabulary and concept maps, and strategies to support reading comprehension are a few examples of LTM's support for literacy learning.
   (2) Short-term memory (STM) is the temporary store for phonological or orthographic information and has practical implications for literacy learning. For example, a child learning to decode words must hold in short-term phonological memory sounds to be blended, or a student reading text must briefly hold in phonological STM an embedded sentence clause in order to extract its meaning.
   (3) Working memory (WM) is the mind's capacity to manipulate information held in temporary store. Language and literacy-related tasks relying on phonological WM include, for example:

(a) Phonological awareness task = "Say 'split' without the /p/ sound."
(b) Syntax task = "Form a sentence beginning with the word 'While'."
(c) WM can be conceptualized to be a central executive system supported by two support systems—a phonological loop and a visual-spatial sketch pad that support literacy learning.
- Central executive system employs executive functioning to coordinate the operations of WM.
- Phonological loop, also termed phonological or verbal rehearsal, refreshes phonological information in STM.
- Visual-spatial sketch pad refreshes visual and orthographic information in STM.
- Effective practices for literacy instruction and intervention involve uses of strategies for scaffolding WM.

6. Chall's Stage Theory is perhaps the most widely referenced theory for reading acquisition and is representative of most approaches to describing children's development of reading skills. According to this theory, each stage is qualitatively different from the next, with distinctive goals addressed during each of the six stages. Each stage relies heavily on children's acquisition of knowledge and skills gained in previous stages (Table 9-1).
   a. Chall's theory has both strengths and weaknesses.
      (1) Strengths of Chall's Stage Theory are its recognition of:
         (a) The importance of early speech and language development prior to the child's exposure to formal literacy instruction in school.
         (b) The reader's mastery of the written language coding as a prerequisite for gaining meaning from print.
      (2) Weaknesses of Chall's Stage Theory are that it does not adequately recognize:
         (a) The importance of ongoing exposure to and development of rich oral language and higher-order thinking skills during the early grades.
         (b) The developmental trajectory for spelling and written language formulation skills.

Table 9-1

Chall's Stage Theory

STAGE	AGES (IN YEARS)	CHARACTERISTICS
Stage 0 "Preliteracy Stage"	0–6	Development of basic receptive and expressive language (phonology, morphology/syntax, semantics, pragmatics/discourse). Development of rudimentary phonological awareness, gross concepts of print, early letter knowledge and book awareness.
Stage 1 "Cracking the Code" or "Decoding/ Encoding"	6–7	Development of alphabetic, sound-symbol correspondence. Development of phonic word attack strategies (decoding). Development of phonic spelling strategies (encoding). Recognition of high-frequency sight words.
Stage 2 "Ungluing from Print"	7–8	Development of automaticity—speed and accuracy of word recognition. Development of fluency of text level decoding—involves speed, accuracy and intonational proficiency.
Stage 3 "Reading to Learn"	8–13	Focus is on learning new information from text. Expository text predominates and the focus is on higher-order thinking skills—involving understanding the main idea, summarizing, inferencing and predicting.
Stage 4 "Multiple Viewpoints"	13–18	Focus is on analyzing and synthesizing information from multiple perspectives.
Stage 5 "Construction and Reconstruction"	18+	Creation of new theories based on analysis, synthesis and evaluation of existing sources of information.

Assessment of Literacy Skills

Types of Assessments: Screening, Diagnostic, Progress Monitoring and Outcomes

1. Although many tests can serve more than one purpose, the goal is to find the most effective and efficient battery.
2. Screening assessments are typically administered to all children to identify those who are at risk for failure and need additional assessment. Screenings allow for the implementation of extra instructional supports.
3. Diagnostic assessments are used to determine at-risk students' specific patterns of strengths and weaknesses

and their instructional needs. These tests are often individually administered and require lengthy testing sessions.
  4. Progress monitoring assessment, also called formative or dynamic assessment, is used to determine whether or not intervention techniques are effective or need to be modified.
     a. Progress monitoring typically occurs throughout the year to ensure that adequate progress in reading growth is being achieved.
     b. These formative measures of progress are typically criterion-referenced—related to the actual material being taught. These tests may be based on a specified benchmark (an expected level of performance).
     c. Data from progress monitoring is critical for determining a student's "response to intervention" (RTI).
  5. Outcomes assessment is typically summative in nature and designed to evaluate overall reading/writing achievement.
     a. Students are often compared to a standard to determine overall progress in comparison to other students in the same grade.
     b. Outcome assessment typically involves use of group-administered, norm-referenced achievement tests or "high-stakes tests" designed at the state level.

Preschool and School-Age Identification of Children at Risk

1. Numerous studies have helped to identify factors that can successfully predict young children's school-age literacy performance early, prior to formal instruction in school.
   a. Parental histories of dyslexia predict with 40%–50% accuracy the likelihood that a child will have a reading disability.
   b. Postnatal assessment of speech perception using elicited response potentials (ERP) paradigms can predict with 80%–90% accuracy which children will fail at word recognition in grade school.
   c. With respect to early preschool predictors, National Early Literacy Panel (2008) meta-analyses have indicated six variables that have medium to large predictive relationships with later literacy performance, independent of IQ or socioeconomic status (SES).
      (1) Alphabetic knowledge of letter names and grapheme-phoneme associations.
      (2) Phonological awareness of syllables and phonemes.
      (3) Rapid automatic naming (RAN) for letters or digits, which involves the ability to rapidly name a sequence of systematically randomized rows of letters or digits.
      (4) RAN for objects or colors.
      (5) The ability to write letters in isolation on request or to write one's own name.
      (6) Phonological memory.
   d. Additional early literacy skills that correlate moderately with at least one of several literacy achievement variables include:
      (1) Concepts of print, referring to the child's knowledge of print conventions (e.g., left–right, front–back directionality) and concepts (book cover, author, text).
      (2) Oral language, including vocabulary and grammar.
      (3) Visual processing—the ability to match or discriminate visually presented symbols.
2. For children in kindergarten, predictors of early grade school word-recognition skills:
   a. Family reading practices.
   b. Letter identification.
   c. Phonological awareness.
   d. Rapid naming.
   e. Phonological memory (digit span, nonword repetition).
3. Kindergarten and first-grade predictors of mid- and later-grade school text reading fluency include rapid naming (objects, letters, digits), as well as speed and accuracy of scanning for letter and non-letter shapes.
4. Kindergarten and first-grade predictors of grade school reading comprehension:
   a. Prior informational knowledge.
   b. Higher-order thinking skills (concept knowledge, inferential skills, figurative language).
   c. Receptive and expressive (oral) vocabulary.
   d. Receptive and expressive (oral) sentence processing.
   e. Narrative retell skills.
   f. Deficits in earlier mentioned predictors of word recognition and reading fluency. Deficient decoding and decoding fluency reduces children's abilities to access meaning in text, even in children with strong underlying language skills.
      (1) This diagnostic pattern has been referred to as a "decoding bottleneck."
5. Key areas to address when conducting a literacy assessment are underlying spoken language skills, reading and writing skills, underlying processing skills, as well as cultural context.
   a. Underlying language testing should examine skills and metalinguistic awareness in morphology, syntax, semantics and discourse.
   b. Assessment of reading and writing should examine both accuracy and automaticity of skills.

(1) Testing should determine the individual's accurate use of knowledge and skills in the areas of letter-sound correspondence, word identification, word attack, sight-word reading and passage comprehension.
(2) Automaticity and fluency assessment should address reading of real words and nonwords, oral reading of paragraphs, as well as silent reading speed.
c. Assessment of spelling should address competency with spelling regular and irregular words, application of phonic rules, as well as knowledge of spelling generalizations.
d. Testing of written expression should determine the child's sentence and discourse-level formulation skills.
(1) Application of strategies for sentence elaboration as well as sentence combining should be examined.
(2) Basic assessment of writing should gather both unedited and self-edited samples of narrative and expository texts.
e. For informal assessment of writing, writing rubrics allow holistic, criterion-related scoring to determine general level of mastery (e.g., Emerging → Adequate → Proficient → Expert).
(1) Rubrics vary according to general type of writing (narrative or expository); criteria for grade school writing vary according to students' developmental levels.
 (a) Narrative: Student employs basic story elements (setting with place and characters, initiating event/problem, character's internal response, character's attempt/solution, consequence and emotional reaction); uses specific vocabulary and well-formed sentences; and employs correct mechanics (spelling, capitalization, punctuation, handwriting).
 (b) Expository: Student addresses the prompt, communicates goals, organizes ideas, uses specific vocabulary and well-formed sentences, provides and elaborates on rationales and employs correct mechanics (spelling, capitalization, punctuation, handwriting).
f. Cognitive processing abilities.
(1) Phonological processing assessment should address phonological awareness, phonological short-term and working memory, as well as rapid naming.
(2) Visual and orthographic processing can be assessed through standardized tests and/or can be studied informally through comparison of the student's spelling of regular versus irregular words.
(3) Additional cognitive processing factors such as attention, WM and executive functioning can be measured directly or inferred through informal analysis of test behaviors.
 (a) In the case of noteworthy concerns regarding any of these factors, referral for neuropsychological assessment should be considered.
g. Cultural context assessment should target extrinsic factors associated with literacy learning.
(1) Determining the language of the home will provide useful information about bi- or multilingual factors.
 (a) In bilingual language learners, it is critical to assess status of first-language (L1) mastery level. L1 mastery is a key predictor of degree of success at L2 language learning in both oral and written domains.
 (b) Assessment of L1 proficiency should be done by a professional with native or near-native proficiency in all aspects of the first language.
(2) Degree of access to reading materials as well as literacy practices in the home should be determined because they are crucial factors that influence literacy learning.
(3) The child's history of formal schooling can provide valuable information about quantity and quality of previous language instruction.
(4) Economic well-being is a general factor associated with lags in language and literacy learning, because basic resources such as food, clothing and shelter provide foundational security for learning to take place.
 (a) Direct or indirect determination of the child's economic context can help the tester to understand the extent to which the child's basic needs are being met.
h. "Exclusionary factors" to rule out in a differential diagnosis of a specific reading/writing disability:
(1) Peripheral sensory deficits in hearing and/or vision.
(2) Global cognitive delay.
(3) Primary emotional disturbance.
(4) Neurological insult, such as stroke or traumatic brain injury.
(5) Environmental exposure to language and literacy learning.
(6) Confirmatory identification of these exclusionary factors may require participation of professionals from multiple disciplines, such as psychiatry, neurology, ophthalmology and neuropsychology.

Reading- and Writing-Related Disorders

Language Learning Disability

1. Language Learning Disability (LLD) is often characterized by difficulties in underlying language skills (deficits in vocabulary, morphology, syntax, discourse).
2. In some cases, coexisting difficulties with word recognition and spelling (orthographic and phonological deficits) are present.
3. In younger children who have not yet received formal reading or writing instruction, the LLD categorization is often replaced by a diagnosis of "Specific Language Impairment" (SLI).

Dyslexia

1. Weaknesses in word recognition and spelling, with deficits in phonological and orthographic processing.
2. Relative strengths in underlying language skills, with typically average or above-average abilities in the areas of vocabulary, morphology, syntax and discourse.

Hyperlexia

1. Deficits in underlying language skills such as vocabulary, morphology, syntax and discourse.
2. Relative strengths with word recognition and spelling (orthographic and phonological deficits).

Attention Deficit/Hyperactivity Disorder

1. Attention Deficit/Hyperactivity Disorder (ADHD) is characterized by behaviors associated with inattention and/or hyperactivity-impulsivity.
2. ADHD is co-morbid in roughly 30%–40% of cases of reading disabilities.
3. The degree of overlap between ADHD and reading disability varies depending on diagnostic criteria and cutoff scores employed for defining reading impairment (LLD or dyslexia) and ADHD.

General Considerations for Reading and Writing Instruction

"Top-Down" versus "Bottom-Up" Approaches

1. Debate regarding "top-down" versus "bottom-up" or "phonics" approaches to reading and writing instruction.
2. Top-down, or whole-language, approaches to reading and/or writing emphasize exposure to authentic literature and leveraging of discourse contexts.
   a. A top-down approach to word-level reading would emphasize reading unfamiliar words through contextual guessing.
   b. A top-down approach to spelling instruction might stress remembering the global shape of words.
   c. With respect to written formulation, a top-down or whole-language approach might emphasize exposing students to rich, authentic texts with the expectation that they would infer sentence and discourse-level writing skills through incidental exposure to texts.
3. Bottom-up approaches to reading, spelling and written language formulation emphasize graduated, systematic instruction that is patterned and multi-modal, involving listening, speaking, reading and writing practice.
   a. A frequently employed bottom-up progression for teaching reading is: phonological awareness → grapheme-phoneme relationships → syllable structure recognition → morphological analysis → text-level decoding fluency.
   b. A frequently employed bottom-up approach to spelling instruction follows a progression of types of words: regular for reading and for spelling → regular for reading but not for spelling → rule-based → irregular for reading and for spelling.
   c. A bottom-up approach to writing formulation might involve multi-modal instruction that systematically follows a progression such as: word → phrase → simple sentence → complex sentence → paragraph → essay.

4. Many professionals advocate for a "balanced approach" to reading that incorporates both bottom-up and top-down methods.
   a. At issue with a balanced approach is a lack of nuanced developmental perspective on when and how much bottom-up versus top-down methodology should be employed and how that balance should vary depending on the child's needs.

Effective Literacy Practices

1. Response to Instruction (RTI) refers to a three-tiered approach to instruction that in theory accommodates the needs of all learners in the classroom according to their changing instructional needs (Table 9-2).
   a. While the RTI model has been adapted to varying degrees across the United States, there are challenges to its efficacy.
      (1) There is not uniform agreement as to what comprises "research-based" instructional methods for reading intervention.
      (2) Lack of regular educators' teacher preparation in research-based literacy methods may result in children receiving inadequate instruction in Tiers One and Two.
      (3) Delayed detection of children for whom Tier One or Tier Two instruction is insufficient may result in months of time passing before individualized Tier Three instruction is provided. This has resulted in some persons calling RTI a "wait until they fail" approach.
2. At-risk readers require a hierarchically structured, systematic approach to reading that is developmentally attuned to their specific reading needs.
   a. Students with dyslexia typically benefit from bottom-up, phonics approaches to word recognition, decoding fluency, spelling and writing.
   b. In addition to receiving systematic instruction in phonics, students with LLDs who display concomitant deficits in both word recognition and underlying language should receive parallel oral language enrichment and instruction that increases their prior knowledge and improves their vocabulary, sentence and discourse-level language skills.
   c. Effective instruction for struggling readers or writers incorporates Multisensory Structured Language (MSL) Principles.
      (1) Teaching should be multi-sensory, involving visual, auditory-oral and tactile-kinesthetic ("V-A-K") modalities.
      (2) Instruction should be systematic, structured and hierarchical, introducing skills incrementally and cumulatively.

Table 9-2

Response to Instruction	
Tier One	Designed to provide for the majority of students' instructional needs. A research-based core reading program in regular education classroom (90 min/day, five components of reading). Benchmark testing of students to determine instructional needs at least three times per year. Ongoing professional development of the classroom teacher.
Tier Two	For those students for whom Tier One instruction is insufficient. Programs, strategies and procedures designed and employed to supplement, enhance and support Tier One. Students in Tier Two receive specialized, scientifically-based reading instruction emphasizing the critical elements of beginning reading. Tier Two instruction includes a minimum of 30 minutes of small-group instruction in addition to 90 minutes of core reading instruction. Children are included in Tier Two instruction for 10–12 weeks, with progress reviewed periodically. Based on progress monitoring, decisions are made about which tier of instruction is most suitable.
Tier Three	Intervention is intensive, strategic and supplemental. Research-based instruction is considerably longer in duration than the 10 to ~20 weeks of supplemental instruction provided in Tier Two. Two 30-minute small-group reading instruction periods/days in addition to 90-minute literacy block for Tiers One and Two. Special instruction to be provided by a qualified provider, typically a specialist in multi-sensory structured language intervention.

      (3) Teach to success—teach within the student's zone of proximal development, ensuring automaticity (promptness and accuracy) of targeted skills before introducing new skills.
      (4) "Spiral" back—revisit and ensure mastery of skills at different levels of language complexity.
         (a) Spiraling might employ practice and mastery of the hard versus soft "c" rule [co-, ca-, cu- = /k + vowel phoneme/; ce, cy, ci = /s + vowel phoneme/] at the following levels: grapheme-phoneme → syllable → word → phrase → sentence → discourse.
3. Effective instruction for all students struggling with literacy learning employs a Gradual Release of Responsibility Model (GRRM).
   a. Initial instruction involves extensive teacher monitoring and modeling, with heavily scaffolded, or supported, practice.
   b. Responsibility for practice, learning and application transition to the student incrementally,

with the final stage involving the student's independent application of target reading or writing skills.
4. Efficacy levels of approaches to reading vary depending on the student's developmental level.
   a. National Early Literacy Panel (2008) meta-analyses of preschool literacy research indicate the following effects of different approaches on children's preliteracy skills and different aspects of writing:
      (1) Moderate to large positive effects on children's conventional literacy skills for code-focused interventions (alphabetic knowledge, word-level decoding/encoding).
      (2) Large effects on oral language skills for language-enhancement interventions.
      (3) Moderate effects on children's print knowledge and oral language skills for book-sharing interventions.
      (4) Moderate to large effects on children's oral language skills and general cognitive abilities for parent training in use of home language and cognitive stimulation.
   b. The National Reading Panel meta-analyses indicate the following intervention effects for methods for improving grade-school-age children's reading skills (2000):
      (1) Moderate effects for phonological awareness intervention, particularly when linked to letter awareness.
      (2) Moderate to large effects for systematic, structured word attack and word identification instruction.
      (3) Small to moderate effects for repeated readings to enhance text-level reading fluency.
      (4) Positive effects for systematical vocabulary and summary writing to enhance reading comprehension skills.
   c. Efficacious approaches for enhancing school-age writing.
      (1) In the area of spelling:
         (a) Systematic teaching of phonic spelling (encoding) and spelling rules improves accuracy.
      (2) In the area of written composition:
         (a) Sentence combining practice enhances the quantity and quality of text produced.
         (b) Strategy instruction improves the form and content of both expository and narrative texts.

The Individuals with Disabilities Education Act (IDEA)

Support for Persons with Reading and Writing Disabilities

1. The Individuals with Disabilities Education Act (IDEA, 2004) is a critical support for persons who struggle with reading and writing difficulties.
2. The law defines "Specific Learning Disability" so as to include ". . . processes involved in understanding or using language, spoken or written . . . ."
   a. For the child to qualify as having a Specific Learning Disability there must be evidence that the learning impairments undermine the child's performance in school.
3. IDEA 2004 addresses issues around evaluation or assessment and identification of learning disabilities related to ". . . written expression, basic reading skill, (and) reading comprehension . . . ."
4. In addition, the law addresses response to intervention (RTI) in noting the local educational agency's role in using "a process that determines if the child responds to scientific, research-based intervention as a part of the evaluation procedures . . . ."
5. Under IDEA, the child with a qualifying learning disability is entitled to an Individualized Education Program (IEP) that meets the child's needs. The IEP process must include:
   a. An initial meeting in which a determination of the child's eligibility for special education.
   b. Provision for an independent evaluation if requested by the parents.
   c. An annual meeting in which the school representatives develop the child's educational plan.
   d. A detailed written description of the child's educational program, including specific training requirements for the person providing specialized education.
   e. Adherence to a strict timeline for steps in the process.
6. The IEP is a legal contract signed by the school and parents that must include several key kinds of information:
   a. The child's present "academic achievement and functional performance."
   b. "Measurable annual goals" that address the child's specific educational needs.

c. A description of the setting and services required to provide the child with a "free and appropriate public education" ("FAPE") in the "least restrictive environment" (LRE).

d. Considerations for vocational and work placements for children who are 16 or older.

e. The parents' right to dispute their child's placement in the school district and take that dispute to an independent party for resolution.

References

The foundational references below reflect a selection of references from key sources, including the American Speech-Language-Hearing Association's (2002) *Knowledge and Skills Needed by Speech-Language Pathologists with Respect to Reading and Writing in Children and Adolescents* as well as the International Dyslexia Association's (2011) policy document *Knowledge and Practice Standards for Teachers of Reading*.

Aaron, P. G., Joshi, R. M., Gooden, R., & Bentum, K. (2008). Diagnosis and treatment of reading disabilities based on the component model of reading: An alternative to the discrepancy model of LD. *Journal of Learning Disabilities*, 41, 67–84.

Adams, M. J. (1990). *Beginning to Read: Thinking and Learning about Print*. Cambridge, MA: MIT Press.

Adams, M., Foorman, B. R., Lundberg, I., & Beeler, T. (Spring/Summer, 1998). The elusive phoneme: Why phonemic awareness is so important and how to help children develop it. *American Educator*, 22(1 & 2), 18–29.

American Speech-Language-Hearing Association. (1997). *Preferred Practice Patterns for the Profession of Speech-Language Pathology*. Rockville, MD: Author.

American Speech-Language-Hearing Association. (1999). *Guidelines for the Roles and Responsibilities of the School-Based Speech-Language Pathologist*. Rockville, MD: Author.

American Speech-Language-Hearing Association. (2001). *Scope of Practice for Speech-Language Pathology*. Rockville, MD: Author.

American Speech-Language-Hearing Association. (2002). *Knowledge and Skills Needed by Speech-Language Pathologists with Respect to Reading and Writing in Children and Adolescents* [Knowledge and Skills]. Available from www.asha.org/policy.

Apel, K., & Swank, L. K. (1999). Second chances: Improving decoding skills in the older student. *Language, Speech, and Hearing Services in Schools*, 30, 231–242.

Ball, E. W., & Blachman, B. A. (1988). Phoneme segmentation training: Effect on reading readiness. *Annals of Dyslexia*, 38, 208–224.

Bashir, A., & Hook, P. (2009) Fluency: A key link between word identification and comprehension, *Language, Speech and Hearing Services in the Schools*, 40(2), 196–200.

Bashir, A., Conte, B. M., & Heerde, S. M. (1998). "Language and School Success: Collaborative Challenges and Choices" in D. D. Merritt & B. Culatta (Eds.), *Language Intervention in the Classroom*. San Diego, CA: Singular, pp. 1–36.

Bear, D., Invernizzi, M., Templeton, S., & Johnston, P. (2000). *Words Their Way*, 2nd ed. Columbus, OH: Merrill.

Beck, I. L., & McKeown, M. G. (2006). *Improving Comprehension with Questioning the Author: A Fresh and Expanded View of a Powerful Approach*. New York: Scholastic.

Beck, I. L., McKeown, M. G., & Kucan, L. (2002). *Bringing Words to Life: Robust Vocabulary Instruction*. New York: Guilford Press.

Bereiter, C., & Scardamalia, M. (1987). *The Psychology of Written Composition*. Hillsdale, NJ: Erlbaum.

Berninger, V. W., & Amtmann, D. (2003). "Preventing Written Expression Disabilities through Early and Continuing Assessment and Intervention for Handwriting and/or Spelling Problems: Research into Practice" in H. L. Swanson, K. R. Harris, & S. Graham (Eds.), *Handbook of Learning Disabilities*. New York: Guilford Press, pp. 345–363.

Berninger, V., & Wolf, B. (2009). *Teaching Students with Dyslexia and Dysgraphia*. Baltimore: Brookes.

Berninger, V., Vaughan, K., Abbott, R., Brooks, A., Begay, K., Curtin, G., Byrd, K., & Graham, S. (2000). Language-based spelling instruction: Teaching children to make multiple connections between spoken and written words. *Learning Disability Quarterly*, 23, 117–135.

Bickart, T. (1998). *Summary Report of Preventing Reading Difficulties in Young Children* (National Academy of Sciences). Washington, DC: U.S. Department of Education.

Biemiller, A. (1999). "Language and Reading Success" in J. Chall (Ed.), *From Reading Research to Practice, A Series for Teachers*. Cambridge, MA: Brookline Books.

Biemiller, A. (2005). "Size and Sequence in Vocabulary Development: Implications for Choosing Words for Primary Grade Instruction" in E. H. Hiebert and M. L. Kamil (Eds.), *Teaching and Learning Vocabulary: Bringing Research to Practice*. Mahwah, NJ: Erlbaum.

Birsh, J. (Ed.). (2005). *Multisensory Teaching of Basic Language Skills*, 2nd ed. Baltimore: Brookes.

Blachman, B. A., Schatschneider, C., Fletcher, J. M., Francis, D. J., Clonan, S., Shaywitz, B., et al. (2004). Effects of intensive reading remediation for second and third graders. *Journal of Educational Psychology*, 96, 444–461.

Brady, S., & Shankweiler, D. (Eds.). (1991). *Phonological Processes in Literacy: A Tribute to Isabelle Y. Liberman*. Hillsdale, NJ: Lawrence Erlbaum Associates.

Burns, S. M., Griffin, P., & Snow, C. E. (1999). *Starting Out Right: A Guide to Promoting Children's Reading Success*. Washington, DC: National Academy Press.

Carlisle, J., & Rice, M. S. (2003). *Reading Comprehension: Research-Based Principles and Practices*. Baltimore: York Press.

Carreker, S. (2005). "Teaching Reading: Accurate Decoding and Fluency" in J. Birsh (Ed.), *Multisensory Teaching of Basic Language Skills*, 2nd ed.. Baltimore: Brookes, pp. 213–255.

Catts, H. W. (1993). The relationship between speech-language impairments and reading disabilities. *Journal of Speech and Hearing Research*, 36, 948–958.

Catts, H. W., & Kamhi, A. G. (1999). *Language and Reading Disabilities*. Boston: Allyn & Bacon.

Catts, H. W., Fey, M. E., Zhang, X., & Tomblin, J. A. (1999). Language basis of reading and language disabilities: Evidence from a longitudinal investigation. *Scientific Studies of Reading*, 3, 331–361.

Catts, H. W., Hogan, T. P., & Adlof, S. M. (2005). "Developmental Changes in Reading and Reading Disabilities" in H.W. Catts & A. Kamhi (Eds.), *The Connections Between Language and Reading Disabilities*. Mahwah, NJ: Erlbaum, pp. 25–40.

Catts, H., Fey, M., Zhang, X., & Tomblin, J. B. (2001). Estimating the risk of future reading difficulties in kindergarten children: A research-based model and its clinical implementation. *Language, Speech, Hearing Services in Schools*, 32, 38–50.

Clark, D., & Uhry, J. K. (1995). *Dyslexia: Theory and Practice of Remedial Instruction*. Baltimore: York Press.

Cornoldi, C., & Oakhill, J. (Eds.). (1996). *Reading Comprehension Difficulties: Processes and Intervention*. Mahwah, NJ: Erlbaum.

Crawford, E. C., & Torgesen, J. K. (2006, July). *Teaching All Children to Read: Practices from Reading First Schools with Strong Intervention Outcomes*. Presented at the Florida Principal's Leadership Conference, Orlando. Retrievable from http://www.fcrr.org/science/sciencePresentationscrawford.ht.

Cunningham, A. E., & Stanovich, K. E. (1997). Early reading acquisition and its relation to reading experience and ability ten years later. *Developmental Psychology*, 33, 934–945.

Cutting, L. E., & Scarborough, H. S. (2006). Prediction of reading comprehension: Relative contributions of word recognition, language proficiency, and other cognitive skills can depend on how comprehension is measured. *Scientific Studies of Reading*, 10, 277–299.

Denton, C. A, Fletcher, J. M., Anthony, J. L., & Francis, D. J. (2006). An evaluation of intensive intervention for students with persistent reading difficulties. *Journal of Learning Disabilities*, 39, 447–466.

Denton, C. A., Foorman, B., & Mathes, P. (2003). Schools that "Beat the Odds": Implications for reading instruction. *Remedial and Special Education*, 24, 258–261.

Denton, C. A., Vaughn, S., & Fletcher, J. (2003). Bringing research-based practice in reading intervention to scale. *Learning Disabilities Research and Practice*, 18, 201–211.

Dickinson, D., & Tabors, P. O. (Eds.). (2001). *Beginning Literacy*. Baltimore: Brookes.

Dickson, S. V., Simmons, D. C., & Kameenui, E. J. (1998). "Text Organization: Research Bases" in D. C. Simmons & E. J. Kameenui (Eds.), *What Reading Research Tells Us about Children with Diverse Learning Needs: Bases and Basics*. Mahwah, NJ: Erlbaum, pp. 239–278.

Ehri, L. (2000). Learning to read and learning to spell: Two sides of a coin. *Topics in Language Disorders*, 20(3), 19–36.

Ehri, L., & Snowling, M. (2004). "Developmental variation in word recognition" in A. C. Stone, E. R. Silliman, B. J. Ehren, & K. Apel (Eds.), *Handbook of Language and Literacy: Development and Disorders*. New York: Guilford Press, pp. 443–460.

Fletcher, J. M., Lyon, G. R., Fuchs, L. S., & Barnes, M. A. (2007). *Learning Disabilities: From Identification to Intervention*. New York: Guilford Press.

Genesee, F., Paradis, J., & Crago, M. (2004). *Dual Language Development & Disorders: A Handbook on Bilingualism & Second Language Learning*. Baltimore: Brookes.

Gersten, R., & Baker, S. (2001). Teaching expressive writing to students with learning disabilities: A metaanalysis. *Elementary School Journal*, 101, 251–272.

Good, R. H., Simmons, D. C., & Kame'enui, E. J. (2001). The importance and decision-making utility of a continuum of fluency-based indicators of foundational reading skills for third-grade high-stakes outcomes. *Scientific Studies of Reading*, 5(3), 257–288.

Graham, S., McArthur, C.A., & Fitzgerald, J. (Eds.). (2007). *Best Practices in Writing Instruction*. New York: Guilford Press.

Graves, D. H. (1983). *Writing: Teachers and Children at Work*. Portsmouth, NH: Heinemann.

Gutierrez-Clellan, V. F. (1999). Mediating literacy skills in Spanish-speaking children with special needs. *Language, Speech, and Hearing Services in Schools*, 30, 285–292.

Gutierrez-Clellan, V. F. (2000). Dynamic assessment: An approach to assessing children's language-learning potential. *Seminars in Speech and Language*, 21, 215–222.

Hart, B., & Risley, T. R. (1995). *Meaningful Differences in the Everyday Experience of Young American Children*. Baltimore: Brookes.

Haynes, C., & Jennings, T. (2006/2011). Listening and speaking: Essential ingredients for teaching struggling writers. *Perspectives*, 32(2, Spring, 12-16), republished in M. Joshi & L. Moats (Eds.). *Expert Perspectives on Intervention with Reading Disabilities: An Anthology from Publications of the International Dyslexia Association*. International Dyslexia Association: Towson, MD.

Henry, M. (2003). *Unlocking Literacy*. Baltimore: Brookes.

Hiebert, E. H. (1993). "Young Children's Literacy Experiences in Home and School" in S. R. Yussen & M. C. Smith (Eds.), *Reading Across the Lifespan*. New York: Springer-Verlag, pp. 33–55.

Hirsch, E. D. (2001). Overcoming the language gap. *American Educator*, 25(2), 4, 6–7.

Hirsch, E. D. (2006). Building knowledge: The case for bringing content into the language arts block and for a knowledge-rich curriculum core for all children. *American Educator*, 30(1), 8–21, 28–29, 50–51.

Hirsch, E. D. (2006). *The Knowledge Deficit: Closing the Shocking Education Gap for American Children*. Boston: Houghton Mifflin.

Hook, P., & Haynes, C. (2009). "Reading and Writing in Child Language Disorders" in R. Schwartz (Ed.), *Handbook of Child Language Disorders*. New York: Psychology Press.

Hulme, C., & Snowling, M. (2009) *Developmental Disorders of Language, Learning, and Cognition*. Oxford, England: Wiley-Blackwell.

Joshi, M., Treiman, R., Carreker, S., & Moats, L. C. (2008/2009). How words cast their spell: Spelling is an integral part of learning the language, not a matter of memorization. *American Educator*, 32(4), 6–16, 42–43.

Juel, C. (1988). Learning to read and write: A longitudinal study of 54 children from first through fourth grades. *Journal of Educational Psychology*, 80, 437–447.

Kameenui, E. J. (Ed.) (1997). *Effective Teaching Strategies That Accommodate Diverse Learners*. Upper Saddle River, NJ: Prentice Hall.

Kamil, M. (2004). "Vocabulary and Comprehension Instruction: Summary and Implications of the National Reading Panel Findings" in P. McCardle & V. Chhabra (Eds.), *The Voice of Evidence in Reading Research*. Baltimore: Brookes, pp. 213–234.

Katzir, T., Kim, Y., Wolf, M., O'Brien, B., Kennedy, B., Lovett, M., et al. (2006). Reading fluency: The whole is more than the parts. *Annals of Dyslexia*, 56(1), 51–82.

Kintsch, E. (2005). Comprehension theory as a guide for the design of thoughtful questions. *Topics in Language Disorders*, 25(1), pp. 51–64.

Koppenhaver, D. A., & Yoder, D. E. (1993). Classroom literacy instruction for children with severe speech and physical impairments (SSPI): What is and what might be. *Topics in Language Disorders*, 13(2), 1–15.

Leach, J. M., Scarborough, H. S., & Rescorla, L. (2003). Late-emerging reading disabilities. *Journal of Educational Psychology*, 95, 211–224.

Leonard, L. B. (1998). *Children with Specific Language Impairment*. Cambridge, MA: MIT Press.

Lovett, M. W., Barron, R. W., & Benson, N. J. (2003). "Effective Remediation of Word Identification and Decoding Difficulties in School-Age Children with Reading Disabilities" in H. L. Swanson, K. R. Harris, & S. Graham (Eds.), *Handbook of Learning Disabilities*. New York: Guilford Press, pp. 273–292.

Lovett, M. W., Lacerenze, L., & Borden, S. L. (2000). Putting struggling readers on the PHAST track: A program to integrate phonological and strategy-based remedial reading instruction and maximize outcomes. *Journal of Learning Disabilities*, 33, 458–476.

Lyon, R., Shaywitz, S., & Shaywitz, B. (2003). A definition of dyslexia. *Annals of Dyslexia*, 53, 1–14.

MacArthur, C. A. (2000). New tools for writing: Assistive technology for students with writing difficulties. *Topics in Language Disorders*, 20(4), 85–100.

MacArthur, C. A., Schwartz, S. S., & Graham, S. (1991). A model for writing instruction: Integrating word processing and strategy instruction into a process approach to writing. *Learning Disabilities Research and Practice*, 6, 230–236.

Mahfoudhi, A., & Haynes, C. (2009). "Phonological Awareness in Reading Disabilities Remediation: Some General Issues" in G. Reid, G. Elbeheri, and J. Everatt (Eds.), *International Handbook of Dyslexia*. New York, NY: Routledge Press.

Masterson, J., & Apel, K. (2000). Spelling assessment: Charting a path to optimal intervention. *Topics in Language Disorders*, 20(3), 50–66.

McCardle, P., & Chhabra, V. (2004). *The Voice of Evidence in Reading Research*. Baltimore: Brookes.

Meyer, M. S., & Felton, R. H. (1999). Repeated reading to enhance fluency: Old approaches and new directions. *Annals of Dyslexia*, 49, 293–306.

Michaels, S. (1981). Sharing time: Children's narrative styles and differential access to literacy. *Language in Society*, 10, 423–442.

Moats, L. C. (1995). *Spelling: Development, Difficulty, and Instruction*. Baltimore: York Press.

Moats, L. C. (2000). *Speech to Print: Language Essentials for Teachers*. Baltimore: Brookes.

Moats, L. C., & Dakin, K. (2007). *Basic Facts about Dyslexia*. Baltimore: The International Dyslexia Association.

National Reading Panel. (2000). *Teaching Children to Read: An Evidence-Based Assessment of the Scientific Research Literature on Reading and Its Implications for Reading Instruction*. Washington, DC: National Institutes of Health.

Nelson, N. W. (1998). *Childhood Language Disorders in Context: Infancy Through Adolescence*, 2nd ed. Boston: Allyn & Bacon.

Newman, S. B., & Dickinson, D. K. (2001). *Handbook of Early Literacy Research*. New York: Guilford Press.

Olson, R. K. (2004). SSSR, environment, and genes. *Scientific Studies of Reading*, 8(2), 111–124.

Paul, R. (2007). *Language Disorders from Infancy Through Adolescence: Assessment and Intervention*, 3rd ed. St. Louis, MO: Mosby.

Pennington, B. (2009). *Diagnosing Learning Disorders*, 2nd ed. New York: Guilford Press.

Prelock, P. A., Miller, B. L., & Reed, N. L. (1995). Collaborative partnerships in a language in the classroom program. *Language, Speech, and Hearing Services in Schools*, 26, 286–292.

Rayner, K., Foorman, B. F., Perfetti, C. A., Pesetsky, D., & Seidenberg, M. S. (2002). How should reading be taught? *Scientific American*, 286(3), 84–91.

Roth, F. P. (2000). Narrative writing: Development and teaching with children with writing difficulties. *Topics in Language Disorders*, 20(4), 15–28.

Ruddell, R. B., Ruddell, M. R., & Singer, H. (Eds.). (1994). *Theoretical Models and Processes of Reading*, 4th ed. Newark, DE: International Reading Association.

Samuels, S. J. (1997). The method of repeated readings. *The Reading Teacher*, 50, 76–81.

Samuels, S. J., & Flor, R. F. (1997). The importance of automaticity for developing expertise in reading. *Reading and Writing Quarterly: Overcoming Learning Difficulties*, 13, 107–121.

Scarborough, H. S. (2001). "Connecting Early Language and Literacy to Later Reading (Dis)Abilities: Evidence, Theory, and Practice" in S. B. Neuman & D. K. Dickinson (Eds.), *Handbook of Early Literacy Research*. New York: Guilford Press, pp. 97–110.

Scarborough, H. S. (1998). "Early Identification of Children at Risk for Reading Disabilities: Phonological Awareness and Some Other Promising Predictors" in B. K. Shapiro, P. J. Accardo, & A. J. Capute (Eds.), *Specific Reading Disability: A View of the Spectrum*. Timonium, MD: York Press, pp. 75–119.

Scardamalia, M., & Bereiter, C. (1986). "Research on Written Composition" in M. C. Wittrock (Ed.), *Handbook of Research on Teaching*. New York: Macmillan, pp. 778–803.

Scott, C. M. (2000). Principles and methods of spelling instruction: Applications for poor spellers. *Topics in Language Disorders*, 20(3), 66–82.

Scott, C. M. (2004). "Syntactic Contributions to Literacy Development" in C. Stone, E. Stillman, B. Ehren, & K. Apel (Eds.), *Handbook of Language & Literacy*. New York: Guilford Press, pp. 340-362.

Scott, C. M. (1999). "Learning to Write" in H. W. Catts & A. G. Kamhi (Eds.), *Language and Reading Disabilities*. Boston: Allyn & Bacon, pp. 224-258.

Scott, C. M., & Brown, S. (2001). Spelling and the speech-language pathologist: There's more than meets the eye. *Seminars in Speech and Language*, 22, 197-298.

Shankweiler, D., Lundquist, E., Katz, L., Stuebing, K. K., Fletcher, J. M., Brady, S., et al. (1999). Comprehension and decoding: Patterns of association in children with reading difficulties. *Scientific Studies of Reading*, 31, 24-35, 69-94.

Shaywitz, S. (2003). *Overcoming Dyslexia: A New and Complete Science-Based Program for Reading Problems at Any Level*. New York: Knopf.

Silliman, E. R., Jimerson, T. L., & Wilkinson, L. C. (2000). A dynamic systems approach to writing assessment in students with language learning problems. *Topics in Language Disorders*, 20(4), 45-64.

Simmons, D. C., & Kameenui, E. J. (Eds.). (1998). *What Reading Research Tells Us About Children with Diverse Learning Needs: Bases and Basics*. Mahwah, NJ: Erlbaum.

Snow, C. E., Burns, M. S., & Griffin, P. (Eds.). (1998). *Preventing Reading Difficulties in Young Children*. Washington, DC: National Academy Press.

Snow, C. E., Griffin, P., & Burns, S. (2006). *Knowledge to Support the Teaching of Reading*. San Francisco: Jossey-Bass.

Spear-Swerling, L. (2004). "A Road Map for Understanding Reading Disability and Other Reading Problems: Origins, Intervention, and Prevention" in R. Ruddell & N. Unrau (Eds.), *Theoretical Models and Processes of Reading: Vol. 5*. Newark, DE: International Reading Association.

Spear-Swerling, L. (2008). "Response to Intervention and Teacher Preparation" in E. Grigorenko (Ed.), *Educating Individuals with Disabilities: IDEA 2004 and Beyond*. New York: Springer, pp. 273-293.

Spear-Swerling, L., & Sternberg, R. J. (2001). What science offers teachers of reading. *Learning Disabilities Research & Practice*, 16, 51-57.

Speece, D. L., & Ritchey, K. D. (2005). A longitudinal study of the development of oral reading fluency in young children at risk for reading failure. *Journal of Learning Disabilities*, 38(5), 387-399.

Stahl, K.A.D. (2004). Proof, practice, and promise: Comprehension strategy instruction in the primary grades. *The Reading Teacher*, 57, 598-609.

Stahl, S. A., & Heubach, K. (2005). Fluency-oriented reading instruction. *Journal of Literacy Research*, 37, 25-60.

Stahl, S. A., & Nagy, W. E. (2006) *Teaching Word Meanings*. Mahwah, NJ: Erlbaum.

Stanovich, K. E. (2000). *Progress in Understanding Reading: Scientific Foundations and New Frontiers*. New York: Guilford Press.

Sterne, A., & Goswami, U. (2000). Phonological awareness of syllables, rhymes, and phonemes in deaf children. *Journal of Childhood Psychology and Psychiatry*, 41, 609-625.

Stone, A. C., Silliman, E. R., Ehren, B. J., & Apel, K. (Eds.). (2004). *Handbook of Language and Literacy: Development and Disorders*. New York: Guilford Press.

Tabors, P. O., & Snow, C. E. (2001). "Young Bilingual Children and Early Literacy Development" in S. B. Neuman & D. K. Dickinson (Eds.), *Handbook of Early Literacy Research*. New York: Guilford, pp. 157-178.

Torgesen, J. K. (1999). "Assessment and Instruction for Phonemic Awareness and Word Recognition Skill" in H. W. Catts & A. G. Kamhi (Eds.), *Language and Reading Disabilities*. Boston, MA: Allyn & Bacon, pp. 128-153.

Torgesen, J. K. (2004). "Lessons Learned from Research on Interventions for Students Who Have Difficulty Learning to Read" in P. McCardle & V. Chhabra (Eds.), *The Voice of Evidence in Reading Research*. Baltimore: Brookes, pp. 355-381.

Trieman, R. (1993). *Beginning to Spell: A Study of First Grade Children*. New York: Oxford University Press.

Van Kleeck, A. (1990). Emergent literacy: Learning about print before learning to read. *Topics in Language Disorders*, 10, 25-45.

Vaughn, S., & Klingner, J. K. (1999). Teaching reading comprehension through collaborative strategic reading. *Intervention in School and Clinic*, 34, 284-292.

Vellutino, F. R., Tunmer, W. E., Jaccard, J. J., & Chen, R. (2007). Components of reading ability: Multivariate evidence for a convergent skills model of reading development. *Scientific Studies of Reading*, 11(1), 3-32.

Wallach, G. P., & Butler, K. G. (Eds.). (1994). *Language Learning Disabilities in School-Aged Children and Adolescents*. Boston: Allyn & Bacon.

Westby, C. E. (2004). "A Language Perspective on Executive Functioning, Metacognition, and Self-regulation in Reading" in C. A. Stone, E. R. Silliman, B. J. Ehren, & K. Apel (Eds.), *Handbook of Language and Literacy: Development and Disorders*. New York: Guilford Press, pp. 398-427.

Westby, C. E. (1994). "The Effects of Culture on Genre, Structure, and Style of Oral and Written Texts" in G. P. Wallach & K. G. Butler (Eds.), *Language Learning Disabilities in School-Aged Children and Adolescents*. Boston: Allyn & Bacon, pp. 180-218.

Westby, C. E. (1999a). "Assessing and Facilitating Text Comprehension Problems" in H. W. Catts & A. G. Kamhi (Eds.), *Language and Reading Disabilities*. Boston: Allyn & Bacon, pp. 154-223.

Wolf, M. (2007). *Proust and the Squid: The Story and Science of the Reading Brain*. New York: Harper Collins.

Wolf, M., & Bowers, P. G. (1999). The double-deficit hypothesis for the developmental dyslexias. *Journal of Educational Psychology*, 91, 415-438.

Wong, B. Y. L. (2000). Writing strategies instruction for expository essays for adolescents with and without learning disabilities. *Topics in Learning Disorders*, 20(4), 29-44.

Yopp, H. K. (1992). Developing phonemic awareness in young children. *The Reading Teacher*, 45, 696-703.

10

Autism Spectrum Disorders

GAIL J. RICHARD, PhD

Chapter Outline

- Background Information, 226
- Definitions, 226
- Etiological Information, 230
- Behavioral Characteristics, 231
- Role of the Speech-Language Pathologist in Autism Spectrum Disorder (ASD), 232
- Assessment, 233
- Treatment, 235
- Intervention Methodologies, 237
- Related Services, 239
- References, 240

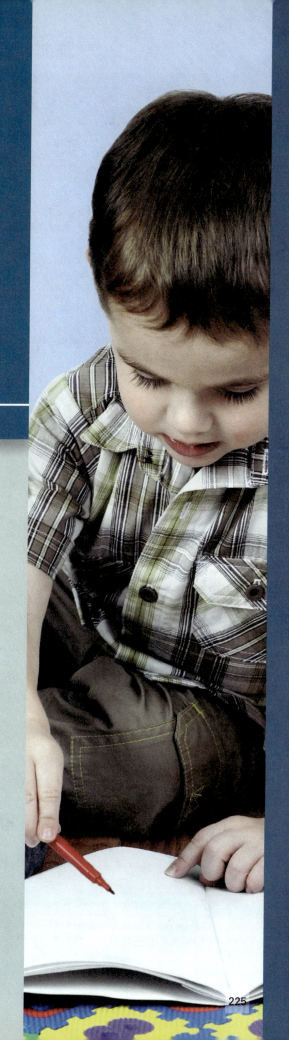

Background Information

Dr. Leo Kanner

1. Introduced the disorder called autistic disturbances of affective contact in 1943.
   a. Autism means *self*, indicating self-absorbed isolation observed in individuals.
   b. Primarily a disorder of difficulty relating to the environment, themselves and other people.
2. Kanner's core shared features observed among all children with the disorder.
   a. Obsessive.
      (1) Persistent, intense, consuming focus on something.
   b. Stereotypic behaviors.
      (1) Rhythmic repetitive motor movements or behaviors.
   c. Echolalia.
      (1) Repeating verbal utterances produced by others.
   d. Purposeful relationship to objects.
   e. Desire for aloneness (isolation) and sameness (routines).
   f. Lack of affective interaction, awareness and contact with people.

Genetic Basis for Physical Disorder

1. Abnormalities in the genetic code for brain development results in cognitive and behavioral differences.
2. Biochemical differences in the brain that negatively impact neurologic development.
3. Deficits in neural connections within and between neural systems during brain development.
4. Neurobiological differences in brain development result in behavioral differences.

Spectrum Disorder

1. Three primary symptoms:
   a. Impaired development of reciprocal social interaction.
   b. Impaired development of speech and language for verbal and nonverbal communication.
   c. Abnormal behavioral patterns and interactions with objects.
2. Severity of symptoms on a continuum from mild to severe.
3. Onset of developmental delays and differences noted by 12–24 months.
4. Disorder genetically predisposed and present throughout life.

Incidence and Prevalence Figures

1. Present in approximately 1% of children in the United States between 3 and 17 years of age (Autism Society of America).
2. Prevalence reported at approximately 1 in 88 (Center for Disease Control).
3. Occurs more frequently in males, with approximately a 3:1 male-to-female ratio.
4. Increased prevalence in siblings, as high as 19% chance of autism exists in siblings.
5. Increased risk in twins, especially monozygotic twins versus dizygotic twins.
6. Reported to occur in all racial, ethnic and social populations.
   a. Prevalence across children in various populations in the United States.
      (1) White, non-Hispanic ranged from 3.4 to 14.8 per 1,000.
      (2) Black, non-Hispanic ranged from 1.6 to 12.9 per 1,000.
      (3) Hispanic ranged from 0.6 to 8.3 per 1,000.
   b. Prevalence in South Korea is very high, with a reported 2.6% of children affected.
   c. Prevalence in England ranges from 0.7 to 1.8% of the population, commensurate with U.S. and Australia reported rates.

Definitions

Diagnostic and Statistical Manual of Mental Disorders–5th Edition (*DSM-5*; APA, 2013) Definitions

1. Autism spectrum disorder (see Figure 10-1).
   a. Persistent deficits in social communication and social interaction across multiple contexts (the severity must be specified).
      (1) Deficits in social-emotional reciprocity (e.g., fail to initiate or respond to social interactions; poor conversational turn taking).

Autism Spectrum Disorder

A. Persistent deficits in social communication and social interaction across multiple contexts, as manifested by the following, currently or by history (examples are illustrative, not exhaustive):
 1. Deficits in social-emotional reciprocity, ranging, for example, from abnormal social approach and failure of normal back-and-forth conversation, to reduced sharing of interests, emotions or affect, to failure to initiate or respond to social interaction.
 2. Deficits in nonverbal communicative behaviors used for social interaction, ranging, for example, from poorly integrated verbal and nonverbal communication, to abnormalities in eye contact and body language or deficits in understanding and use of gestures, to a total lack of facial expressions and nonverbal communication.
 3. Deficits in developing, maintaining and understanding relationships, ranging, for example, from difficulties adjusting behavior to suit various social contexts, to difficulties in sharing imaginative play or in making friends, to absence of interest in peers.
 4. *Specify current severity of these social communication deficits.*
B. Restricted, repetitive patterns of behavior, interests, or activities, as manifested by at least two of the following, currently or by history (examples are illustrative, not exhaustive):
 1. Stereotyped or repetitive motor movements, use of objects, or speech (e.g., simple motor stereotypies, lining up toys or flipping objects, echolalia, idiosyncratic phrases).
 2. Insistence on sameness, inflexible adherence to routines or ritualized patterns of verbal or nonverbal behavior (e.g., extreme distress at small changes, difficulties with transitions, rigid thinking patterns, greeting rituals, need to take same route or eat same food every day).
 3. Highly restricted, fixated interests that are abnormal in intensity or focus (e.g., strong attachment to or preoccupation with unusual objects, excessively circumscribed or perseverative interests).
 4. Hyper- or hyporeactivity to sensory input or unusual interest in sensory aspects of the environment (e.g., apparent indifference to pain/temperature, adverse response to specific sounds or textures, excessive smelling or touching of objects, visual fascination with lights or movement).
 5. *Specify current severity of these repetitive behaviors.*
C. Symptoms must be present in the early developmental period (but may not become fully manifest until social demands exceed limited capacities, or may be masked by learned strategies in later life).
D. Symptoms cause clinically significant impairment in social, occupational or other important areas of current functioning.
E. These disturbances are not better explained by intellectual disability (intellectual developmental disorder) or global developmental delay. Intellectual disability and autism spectrum disorder frequently co-occur; to make comorbid diagnoses of autism spectrum disorder and intellectual disability, social communication should be below that expected for general developmental level.
F. *Specify if these symptoms occur:*
 With or without accompanying intellectual impairment.
 With or without accompanying language impairment.
 Associated with a known medical or genetic condition or environmental factor.
 Associated with another neurodevelopmental, mental, or behavior disorder.
 With catatonia.

Figure 10-1 DSM-5 Characteristics of Autism Spectrum Disorder

Adapted from American Psychiatric Association. (2013). *Diagnostic and statistical manual of mental disorders*, 5th ed. Washington, DC: APA.

Table 10-1

Severity Levels for Autism Spectrum Disorder

SEVERITY LEVEL	SOCIAL COMMUNICATION	RESTRICTED, REPETITIVE BEHAVIORS
Level 3 Requires very substantial support	Severe deficits in verbal and nonverbal social communication skills. Severe impairment in social functioning, very limited initiation and minimal response in social interaction.	Inflexible behavior, extreme difficulty coping with change. Restricted, repetitive behaviors significantly interfere with functioning. Great distress with changes in action or focus.
Level 2 Requires substantial support	Marked deficits in verbal and nonverbal social interaction and initiation. Abnormal responses in social exchanges.	Inflexible behavior and difficulty coping with change. Restricted repetitive behaviors obvious to casual observers and interfere with functioning.
Level 1 Requires support	Deficits in social communication cause noticeable impairments. Problems initiating social interactions; decreased interest in social interactions.	Inflexible behavior causes interference with functioning in one or more contexts. Difficulty switching activities. Problems in organization and planning restrict independence.

Adapted from American Psychiatric Association. (2013). *Diagnostic and statistical manual of mental disorders*, 5th ed. Washington, DC: APA.

   (2) Deficits in nonverbal communication behaviors used for social interaction (e.g., abnormalities in eye contact, body posture, gestures; lack of facial expression).
   (3) Deficits in developing, maintaining and understanding relationships (e.g., difficulty adjusting social behavior in various contexts, reduced interest in peer relationships and friendships).
  b. Restricted, repetitive patterns of behavior, interests or activities (the severity must be specified).
   (1) Stereotyped or repetitive motor movements, use of objects or speech (e.g., echolalia, lining up objects).
   (2) Insistence on sameness, inflexible adherence to routines or ritualized patterns of verbal or nonverbal behavior (e.g., difficulty with transitions or changes in routine; impose ritualistic sameness in actions or activities).
   (3) Highly restricted, fixated interests that are abnormal in intensity or focus (e.g., perseverative interests, obsessive attachment to objects).
   (4) Hyper- or hyporeactivity to sensory input or unusual interest in sensory aspects of the environment (e.g., adverse reactions to touching and/or auditory stimuli; visual fixation on lights or spinning movements).
  c. Symptoms must be present in the early developmental period.
  d. Symptoms cause clinically significant impairment in social, occupational or other important areas of functioning.
  e. These disturbances are not better explained by intellectual disability or global developmental delay.
   (1) Any comorbidities must be specified (e.g., with or without accompanying intellectual impairment, language impairment, known medical or genetic condition).

2. Severity levels for autism spectrum disorders (see Table 10-1).
  a. Three levels of severity, with 1 being the least level of support and 3 requiring the most intense support.
  b. Social communication severity levels.
   (1) Level 1.
    (a) Noticeable deficits in social communication without supports in place.
    (b) Difficulty initiating and decreased interest in social interactions.
    (c) Attempts to make friends and engage with others are odd and unsuccessful.
   (2) Level 2.
    (a) Marked deficits in verbal and nonverbal social communication that are apparent even with supports in place.
    (b) Reduced or abnormal responses to social overtures.
   (3) Level 3.
    (a) Severe deficits in verbal and nonverbal social communication.
    (b) Very limited social interaction and response to social overtures.
  c. Restricted, repetitive behaviors severity levels.
   (1) Level 1.
    (a) Inflexible behaviors cause significant interference with functioning.
    (b) Difficulty switching between tasks.
    (c) Problems with organization and planning that negatively impact independence.
   (2) Level 2.
    (a) Inflexible behavior and restricted repetitive behaviors are obvious to the casual observer and interfere with functioning in a variety of contexts.
    (b) Distressed behavior is noted when changing focus or activity.

> **Asperger's Disorder**
>
> A. Qualitative impairment in social interaction, as manifested by at least two of the following:
>   1. Marked impairment in the use of multiple nonverbal behaviors such as eye-to-eye gaze, facial expression, body postures and gestures to regulate social interaction.
>   2. Failure to develop peer relationships appropriate to developmental level.
>   3. A lack of spontaneous seeking to share enjoyment, interests, or achievements with other people (e.g., by a lack of showing, bringing, or pointing out objects of interest to other people).
>   4. Lack of social or emotional reciprocity.
> B. Restricted repetitive and stereotyped patterns of behavior, interests and activities, as manifested by at least one of the following:
>   1. Encompassing preoccupation with one or more stereotyped and restricted patterns of interest that is abnormal either in intensity or focus.
>   2. Apparently inflexible adherence to specific, nonfunctional routines or rituals.
>   3. Stereotyped and repetitive motor mannerisms (e.g., hand or finger flapping or twisting, or complex whole-body movements).
>   4. Persistent preoccupation with parts of objects.
> C. The disturbance causes clinically significant impairment in social, occupational or other important areas of functioning.
> D. There is no clinically significant general delay in language (e.g., single words used by age 2 years, communicative phrases used by age 3 years).
> E. There is no clinically significant delay in cognitive development or in the development of age-appropriate self-help skills, adaptive behavior (other than in social interaction), and curiosity about the environment in childhood.
> F. Criteria are not met for another specific pervasive developmental disorder or schizophrenia.

Figure 10-2 *DSM-IV-TR* **Characteristics of Asperger's Disorder**

Adapted from American Psychiatric Association. (2000). *Diagnostic and statistical manual of mental disorders,* 4th ed., text revised. Washington, DC: APA.

(3) Level 3.
  (a) Inflexible behavior creates extreme difficulty in coping with change.
  (b) Restricted, repetitive behaviors markedly interfere with functioning.
  (c) Significant distress in response to changing focus or activity.
 d. Severity may fluctuate over time and vary in specific contexts.
3. Asperger's disorder.
 a. Previously defined as an independent disorder (*DSM-IV*, APA, 1994; *DSM-IV-TR*, APA, 2000); however, now classified as autism spectrum disorder.
 b. Characteristics (see Figure 10-2).
  (1) Normal to above average intellectual/cognitive function and language skills.
  (2) Deficits in the social domain, lack of reciprocity and empathy.
  (3) Extreme interests and routines.
  (4) Pedantic, unusual prosody.
  (5) Limited development of executive function skills, similar to nonverbal learning disorder characteristics.
  (6) Deficits in "theory of mind."
   (a) Lack the ability to relate to other persons' perspective.
  (7) Well-developed vocabulary, but one-sided monologue in conversation.

Educational Definition

1. Individuals with Disabilities Education Act (IDEA, 2004; see Figure 10-3).
 a. Federal law ensures services to children with disabilities.
 b. Guidelines for states to provide early intervention, special education and related services.
 c. Autism is 1 of 13 disability levels that qualify for educational support services.
 d. Educational label can be introduced by a member of the multidisciplinary team with an appropriate knowledge of and experience with autism spectrum disorder (ASD), including the speech-language pathologist (SLP).
 e. Educational eligibility label of autism is similar to pervasive developmental disorder (PDD) category in the *DSM-IV*.
  (1) Broad category label of ASD, not differential label under PDD of Autistic Disorder in *DSM-IV*.
  (2) All subtypes of ASD qualify for services under the one eligibility label.
  (3) Educational definition parallels *DSM-V* definition description.

> **Individuals with Disabilities Education Act (2004), Regulations Section 300.8.c.(1) i**
>
> Autism means a developmental disability significantly affecting verbal and nonverbal communication and social interaction, generally evident before age three, that adversely affects a child's educational performance. Other characteristics often associated with autism are engagement in repetitive activities and stereotyped movements, resistance to environmental change or change in daily routines, and unusual responses to sensory experiences.

Figure 10-3 IDEA (2004) Definition of Autism Spectrum Disorder

Etiological Information

Background Information

1. No clearly substantiated cause for autism.
2. Presumed abnormality in brain structure of function during development.
   a. Underdevelopment of neural connections.
   b. Subtle differences in the number, connectivity and complexity of neural branches.
3. Theorize a genetic predisposition to autism of unknown etiology.
4. Possible interaction between multiple genes and environmental factors.
5. Understanding multiple variants or subtypes of ASD will lead to better treatment.
6. Several main emphasis areas of research to investigate possible causes.

Genetic Research

1. Genetic theories and research evidence to account for autism suggest four to six genes interacting.
   a. Chromosome 5.
      (1) Genes involved in development of brain circuitry in early childhood.
   b. Chromosome 7.
      (1) Possible biological differences in male vs. female autism, also involved in language development.
   c. Chromosome 11.
      (1) Group of genes involved in communication between neurons during brain development.
   d. Chromosome 15.
      (1) Duplication on part of chromosome associated with intellectual impairment.
   e. Chromosome 16.
      (1) Small deletion associated with ASD, responsible for cell-to-cell signaling and interaction.

Neurochemical Research

1. Neurochemical studies explore the roots of ASD by measuring several different variables.
   a. Oxidative stress.
      (1) Measured by reduced cerebral blood flow.
         (a) Abnormal blood vessel function in the brain.
         (b) Behavioral symptoms improve after taking antioxidants.
   b. Brain inflammation.
      (1) Linked with changes in immune system responses.
      (2) Introduce anti-inflammatory antibiotic to treat regressive ASD.
   c. Autoimmunity.
      (1) Increased food sensitivity (e.g., gluten, casein, food dye, preservatives).
      (2) Carefully manage diet and nutritional intake.
   d. Antibodies in maternal blood supply.
      (1) Antibodies interrupt later healthy brain development for the fetus.

Environmental Theories

1. Toxins present in the environment (e.g., lead, chemicals in groundwater, chemicals in fertilizer and food products).
2. Vaccines are NOT substantiated as a cause of ASD.
   a. Thimerosal, a mercury-based preservative, implied as the basis of ASD onset in children.
   b. Thimerosal was eliminated from childhood vaccines by 2001 in the United States.
   c. Multiple studies in several countries refute vaccines as ASD cause; similar incidence of ASD in vaccinated and nonvaccinated children.

d. Nonvaccinated children are at greater risk to contract viral infections (e.g., measles, mumps, polio, rubella) with no immunity to prevent significant life-long consequences.
e. Estimate 1 in 4 children are out of compliance with U.S. vaccination guidelines due to fear of ASD onset.

Risk Factors for ASD

1. Paternal age.
   a. If a father is 40 years or older, there is a 6 times greater risk of having a child with autism.
2. Maternal factors.
   a. Maternal use of antidepressants during pregnancy leads to a greater risk of ASD.

Behavioral Characteristics

Primary Characteristics

1. Core features shared by ASDs vary in severity and presentation.
2. Primary behavioral symptoms revolve around isolation, withdrawal and a desire for solitary focus that is characteristic of ASDs.
3. Three diagnostic areas of behavioral symptom deficits:
   a. Reciprocal social interaction.
   b. Communication.
   c. Restricted, repetitive, stereotyped patterns of behavior.
4. Examples of reciprocal social interaction deficits.
   a. Eye contact is often averted or indirect, with a reliance on peripheral vision.
   b. Facial expression is minimal and incongruent with events occurring or with words spoken.
   c. Body posture is rigid and uncomfortable when engaged in interaction.
   d. Gestures accompanying verbalization may be absent or very exaggerated and animated.
   e. Lack of initiation for interaction with people (i.e., avoids or ignores initiation from others).
   f. Limited ability to relate to peers and an absence of friends.
   g. Failure to share interests or achievements with others.
   h. Lack of interest in activities, emotions or focus of others.
   i. Verbal and social interactions are egocentric or self-focused (i.e., one-sided monologue rather than reciprocal, shared dialogue).
   j. Lack of joint attention or focus on others (i.e., oblivious to the interests of other people).
5. Examples of communication deficits.
   a. Significant delays in acquisition of spoken language skills.
   b. Childhood apraxia of speech.
      (1) An inability to voluntarily program neurologic sequences for verbal speech production.
   c. Echolalia.
      (1) Repetition of utterances spoken by others; can be immediate or delayed.
   d. Verbal perseveration.
      (1) Continuous repetition of a sound, word or phrase.
   e. Monotone, robotic or pedantic vocal prosody in expressive language.
   f. Jargon or idiosyncratic speech production that is nonmeaningful to others.
   g. Lack discourse skills to initiate, maintain or terminate conversation with others in an appropriate manner.
   h. Lack of imaginative play or social imitative play, with a tendency to demonstrate parallel or repetitive play patterns.
   i. Failure to develop abstract language (e.g., concepts, inference, idioms, etc.) and remain very literal and concrete in language interpretation.
   j. Failure to comprehend or express nonverbal aspect of communication, such as gestures, body language, humor, sarcasm or teasing.
6. Examples of restricted, repetitive patterns of behavior.
   a. Self-stimulatory behaviors.
      (1) Rhythmic, repetitive motor movements, such as hand-flapping, twirling or finger tapping.
   b. Repetitive, ritualistic interaction with objects, such as lining items up or spinning the wheels on a toy car.
   c. Motor perseveration.
      (1) Doing a motor activity over and over, such as putting a puzzle together or climbing up and down a slide.
   d. Inflexible reliance on routines or rituals, such as adhering to a specific order of activities to get

      dressed in the morning, taking a designated route to drive to school, walking a specific path in the backyard or keeping an order for toys to be put away.
- e. Fascination with mechanical movement and objects, such as watching a ceiling fan twirl or toilet flush, turning on and off lights or inserting and ejecting DVDs.
- f. Obsessive preoccupation with particular interests or items, such as dinosaurs, insects, the weather, maps or certain cartoon characters.
- g. Excessive sustained attachment to certain objects, such as stuffed animals, Legos or clothing items.
- h. Perimeter walking.
  - (1) Moving to the outer edge of a room or environment to avoid interaction.

Other Characteristic Features

1. Cognitive or intellectual deficits.
   a. Estimates of intellectual impairment as a component of ASD vary from normal curve distribution to as high as 70% with comorbid IQ deficits.
   b. Difficult to determine exact figures due to challenges in reliability and validity issues in assessing intelligence in ASD individuals.
   c. Primary features of ASD (i.e., impairment in social interaction, communication and stereotyped behaviors) compromise assessment.
      (1) Evaluation requires responses in a socially interactive setting.
      (2) Many tasks are dependent on language/communication.
      (3) Restricted and repetitive behaviors interfere with standardized scoring and timing constraints.
   d. Variability in the diagnosis of ASD, particularly in high-functioning individuals, skews the data negatively (i.e., more impaired individuals are likely to be identified while more functional individuals are not labeled).

2. Sensory integration disorder or dysfunction.
   a. Hyper- and/or hyporesponsiveness to sensory stimuli can trigger aberrant behavioral responses.
      (1) Tactile defensiveness.
         (a) Not liking to be touched, sensitive to clothing textures.
      (2) Auditory sensitivity or hyperacusis.
         (a) Negative reaction to loud noises and noisy environments (e.g., hallways, cafeterias, gymnasiums or sporting events).
      (3) Picky eating patterns.
         (a) Food sensitivity contributes to a restricted diet, based on intolerance to taste, smell and/or texture of some foods.
   b. Problems with self-regulation in response to sensory stimuli.
      (1) Fail to modulate volume in response to environmental expectations, such as at a movie theater, library, church or restaurant.
      (2) Seek inappropriate amounts and types of sensory stimulation to satisfy needs, such as sucking on strings and clothing or rubbing the skin until chapped and raw.
   c. Hyperlexia.
      (1) Fascination with letters, numbers and words that begins at a very young age.
      (2) Precocious decoding skills in the absence of comprehension.
   d. Motor deficits.
      (1) Hypotonia.
         (a) Low muscle tone contributes to flaccid limbs and poor posture.
      (2) Fine motor deficits negatively impact self-help skills for feeding, dressing, toileting and handwriting.
      (3) Gross motor delays compromise coordination for activities such as riding a bicycle, athletics and sequenced fitness exercises.
      (4) Some individuals with ASD demonstrate excellent balance and coordination that exceeds development in typical peers, such as children with gifted artistic or musical talent.

Role of the Speech-Language Pathologist in Autism Spectrum Disorder (ASD)

General Factors for SLPs

1. Autism is a social communication disorder with significant challenges for the SLP.
2. Two core features (impairment in reciprocal social interaction and verbal/nonverbal communication deficits) are within the scope of practice for SLPs.
3. SLPs are involved in the screening, diagnosis and intervention.

Table 10-2

Responsibilities of the SLP in Autism Spectrum Disorders

RESPONSIBILITY	DESCRIPTION
Screening	Facilitate early identification of children at risk for ASD and make referrals for appropriate diagnosis and intervention.
Diagnosis	Acquire knowledge and skills to function as a contributing member of multidisciplinary team to appropriately diagnose ASD.
Assessment and intervention	Utilize evidence to engage in appropriate assessment and intervention for social communication and speech-language issues, including verbal, nonverbal, academic and vocational concerns.
Working with families	Provide education, counseling, training, service coordination and assistance for family members.
Collaboration	Work cooperatively with families, other professionals, support personnel and colleagues to ensure appropriate services and functional outcomes.
Professional development	Participate in providing and attending continuing education seminars to remain current in knowledge and skills necessary for effective services.
Research	Stay informed of current developments and participate in advancing the knowledge base in ASD.
Advocacy	Promote participation in activities that promote each individual achieving appropriate functional outcomes.

4. Speech-language services are critical to address the pervasive communication deficits in ASD (see Table 10-2).

Determination of Eligibility for SLP Services

1. Avoid criterion referencing (i.e., discrepancy between cognitive ability and language-functioning level).
   a. Evaluate the child's current intellectual/cognitive age and compare it to assessment results indicating language developmental age.
   b. If the cognitive level and language level scores are relatively commensurate, then some professionals advocate that the lack of discrepancy means there is no need for speech-language services.
      (1) This is not considered best practice for treatment decisions.
   c. Measurement of cognitive ability is often significantly impaired and negatively influenced by language ability, minimizing a child's potential for improvement in response to intervention.
2. Include both formal and informal procedures in evaluation process.
   a. Formal assessment results may not be an accurate reflection of a child's abilities.
   b. Informal observation of behavioral characteristics and abilities is critical.
   c. Diagnostic label may not be accurate, due to the heterogeneity in the ASD population.
3. Make independent decisions regarding the provision of services.
   a. Determine goals with a consideration of the core features of ASD.
   b. Prioritize goals based on functional outcomes to enhance social communication.
   c. Intervention objectives should be congruent with the individual's needs, family goals and cultural contexts.
   d. Consider and incorporate classroom curricular expectation.
   e. Review any available evidence to guide treatment methodologies.
4. The SLP assumes multiple roles in meeting the needs of ASD clients.

Assessment

General Information on Assessment

1. There is no definitive medical test or biological marker for an ASD diagnosis.
2. Diagnosis should rely on careful observation of behavioral characteristics.
3. The median age of diagnosis in the United States is 4 years of age.
4. Recently, there have been efforts to increase routine screenings and identify early behavioral indicators.

> **National Institute of Child Health and Human Development (NICHD)**
>
> **Five Warning Behaviors for ASD Evaluation**
>
> - Does not babble or coo by 12 months.
> - Does not gesture (point, wave, grasp) by 12 months.
> - Does not say single words by 16 months.
> - Does not say two-word phrases on his/her own by 24 months.
> - Has any loss of any language or social skills at any age.

Figure 10-4 NICHD Warning Behaviors for ASD Evaluation

Screening for ASD

1. Pediatricians do not routinely screen for ASD as part of well-child check-ups.
   a. There is no blood, medical or genetic-based definitive test for ASD.
   b. Physicians are exploring the presence of typical and atypical behaviors as milestones of normal development.
2. Most referrals for ASD testing are initiated by parents who notice developmental differences (see Figure 10-4).
3. Early warning signs of possible ASD can be observed by 12–15 months, and a diagnosis of ASD can occur by 24 months (see Table 10-3).
4. Screening instruments for ASD can be completed by parents and health providers.
   a. First Year Inventory (FYI, 2003).
      (1) Purpose is to identify children at risk for ASD or related developmental disorders.
      (2) Explores two developmental domains—social communication and sensory regulatory function.
   b. Checklist for Autism in Toddlers (CHAT, 2000) and Modified Checklist for Autism in Toddlers (M-CHAT, 2001).
      (1) The CHAT was designed to be used as a screening tool at an 18-month check-up.
      (2) There are 14 items on the checklist.
         (a) Nine items are filled out by parents.
         (b) Five items are filled out by health care professionals.
      (3) The M-CHAT expands on the CHAT with 23 questions and targets diagnosis by 24 months.
   c. Communication and Symbolic Behavior Scales Developmental Profile (CSBS DP, 2002) and Systematic Observation of Red Flags (SORF, 2004).
      (1) The CSBS DP identifies communication and symbolic play deficits that are not specific to ASD, but are sensitive to the core behaviors.
      (2) The SORF rates specific "red flags" for ASD from the CSBS DP screening procedures.
   d. Social Communication Questionnaire (SCQ, 2003).
      (1) A 40-item parent questionnaire to screen for autism.
      (2) Intended for older children (i.e., 4 years and older).
   e. Earlier diagnosis allows for initiation of treatment to address differences in development.

Table 10-3

ASD Social-Communication Warning Signs

9–12 MONTHS	18 MONTHS	24 MONTHS
Lack of response to name	Lack of response to name	Lack of responsiveness
Lack of social smile	Lack of shared joy	Lack of shared enjoyment
Poor mutual attention	Poor joint attention	Lack of facial expression
Limited gestures	Minimal pointing or gesturing	Lack of pointing to share interest
Poor imitation	Unusual prosody to speech	Poor imitation; delayed speech
Poor eye contact	Lack of appropriate gaze	Abnormal eye contact
Limited affective range	Lack of shared interest	Limited interest in shared games
Extreme passivity	Repetitive body movements	Over or under sensory reactions
Poor visual orientation to stimuli	Repetitive movement with objects	Unusual visual interests; unusual play with objects

Diagnostic Procedures in ASD

1. Procedures should include a compilation of information and an evaluation of the individual.
   a. Review background information and developmental records and reports.
   b. Interview the parent/caregiver to explore family history, the child's general health and medical background, behavior and developmental progression in speech-language, motor, sensory and social interaction.
   c. Conduct an observation, behavioral evaluation and interaction with the individual.
   d. Administer appropriate assessment tools for a normative comparison in developmental areas, particularly communication skills.
   e. Diagnostic instruments for ASD determination.
      (1) Autism Diagnostic Observation Schedule (ADOS, 2000).
         (a) Considered the gold standard in the diagnosis of ASD.
         (b) Evaluates ASD and other PDD from early childhood to adult ages.
         (c) Four modules to evaluate:
            - Communication.
            - Reciprocal social interaction.
            - Stereotypic behaviors and interests.
            - Play.
      (2) Autism Diagnostic Interview-Revised (ADI-R, 2003).
         (a) Evaluates three domains of autism:
            - Language/communication.
            - Reciprocal social interaction.
            - Restricted, repetitive, stereotyped behaviors.
         (b) Interview caregivers to probe for ASD behaviors.
         (c) Assesses children through adult ages.
      (3) Childhood Autism Rating Scale, 2nd Edition (CARS-2, 2011).
         (a) Evaluates ages 2 years and older, using an observation instrument.
         (b) Determines the severity of ASD symptoms using a rating scale to evaluate presenting behaviors.
      (4) Gilliam Autism Rating Scale, 2nd Edition (GARS-2, 2011).
         (a) Checklist normed from ages 3 to 22 years.
         (b) Categorizes observed behavioral deficits into stereotyped behaviors, communication and social interaction.
         (c) Results in an autism quotient that designates the risk of ASD.

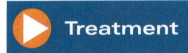

Treatment

National Research Council

1. The National Research Council's (NRC, 2001[RC11]) review of evidence resulted in recommendations for essential aspects of intervention for children with ASD.
   a. Identify ASD and begin intervention as early as possible.
      (1) Intervention initiated by age 3 years significantly improves outcomes.
   b. Provide intensive intervention that promotes active engagement (i.e., minimum of 5 hours a day, 5 days a week) through collaboration with family and teachers to structure teaching opportunities in natural learning environments.
   c. Provide systematic, repeated, instructional activities in brief, focused time intervals.
   d. Train family members to implement teaching strategies to reinforce learning and minimize disruptive behaviors.
   e. Individual instruction and low student-to-teacher ratio improves the efficacy of instructional strategies.
   f. Maintain ongoing assessment data to prompt modifications in program objectives, based on regular review of client progress.
   g. Instructional priorities for individuals with ASD, specified by NRC.
      (1) Functional, spontaneous communication.
      (2) Social skills addressed in various environments.
      (3) Peer interaction and play skills
      (4) New skills generalized and maintained in natural contexts.
      (5) Functional assessment and support to address problematic behaviors.
      (6) Functional academic skills.

Intervention Goals

1. Intervention goals should be derived from multiple assessment procedures.
   a. Avoid criterion referencing in interpretation of results.
   b. Carefully evaluate validity of performance results.

c. Consider the clinical impressions during assessment as well as resulting scores.
2. Impressions from informal observation and interaction.
   a. Core features of social pragmatic competence are difficult to assess in formal procedures.
   b. Consider the strengths and weaknesses, as well as adaptive and maladaptive behaviors.
   c. Evaluate communication in different settings and with different people.
   d. Include both verbal and nonverbal communication impressions.
3. Reports from parents, caregivers and teachers.
   a. Identify learning objectives designated by the classroom curriculum.
   b. Identify family priorities, typical environments and communication partners.
   c. Be sensitive to cultural expectations and concerns.

Language Impairments within ASD

1. Pragmatic language (use of language in social contexts) is the primary impairment in all types and severity levels of ASD.
   a. Young children require basic pragmatic skill instruction (e.g., turn taking, sharing, joint attention, polite requests and responses).
   b. School-age children require pragmatic skills consistent with peer interaction (e.g., considering others' feelings, sharing interests, expressing preferences politely, shared attention).
   c. Adolescents and adults require more complex pragmatic skills involved in executive functions and nonverbal messages (e.g., reading others' intentions, making decisions, problem solving, determining appropriate verbal questions and responses, understanding others' feelings and perspectives).
2. Semantic language (word meanings) is usually impaired in all types of ASD.
   a. Young children limit vocabulary to items of interest and words gained through functional experience.
      (1) Goals should address conceptual terms necessary for academic learning, such as quantity, quality and positional prepositions.
   b. School-age children need to transition from literal to abstract and metalinguistic aspects of semantics, such as multiple meanings, idiomatic expressions and figurative language.
   c. Adolescents and adults lack comprehension of semantic nuances, such as inferred meaning, humor, sarcasm, discourse/conversational rules, as well as vocabulary consistent with adult independent living expectation (i.e., hygiene, health, banking, transportation).
3. Syntax and morphology (grammar rules for word and sentence construction) are impaired when language deficits present.
   a. Young children speak telegraphically and omit articles, verb conjugations and small connective words.
   b. School-age children struggle with pronouns, preferring to use concrete reference and proper nouns, and morphological markers, such as plurals, possessives, verb conjugations and conjunctions.
4. Phonology (rules of sound combinations) and articulation (oral motor sound production) are impaired when childhood apraxia of speech or significant expressive speech delays are present.
   a. Young children may produce jargon and echolalia, but not be able to program or produce spontaneous voluntary speech.
   b. Goals should establish basic power words for immediate environmental impact, such as *no, stop, help, want*, etc.
   c. Augmentative and alternative communication (AAC) techniques supplement and facilitate speech production attempts.

ASHA Guidelines for ASD Intervention

1. ASHA produced guidelines (2006a, b) that specify major domains and sample goals for SLP intervention with ASD (refer to Figures 10-1 and 10-5).
   a. Joint attention.
   b. Social reciprocity.
   c. Language and related cognitive skills.
   d. Behavior and emotional regulation.

Guidelines for Goal Prioritization

1. Establish a functional, meaningful, independent vehicle for communication.
   a. Allow the individual to express basic wants and needs.
   b. Alleviate frustration and decrease behavioral outbursts.
   c. Can be expressive, gestural or augmented (AAC).
2. Continually evaluate receptive comprehension of language.
   a. Facilitate determination of educational curriculum expectations.
   b. Provide parents and teachers with guidance for expressive language input that the individual can understand.

```
Joint attention
Turn-taking/reciprocity
Initiation
Play
Topicalization
Communicative functions
Conversational discourse
  • Negotiation
  • Persuasion
  • Narration
  • Humor
  • Empathy
Nonverbal communication
  • Facial expression
  • Body language/gesture
  • Paralinguistics
  • Proxemics
Presupposition
```

Figure 10-5 Sample Goal Hierarchy for Social Pragmatics

c. Revise treatment goals to progressively increase functional comprehension.
3. Focus on increased appropriate social engagement and interaction.
   a. Joint attention and social engagement are critical features for learning.
   b. Appropriate social behavior improves access to diverse environments and opportunities for learning.
   c. Future vocational and occupational options are increased with appropriate reciprocal social communication skills.
4. Adjust treatment goals to level of language competence and potential.
   a. Initiate goals with objectives to establish functional, concrete competence.
   b. Progress in goal areas, guided by treatment data, to complex abstract levels.

Intervention Methodologies

Variety of Intervention Methodologies

1. The SLP must consider several factors when choosing a treatment method.
   a. Review the research to explore the evidence base to support efficacy.
   b. Consider the unique needs and characteristics of the individual with ASD.
   c. Critically evaluate the advantages/disadvantages and core features of the intervention method.
   d. Reconcile philosophical beliefs with realistic parameters for best practice principles.
   e. Categorize treatment methodologies by primary emphasis:
      (1) Behavioral.
      (2) Developmental.
      (3) Naturalistic.
      (4) Affective or relationship-based.
   f. Maintain focus on the core characteristics of ASD and essential outcomes.
2. ASHA Guidelines (2006a, b) present several types of intervention strategies that capitalize on strengths within ASD (see Table 10-4).

Classification System for Intervention

1. Proposed by the National Standards Project (National Autism Center, 2009a, b).
   a. Reviewed research to establish an evidence base for intervention decisions in ASD.
   b. Created a merit-based rating scale to evaluate treatment effects reported in research articles.
   c. Classification system placed treatment methods in efficacy categories in regards to ASD (see Table 10-5).
      (1) Established.
         (a) Sufficient research evidence to suggest a favorable outcome.
      (2) Emerging.
         (a) Appears favorable, but not consistently showing research-based conclusive evidence.
      (3) Unestablished.
         (a) Little or no evidence to form conclusion on treatment effectiveness; may be effective, ineffective or harmful.
      (4) Ineffective/harmful.
         (a) Research evidence determines treatment as detrimental or ineffective.

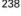

Table 10-4

Description of Intervention Approaches to ASDs

INTERVENTION TYPE	DESCRIPTION/EXAMPLE
Environmental arrangements and structure	Use preferred materials, sabotage to promote interaction, space designed for visual clarity
Picture schedules and visual supports	Picture sequences for activity, steps to complete, pictured choices, visual prompts
Written scripts and social stories	Cue cards, prompts for initiation, practice script until generalized, identification of relevant aspects of activity, thought bubbles
Video modeling	Recorded highlight of critical features within situation, visual feedback and example of desired behavior, relate better to video/object
Computerized instruction	Teach focused communication aspects, nonsocial nature of computer beneficial
Previewing learning context and activity	Prepare for coming events, decrease anxiety behaviors
Strategies to promote generalization	Transfer new skill to natural environment, use parents, caregivers, field trips
Strategies to promote self-generalization	Increase control and independence, make decisions, express preferences

Table 10-5

Treatment Techniques in Efficacy Categories

ESTABLISHED	EMERGING	UNESTABLISHED	HARMFUL/INEFFECTIVE
• Antecedent package • Behavioral package • Comprehensive behavioral treatment • Joint attention • Modeling • Naturalistic teaching • Peer teaching • Pivotal response • Schedules • Self-management • Story-based intervention	• Augmentative and alternative communication • Cognitive behavioral intervention • Developmental relationship • Exercise • Exposure package • Imitation interaction • Imitation training • Language training • Massage/touch • Music therapy • Peer-mediated instruction • Picture exchange communication system • Scripting • Sign instruction • Social communication • Social skills • Structured teaching • Technology • Theory of mind	• Academic interventions • Auditory integration training (AIT) • Facilitated communication (FC) • Gluten- and casein-free diets • Sensory integration	• None

d. The classification system is a beneficial effort to guide ASD intervention, but there are some limitations.
   (1) Behavioral treatments show the strongest efficacy.
      (a) Concrete, measurable, clean administration.
      (b) Able to quantify results using research standards.
   (2) Nonbehavioral treatments are valuable, despite weak support.
      (a) Difficult to quantify in measurable research terms.

(b) Individualized functional outcomes are important.
(c) More research is needed on this type of intervention.

Description of Selected ASD Intervention Techniques

1. Applied behavioral analysis (ABA) and discrete trial teaching (DTT).
   a. Principle of behavior modification through operant conditioning.
   b. Teach skills through carefully sequenced steps of objectives.
   c. Intense focus training with prompts and rewards.
   d. Teaching segment one-on-one with three primary components.
      (1) Antecedent.
         (a) Instruction or request for specific action.
      (2) Behavior.
         (a) Response from the child.
      (3) Consequence.
         (a) Trainer's reaction (e.g., reinforcement, praise).
2. Augmentative and alternative communication (AAC).
   a. Improvement noted in three areas:
      (1) Behavior and emotional regulation.
      (2) Speech, expressive language and social communication.
      (3) Receptive language development and comprehension.
   b. Low-tech (pictures, graphic symbols, written cues) to high-tech options (computer, AAC devices, voice output).
3. Floor time.
   a. Engage in spontaneous, interactive, pleasurable activity with the child.
   b. Follow the child's interest while providing semistructured play.
   c. Natural learning situation tailored to developmental level.
4. Peer and play mediation.
   a. Promote natural interaction and carryover.
   b. Peers provide a model to imitate.
   c. Social interaction opportunities are increased.
   d. Incorporate items of interest to motivate social engagement.
   e. Responsive teaching in a play setting.
5. Picture exchange communication system (PECS).
   a. Establish a functional reciprocal picture communication system within a social context.
   b. A picture of a desired item is exchanged with a communication partner.
   c. A form of AAC that also incorporates ABA principles with focused teaching, motivation and reinforcement.
6. Social stories.
   a. Teach social skills through a story format.
   b. Specific to the child and problem situation.
   c. Story sequence describes relevant aspects of situation and appropriate social responses, both verbal and nonverbal.
   d. Introduce story repetitively until it becomes a routine social response.
7. Theory of mind.
   a. Teach the individual to understand mental states—how others think and feel.
   b. Mindblindness.
      (1) Inability to understand perceptions and beliefs from another person's perspective.
   c. Associated with executive function deficits evidenced in Asperger's disorder.

Related Services

Interdisciplinary Approach

1. Collaborative effort among professionals and parents required to successfully address ASD (see Table 10-6).
2. Team focus on the whole child, not isolated skill deficits.
3. Multidisciplinary intervention enhances progress and future prognosis.
4. Cross-disciplinary consistent reinforcement of treatment objectives is critical for generalization of goals.

Table 10-6
Other Professionals and Their Role in ASD

PROFESSIONAL TEAM MEMBER	PRIMARY RESPONSIBILITIES
Administrator	• Liaison among team members and family • Funding/paperwork oversight
Behavior consultant	• Evaluate dysfunctional behavior patterns • Coordinate replacement/modification of problematic behaviors
Occupational therapist	• Sensory integration assessment and treatment • Fine motor skills (e.g., handwriting, self-help)
Physical therapist	• Gross motor skills • Motor movement and strength
Physician	• General overall health • Prescribe and monitor medications
Psychologist	• Cognitive assessment • Psychometric achievement assessment • Monitor mental health and well-being
Social worker	• General background information and health history • Support network for family • Investigate funding options for family
Speech-language pathologist	• Assessment and treatment of communication and social skills • Integration of treatment goals into classroom and home environments
Teacher	• Academic achievement assessment • Curricular teaching • Integration of social and communication skills

References

American Psychiatric Association. (1994). *Diagnostic and Statistical Manual of Mental Disorders*, 4th ed. Washington, DC: APA.

American Psychiatric Association. (2000). *Diagnostic and Statistical Manual of Mental Disorders*, 4th ed., text revised. Washington, DC: APA.

American Psychiatric Association. (2013). *Diagnostic and Statistical Manual of Mental Disorders*, 5th ed. Washington, DC: APA.

American Speech-Language-Hearing Association. (2006a). *Guidelines for Speech-Language Pathologists in Diagnosis, Assessment, and Treatment of Autism Spectrum Disorders Across the Life Span*. Rockville, MD: ASHA. Available from http://www.asha.org.

American Speech-Language-Hearing Association. (2006b). *Roles and Responsibilities of Speech-Language Pathologists in Diagnosis, Assessment, and Treatment of Autism Spectrum Disorders Across the Life Span: Position statement*. Rockville, MD: ASHA. Available from http://www.asha.org.

Kanner, L. (1943). Autistic disturbances of affective contact. *Nervous child*, 2, 217–250.

National Autism Center. (2009a). *Evidence-Based Practice and Autism in the Schools: A Guide to Providing Appropriate Interventions to Students with Autism Spectrum Disorders*. Randolph, MA: National Autism Center, Inc.

National Autism Center. (2009b). *Findings and Conclusions of the National Standards Project: Addressing the Need for Evidence-Based Practice Guidelines for Autism Spectrum Disorders*. Randolph, MA: National Autism Center, Inc.

National Autism Center. (2009c). *National Standards Report: National Standards Project—Addressing the Need for Evidence-Based Practice Guidelines for Autism Spectrum Disorders*. Randolph, MA: National Autism Center, Inc.

Powers, M. (2000). *Children with Autism: A Parent's Guide*, 2nd ed. Bethesda, MD: Woodbine House.

Prelock, P. (2009). Assessment and intervention in autism spectrum disorders: The role of the SLP. ASHA Autism online conference.

Richard, G., & Veale, T. (2009). *The Autism Spectrum Disorders IEP Companion*. East Moline, IL: LinguiSystems.

Wetherby, A., Woods, J., Allen, L., Clearly, J., Dickinson, H., & Lord, C. (2004). Early indicators of autism spectrum disorders in the second year of life. *Journal of Autism and Developmental Disorders* 34, 473–493.

11
Stuttering and Other Fluency Disorders

DEREK E. DANIELS, PhD
AND ALEX F. JOHNSON, PhD

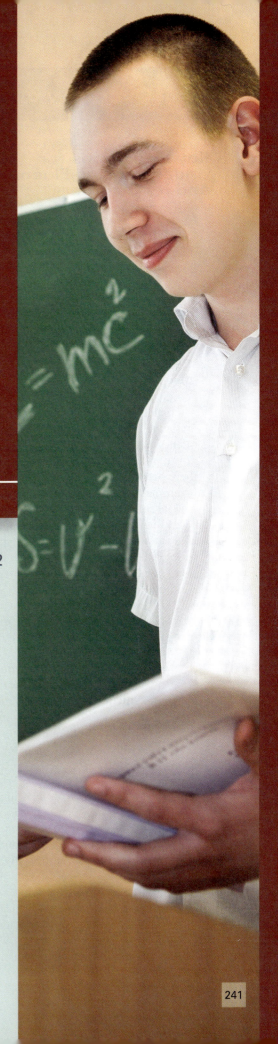

Chapter Outline

- Overview of Stuttering and Its Characteristics, 242
- Other Types of Fluency Disorders, 244
- Assessment in Stuttering, 245
- Treatment of Stuttering, 248
- References, 251

Overview of Stuttering and Its Characteristics

Key Definitions for Understanding Fluency and Its Disorders

1. *Fluency* refers to the forward, continuous flow of speech. A speaker who is fluent typically speaks with minimal physical or mental effort.
2. *Disfluency* refers to interruptions in the forward movement, and these can be either typical (those seen in all speakers) or atypical (those seen primarily in people with speech disturbances).
   a. Typical disfluencies can include phrase repetitions, multisyllabic word repetitions, phrase revisions and nongrammatical interjections (see Table 11-2).
   b. Atypical disfluencies are more commonly seen in individuals who stutter (see Table 11-3 for characteristics of stuttering).
3. *Stuttering* can be defined as an abnormally high frequency and/or duration of stoppages in the forward flow of speech. When stuttering is considered further, there are several additional defining considerations (examples are provided in Table 11-3).
   a. Core stuttering behaviors.
      (1) Include atypical speech disfluencies occurring at a higher frequency than typical disfluencies.
   b. Secondary behaviors.
      (1) Are understood as attempts to control the core stuttering movements.
      (2) Include a variety of adjustments in word choice, changes in speech and motoric behaviors.
      (3) Can be classified as either escape or avoidance behaviors.
         (a) Escape behaviors are attempts to stop the moment of stuttering and finish a word or sentence. Examples include eye blinks, head nods or other motor adjustments made to "get out" of the moment of stuttering.
         (b) Avoidance behaviors are learned behaviors that are associated with the anticipation of a moment of stuttering. Thus, when an individual fears that they will stutter on a sound or a word, they may choose to substitute a different sound or word. There are many different types of avoidance.
4. Over time, persons who stutter (PWS) also commonly develop a number of specific attitudes and feelings in response to their stuttering.
   a. Feelings are emotional reactions that an individual experiences in reaction to his/her stuttering. Common feelings that individuals who stutter report include shame, embarrassment and guilt.
   b. Attitudes are beliefs that are formed over time. This cognitive component of stuttering is especially evident in older children and adults as they have more negative experience with stuttering. Negative beliefs about oneself can be acquired through a variety of experiences and are sometimes reflections of the beliefs of others in the environment.
5. The World Health Organization (2001) has adopted a model for considering the impact of a condition on one's life situation. Applied to stuttering, the concept of *disability* includes the limitations on communication and struggles with speech that are experienced by the PWS (e.g., disfluencies, secondary behaviors).
   a. More significantly, when an individual allows stuttering to interfere with important life issues (i.e., education, employment, interpersonal relationships, participation in the community), it can be described as a *handicap*.

Developmental Stuttering

1. Developmental stuttering is the most common type of fluency disorder.
2. Developmental stuttering is the speech disorder that most individuals refer to when they use the term "stuttering." Other disorders of fluency (neurogenic stuttering, cluttering, psychogenic stuttering) will be described later in this chapter. Developmental stuttering is observed in all languages and cultures.
3. Onset and occurrence of stuttering.
   a. Stuttering typically emerges between the ages of 2 and 5 years, with more males than females exhibiting stuttering.
   b. At onset, the male to female ratio is 2:1, and by adulthood the ratio is about 5:1.
   c. About 80% of children who exhibit stuttering at an early age will recover from stuttering. As children mature, the likelihood of spontaneous recovery diminishes.
   d. Stuttering can co-occur with a variety of other communication problems (e.g., phonological disorders, language impairment) and is often seen in a number of developmental conditions (e.g., Tourette's syndrome, Down syndrome).
   e. Overall, stuttering occurs in about 1% of the population, and about 55 million people worldwide stutter.
      (1) Approximately 5% of the population is believed to have stuttered at some point in their life.
4. Speech characteristics of people who stutter.

a. In addition to the prolongations, repetitions and blocks described earlier, there are some patterns observed that are useful for the speech-language pathologist (SLP) to consider.
   (1) Stuttering is more likely to occur upon initiation of words, phrases and sentences. It is more likely to be found in longer, more grammatically complex utterances than in shorter ones. Stuttering occurs more on stressed syllables than unstressed.
   (2) There are certain conditions that increase stuttering:
      (a) Pressure around time.
      (b) Speaking in situations that the PWS perceives as threatening or stressful.
      (c) Speaking on the telephone.
   (3) There are also conditions that can diminish stuttering:
      (a) Singing, speaking or reading in unison.
      (b) Delayed auditory feedback.
      (c) Speaking in less stressful situations (e.g., speaking with young children or with animals).
b. Observation of people who stutter in a variety of speaking conditions has demonstrated effects that are important to understand because they appear to explain some of the variability seen among PWS. Additionally, some approaches to treatment can be understood as using these variations in improving fluency and overall communication.
   (1) In successive speaking attempts of the same material, PWS are likely to stutter on the same words (consistency effect).
   (2) PWS are also able to predict (anticipate) those words on which they are most likely to stutter (anticipation effect).
   (3) The overall amount of disfluency decreases with repeated successive readings (adaptation effect).
      (a) This is also observed in rehearsed practices of a script or common conversation.
   (4) Individuals who stutter also produce different rates of stuttering in different social environments, among different conversational partners, and in differing linguistic contexts.
c. Biological, physical and emotional considerations are all part of the ongoing discussion about stuttering and its causes.
   (1) There has been extensive work addressing the possible underlying causes of developmental stuttering. Attempts to identify biological markers, learned or psychodynamic causes and neurophysiologic patterns continue.
      (a) Despite the lack of establishment of a definitive cause of stuttering, there have been important findings that contribute to the understanding of this condition.
   (2) It is well established that stuttering has been observed in some families. This has led to research describing these trends and specific genetic mutations have been identified to explain some familial stuttering, but not all.
   (3) Studies of twins, children who were adopted at a very early age, siblings and family lines have all contributed to the understanding of stuttering as having some hereditary component.
      (a) It is important to note that heredity is not a single likely cause in all cases of stuttering.
   (4) Neurophysiology has also been studied extensively in PWS. There is evidence of increased right hemisphere activation in PWS over typical speakers.
      (a) Studies using blood flow measures have demonstrated this pattern of activation and also shown tendency for increased activation of the left hemisphere when PWS become more fluent.
      (b) Imaging studies have also demonstrated some physical differences between the right and left hemisphere structures that support speech and language between PWS and typical speakers.
   (5) Other indicators of underlying processing differences between stutterers and nonstutterers can be seen in central auditory processing functions, reaction times to speech and nonspeech stimuli and a variety of auditory feedback measures.
   (6) The development of stuttering is aligned with the development of language in young children. Given the evidence for left hemisphere differences in PWS, it is likely more than coincidental that a variety of semantic and syntactic variables can be associated with manipulation of stuttering frequency.
      (a) It has also been observed that when language complexity is reduced (e.g., simplified grammar), stuttering occurrence is also reduced.
   (7) There has also been considerable attention given to issues of autonomic arousal, anxiety and temperament in children who stutter.
      (a) The research to date suggests that in some cases, individuals who stutter may have heightened sensitivity to the environment. This observation justifies some treatment approaches that focus on reducing this sensitivity by "unlearning" feared conditions.
   (8) At younger ages, the sex ratio for stuttering is about equal.
      (a) Young girls who stutter are more likely to demonstrate more typical fluency within 2 years, and these ratios then change to about 3:1 in early elementary school.

(9) Risk factors that have been described for persisting in stuttering include:
  (a) Being male.
  (b) Positive family history for stuttering.
  (c) Weak phonological abilities.
d. Important theories of developmental stuttering have contributed to the evolving understanding of stuttering and attempt to explain this disorder and its associated phenomena.
  (1) Given the complexity of stuttering from a developmental, biological and psychological perspective, there have been numerous attempts to generate explanatory theoretical models to explain this communication disorder.
  (2) Guitar (2014) has proposed a comprehensive and integrated theoretical model of stuttering that attempts to account for the many different findings that have been consistently observed. His model includes two major components or stages.
    (a) The first part of this model (primary stuttering) includes the earliest developmental symptoms of stuttering (speech disfluencies).
    (b) The second part of this model (secondary stuttering) includes those features (tension, struggle, escape, avoidance) that are reactions to the primary features.
    (c) In this model, primary stuttering is associated with those constitutional factors that have led to the disruptions in the speech and language process.
    (d) Secondary stuttering, as proposed, is associated with the individual's reactive temperament.
  (3) There are several other theories, proposed much earlier in the historical discussion of stuttering, that have had considerable influence on the practice of stuttering treatment. These theories include attempts to focus on the interpersonal (parent-child) and learning component in developmental stuttering.
  (4) The prevalent thinking at this time considers multiple factors as being necessary for stuttering to occur.
    (a) Physiological and developmental predisposition (which in many cases can be genetic) along with important environmental interactions appear to account for most developmental stuttering.

Other Types of Fluency Disorders

Cluttering, Neurogenic Stuttering and Psychogenic Stuttering

1. Table 11-1 provides a summary of other types of fluency disorders.
2. Cluttering.
   a. Cluttering is a low-incidence fluency disorder that is characterized by several distinct features including:
     (1) Abnormally rapid and irregular rate of speech, and one or more of the following features:
       (a) Excessive accompanying disfluencies that are not typical of developmental stuttering.
       (b) Abnormal prosody and pausing.
       (c) Excessive errors of coarticulation with more difficulty observed on multisyllabic words.
     (2) Cluttering typically occurs with other disorders (e.g., articulation, language, ADHD, other learning problems).
     (3) Another feature commonly described in the literature is reduced self-awareness of the speech errors in the person who clutters.
       (a) This is in contrast to the particular sensitivity and self-consciousness seen in most PWS.
3. Neurogenic stuttering.
   a. A form of acquired stuttering (as opposed to developmental stuttering) that is seen most commonly in adults with brain injury or neurologic diseases.
   b. Key characteristics of these patients include:
     (1) Patient awareness (but not anxiety) about the disfluency.
     (2) Disfluencies occur equally on both content and function words.
     (3) Disfluencies occur throughout the utterance (not just on initiation).
     (4) Secondary behaviors do not occur in conjunction with moments of stuttering.
     (5) Adaptation does not occur.
   c. Neurogenic stuttering is reported to be quite variable.
     (1) It may develop abruptly or slowly, may resolve over time, and there are a number of reports of successful treatments with therapies similar to those used in developmental stuttering treatment.
4. Psychogenic stuttering.
   a. A fluency disorder that is seen in patients later in development, usually in the late teens or as an adult. It is reported to emerge after a prolonged period of stress or emotional trauma.

Table 11-1

Differentiations of the Four Major Types of Fluency Disorders

	DEVELOPMENTAL STUTTERING	CLUTTERING	NEUROGENIC STUTTERING	PSYCHOGENIC STUTTERING
Age of Onset	Age 2 to 6, occasionally later	Similar period, more notable as language and speech skills develop in school years	Usually after early childhood and associated with a neurologic event or condition	Usually after early childhood and more common in adolescents and adults
Key Causal Factors	Neurophysiologic factors plus environmental conditions	Neurologic causes	Stroke, traumatic brain injury, tumors, and other neurologic conditions	Disfluency develops in reaction to stressful or emotional situations or a traumatic event
Speech	Prolongations, repetitions, blocks, secondary behaviors are present; variable fluency under different conditions	High frequency of disfluency, rapid and irregular speech rate	Few or no secondary behaviors, attempts to modify speech are less successful	Stuttering behaviors may be atypical and unusual; short-term therapy may produce a dramatic improvement
Self-Awareness	Very aware, especially 1 to 2 years after onset; fear and embarrassment	Often (not always) unaware or not concerned	Varies; less likely to be embarrassed	Variable; may show exaggerated concern

(1) Mahr and Leith (1992) and others have described psychogenic stuttering as a form of conversion symptom.
   (a) Conversion disorders are different from malingering (faking), a symptom for some secondary gain. Rather, the patient's symptoms are not volitional.

(2) Additional characteristics that can help to confirm psychogenic stuttering include:
   (a) An absence of neurologic factors associated with the onset.
   (b) Rapid improvement with trial therapy.
   (c) Resistance to change during fluency enhancing situations.
   (d) Bizarre secondary behaviors.

Assessment in Stuttering

Approach to Assessment

1. Assessment of stuttering is a critical skill that involves knowledge of the indicators of development of stuttering in the context of speech and language development, knowledge of appropriate tools and procedures across the lifespan and skills in differential diagnosis.
2. When considering developmental stuttering, a useful set of descriptors involves describing the developmental characteristics, which can ultimately provide important guidance in planning treatment.
   a. While a number of developmental approaches have been specified, Guitar (2014) presented a comprehensive model that is frequently used for purposes of staging the stuttering experience of the PWS, ranging from a stage of normal disfluency in early development to advanced stuttering. This model of stuttering development is useful as an overarching framework that is especially useful as an overview. The components of Guitar's model include:
(1) Normal disfluency is observed in many typically developing children early in their language development years. The speech characteristics include:
   (a) Observed disfluencies occurring on less than 10% of the words produced.
   (b) Mild easy disfluencies.
   (c) Typical disfluencies of the type observed in Table 11-2.
   (d) Children at this stage do not show any of the secondary behaviors seen in more advanced stuttering. It is rare for a child at this stage to notice his/her disfluencies.
(2) Borderline stuttering also occurs in younger children. It is difficult to differentiate from the

Table 11-2

Typical Disfluencies (Seen in Most Speakers)	
TYPE OF DISFLUENCY	**EXAMPLE**
Simple phrase repetitions	I want-**I want** a piece of candy.
Simple phrase revisions	I want-I **need** a drink of water.
Grammatical interjections of one iteration	I am **you know** feeling pretty tired.
Nongrammatical repetitions	I am **umm** feeling pretty tired.

normal disfluency stage, but the distinguishing characteristics at this stage are:
   (a) Occurrence of disfluency is greater than 10% of words produced.
   (b) The child may begin to use some of the more atypical (stuttering-like) speech disfluencies listed in Table 11-3, however struggle behaviors are not observed.
   (c) There may be greater than two units of repetition.
   (d) These children show little awareness or concern.
(3) Beginning stuttering occurs when the child's disfluencies become more stuttering-like and he or she begins to show more secondary behaviors (tension and struggle) in speech.
   (a) Escape devices and starters become obvious at this stage, as do the initial signs of frustration with difficulty talking.
   (b) Children at this stage show these first signs of feeling surprised or threatened (indicating awareness).
(4) Intermediate stuttering is evident when the child (usually in elementary or middle school) is frankly afraid of his or her stuttering and beginning to use various methods of avoidance. It has been hypothesized that this avoidance is the result of reactions from the environment and the child's repeated negative experiences with speaking and stuttering.
   (a) Children at this stage begin to show blocks in addition to repetitions and prolongations.
   (b) The child can also show anticipation of stuttering and so tension before a block becomes evident.
   (c) Because of experience with embarrassment or other reactions from listeners, the child may develop more complex forms of avoidance (avoiding situations completely).
   (d) Fear is more prominent at this stage.
(5) Advanced stuttering refers to older adolescents and adults who stutter. In some ways, this is an age difference more than a type difference, based on the other features described. Blocks continue to be obvious and the individual may show signs of tremors, as an attempt to control moments of stuttering. Repetitions and prolongations are present as well.
   (a) Some individuals at this advanced stage have developed sophisticated forms of avoidance and have no obvious blocks. These individuals (sometimes called covert stutterers) may experience the same attitudes and feelings as other PWS.

Table 11-3

Features of Stuttering: Core and Secondary Behaviors, Feelings and Attitudes		
	FEATURE	**EXAMPLE**
Core Behaviors	Sound or syllable **repetitions** of greater than three iterations	I want a piece of **c-c-c** candy.
	Word **repetitions** of greater than three iterations	I **want-want-want** a piece of candy.
	Sound (phoneme) **prolongations** longer than 1 second	I **wwwww**want a piece of candy.
	Blocks lasting longer than one second	I want a **p........iece** of candy.
Secondary Behaviors	Circumlocutions (talking around a troublesome word)	I want a piece of that red sweet stuff.
	Physical (motor) actions	Excessive eye blinks, long eye movements of face and arms, muscle tension
	Other speech changes	Changes in voice or articulation
Feelings (Emotional Reactions)	Affective responses to stuttering by the PWS	Shame, embarrassment, guilt, anger
Attitudes (Beliefs About Oneself)	Cognitive response to stuttering by the PWS	"I can't talk on the telephone." "My parents are sad because I stutter." "I stutter because I am a shy, anxious person."

(b) At this stage, emotions of fear, shame and embarrassment are strong. The PWS who has developed to this stage has very strong feelings of helplessness when he or she stutters.
b. It is important to note that this developmental model of stuttering is a guide for considering where to begin treatment. Some individuals, regardless of age, may never advance to the most serious levels. Conversely, some children with severe stuttering problems can quickly advance to the intermediate level of stuttering.

Procedures for Assessment

1. Assessment of stuttering also involves the use of a number of procedures for understanding the individual's communication needs and demands, eliciting a variety of speech samples and observing communication in as natural a manner as possible.
2. The tools and approaches for individuals of different ages require a variety of different considerations. However, for all PWS regardless of age, the diagnostic approach is to determine the presence of stuttering (or not), to differentiate the type of fluency disorder, to obtain a careful history, and if the individual does stutter, to describe the core and secondary behaviors, determine their severity and also understand the individual's attitudes and beliefs about his/her stuttering and about communication.
3. Table 11-4 provides a summary of considerations for this general approach to all PWS.

Table 11-4

General Considerations for Evaluation of Stuttering

- Are significant history and background information (including family history of fluency disorder) available?
- How does the parent or client describe the problem?
- Is there a fluency disorder present?
- If there is a fluency disorder, is it developmental stuttering or another fluency disorder (cluttering, psychogenic, neurogenic)?
- If it is typical stuttering, what is the developmental level?
- Are there any specific cultural, health, language, or psychological factors that are of particular concern?
- What are the core behaviors present? Frequency of occurrence? Severity?
- Are there secondary behaviors present? Frequency of occurrence? Severity?
- What are the individuals' attitudes and feelings about communication? About stuttering?
- What environmental features contribute to the problem? Excessive demands on communication? Reduced capacity to support communication?

4. Assessment of young (preschool) children.
    a. Initially directed at determining whether or not the child has a speech disorder (stuttering) or is exhibiting normal disfluencies.
    b. Using the developmental model described above, it is most likely that a child at this stage, if stuttering, will be at either the borderline or beginning level of stuttering.
    c. As noted earlier, this is accomplished through obtaining a history, eliciting (and recording) speech samples that allow for determination of the types of disfluencies present and their frequency (per 100 words), units of repetition and prolongation, and any secondary behaviors or word avoidances.
    d. Elicitation of the speech sample by observing the parent in interaction with the child can improve reliability.
    e. With a preschool child, assessment (or at least a thorough screening) should be completed for other aspects of speech and language development.
5. Assessment of school-age children.
    a. Focused on the level of stuttering present, the type and severity of disfluencies (core) and secondary behaviors.
    b. By the time a child is in elementary school, stuttering, if it exists, has been identified. Thus, careful description of the features that are most predictive of treatment needs and type is the focus of the evaluation.
    c. Identification of early risk factors and family history of stuttering should be elicited, although a child who is stuttering into the elementary school years is a candidate for treatment.
    d. In addition to the assessment of the child, it is critical to obtain a complete parent interview and also an interview with the child's teacher.
    e. In addition to appreciating the impact of the child's speech problem on his social interactions, it is essential to determine any effect on school performance. Of course, if the assessment is being completed in the school setting, the requirements are established through regulations specified by public law.
6. Assessment with adolescents and adults.
    a. Focused on determining the effect of stuttering on the individual's daily activities, communication and quality of life.
    b. Additionally, degree of severity, frequency and type of stuttering and secondary behaviors are all assessed.
    c. A number of self-assessment tools are commercially available to assess the attitudes, avoidances, speaking goals and other important areas for the client who stutters. In adolescents and adults, it is critical to bring in the patient's own perspective on their stuttering problem.

Treatment of Stuttering

Treatment Decisions

1. Stuttering treatment decision-making is always informed by a number of important variables, including:
   a. Specific client/patient/family variables.
      (1) Age.
      (2) Culture.
      (3) Linguistic background.
      (4) Educational level.
      (5) Developmental stage of stuttering.
      (6) Motivation for treatment at this time.
   b. Clinical variables.
      (1) Developmental stuttering stage.
      (2) Severity.
      (3) Other speech-language or developmental concerns.
      (4) Client/family preferences and expectations.
   c. Environmental variables.
      (1) Family issues or availability.
      (2) Setting for service delivery (school, clinic, other).
2. In general, therapy approaches for PWS can be described by three characteristics.
   a. Degree of focus on the client or the environment (parent, teacher, etc.).
      (1) This really is related to the directness of the approach that is being taken.
   b. Degree of focus on achieving natural effortless speech and whether the method utilized is targeted at fluency shaping or stuttering modification.
   c. Degree of focus on counseling and interpersonal issues.

Treatment Approaches

1. There are a number of specific treatment approaches available for use with PWS. The choice of treatment approach is based on the various decisions outlined above; however, the primary decision about the appropriate range of approaches is guided by the age and stuttering stage of the client.
2. Some common clinical scenarios follow. While these prototype examples are useful for appreciating the range of options available for treatment in stuttering, the always important consideration of the unique features presented and the client's background are critical to best practice in management of stuttering.
3. Young child (2–5 years) with normal disfluency or beginning stuttering.
   a. It is common for parents of young children to take note of disfluency in the speech of their children and to seek assistance.
   b. As noted earlier, most children who show disfluency at this stage will emerge as fluent speakers. Having said that, factors that increase the risk for advancing to more significant difficulties include:
      (1) Increased stress around speech for the child or the parents.
      (2) Any negative feedback to the child about speech or stuttering.
   c. Additionally, children who exhibit concomitant speech and language disorders, or a higher frequency of disfluencies (even those that are not stuttering-like) will likely benefit from assistance.
      (1) Indirect treatment approaches for young children are frequently used as an approach to managing concerns about disfluencies.
         (a) The primary goal of intervention at this stage is to reduce the likelihood that the child will advance to beginning or intermediate stuttering.
         (b) Indirect treatment approaches include features of parent education and counseling, modeling (with the parent) and reinforcing relaxed speech, slower rates and less linguistic complexity.
         (c) The desired outcome is a reduction in the amount of stuttering-like disfluencies (if present) and reduction of overall percentage of disfluent speech.
         (d) Variations on this basic approach are seen in a number of established treatment approaches that have been published in the literature (see Table 11-5).
      (2) Direct treatment approaches for young children are also frequently described in the literature on treatment.
         (a) These more direct approaches include skills in teaching the child how to respond to disfluencies, developing the ability to demonstrate fluency skills and/or using operant methods or other feedback to reinforce fluent productions.
         (b) Even in the direct approaches, it should be noted that parents are a focus of treatment along with the child who stutters.

Table 11-5

Sample Therapy Approaches: Young Children (Preschool) Who Stutter (Normal Disfluency and Beginning Stuttering)

REFERENCE	BRIEF DESCRIPTION OF APPROACH
Richels, C. G., & Conture, E. G. (2009). "An Indirect Treatment Approach for Early Intervention for Childhood Stuttering," in E.G. Conture & R.F. Curlee (Eds.), *Stuttering and Related Disorders of Fluency*. New York: Theime Medical Publishing.	• Uses family-centered, indirect treatment, with separate parent and child groups. • Focuses on the documented effect of increased linguistic/communicative complexity and time demands on stuttering in young children. • Focuses on emotional regulation and adaptability. • Measures change in stuttering like disfluencies and overall percentage of disfluency. • Models easy, simple, stress-free speech in group activities. • Reports a 17% decrease overall in disfluencies and a 31% decrease in stuttering-like disfluencies.
Guitar, B. (2006). *Stuttering: An Integrated Approach to Its Nature and Treatment*. Philadelphia: Lippincott, Williams, and Wilkins Co.	• Program uses indirect treatment, family centered. • Goal is to achieve spontaneous fluency. • Focus is on modifying child-parent communication interaction. • If child's speech worsens or there are signs of anxiety in the child, then Guitar moves to a more direct approach. • No results are reported.
Gregory, H. (2003). *Stuttering Therapy: Rationale and Procedures*. Boston: Allyn and Bacon.	• Individual and group therapy • Program is parent and child focused • Clinician models relaxed, slow speech and gradually increases language complexity. • Parent focus is on education. • Therapy program lasts 8–12 months. • Up to 5% of children persist with problems that require additional treatment.
Onslow M., Packman, A., and Harrison, E. (2003). *The Lidcombe Program of Early Stuttering Intervention: A Clinician's Guide*. Austin, TX: Pro-Ed.	• Goal is to provide extensive, repeated, positive fluent speaking experiences • SLP trains the parent to reinforce fluent speech and then respond to stuttering when it occurs. • Operant conditioning is used in weekly sessions, and parent learns to do daily sessions at home. • Numerous outcome studies have been reported; all indicate positive results in eliminating stuttering in young children at early stages of stuttering.

(c) The most frequent approaches to attaining fluency in these methods are achieved through modeling natural, relaxed speech and providing adequate time for children to respond or initiate.

(d) One program in particular, the Lidcombe Program (Onslow et al., 2003), used a randomized control trial to demonstrate effectiveness.
- However, there are numerous single-subject and small-group studies that support positive outcomes when working with preschool children who stutter.

(e) Table 11-5 provides a summary of documented approaches for PWS at the normal disfluency and beginning stuttering levels.

4. School-age children who stutter (intermediate stuttering).
   a. By the time that children who stutter are enrolled in elementary school, they are likely experiencing symptoms of struggle, including blocks, along with their repetitions and prolongations.
   b. They are also likely to be experiencing some of the attitudes and feelings that have been described.
   c. Negative experiences with communication, bullying at school and failed attempts at correcting the problem are all unfortunate, but common features of the experience of stuttering in this age group.
   d. Approaches to treatment may be focused on developing fluent speech, modifying stuttering and equipping the child for success in a variety of social and academic situations.
   (1) Stuttering modification focus.
      (a) Traditional approaches to stuttering treatment include a focus on reducing tension at the moment of stuttering, developing healthy communication attitudes and equipping the child who stutters for a variety of speaking situations.
         • Approaches to tension reduction frequently include learning to describe what is happening during stuttering, relaxing the speech musculature and differentiating degrees of muscular effort/tension.

Table 11-6

Sample Therapy Approaches: School-Age Children (Intermediate Level)

REFERENCE	BRIEF DESCRIPTION OF APPROACH
Guitar, B. (2006). *Stuttering: An Integrated Approach to Its Nature and Treatment.* Philadelphia: Lippincott, Williams, and Wilkins Co.	• Help the child explore his/her stuttering in terms of beliefs, core behaviors, secondary behaviors, and feelings. • Build fluency skills and then master them. • Desensitize to fluency disruptions. • Reduce fear. • Deal with bullying and teasing. • Work with parents and teachers.
Ramig, P., & Dodge, D. (2005). *The Child and Adolescent Treatment and Activity Resource Guide.* Clifton Park, NY: Thomson Delmar.	• Uses very focused resources for school-age children and teens. • Supplies resources to support individual education plan development. • Supplies therapy materials that can augment various approaches. • Uses child-friendly materials/handouts. • Resources in Spanish and English.
Langevin, M., Kully, D., & Ross-Harold, B. (2009). "The Comprehensive Stuttering Program for School-Age Children with Strategies for Bullying and Teasing" in E. G. Conture & R.F. Curlee (Eds), *Stuttering and Related Disorders of Fluency.* New York: Thieme Medical Publishing.	• Addresses both attitudinal and behavioral aspects of stuttering. • Uses fluency-enhancing skills, involvement of parents and family, and home practice. • Deals specifically with helping the child learn to cope with teasing and bullying with specific conflict resolution approaches.

- Another aspect of this approach includes exploring feelings associated with stuttering, and this can be done in a number of ways. For some children it is not easy to do this verbally, and they may benefit from drawings or other creative activities to assist with expression of these emotions.
- Cancellation of stuttering involves repeating a stuttered word in a more fluent way. Voluntary stuttering involves practicing one's stuttering as a method to decrease fear. These two techniques are common in speech modification approaches.
- As the child learns to use these modifications more reliably, practice is extended to more meaningful communication situations.
- Environmental focus addresses important work with teachers, parents, classmates and other people who are important to the child.

(2) Fluency shaping focus.
  (a) In fluency-shaping approaches, the goal of the client is to replace stuttered speech with fluent speech.
  (b) Many different techniques have been developed to achieve fluent speech in people who stutter. Of these, a few approaches are most often described:
   - Rate modification, especially at the initiation of speech.
   - Easy onset of phonation as a method of reducing hard glottal attack at speech onset.
   - Light contact of the articulators.
   - Continuous phonation.

  (c) These techniques are often delivered through modeling in an exaggerated manner and then shaping the behavior toward a more standard production. Operant conditioning techniques are often used to help establish and generalize the speaking behavior.
  (d) Once the behaviors are established in structured settings, then the "new" speaking skills are transferred to real world contexts.
  (e) Table 11-6 provides a summary of documented approaches for PWS at the intermediate level.

5. Adolescents and adults who stutter (advanced stuttering).
  a. Frequently come to the treatment experience having had previous therapy.
  b. Building a trusting relationship and allowing open discussion of thoughts and feelings about these experiences (as well as stuttering) becomes an important part of the treatment paradigm.
  c. When individuals have experienced stuttering throughout development as it has persisted to adulthood, unique treatment challenges are presented for both the client and the clinician.
  d. In general, the same approaches as in intermediate stuttering (previous section) are available to the clinician to use with the older client.
  e. The major difference is the necessity to approach the more mature individual as an adult, allowing for open discussion and reflection and developing an expectation for independent use of treatment skills outside of therapy.
  f. Regardless of which major approach is used (fluency shaping or stuttering modification or combination), there are a few unique features that are often discussed as important features of therapy with adults:

Table 11-7

Sample Therapy Approaches: Adolescents and Adults Who Stutter (Advanced Level)

REFERENCE	BRIEF DESCRIPTION OF APPROACH
Gregory, H. (2003). *Stuttering Therapy: Rationale and Procedures.* Boston: Allyn and Bacon.	• Uses integrated approach. • Includes use of relaxation plus stuttering modification and fluency shaping. • Addresses attitudes and beliefs and education about stuttering. • Implements a specific speaking style referred to as ERA-SM (easy relaxed approach with smooth movement) as a transition to more fluent production.
Kully, D. and Langevin, M. (1999). "Intensive treatment for stuttering adolescents," in R. Curlee (ed.), *Stuttering and Related Disorders of Fluency*, 2nd ed. New York: Thieme Medical Publishing.	• Program is delivered over 3-week period. • Program uses fluency-shaping techniques to build initial skill. • Once clients move to a normal speech rate, they learn speech modifications. • Cognitive behavioral therapy is used to develop comfort in challenging situations and to reduce avoidance. • Collaboration with support groups is encouraged, and follow-up with clients is maintained after the intensive program concludes.
O'Brian, S., Onslow, M., Cream, A., & Packman, A. (2003). "The Camperdown Program: Outcomes of a New Prolonged Speech Treatment Model." *Journal of Speech-Language-Hearing Research*, 46, 933–946.	• Unique program that uses a videotaped speech sample to provide a model for prolonged speech without additional fluency-shaping instruction. • Clients are taught to use a 9-point self-rating scale of stuttering severity as a method for monitoring and self-management. • Clients are seen in a group for 1 full day of practice and then followed individually. • Results are reported as a mean pretreatment 7.9% SS to 0.4% at 12 months posttreatment.
Guitar, B. (2014). *Stuttering: An Integrated Approach to Its Nature and Treatment.* Philadelphia: Lippincott, Williams, and Wilkins Co.	• Uses many of his same principles from intermediate stuttering. • Particular attention paid to fear reduction, self-understanding of stuttering by the client, and discussing stuttering openly. • Replaces avoidance behaviors with approach behaviors.

(1) Assuring that the individual's beliefs and attitudes about stuttering are addressed as a method for reducing speaking fears and avoidance.
(2) Development of client competence in self-management of therapy, including self-measurement of change.
(3) Development of highly specific strategies for generalizing desired speech changes to situations, especially those that are self-identified as most challenging.
(4) Table 11-7 provides a summary of documented approaches for PWS at the advanced level.

References

Bennett, E. M. (2006). *Working with People Who Stutter: A Lifespan Perspective.* Upper Saddle River, NJ: Pearson Education, Inc.

Bloodstein, O., & Bernstein Ratner, N. (2008). *A Handbook on Stuttering*, 6th ed. Clifton Park, NY: Delmar.

Conture, E., & Curlee, R. F. (2007). *Stuttering and Related Disorders of Fluency*, 3rd ed. New York, NY: Thieme.

Gregory, H. H. (2003). *Stuttering Therapy: Rationale and Procedures.* Boston, MA: Pearson Education, Inc.

Guitar, B. (2006). *Stuttering: An Integrated Approach to Its Nature and Treatment.* Philadelphia: Lippincott, Williams, and Wilkins Co.

Guitar, B. (2014). *Stuttering: An Integrated Approach to Its Nature and Treatment*, 4th ed. Baltimore, MD: Lippincott Williams & Wilkins.

Guitar, B., & McCauley, R. J. (2010). *Stuttering Treatment: Established and Emerging Approaches.* Baltimore: Lippincott Williams & Wilkins.

Langevin, M., Kully, D., & Ross-Harold, B. (2009). "The Comprehensive Stuttering Program for School-Age Children with Strategies for Bullying and Teasing" in E. G. Conture & R.F. Curlee (Eds), *Stuttering and Related Disorders of Fluency.* New York: Thieme Medical Publishing.

Mahr, G., & Leith, W. (1992). Psychogenic stuttering of adult onset. *Journal of Speech-Language-Hearing Research*, 35, 283–286.

Manning, W. H. (2010). *Clinical Decision Making in Fluency Disorders*, 3rd ed. Clifton Park, NY: Delmar.

O'Brian, S., Onslow, M., Cream, A, & Packman, A (2003). "The Camperdown Program: Outcomes of a New Prolonged Speech Treatment Model." *Journal of Speech-Language-Hearing Research*, 46, 933–946.

Onslow M., Packman, A., and Harrison, E. (2003). *The Lidcombe Program of Early Stuttering Intervention: A Clinician's Guide.* Austin, TX: Pro-Ed.

Ramig, P., & Dodge, D. (2005). *The Child and Adolescent Treatment and Activity Resource Guide.* Clifton Park, NY: Thomson Delmar.

Richels, C. G., & Conture, E. G. (2009). "An Indirect Treatment Approach for Early Intervention for Childhood Stuttering," in E.G. Conture & R.F. Curlee (Eds.), *Stuttering and Related Disorders of Fluency.* New York: Theime Medical Publishing.

Ward, D. (2006). *Stuttering and Cluttering: Frameworks for Understanding and Treatment.* New York, NY: Psychology Press.

World Health Organization. (2001). *International Classification of Functioning, Disability and Health: ICF.* Geneva, Switzerland: World Health Organization.

Yairi, E., & Seery, C. H. (2014). *Stuttering: Foundations and Clinical Applications*, 2nd ed. Upper Saddle River, NJ: Pearson Education, Inc.

SECTION III

Acquired Communication Disorders

Section Outline

- **Chapter 12:** Acquired Language Disorders: Aphasia, Right-Hemisphere Disorders and Neurodegenerative Syndromes, 255
- **Chapter 13:** Motor Speech Disorders, 299

12

Acquired Language Disorders: Aphasia, Right-Hemisphere Disorders and Neurodegenerative Syndromes

MARJORIE NICHOLAS, PhD

Chapter Outline

- Aphasia and Related Terms, 256
- Neuroanatomical Bases of Aphasia, 258
- Assessment of Aphasia, 261
- Classification of Aphasia, 266
- Psychosocial Effects of Aphasia on the Individual and the Family, 269
- Treatment of Aphasia, 270
- Recovery from Aphasia, 284
- Communication Disorders Associated with Right-Hemisphere Brain Damage (RBD), 285
- Neurodegenerative Syndromes Affecting Language and Cognition, 286
- Multicultural Considerations in Working with People with Dementia, 295
- References Cited, 295
- References from the ANCDS: Guidelines for Treatment of Cognitive-Communication Disorders of Dementia, www.ancds.org, 297

Aphasia and Related Terms

Aphasia Defined

1. Aphasia is a language disorder caused by acquired brain damage.
2. *Important:* it is language impairment and not speech impairment that is the critical feature of aphasia.
3. Motor speech disorders such as dysarthria or apraxia of speech may accompany the aphasia but are separate from the aphasia.
4. Other cognitive disturbances may accompany aphasia but generally it is the language impairment that most affects communication.
   a. Many person(s) with aphasia (PWA) have intact nonverbal cognition and their thinking abilities and intelligence are for the most part intact.
   b. Other PWA may have additional deficits in selected areas of cognition that will interact with their ability to use language and perhaps may limit their response to treatment.

Components of Language Affected by Aphasia

1. Lexical retrieval refers to the ability to access the words within one's lexicon for communicating content.
   a. Lexical retrieval deficits will affect both verbal expression and writing.
   b. Anomia is difficulty finding words and it is a core feature of every aphasia syndrome.
   c. Anomia comes in many severity levels, from total inability to retrieve desired words for verbal expression or writing to mild, occasional failures to retrieve a desired word during conversation.
2. Grammatical competence refers to the expression and comprehension of the formal grammatical aspects of language (syntax and morphology).
   a. Agrammatism is difficulty with the expression and/or comprehension of the grammatical units of language.
   b. Patterns of agrammatism are variable depending on the characteristics of the language used by the PWA but also show patterns that are consistent across languages.
   c. In English, agrammatism in PWA manifests by:
      (1) Omission of functor words such as articles, prepositions, auxiliary verbs and pronouns when speaking.
      (2) Omission or errors on grammatical markers in affixes such as the plural –s, past tense –ed when speaking.
      (3) Inability to comprehend passive constructions and other non-canonical, less frequent grammatical structures.
3. Auditory comprehension (A/C) of single words or longer linguistic units refers to the ability to attach meaning to the words spoken by others.
   a. Impairments of A/C are common in aphasia and help to distinguish among the varieties of aphasia.
   b. A/C impairments range in severity from near total inability to understand spoken language to a mild comprehension difficulty that barely impacts functional communication.
4. Verbal repetition of words spoken by the examiner is used to differentiate the aphasia syndromes and may be relatively preserved or relatively impaired compared to other language skills.
   a. *Verbal short-term memory* and *verbal working memory* are terms used to describe functions that are also required in the repetition task.
5. Reading and writing deficits are also common in aphasia.
   a. Alexia is an aphasic reading disorder.
   b. Deep dyslexia.
      (1) A person with deep dyslexia cannot access grapheme-to-phoneme (letter-to-sound) conversion rules, so they cannot "sound out" words from written form.
      (2) They are only able to use the "whole-word," also known as "lexical," reading route.
      (3) They produce semantic paralexic errors in oral reading, substituting a semantically related word for the target word (e.g., reading *doctor* as "nurse").
      (4) They cannot read nonwords (e.g., *flamp*) or semantically empty functor words (e.g., *for, by, to*).
   c. Surface dyslexia.
      (1) Surface dyslexia is a syndrome that is almost the reverse of deep dyslexia.
      (2) People with surface dyslexia have limited access to meaning on a whole-word basis and are only able to use the grapheme-to-phoneme mapping route.
      (3) This strategy works for words with regular spelling but not for irregular words.
      (4) People with surface dyslexia attempt to understand words by sounding out the letters (e.g., the irregularly pronounced word *pint* would be read aloud as /pɪnt/, rhyming with the word *mint*).

(5) They have good ability to read aloud pseudowords (e.g., *blix*).
d. Pure alexia without agraphia.
   (1) People with this disorder have a complete inability to read aloud; they cannot recognize letters or words.
   (2) They can write normally, yet cannot read back what they wrote.
   (3) They are able to understand tactile spelling on their skin and may be able to access letter information by tracing letter forms with their fingers.
   (4) Pure alexia is caused by a loss of specifically visual input into the language areas due to a disconnection of bilateral occipital pathways into the language areas of the left hemisphere.
e. Letter-by-letter (LBL) reading.
   (1) LBL reading is a less severe form of a visual-input-based reading disorder.
   (2) There is preservation of individual letter reading but LBL readers cannot read words as a whole.
   (3) LBL readers tend to read each letter aloud and then construct internally what the word is by using their comprehension of oral spelling (e.g., "f-a-t-h-e-r... oh, it's father.").
f. Agraphia is an aphasic writing disorder.
   (1) Typical aphasic agraphia is characterized by difficulty retrieving words for writing and by various spelling errors.
      (a) The severity and form of agraphic errors often mirrors the characteristics of spoken output in PWA.
      (b) Agraphia is caused by the linguistic disorder, not by the fact that the PWA may be using their nondominant hand.
      (c) Agraphia can be seen when writing with pen/pencil on paper or when using a keyboard.
   (2) Pure agraphia is a rare syndrome characterized by inability to write but no other language problems.
      (a) In this disorder, the PWA seems to have lost the memories of the motor engrams needed for writing letters and words.

Other Disorders Commonly Accompanying Aphasia

1. Perseveration is the inappropriate repetition of a response or continuation of a behavior when it is no longer required or appropriate. Perseveration is common in PWA and can take several different forms.
   a. Recurrent perseveration is the production of a previously made response after a filled delay (e.g., carrying over some of the phonemes from a previous response on a naming test into a subsequent response, or a complete repetition of an entire previous response).
   b. Continuous perseveration is the immediate repetition of the same response that was just made; the person cannot stop making the same response.
   c. Stuck-in-set is an inability to shift response set when it is required (e.g., the PWA continues to count when asked to recite the alphabet after having just completed a counting task).
2. Apraxia is a disorder of the execution of learned movement that is not caused by motor weakness, incoordination, or sensory loss and is not due to failure to understand the command.
   a. The most common form of apraxia, known as ideomotor apraxia, is particularly seen in left-hemisphere strokes.
      (1) Ideomotor apraxia may affect limb or oral-facial movements, or both.
      (2) It refers to difficulty with the selection, sequencing and spatial orientation of movements for gestures.
      (3) Hugo Liepmann wrote about apraxia in the early 1900s and described it as if the person with apraxia knows the idea of the movements they want to perform (ideo) but cannot get the body (motor) to perform them correctly due to a disconnection in neuroanatomical pathways.
   b. Apraxia of speech (AOS) is a sensorimotor speech disorder with symptoms of impaired volitional production of articulation and prosody that does not result from abnormal muscle strength, tone or timing; nor does it arise from aphasia, confusion, generalized intellectual impairment or hearing loss.
      (1) AOS results from impairment of neural programming of skilled movements.
      (2) AOS may also be seen in PWA. Some people believe that AOS is necessarily part of the nonfluent syndrome of Broca's aphasia.
      (3) See Chapter 13 on motor speech disorders for further information on AOS.
3. Agnosias are disorders of recognition of objects, people, sounds, colors, etc. that are not a result of primary sensory deficits.
   a. Agnosias are generally associated with cortical brain damage in regions of the parietal, temporal and occipital lobes.
   b. Visual agnosia is the inability to recognize what visual objects or pictures of objects are. It is not

simply a failure to name them but rather to understand the "meanings" of them.
   c. Prosopagnosia is the inability to recognize faces.
   d. Anosognosia is the inability to recognize one's own illness, to be aware that one has an illness.
4. Nonverbal cognitive impairments are also common in some PWA. Frontal lobe lesions are likely to result in some degree of executive system impairment, causing problems in numerous cognitive functions.

History of Modern Aphasiology

1. The history of modern aphasiology is generally acknowledged as beginning in the latter half of the 19th century.
2. Paul Broca was a French neurologist who studied PWA in life and subsequently examined their brains postmortem.
   a. In 1861, he reported that a region of the frontal lobe (third frontal convolution, now called Broca's area) was implicated in disorders of speech production.
   b. In 1865, Broca established the association between language disorders and damage specifically to the left hemisphere of the brain.
      (1) Marc Dax had discovered the relationship between language disorders and damage to left-hemisphere brain regions 30 years earlier in 1836.
      (2) However, Broca publicized this to the scientific community.
      (3) Broca also suggested the possibility that the right hemisphere could take over function in the recovery process.
3. Carl Wernicke (1874) was a German neurologist who also studied PWA and together with Hugo Lichtheim wrote about many other forms of aphasia. The Wernicke-Lichtheim model is the basis for many classification systems that are still in use today.
   a. Wernicke wrote about a second major variety of aphasia (now known as Wernicke's aphasia) that was characterized by auditory comprehension deficit and was associated with lesions in an area of the temporal lobe now called Wernicke's area.
   b. He also wrote about what are now termed classic connectionist models and suggested that information could be transmitted within the brain from one region to another.
   c. He predicted the existence of a third form of aphasia called conduction aphasia.
      (1) Conduction aphasia would be caused by a disconnection in the neural pathways between the auditory comprehension area in the temporal lobe and the verbal expression area in the frontal lobe.
      (2) He predicted that verbal repetition would be particularly poor in this form of aphasia because of this disconnection.

Neuroanatomical Bases of Aphasia

Language Zone Region of the Brain

1. The language zone region of the left hemisphere is depicted in Figure 12-1. Brain damage to structures within this region is likely to result in some degree of language impairment.
2. The language zone includes cortical as well as subcortical regions in the frontal, parietal and temporal lobes of the left hemisphere.
3. The region of the language zone is fed almost entirely by the left middle cerebral artery (MCA); therefore, aphasia is typically caused by a stroke within the territory of the left MCA. See Figure 12-2.
4. The language zone includes Broca's area in the left frontal lobe, which is important for the verbal expression of language and for grammatical competence.

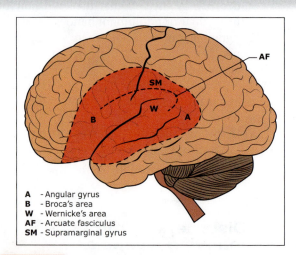

A - Angular gyrus
B - Broca's area
W - Wernicke's area
AF - Arcuate fasciculus
SM - Supramarginal gyrus

Figure 12-1 The language zone of the left hemisphere, showing Broca's and Wernicke's areas, the angular and supramarginal gyri, and the arcuate fasciculus.

Based on *Manual of Aphasia and Aphasia Therapy*, 2nd ed., by Nancy Helm-Estabrooks and Martin L Albert, Austin, TX: Pro-ed., 2004.

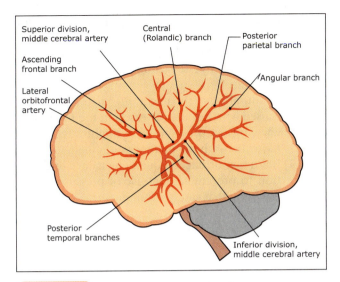

Figure 12-2 The middle cerebral artery territory.

Based on *Manual of Aphasia and Aphasia Therapy,* 2nd ed., by Nancy Helm-Estabrooks and Martin L Albert, Austin, TX: Pro-ed., 2004.

5. The language zone includes Wernicke's area in the left temporal lobe, which is important for the auditory comprehension of language.
6. The language zone also includes the left angular gyrus and the supramarginal gyrus in the border zone regions between the parietal and temporal lobes.
7. The language zone also includes white matter pathways beneath these regions, particularly the arcuate fasciculus and the superior longitudinal fasciculus.

Neuroanatomy and Aphasia

1. Classification of aphasia syndromes is discussed in a later section but basic facts related to lesion location and aphasia are:
   a. Anterior lesions lead to nonfluent aphasias. In general, if a PWA has had a stroke or brain injury affecting only anterior structures of the language zone in the left hemisphere (i.e., anterior to the central sulcus), the PWA will most likely have a nonfluent type of aphasia.
      (1) In general, if the brain damage involves the left precentral sulcus, also called the motor strip, or subcortical regions deep to this area, the PWA is likely to have some degree of right hemiparesis.
         (a) Right hemiparesis is impairment of motor functioning on the right side of the body, ranging from mild to severe, affecting various regions of foot, leg, arm and face, depending on the location of the damage to the motor strip.
         (b) Right hemiplegia is paralysis on the right side of the body.
   b. Posterior lesions lead to fluent aphasias. In general, if a PWA has had a stroke or brain injury that is restricted to the posterior structures of the language zone in the left hemisphere (i.e., posterior to the central sulcus), the PWA will most likely have a fluent type of aphasia.
      (1) There will NOT be any concomitant motor impairment.
      (2) If the brain damage affects the postcentral sulcus in the parietal lobe, also called the sensory strip, the PWA is likely to have some sensory impairment on the right side of the body.
   c. Brain damage that affects both anterior and posterior regions of the language zone of the left hemisphere is likely to result in a severe aphasia with a concomitant right hemiparesis.

Cerebral Dominance for Language

1. Cerebral dominance refers to the fact that, for most people, the left hemisphere is dominant for language processing.
2. Among right-handers 99% are left-hemisphere-dominant for language. Approximately 70% of left-handers are also left-hemisphere-dominant for language.
3. Only about 1% of right-handers and 30% of left-handers do not show the typical pattern; this is referred to as anomalous dominance.
   a. Right-handed people who develop aphasia from a right-hemisphere stroke are given the label *crossed aphasia* because the condition is so rare.
4. Anomalous dominance may mean that the right hemisphere is dominant for language (a reverse or mirror-image pattern of the typical) or it may mean that language is controlled by both hemispheres (i.e., no single hemisphere is dominant).
5. People with anomalous dominance may show better or atypical patterns of recovery from aphasia if they have had a left-hemisphere stroke.

Common Etiologies of Aphasia

1. Cerebrovascular disease that damages the language zone of the left hemisphere.
2. Traumatic brain injuries that damage the language zone of the left hemisphere.
3. Brain tumors that affect the tissue or functioning of the language zone.
4. Neurodegenerative disorders that affect the left hemisphere.
5. Cerebrovascular disease is the leading cause of aphasia and is responsible for approximately 50% of the cases of aphasia.

a. Risk factors for cerebrovascular disease include high cholesterol, diabetes, smoking, hypertension and heart disease.
b. A transient ischemic attack (TIA) is a temporary loss of neurological function caused by an interruption of blood flow to a brain region.
  (1) A TIA is viewed as a "warning sign" for stroke and the person should be thoroughly evaluated by a neurologist if a TIA is suspected.
  (2) Symptoms of a TIA are variable and include difficulty speaking (dysarthria or word-finding blocks), clumsiness in one hand or arm, numbness or tingling in a limb or on one side of the face and visual disturbances.
  (3) F.A.S.T. = Face, Arm, Speech, Time. The FAST acronym is a way for the layperson to remember the warning signs of stroke (facial droop, arm motor difficulties, speech abnormalities) and that emergency medical attention should be obtained immediately (time).
c. Cerebrovascular accident (CVA, or stroke) is the most common cause of aphasia.
  (1) An occlusive stroke may be caused by an embolus or a thrombosis or a combination of the two.
    (a) Embolus is a clot formed in another body area (often the heart) that can travel up to the brain and then interrupt blood flow.
    (b) Thrombosis is a clot that can form in the blood vessels of the brain and results in a blockage but has not travelled from another region.
    (c) Thrombo-embolic stroke is a combination of an embolus and a thrombus or a stroke that could possibly be caused by either.
  (2) Occlusive strokes may be treated emergently with "clot-busting" drugs such as Tissue Plasminogen Activator (TPA) to prevent long-term brain damage.
    (a) The individual must be medically evaluated within a short window of time post onset—approximately 3 to 5 hours.
    (b) Cerebral hemorrhage must be ruled out first, usually via neuroimaging studies prior to administration of TPA.
    (c) Administration of TPA may prevent permanent neurological damage from the stroke or may reduce the severity of the stroke.
d. A hemorrhagic CVA results when there is a rupture of the vessels in the brain rather than a blockage of blood flow.
  (1) A ruptured aneurysm is a ballooned-out area of a blood vessel wall that becomes very thin and subsequently breaks.
  (2) An arteriovenous malformation (AVM) is a tangled mass of brain blood vessels that is often congenital and that subsequently ruptures or leaks.
  (3) An intracerebral hemorrhage is caused by a rupture of a vessel within the neural tissue of the brain.
  (4) Subdural or subarachnoid hemorrhage is caused by a rupture of vessels in the meningeal coverings of the brain that might affect brain tissue beneath the meninges.
  (5) Brain hemorrhages require emergency intervention to prevent an increase of pressure within the brain that can result in death.
    (a) Craniotomy is opening up the skull to relieve pressure and to drain excess blood resulting from the hemorrhage.
6. Traumatic brain injuries (TBI) that damage the language zone of the left hemisphere are the second most common cause of aphasia in adults.
  a. The specific linguistic and cognitive symptoms seen in TBI will depend on the brain regions affected by the TBI and may be somewhat different from symptoms seen in aphasia from stroke.
  b. Symptoms may arise from either focal (localized to a specific area) or diffuse (widespread) injury or a combination of both focal and diffuse brain damage.
    (1) Focal injuries sometimes have both coup (site of impact) and contrecoup (opposite the site of impact) components, caused by the brain impacting different areas of the skull depending on how the TBI occurs.
    (2) Diffuse damage includes diffuse axonal injury (DAI), often occurring in high-speed motor vehicle accidents, where many long branches of axons within the brain become damaged, often resulting in significant motor and cognitive difficulties.
  c. TBI may result in damage to subcortical structures in the limbic system, causing significant memory problems and emotional regulation difficulties.
  d. A common site of damage in TBI is either unilateral or bilateral prefrontal damage resulting in significant problems with emotional and behavioral regulation and executive functioning impairments.
  e. Causes of TBI.
    (1) Motor vehicle accidents are a common cause of TBI, particularly in young adult males.
    (2) Falls resulting in brain injuries are more common in young children and elderly adults.
    (3) Blows to the head causing injury to the brain such as in assaults are also more common in young adult males.
    (4) Chronic traumatic encephalopathy (CTE) is the name given to multiple concussions and more serious head injuries sustained primarily

by professional and amateur athletes such as boxers, football players and soccer players.
(5) Blast injuries from improvised explosive devices (IEDs) resulting in brain injuries, such as those sustained by soldiers and civilians in war-torn areas, have become much more numerous in recent years due to the Iraq and Afghanistan wars.
(6) Gunshot wounds and stab wounds to the head that affect the left hemisphere may also result in aphasia. These are known as penetrating head injuries.
(7) Closed head injuries (CHI): many head injuries do not involve the penetration of an object through the skull or the breakage of the skull itself.
7. Brain tumors that affect the tissue of the language zone may also result in aphasia.
   a. Specific linguistic and cognitive symptoms will depend on the region affected by the tumor and may be different from symptoms seen in aphasia from stroke.
   b. Tumors may arise from the neural tissues of the brain itself, such as a glioma, or from the protective meninges, such as a meningioma.
   c. Tumors may also originate elsewhere in the body as a metastatic tumor.
   d. Aphasia may worsen as the tumor grows or may improve if the tumor is removed or treated via medication or surgery to decrease its size.
   e. Cognitive and linguistic processing may also be affected by medical treatments for the brain tumor (chemotherapy, surgical resections) and the speech-language pathologist (SLP) needs to consider this when planning the assessment or treatment for a person with a brain tumor.
8. Neurodegenerative disorders that affect the left hemisphere may also result in aphasia. (*Note*: See the later section on dementia syndromes in this chapter.)
   a. Dementia is a progressive neurodegenerative brain disorder affecting multiple domains of cognition, including memory, language, visuospatial skills and behavior.
   b. Dementia syndromes that also have significant language deficits as part of the behavioral profile include:
   (1) Alzheimer's disease (AD).
   (2) Frontotemporal dementia (FTD) and the subtypes of FTD known as primary progressive aphasia (PPA).
   (3) Vascular dementia (VaD).
   (4) Dementia with Lewy bodies (DLB).

Assessment of Aphasia

Thorough Examination of All Language Components

1. Language assessment of aphasia by an SLP requires a thorough examination of all components of language, including auditory comprehension and many aspects of speaking, reading and writing.
2. Standardized formal measures that can be used to evaluate language and communication include (among others not listed):
   a. Boston Diagnostic Aphasia Examination (BDAE-3) by Harold Goodglass, Edith Kaplan, and Barbara Barresi, 3rd edition (2001).
      (1) The BDAE provides an aphasia profile on the Rating Scale Profile of Speech Characteristics that can be compared to profiles consistent with one of the seven aphasia syndromes.
      (2) The examiner also assigns a "subjective" Aphasia Severity Rating (ASR) from 0 to 5.
      (3) The BDAE is a comprehensive assessment tool that includes both standard and extended testing subtests.
      (4) Depending on the individual, it may take 2 to 6 hours to administer the test in its entirety.
   b. Boston Naming Test (BNT), published as part of the BDAE, is a 60-item test of picture confrontation naming ability.
   c. Western Aphasia Battery-Revised (WAB-R) by Andrew Kertesz (2006).
      (1) The WAB subtests assess similar language abilities as the BDAE but it is somewhat quicker to administer than the BDAE.
      (2) Test scores result in an Aphasia Quotient, a Cortical Quotient, an Auditory Comprehension Quotient, a Verbal Expression Quotient, a Reading Quotient and a Writing Quotient.
   d. Aphasia Diagnostic Profiles (ADP) by Nancy Helm-Estabrooks (1992) result in diagnostic profiles similar to BDAE or WAB.
      (1) Profiles that can be analyzed from results include the Aphasia Classification Profile, the Aphasia Severity Profile, the Alternative Communication Profile, Error Profiles and the Behavioral Profile.

e. Cognitive Linguistic Quick Test (CLQT) by Nancy Helm-Estabrooks (2001) provides assessment of language ability as well as assessments of nonverbal cognitive abilities in attention, memory, executive functioning and visuospatial skills.
f. Porch Index of Communicative Abilities Revised (PICA-R) by Bruce Porch (2001).
   (1) A battery of 18 subtests samples gestural, verbal and graphic abilities at different levels of difficulty.
   (2) Known for its multidimensional scoring system that describes accuracy, responsiveness, completeness, promptness and efficiency of response.
g. Minnesota Test for the Differential Diagnosis of Aphasia (MTDDA) by Hildred Schuell (1965).
   (1) The MTDDA was one of the first comprehensive assessments for aphasia.
   (2) It is no longer in print.
3. Nonstandardized assessments are also commonly conducted by SLPs in many settings, but an attempt to evaluate verbal expression, auditory comprehension, reading comprehension and writing should be part of every aphasia examination.
4. The assessment provides a detailed profile of the individual's strengths and weaknesses within each language modality.
5. These profiles are subsequently used to develop personalized treatment plans and to aid in determining an aphasia diagnosis (i.e., an aphasia syndrome label) if desired.
6. Formal tools also exist to measure specifically functional communication abilities. Some of the more commonly used tools include:
a. Communication Activities of Daily Living, 2nd edition (CADL-2), by Audrey Holland, Carol Frattali, and Davida Fromm (1999).
   (1) Assesses communication activities in seven areas: reading, writing, and using numbers; social interaction; divergent communication; contextual communication; nonverbal communication; sequential relationships; and humor/metaphor/absurdity.
b. Functional Assessment of Communication Skills for Adults (ASHA FACS) by Carol Frattali, Audrey Holland, Cynthia Thompson, Cheryl Wohl, and Michelle Ferketic (2003).
   (1) ASHA FACS is a 43-item test completed by interviewing the PWA and family members/caregivers to determine functional communication in several domains.
   (2) Items are rated on a 7-point scale of independence.
c. Communicative Effectiveness Index (CETI) by Jonathan Lomas and colleagues (1989) is a checklist filled out by caregivers that asks questions referring to 16 different communication situations.
d. Boston Assessment of Severe Aphasia (BASA) by Nancy Helm-Estabrooks, Gail Ramsberger, Alisa Morgan, and Marjorie Nicholas (1989).
   (1) The BASA is a 60-item assessment tool specifically for people with severe aphasia that is designed to capture islands of preserved ability.
   (2) The scoring system captures both verbal and nonverbal (gestural) responses to a variety of stimuli.
7. Many clinicians use a process approach to assessment, which is associated with the neuropsychologist Edith Kaplan.
a. A process approach allows for a more thorough understanding of the PWA than simply recording right or wrong on the test booklet.
b. An examiner following the process approach should:
   (1) Record exact error responses and behaviors made by the PWA during the assessment.
   (2) Note and record all off-task behaviors produced by the PWA during the assessment, such as noting whether the PWA was distracted by activities in the environment.
   (3) Note any self-cueing attempts as well as responses to cues provided by the examiner.
   (4) Conduct a qualitative analysis of error responses after the completion of the test.
   (5) Analyze data obtained from this assessment approach to form hypotheses about the cognitive processes that might underlie partially or fully incorrect responses and associated observed behaviors.
   (6) Use these hypotheses to determine the best approaches to remediation.

Components of a Standardized Language Examination

1. Verbal expression should be evaluated to establish strengths and weaknesses using the following types of tasks:
a. Spontaneous narrative expression, in response to open-ended questions such as "Tell me what happened to you?" or "What kind of work do you do?"
b. Complex picture description tasks in which expected content words are specified by the picture.
c. Retelling a story such as a fable.
d. Responses to simple social greetings such as "What is your name?"
e. Naming of items presented (pictures or objects); may include naming of items in specific categories such as body parts, animals, colors, letters, numbers, tools or actions.

f. Responsive naming, e.g., in response to a question such as "What do we tell time with?"
g. Word list generation, e.g., "Tell me the names of as many animals as you can think of in a minute."
h. Repetition of single words, phrases and sentences that are first spoken by the examiner.
i. Oral reading of single words and longer phrases.
j. Production of automatic overlearned sequences such as the alphabet, counting from 1 to 10, the days of the week, the months of the year and nursery rhymes.
k. Singing familiar songs such as "Happy Birthday."

2. Evaluation of verbal expression task responses. At the completion of the assessment, the examiner should seek to answer the following questions:
   a. Is the verbal output primarily fluent or nonfluent, and what is the typical phrase length produced by the individual?
      (1) Fluent is verbal expression in which the amount of words produced per utterance is similar to or greater than a nonaphasic individual regardless of whether the words make sense or not.
         (a) Generally, 7 words or more are produced in the occasional longest phrase.
         (b) Some PWA are hyperfluent, producing more words than typical. This is referred to as logorrhea or press of speech.
      (2) Nonfluent is verbal expression in which the amount of words produced per utterance is less than a typical nonaphasic individual.
         (a) Severely nonfluent would be 1–2 words or fewer per phrase.
         (b) Moderately nonfluent would be approximately 3–5 words per phrase.
         (c) People who say exclusively verbal stereotypes such as repeating words or syllables (e.g., "si si wa wa…si si…wa wa") are not considered to be fluent; rather, this is considered a severe form of nonfluency and phrase length cannot be calculated for these individuals.
   b. Is there evidence of agrammatism, such as omissions of functor words and simplified syntax within phrases or sentences?
   c. Is there evidence of a word-finding problem with lack of content words or overuse of indefinite terms like "thing" or "that one"?
   d. Are there any obvious category-specific deficits in naming, such as the inability to name animals but good ability to name tools?
   e. How intelligible is the verbal output? Is there evidence of a concomitant dysarthria or apraxia of speech?
   f. What is the prosodic contour or melodic line of the verbal output? Does it sound like normal prosody or is it restricted and spoken in a monotone, word-by-word fashion?
   g. Are there paraphasic errors in the verbal output? Paraphasias are word-substitution errors and may be of several types:
      (1) Semantic paraphasias share elements of meaning with the target word, such as saying "lion" for the target word *tiger*.
      (2) Phonemic paraphasias share elements of phonology with the target, such as saying "piger" for the target word *tiger*.
      (3) Verbal paraphasia unrelated—another real-word substitution that is not semantically or phonemically related, such as saying "auto" for the target word *tiger*.
      (4) Neologism—a nonword with no apparent relation to the target, such as saying "palipon" for the target word *tiger*.
      (5) Mixed paraphasias may be both semantically and phonemically related.
   h. Is repetition relatively preserved or particularly poor compared to narrative expression?
   i. Can the individual produce words better when singing than in spoken language?
   j. Is there preservation of overlearned verbal sequences, such as counting and saying the days of the week?
   k. Is there evidence of perseveration? In which tasks? What types of perseverative errors are made?
   l. Does the individual use other communicative modalities, such as gesturing, drawing or writing when verbal expression fails?

3. Auditory comprehension should be evaluated taking care to use tasks that are as "pure" as possible (i.e., they do not require other language skills such as talking, reading or writing). Typical tasks used to evaluate auditory comprehension include:
   a. Word discrimination: pointing to pictures or objects named by the examiner.
   b. Following commands: using a variety of different commands from short and simple (e.g., "Close your eyes.") to complex (e.g., "Tap your shoulder with two fingers keeping your eyes shut.").
   c. Answering yes/no questions presented in pairs.
      (1) Because there is a 50% chance of answering a yes/no question correctly, questions should be presented in pairs and the evaluation of correctness should be for the pair only.
      (2) Personally relevant biographical questions are most likely to be comprehended well (e.g., "Is your name Bob?" paired with "Is your name Greg?").
      (3) Questions related to the current time and place should also be asked (e.g., "Are we at the VA Hospital?"; "Is it summer now?").

(4) Yes/no questions related to a short story that is read to the PWA will be more difficult and are dependent on verbal memory. Take care to create questions that could not be answered unless the PWA had comprehended the story.
  d. Comprehension of grammatical forms and complex syntactic constructions such as:
     (1) Reversible possessives (e.g., "Point to the ship's captain.").
     (2) Embedded sentences (e.g., "Which picture shows the man wearing the hat holding the pizza?").
  e. Comprehension of geographical place names by pointing to locations named by the examiner on a map.
     (1) Comprehension of geographical place names tends to be relatively preserved even in severe aphasia.
  f. Comprehension of typical conversational discourse.
     (1) Many PWA may appear to comprehend language in conversational discourse better than on standardized testing.
4. Reading comprehension should be assessed to evaluate if the PWA is able to understand written language. Care should be taken to use tasks that are "pure" measures of reading comprehension and do not require speaking, auditory comprehension or writing. Typical tasks to evaluate reading comprehension are:
  a. Word-picture matching: present a picture and a choice of single words from which the PWA must select.
  b. Sentence-picture matching: present a picture and a choice of sentences that describe the picture.
  c. Lexical decision: point to the words that are real words from a selection of both real words and nonwords.
  d. Sentence and paragraph comprehension: read a sentence or a paragraph and answer follow-up written questions about the content.
  e. Functional reading of newspapers, written instructions, forms, etc.
     (1) Note: Oral reading and reading comprehension can be differentially impaired or spared. Poor ability to read aloud does not necessarily imply poor comprehension of written words.
     (2) PWA may also have modality-specific comprehension deficits (e.g., poor auditory comprehension and good reading comprehension or vice versa).
  f. Writing should be assessed in every PWA.
  g. Note: A right-handed PWA who has a hemiparetic right arm and hand should be tested with their nondominant left hand for writing.
     (1) Using the nondominant hand will result in slower and perhaps less legible written output but will not affect the linguistic nature of the writing.
     (2) Spelling errors and word-selection errors in writing are attributable to the aphasic writing disorder alone.
     (3) Aphasic writing disorder = agraphia.
  h. Signature: signing one's name tends to be preserved even in severe agraphia.
  i. Writing overlearned sequences such as the alphabet or the numbers from 1 to 10.
  j. Writing to dictation of primer-level words (e.g., *cat, boy, run*) and longer phrases and sentences.
     (1) Note: This is not a "pure" task of writing. Poor performance may also be caused by deficits in auditory comprehension of the spoken stimulus.
  k. Written confrontation naming: present pictures and ask the PWA to write the names for them.
  l. Written narrative description either to describe a picture or to write a short story or narrative on a topic.
  m. Functional writing tasks such as writing one's address, telephone number or family members' names.
  n. Written production should be evaluated similarly to the way verbal expression was evaluated.
     (1) Is there evidence of lexical retrieval difficulty?
     (2) What types of spelling errors are made?
     (3) Is there evidence of agrammatism in the writing (e.g., omitted functor words, lack of morphological endings, poor syntax)?
     (4) Are there paragraphic errors (written paraphasias)? What types (semantic, phonological, orthographic)?
     (5) Is writing particularly worse or better than oral-verbal expression?

Cognitive Assessment of PWA

1. Cognitive assessment of PWA should also be part of the overall evaluation, and a comprehensive assessment of cognition is usually conducted by a psychologist or neuropsychologist or behavioral neurologist, not by a SLP.
2. Language is an important part of cognition, and it also interacts with other nonlinguistic cognitive functions such as memory, attention, executive functioning and visuospatial functioning.
3. Therefore, assessment of these other areas will greatly enhance understanding of the behavior of a PWA, particularly because, in many instances, PWA also show degrees of impairment in these other areas.
4. Formal measures for the assessment of cognition include the Wechsler Adult Intelligence Scale, 4th edition (WAIS-IV; Wechsler, 2008); the Wechsler Memory Scale, 4th edition (WMS-IV, 2008); the Cognitive Linguistic Quick Test (CLQT; Helm-Estabrooks, 2001); the Ravens

Coloured Progressive Matrices (Raven, Raven, & Court, 2004); and many others.
   a. Many of these formal measures, such as the WAIS, are only available to psychologists.
   b. The CLQT was designed to be used by SLPs as well as other professionals.
5. Patterns of impairments in nonlinguistic functions assessed by these formal measures are highly variable across individuals and depend on numerous factors, including lesion location, additional medical factors or preexisting conditions, personal history of premorbid learning disabilities, etc.
6. Nevertheless, some common patterns of nonlinguistic cognitive impairments and areas of preservation in PWA may be seen:
   a. Some degree of impairment in executive functioning, particularly in those with lesions affecting the frontal lobe.
   b. Relatively intact nonverbal memory functions, although verbal memory may appear to be impaired due to the aphasia.
      (1) PWA often show reduced working memory capacity, particularly for verbal material but also sometimes for visual material.
      (2) Working memory (WM) requires the individual to hold information in memory for a short time period and to perform some manipulation of the information.
         (a) A standard working memory task is "digits backward" where the individual must listen to a series of digits spoken by the examiner and then tell them back in the reverse order.
         (b) PWA may have difficulty with this task due to their verbal expression deficits separate from a deficit in WM.
   c. Visuospatial functioning is relatively preserved but shows a characteristic pattern in visuoconstruction tasks such as drawing.
      (1) Drawings display good outer configurations but may be lacking in internal details (opposite of the pattern seen in those with right-hemisphere strokes).
      (2) PWA who have posterior involvement of visual pathways in the left hemisphere may have either a hemianopsia (right visual field cut) or some degree of visual inattention to the right side of space.

Limb and Oral-Facial Praxis Assessment

1. Assessment of limb and oral-facial praxis should be part of the comprehensive examination because presence of limb and/or oral apraxia may affect performance on a number of tasks especially if the PWA is asked to follow commands.
2. Modalities of assessment.
   a. Verbal command of the examiner, e.g., "Show me how you would wave goodbye."
   b. Imitation of the movement made by the examiner.
   c. Performing the action to command with an actual object.
3. Body regions to assess.
   a. Limb movements involving the arm and hand.
   b. Oral-facial (e.g., "Stick out your tongue"; "Show me how you would blow out a match"; "Show me how you would cough").
   c. Axial (midline or whole-body postures) (e.g., "Lean forward"; "Stand up"; "Stand like a boxer").
      (1) Axial movements tend to be better preserved than other types of movements to command.
4. PWA may have limb apraxia and not oral/facial apraxia or vice versa.
5. The left hemisphere is dominant for praxis just as it is dominant for language; therefore, it is common for PWA to have limb and/or oral-facial apraxia.

Multicultural Considerations for Assessment of Aphasia

1. Approximately 45,000 new bilingual aphasia cases are expected per year in the United States.
2. When working with multilingual PWA, SLPs need to determine what language(s) was their dominant language pre-aphasia.
   a. Ask the PWA to indicate their self-perception of their facility with each language.
   b. Determine what language(s) were used for various daily life activities such as at work, at school, socializing at home, for reading and writing.
   c. If possible, use a formal assessment such as the Bilingual Aphasia Test (BAT) (see below) to ensure an accurate picture of the strengths and weaknesses within each language.
      (1) PWA may be unaware of which of their languages is more impaired after onset of aphasia.
      (2) If the SLP only speaks one of the languages of the PWA, the SLP may wrongly perceive that the other language(s) is either less or more impaired than it really is.
      (3) SLPs should not attribute differences between the languages to brain damage, as they may already have differed premorbidly.
      (4) SLPs need to understand relative deficits across languages to determine which languages to include in therapy and to identify specific goals within each language.

(5) Treatment should be provided in the language requested by PWA and their family.
d. Ideally, an SLP who is fluent in the language being assessed will conduct the assessment.
  (1) Interpreter services may be used in some clinical settings if available.
  (2) It is not recommended that family members be used as language testers, but family impressions of the language of the PWA and reports of language behaviors are valuable.
e. The Bilingual Aphasia Test was developed by Michel Paradis and colleagues (see Paradis, 2001) and is available in many different languages online at: http://www.mcgill.ca/linguistics/research/bat/.
  (1) The BAT consists of three main parts:
    (a) Part A: evaluation of the PWA's multilingual history.
    (b) Part B: systematic and comparable assessment of the language disorder in each language known by the subject.
    (c) Part C: assessment of translation abilities and interference detection in each language.
  (2) The BAT is currently available in 65 languages (Part B) and 160 language pairs (Part C).
  (3) Parts B and C of this test have not simply been translated into different languages, but rather adapted across languages.
f. Versions of other standardized aphasia tests such as the BDAE and the WAB also are available in other languages.
g. Caution should be observed in simply translating a standardized test from one language to another. Language and content need to be culturally appropriate as well.
3. Besides multilingualism, the SLP should remain sensitive to other cultural differences in PWA who are being assessed, such as differences in ethnic background, religion, place of origin, sexual orientation, etc.
4. Adaptations to assessment protocols and procedures may need to be made to address cultural differences.

Classification of Aphasia

The Boston Classification System

1. Numerous classification systems exist for describing the various common syndromes of aphasia. Perhaps the best-known system is the Boston classification system that is described in the BDAE by Goodglass and colleagues.
2. The Boston classification system has seven aphasia syndromes, each determined by a unique profile of three language characteristics: 1) fluency of verbal output (fluent or nonfluent), 2) auditory comprehension (relatively impaired or relatively spared), and 3) verbal repetition abilities (relatively impaired or relatively spared). See Table 12-1 for each of these profiles.
   a. *Important*: The seven syndromes are NOT based on lesion location; rather, they are determined by the linguistic profiles.
   b. There are three nonfluent syndromes: Broca's aphasia, transcortical motor aphasia and global aphasia.
   c. There are four fluent syndromes: Wernicke's aphasia, transcortical sensory aphasia, conduction aphasia and anomic aphasia.
   d. Detailed profiles of the seven syndromes, including typical lesion location and other associated features, are presented in Table 12-2.

Table 12-1

Language Profiles of the Seven Aphasia Syndromes of the Boston Classification System ("Plus" = relatively preserved; "Minus" = relatively impaired.)

SYNDROME	FLUENT (F) OR NONFLUENT (NF)	AUDITORY COMPREHENSION	REPETITION
Broca's Aphasia	NF	+	−
Transcortical Motor Aphasia	NF	+	+
Global Aphasia	NF	−	−
Wernicke's Aphasia	F	−	−
Transcortical Sensory Aphasia	F	−	+
Conduction Aphasia	F	+	−
Anomic Aphasia	F	+	+

Table 12-2

Detailed Profiles of the Seven Aphasia Syndromes of the Boston Classification System

	APHASIA SYNDROME	LANGUAGE FEATURES	COMMON LESION LOCATION AND ASSOCIATED NEUROLOGICAL DEFICITS
Nonfluent	Broca's Aphasia	Nonfluent, effortful, sparse verbal output with short phrase length; agrammatism, telegraphic, omission of functor words; impaired articulation, prosody and melodic line; relatively preserved auditory comprehension, but difficulty with complex syntax; deep dyslexia; poor repetition; aware of errors; range of severities.	A large frontal lobe lesion affecting Broca's area and surrounding cortical regions as well as white matter deep to Broca's area. Often a right hemiparesis. Often has apraxia of speech; May have dysarthria.
	Transcortical Motor Aphasia	Nonfluent, sparse output; difficulty initiating and organizing verbal responses; fair to good articulation; few paraphasias; relatively preserved auditory comprehension; strikingly preserved repetition.	A frontal lobe lesion often anterior and/or superior to Broca's area, sometimes in the territory of the ACA or in border zone between MCA and ACA; may involve supplementary motor area. Motor inertia for nonspeech activities also.
	Global Aphasia	Nonfluent, severely restricted output, phrases of one word or less or verbal stereotypy; may use "swear" words; preservation of vocal intonation for affective expression; poor auditory comprehension; all language modalities impaired; may have no ability to read or write.	A large lesion affecting the frontal, parietal and temporal lobes, or a smaller deep lesion affecting pathways from both anterior and posterior language regions. Usually a right hemiparesis. May have visual deficits if occipital lobe pathways are affected.
Fluent	Wernicke's Aphasia	Fluent, well-articulated, paraphasic, circumlocutory, anomic verbal output results in empty speech; may have neologistic jargon; may have excess (press of) speech; poor auditory comprehension (A/C); may show better reading comprehension (R/C) than A/C; letter-by-letter oral reading; exceedingly poor repetition.	A lesion affecting Wernicke's area in the temporal lobe, often with extension into other temporal regions and parietal lobe. Usually no motor deficits. May have visual deficits if occipital lobe pathways also affected.
	Conduction Aphasia	Fluent, paraphasic output, with primarily phonemic paraphasias; strings of successive attempts to self-correct (conduit d'approche); may seem hesitant and sometimes not fluent as a result; relatively good auditory comprehension; strikingly poor repetition.	Lesion in the supramarginal gyrus region of parietal/temporal lobe junction or deep to it, or in arcuate fasciculus.
	Transcortical Sensory Aphasia	Verbal output similar to Wernicke's except repetition is preserved; fluent, paraphasic, neologistic output; poor auditory comprehension; strikingly preserved repetition; echoes examiner's words; preservation of overlearned material such as Lord's Prayer; rare syndrome.	Border zone regions of the middle cerebral artery-posterior cerebral artery territories, sparing Wernicke's area.
	Anomic Aphasia	Fluent, well-articulated, but anomic output; empty speech with lack of content words; overuse of indefinite terms like "thing" and "place"; relatively preserved auditory comprehension; preserved repetition.	A variety of lesion locations, often in posterior language regions, but sometimes in frontal lobe.

e. An eighth syndrome, known as mixed nonfluent aphasia, refers to a severe nonfluent syndrome in which auditory comprehension has improved beyond the level of global aphasia but is not good enough to qualify as relatively preserved, as in Broca's aphasia.

f. Subcortical aphasia syndromes have also been identified. Unlike the seven cortical syndromes, the subcortical syndromes are named for their lesion locations. See Table 12-3 for more detailed profiles of these four syndromes.
  (1) Anterior capsular-putaminal aphasia.
  (2) Posterior capsular-putaminal aphasia.
  (3) Global capsular-putaminal aphasia.
  (4) Thalamic aphasia.

Table 12-3

The Four Subcortical Aphasia Syndromes

APHASIA SYNDROME	LANGUAGE FEATURES	COMMON LESION LOCATION AND ASSOCIATED NEUROLOGICAL DEFICITS
Anterior Capsular-Putaminal Aphasia	Features of both Broca's aphasia and TCM; sparse output, reduced phrase lengths, severely reduced articulation (these like Broca's aphasia); agrammatism is NOT prominent, relatively good syntax, and preserved repetition (these like TCM); hypophonic (low volume) speech; good auditory comprehension.	Lesion in anterior part of the internal capsule and putamen. Frequently a hemiplegia.
Posterior Capsular-Putaminal Aphasia	Features of both anterior and posterior aphasias because some pathways from cortex of Wernicke's area and motor pathways from motor cortex are interrupted; fluent, poor repetition, poor A/C; good articulatory agility (these features like a posterior aphasia case). Therefore, if PWA comes in with a fluent type of aphasia and yet they are hemiplegic and in a wheelchair, you might suspect a subcortical lesion site in the posterior internal capsule/putamen.	Lesion in the posterior part of the internal capsule and the putamen. Frequently hemiplegia (like an anterior aphasia case).
Global Capsular-Putaminal Aphasia	Global type of aphasia with severe impairments in all language modalities; poor A/C; little or no verbal output. Pathways interrupted from both anterior and posterior cortical language areas.	Lesion in both the anterior and posterior portions of the internal capsule and the putamen. Often hemiplegia (but not always, if motor pathways happen to be spared).
Thalamic Aphasia	Features of transcortical sensory or W's aphasia; generally fluent; repetition relatively good; sometimes see echolalia; semantic paraphasia; way off-target paraphasias as in extended English jargon.; poor word-finding; perseveration; attention deficits. Quick tip: May look like Wernicke's or TCS but with better A/C.	Lesion in the thalamus; more likely a hemorrhage than an occlusive infarct. With or without hemiplegia depending on specific pathways affected.

Expressive Aphasia and Receptive Aphasia

1. An earlier classification system that originated in the 1930s used the dichotomy of expressive aphasia and receptive aphasia. Some professionals still use this terminology, but for SLPs, use of these terms is NOT preferred for these reasons:
   a. Most individuals with aphasia have linguistic deficits involving both expression and reception (comprehension of language).
   b. Two individuals given the label of "expressive aphasia" may be exceedingly different (e.g., the expressive difficulties associated with Broca's aphasia are very different from the expressive difficulties associated with Wernicke's aphasia, yet both involve significant problems in expression of language).
   c. Likewise, two individuals given the label "receptive aphasia" may be exceedingly different.
   d. Thus, these terms tend to obscure rather than clarify the deficit.

Neuropsychological Models Classification

1. In recent years, use of the "syndromes" approach to classification of aphasia described above in the section on the Boston Classification system has received criticism. Why?
   a. Grouping together characteristics of PWA and labeling these as a "syndrome" does not help to explain the underlying cognitive mechanisms of the linguistic disorder.
   b. PWA all grouped under the heading of one syndrome (e.g., Broca's aphasia) may have widely variable profiles of strengths and weaknesses, as well as severities.
   c. Treatment approaches might be individualized in a more meaningful way if the examiner was able to obtain a more thorough understanding of the cognitive processes underlying task performances.
2. Therefore, some clinical and research SLPs have begun using an approach based on cognitive neuropsychological models such as the one in Figure 12-3.
   a. The aim of the assessment is thus to determine which of the cognitive processes depicted in the "boxes" and "arrows" of the model seem to be relatively intact or impaired in the PWA.
   b. If this can be clarified, then there is a rationale for which processes the SLP would target for treatment.
   c. In general, this approach is more successful for individuals with less severe impairments or those who have isolated impairments than it is for those with severe forms of aphasia and multiple impaired cognitive processes.

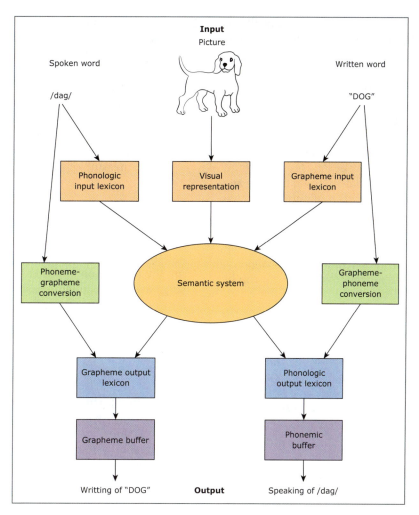

Figure 12-3 Sample neuropsychological model of lexical processing used for tasks of writing to dictation, picture naming and reading aloud in PWA.

Based on Beeson and Hillis, in Chapey, 2001, p. 573.

Psychosocial Effects of Aphasia on the Individual and the Family

Alleviating Havoc Wrought by Aphasia

1. Helping to alleviate some of the havoc wrought by aphasia in the psychosocial sphere needs to be a priority of every clinician.
2. Psychosocial effects may arise from:
   a. Organic causes: the brain damage that causes aphasia also has characteristic effects on emotional/psychological behavior.
      (1) Left-frontal lesions are associated with depression, catastrophic reactions and sometimes indifference/apathy (from prefrontal lesions).
      (2) Left-posterior lesions are associated with unawareness, agitation, occasionally paranoia and very rarely euphoria.
      (3) Left-hemisphere lesions are also associated with catastrophic reactions:
         (a) A behavioral state in which the PWA switches suddenly, and often violently, into a state of intense negativity.
         (b) Catastrophic reactions are not under voluntary control.
         (c) Usually last no more than a few days and are somewhat rare.
         (d) Goldstein (1948) associated catastrophic reactions with a "loss of the abstract attitude" that was seen in PWA.

b. Reactive causes: people with acute onset of illness have emotional/behavioral reactions to their newly acquired disorders.
   (1) Increased egocentrism and what appears to be reduced concern for others.
   (2) Increased concretism and need for routine.
   (3) Withdrawal from social contact that leads to social isolation.
   (4) Emotional lability such that the threshold for emotional spillover may be lowered. If extreme, this may be a sign of bilateral brain damage and is not part of the "reaction" but rather likely has an organic cause.
   (5) Anxiety and fear about having another stroke.
   (6) Frustration, anger or embarrassment.
   (7) Guilt because of life and family role changes.
      (a) Involuntary removal of work, which can be devastating.
      (b) Familial roles may be shifted—who takes care of finances, caretaking, cooking, driving, etc.
      (c) Loss of a conversational partner to talk over events of the day.
      (d) Changes in parent-child relationships. Children may be forced into a caregiver role, rather than being recipients of care.

Assessment of Psychological State in PWA

1. It is often difficult to assess psychiatric and emotional disturbances in people with significant communication disorders because talking and answering questions is often integral to psychological assessment.
2. Visual analog mood scales for different emotions (e.g., sad, happy, angry) have been created to accommodate some of these difficulties.
   a. The scales have a "neutral" schematic face (and accompanying word) at the top of a 100-mm vertical line and a specific "mood" face (and word) at the bottom of the line.
   b. People are asked to indicate how they are feeling by placing a mark on the line, which provides a quantitative measure of the emotional state in mm.

Reactions to Aphasia

1. Reactions to a major change such as a stroke and aphasia may be understood as a period of mourning the loss of one's former life. Stages of mourning suggested by E. Kubler-Ross in mourning the death of a loved one may also apply to PWA as they adjust to their new life.
   a. Denial: The PWA and family members are in shock and often feel numb.
   b. Anger: The PWA feels anger about the events and questions, "Why me?"
   c. Bargaining: The PWA attempts to bargain, "If I just do X, then I will recover."
   d. Depression: Denial and anger have subsided and the reality of the situation sets in.
   e. Acceptance: The PWA is able to acknowledge the reality of the situation and can go on with life.
      (1) The SLP is an important part of the support system to help the PWA and family members reach the acceptance stage.
      (2) Referrals to psychological professionals may be required, however, if there appears to be a persistent depression or other psychological disturbance.

Treatment of Aphasia

General Treatment Considerations

1. Impairment-based vs. non-impairment-based treatment.
   a. Impairment-based treatments are those that target a specific impairment of language and attempt to improve the language skill, thereby lessening the impairment. The majority of treatments for aphasia are of this type (e.g., using Melodic Intonation Therapy [MIT] to increase phrase lengths and word production).
      (1) Some treatment approaches attempt to fix the underlying deficit leading to the communication problem (e.g., directly working on verbal expression of grammatical forms).
      (2) Other treatment approaches compensate for the deficit either because it is unlikely to be "fixable" or a compensatory means to communicate is preferable (e.g., learning to use a system of manual gestures to communicate).
      (3) Both of these are still focused on the impairments associated with the aphasia.

(4) Both fix-it and compensatory approaches may be simultaneously implemented as elements of a treatment plan.
  b. Non-impairment-based treatments seek to improve the communication environment of PWA and their quality of life without directly addressing the language deficits leading to the impairments. (See later section on community-based treatment approaches.)
    (1) Non-impairment-based treatments have gained in popularity over the last 20 years.
    (2) They may also be referred to as indirect treatments.
2. General goals for treatment of aphasia.
  a. Improve communication skills either by fixing the deficit, compensating for it or both.
  b. Maintain achievements once improvements have been achieved.
  c. Facilitate the PWA's psychosocial and emotional adjustment to the new onset of aphasia.
3. When should therapy begin?
  a. For PWA who have just developed aphasia and are in the acute stage, therapy can begin as soon as they are medically stable.
  b. Keep in mind that diaschisis is operating in the acute phase.
    (1) Diaschisis is a temporary loss of function and electrical activity in brain regions remote from the lesion but connected via neural networks (i.e., not actually damaged, but temporarily dysfunctional).
    (2) Deficits in some functions may appear worse than they will be within a few weeks, after diaschisis is over.
  c. Clinicians often try to "harness" spontaneous recovery by treating vigorously in the first 6-month period post onset.
    (1) Spontaneous recovery starts to take place after diaschisis fades.
    (2) Spontaneous recovery implies that most PWA will show some natural recovery of functions even without treatment.
  d. However, research evidence shows PWA will respond to treatment regardless of time post onset (even after many years) if the treatment is appropriately selected and administered.
4. Measuring treatment effectiveness.
  a. SLPs follow the principles of evidence-based practice (EBP) when working with PWA.
    (1) They carefully select which treatments to administer based on prior research evidence, the concerns of the PWA and their family, and their own clinical experiences. See Chapter 4 on evidence-based practice.
    (2) They carefully and objectively measure the effects of the treatment they provide to each PWA.
    (3) SLPs measure performance at baseline, during treatment, and at the completion of treatment using appropriate measures of the desired outcome variables.
5. General descriptions of direct impairment-based treatment approaches.
  a. Multi-modality stimulation and response approaches.
    (1) Multi-modality input with pairing of two modalities followed by fading out of one. The clinician presents a stimulus in two modalities (e.g., spoken and written) then gradually fades out one of the modalities (e.g., written) as performance improves on the other modality.
    (2) Multi-modality output requiring multiple functions per word. The task requires the PWA to produce a response in multiple modalities with the expectation that one modality may stimulate performance in another (e.g., drawing a picture of an item while also attempting to say the name of it).
    (3) Deblocking: An unblocked modality is used to deblock a blocked modality (e.g., asking the PWA to complete a verbal repetition task first, and then asking the patient to name the same items, in the hope that naming may be achieved more easily).
  b. Intersystemic reorganization is a notion from the Russian aphasiologist A.R. Luria (1970) in which an intact function, which is not normally involved in the impaired function, is introduced into the operation of the function.
    (1) Using a written scaffold of three columns on a piece of paper to help a PWA create sentences with a subject (first column), plus a verb (second column) and an object (third column).
    (2) Melodic Intonation Therapy is another example of intersystemic reorganization because it uses intoning and hand tapping to assist verbal expression.
  c. Divergent therapies involve zeroing in on or converging on a specific target word in a treatment task item. Divergent therapies allow the PWA to come up with their own words.
    (1) In a divergent therapy approach, the SLP accepts a wider range of responses from the PWA's own verbal repertoire.
    (2) Research has shown this approach may result in better generalization of treatment effects than convergent therapies.
    (3) Response Elaboration Therapy (RET), for example, by Kearns and colleagues (1985, 1989):
      (a) Targets verbal expression with the goal of increasing phrase lengths and lexical retrieval.

(b) Clinician shows a picture and asks for any related response from the PWA.
  (c) Follow-up with a series of wh-questions to probe for longer and longer chaining of phrases. See Table 12-4.
 d. Pragmatic approaches: A variety of treatment approaches fall under the heading of pragmatic approaches.
  (1) Overall communication is the goal; therefore, encourage any modality of expression by the PWA.
  (2) Compromise on linguistic accuracy if the idea was communicated successfully.
  (3) Change the environment to make communication more successful.
  (4) Concern for transfer outside the clinic is built into the treatment.
  (5) Set up tasks so that they adhere to the four PACE principles: Promoting Aphasics' Communicative Effectiveness (Davis & Wilcox, 1981).
   (a) The clinician and PWA participate equally as senders and receivers of messages.
   (b) There is an exchange of new, previously unknown information by both parties.
   (c) The PWA has a free choice of communication modalities to use for expression (speaking, writing, gesturing, drawing or using a communication assistive device).
   (d) The clinician provides feedback as a receiver that lets the PWA know whether the message was adequately conveyed.

Table 12-4

An Example from the Verbal Expression Treatment Method Called Response Elaboration Therapy (RET)

Present a stimulus picture, for example, a line drawing of a figure kicking a ball.

Clinician:	Tell me what you can about this picture. What does it make you think of?
PWA:	Soccer.
Clinician:	Right! Who is playing soccer?
PWA:	My son...soccer.
Clinician:	Your son played soccer? Tell me more. When was that?
PWA:	High school.
Clinician:	Your son played soccer in high school. Where was his high school?
PWA:	Weymouth.
Clinician:	Oh your son played soccer in high school in Weymouth. Can you try to say that whole thing?
PWA:	Son... soccer... in high school...Weymouth.

Present the next stimulus picture and continue in this fashion.

Multicultural Considerations for Treatment of Aphasia

1. Treatment of PWA who are bilingual or multilingual.
   a. Generally treatment should be provided in the language desired by the PWA and their family, not simply the SLP's most proficient language.
   b. Cross-language generalization of effects from the treated language to untreated language(s) has been seen in research studies.
   c. Future investigations are needed to define, more precisely, factors promoting or inhibiting generalization from one language to another.
   d. In general, SLPs can be reassured that they are not hampering bilingual recovery when providing direct treatment in only a single language.
2. Recovery patterns seen in bilingual and multilingual PWA.
   a. Parallel recovery refers to the pattern seen in approximately 40% of bilingual aphasia cases, in which the extent to which languages recover is consistent with their premorbid patterns: If one language was stronger premorbidly, it would recover to being stronger.
   b. Differential recovery refers to the pattern in which one language recovers to a much greater extent than the other compared to premorbid abilities with the languages.
   c. Antagonistic recovery refers to a pattern in which one language is initially available, yet as the other language recovers, the initially available language becomes less accessible.
   d. Blending recovery refers to a pattern in which there is uncontrolled mixing of words and grammatical constructions of two or more languages when attempting to speak in only one language.
   e. Selective aphasia refers to the rare pattern in which there is language loss in one language with no measurable deficit in the other.
3. Using interpreters in treatment is often required when working with bilingual or multilingual PWA.
   a. An interpreter is a person specially trained to transpose oral or signed text from one language to another.
   b. Good interpreters need to be able to say the same things in different ways, shift styles easily, retain chunks of information while interpreting and have familiarity with medical, educational and professional terminology.
   c. Ideally, professional interpreters should be used rather than friends or family members. Professional interpreters are expected to maintain neutrality, respect confidentiality, interpret faithfully and participate in ongoing learning.

d. Before working with the PWA, the SLP should meet with the interpreter.
   (1) Both parties should discuss the purpose of the session, nature of the case and the format and goals for the session.
   (2) They should agree on the best physical arrangement for the session.
   (3) The interpreter should be made familiar with the test protocols and treatment tasks to be presented and the need to interpret verbal output as close to the original as possible (e.g., identifying phonological errors or instances of agrammatism).
   (4) The clinician should plan for a longer session with the PWA so as to allow time for the interpreting process and subsequent meeting with the interpreter.
   (5) The clinician should brief the interpreter on the different types of communication impairments that may be present.
   (6) When using an interpreter, the SLP should talk directly to the PWA, not the interpreter.
      (a) The SLP should maintain eye contact and use the second person (e.g., "Tell me what problems you are having" rather than "Ask them what problems they are having").
      (b) The SLP should explain to the PWA the reason for using an interpreter in the session.
4. The National Aphasia Association (NAA), www.aphasia.org, has several resources from its Multicultural Task Force available on its website.

Specific Treatments for Improving Verbal Expression

1. Response Elaboration Therapy (RET) (described above and in Table 12-4).
2. Voluntary Control of Involuntary Utterances (VCIU), a method that uses oral reading to improve production of single words to communicate ideas in people with severe aphasia (Helm-Estabrooks & Albert, 2004).
   a. Candidacy for VCIU.
      (1) People with severe nonfluent aphasia who have at least a few real words that they produce spontaneously.
      (2) It is not appropriate for totally nonverbal PWA or those with moderate or mild nonfluent aphasia.
      (3) The PWA can read at least one or two words aloud during the assessment and have some limited preservation of reading comprehension as seen in their ability to match written words to pictures.
   b. Procedures used for VCIU.
      (1) Use words the PWA has been heard to utter as the starting set of stimuli; expand with personally relevant names and emotional words.
      (2) Present a written stimulus word on a card and ask the PWA to try to read it. If the response is correct, keep that word in the VCIU "deck."
      (3) If the response is an error but it is a real word, write down that error and use that as the next stimulus. See Table 12-5.
      (4) Continue to expand the list by repeated trials of new words.
      (5) After the PWA has mastered a set of words, change the task to a confrontation naming task by putting pictures on the back sides of the word cards in the VCIU deck and ask the PWA to name them.
      (6) Build up to a vocabulary set of 100 to 200 words that can be orally read and named to confrontation consistently.
      (7) Proceed to more conversational tasks with the words on the list and, if possible, work on production of 2- to 3-word phrases using words on the list.
3. MIT is a method that uses a combination of intoning of phrases, hand tapping, and verbal repetition to improve verbal output. Sparks, Helm and Albert (1973) were the originators of the method.
   a. MIT is based on clinical observations that some PWA could say words much better while singing over learned songs than when they tried to speak conversationally.

Table 12-5

Sample Initial Session of Voluntary Control of Involuntary Utterances (VCIU)

Task: Present a written word on a card and ask the PWA to read what it is.

WRITTEN STIMULUS	PWA'S RESPONSE	ACTION
man	"mom"	discard man
Mom	"mom"	keep
hi	"hi"	keep
baby	"boy"	discard baby
boy	"boy"	keep
two	"two"	keep
love	"two"	discard love
Boston	"Boston"	keep
beer	"beer"	keep
OK	"OK"	keep
baseball	"Red Sox"	discard baseball
Red Sox	"Red Sox"	keep

Continue in this fashion, trying different words to get a set that the PWA is consistently able to read correctly, while using any real word "errors" produced by the PWA as the next stimulus item.

b. MIT is based on the hypothesis that singing and melody production are primarily controlled by the right hemisphere, which is not damaged, and therefore perhaps this nondamaged function of singing could be exploited to assist the production of meaningful verbal output.
c. Although specific target words and phrases are used, the aim of MIT is not to train production of just those specific stimulus items but rather to stimulate the language system for verbal expression in general.
d. MIT has been the subject of numerous research studies, many of which have shown it to be an effective method for improving verbal output in PWA.
e. Candidacy for MIT. Research has indicated that good candidates have the following characteristics:
   (1) Etiology of stroke and nonfluent aphasia or severely restricted verbal output such as a verbal stereotypy only.
   (2) Relatively good auditory comprehension, poor verbal repetition and poor articulatory agility (i.e., people with Broca's aphasia).
   (3) No lesion in the right hemisphere.
f. Selection of target stimuli.
   (1) High-probability words and phrases as well as emotional words.
   (2) Functionally useful words and phrases (e.g., family names, places).
   (3) Phonologically simple at first (e.g., no consonant clusters, at most two-syllable words).
g. Procedures for initial stimulus presentation.
   (1) Present each target phrase with continuous voicing, using a simple high note and low note pattern (two tones only), presented with the stress pattern of normal speech (i.e., the higher tone should be used for stressed syllables).
   (2) Pick up the PWA's left hand and tap it once on the table for each syllable.
   (3) Control the PWA's behavior with your other hand to let them know when to speak and when to wait.
h. The complete levels and steps of the MIT program are presented in Table 12-6.
4. Treatments for agrammatism in aphasia.
   a. Treatment of Underlying Forms (TUF; Thompson and Shapiro, 2007) is based on the idea that treatment of grammatical deficits should focus on remediation of the underlying linguistic deficit.
      (1) Developed from linguistic theories explaining how surface sentences are derived from underlying "deep" structures.
      (2) Thompson's research shows that if more complex forms are treated first, generalization

Table 12-6

Melodic Intonation Therapy Levels and Steps (C = Clinician; P = PWA)		
ELEMENTARY LEVEL*	**USE SHORT, PHONOLOGICALLY SIMPLE PHRASES**	**POSSIBLE SCORE**
Step 1: Humming	C hums the phrase using only two tones while lifting up and tapping P's hand once for each syllable. P just listens.	Not scored
Step 2: Unison singing	C intones the phrase and asks P to join in; may require a few trials until P produces most of the phrase.	1
Step 3: Unison with fading	Once P has been able to produce the phrase by intoning it, C fades out and asks P to continue the phrase.	1
Step 4: Immediate repetition	C intones the phrase while P just listens. Then P immediately intones it.	1
Step 5: Response to a question	C asks a question such as "What did you say?" and P replies with the intoned target phrase.	1
INTERMEDIATE LEVEL	**USE SLIGHTLY LONGER PHRASES AND IMPLEMENT DELAYS BETWEEN STIMULUS AND RESPONSE**	**POSSIBLE SCORE**
Step 1: Introducing the item	C intones the phrase and asks P to join in; may require a few trials until P produces most of the phrase.	Not scored
Step 2: Unison with fading	Once P has been able to produce the phrase by intoning it, C fades out and asks P to continue the phrase.	1
Step 3: Delayed repetition	C intones the phrase while P just listens. After a delay of 6 seconds of silence, P is asked to intone the phrase.	2 or 1 if a back-up to the previous step is required.
Step 4: Response to a question	C waits 6 seconds in silence and then asks a question such as "What did you say?" P replies with the intoned target phrase.	2 or 1 if a back-up to the previous step is required.

(Continued)

Table 12-6

Melodic Intonation Therapy Levels and Steps (C = Clinician; P = PWA) (Continued)

ADVANCED LEVEL	USE LONGER PHRASES WITH SOME PHONOLOGICAL COMPLEXITY. RETURN TO NORMAL SPEECH PROSODY VIA THE TRANSITIONAL SPRECHGESANG TECHNIQUE.	POSSIBLE SCORE
Step 1: Delayed repetition	C intones the phrase while P just listens. After a delay of 6 seconds of silence, P is asked to intone the phrase.	2 or 1 if a back-up to the previous step is required.
Step 2: Introducing sprechgesang, "Speech Song"	C presents the phrase with exaggerated prosody and continuously changing pitch as in choral speaking. P just listens.	Not scored.
Step 3: Sprechgesang with fading	C presents the phrase in sprechgesang and asks P to join in; once P has mastered the phrase in unison, C fades out and P continues the phrase.	2
Step 4: Delayed spoken repetition	C speaks the phrase using normal intonation and makes P wait 6 seconds before P attempts to repeat the phrase also using normal spoken intonation.	2
Step 5: Response to a question	C waits 6 seconds in silence and then asks a question such as "What did you say?" P replies with the spoken target phrase.	2

Note: If P is unable to complete a step at any level, the item is dropped and a new item is attempted at Step 1 of the current level.

Table 12-7

Procedures Used for a Sample What-Question Item of the Treatment of Underlying Forms Method

Target sentence: "What is Susan baking?"

1. Present entire written underlying form.

    | Susan is baking muffins |

2. Present underlying form on 4 index cards and explain about the verb, the subject noun phrase (NP) and the object noun phrase (NP).

    | Susan | is | baking | muffins |

3. Explain how the object NP (muffins) gets replaced by the word "what" and a question mark gets added.

    | Susan | is | baking | what | ? |

4. Examiner demonstrates subject/auxiliary inversion by moving the cards.

    | is | Susan | baking | what | ? |

5. Examiner demonstrates movement of "What" to sentence-initial position, resulting in the target question.

    | What | is | Susan | baking | ? |

6. PWA reads or repeats the question.
7. Cards are put back into the deep structure order.
8. Question cards are offered.
9. PWA repeats Steps 3–5 with assistance if needed

to simpler forms will be achieved without having to directly treat them.
   (a) This is known as the Complexity Account of Treatment Effectiveness (CATE).
   (b) For example, linguistic theory states that what-questions and who-questions share certain features. Therefore, if what-questions are treated, generalization to who-questions will automatically occur.

(3) The TUF procedure trains production of wh-question forms and other syntactic structures by bringing to conscious awareness the linguistic transformations that derive the sentences from underlying forms to surface structures.

(4) See Table 12-7 for the procedures used for a sample target item for Treatment of Underlying Forms.

Table 12-8

Sentence Types and Sample Items for the Sentence Production Program for Aphasia (SPPA)

SENTENCE TYPE	SAMPLE TARGET PHRASE	LEVEL A PROBE TO ELICIT THE PHRASE	LEVEL B PROBE TO ELICIT THE PHRASE
Type 1: Imperative Intransitive	Dive in.	Ginny doesn't like getting into cold water, so Charles says to her, "Dive in!" What does Charles tell her?	Ginny doesn't like getting into cold water, so what does Charles tell her?
Type 2: Imperative Transitive	Open the window.	It is very hot in the kitchen, so Mary says to Paul, "Open the window." What does Mary say to Paul?	It is very hot in the kitchen, so what does Mary tell Paul to do?
Type 3: Wh-interrogative What and Who Qs	Who is winning?	Frank sees Nick and Billy playing basketball, so he asks, "Who is winning?" What does he ask them?	Frank sees Nick and Billy playing basketball, so what does he ask them?
	What are you making?	Paul is busy in his workshop. Frank drops by and asks, "What are you making?" What does Frank ask?	Paul is busy in his workshop when Frank drops by. What does Frank ask?
Type 4: Wh-interrogative Where and When Qs	Where is the paper?	Mary wants to do the crossword puzzle, so she asks Paul, "Where is the paper?"	Mary wants to do the crossword puzzle, so what does she ask Paul?
	When are you leaving?	Shawna tells her mother that she has to go to softball practice. Her mother asks, "When are you leaving?" What does her mother ask?	Shawna tells her mother that she has to go to softball practice. What does her mother ask?
Type 5: Declarative Transitive	I make coffee.	When friends ask Charles what he does to help with breakfast, he says, "I make coffee." What does he say?	When friends ask Charles what he does to help with breakfast, what does he say?
Type 6: Declarative Intransitive	She works.	Whenever Angela is trying a big case, in the evening she works. What does Angela do in the evening when she has a big case?	When she has a big case, what does Angela do in the evening?
Type 7: Comparative	He's funnier.	Everyone wants Frank, not Ginny, to tell jokes because he's funnier. Why do people want Frank to tell jokes?	Why do people want Frank, and not Ginny, to tell jokes? It's because_____.
Type 8: Yes/No Questions	Is it raining?	Charles asks Ginny for the umbrella, so Ginny asks, "Is it raining?" What does she ask?	Charles asks Ginny for he umbrella, so what does she ask?
	Do you need money?	Frank is getting his wallet out to pay their restaurant bill, so Angela asks, "Do you need money?" What does she ask him?	Frank is getting his wallet out to pay their restaurant bill, so what does Angela ask him?

(5) In 2010, Thompson created a computer-automated version of this method called Sentactics®.

b. Sentence Production Program for Aphasia (SPPA; Helm-Estabrooks & Nicholas, 2000) is for nonfluent PWA who also present with a prominent agrammatism.
  (1) SPPA is based on an earlier research study that looked at the ease of production of 14 different sentence types by PWA.
  (2) Easier sentence types are treated first, before more difficult types.
  (3) SPPA is a structured treatment method to simulate production of sentence-level verbal output and to increase use of selected syntactic constructions.
  (4) Target sentences are presented in story scenarios and elicited first with direct repetition probes and then from memory.
  (5) There are 15 target stimulus items for each of 8 different sentence types. The sentence types and sample treatment items are presented in Table 12-8.

5. Constraint-Induced Language Therapy (CILT).
  a. CILT is also known as Constraint-Induced Aphasia Therapy (CIAT).
  b. It is based on constraint-induced movement therapy (CIMT) for stroke patients receiving physical therapy to improve functioning of a hemiparetic limb.
    (1) In CIMT, the nonparetic "good" limb is constrained from being used for a significant amount of time each day for many days by keeping it in a sling or other means of preventing its use.
    (2) This results in forced use of the "impaired" limb for functional everyday activities and theoretically prevents "learned nonuse" of that limb.

(3) People must have some movement to qualify for CIMT.
(4) Research shows improved functioning of the impaired limb as well as changes in functional brain imaging after CIMT.
c. In CILT, the "constraint" imposed is that the PWA must communicate via verbal expression. They are not allowed to use any compensatory means of expression such as gesturing or drawing.
d. The procedures used in CILT often use pairs or groups of PWA who engage in games like "Go Fish" in a barrier game format so that information must be communicated verbally.
e. The goals are personalized to the individual (e.g., single-word names vs. phrase-length descriptions).
f. Generally, treatment is administered on an intense treatment schedule known as massed practice.
g. Cueing/scaffolding is personalized to the individual's needs.
h. In a meta-analysis of CILT research studies, Cherney and colleagues (2008) concluded that while there was good evidence that CILT was effective, questions remained as to whether this may have been due primarily to the intensity of the treatment.

6. Oral Reading for Language in Aphasia (ORLA) is a method developed by Leora Cherney and colleagues (2004) that uses the task of reading aloud to stimulate improvements in language in PWA.
  a. Results of research studies indicated cross-modal generalization was seen after ORLA treatment: improvements in oral expression, auditory comprehension and written expression in both fluent and nonfluent aphasia.
  b. ORLA uses short phrases and/or sentence stimuli, depending on the needs of the PWA.
  c. For each stimulus there is a structured, step-by-step series of tasks presented in the following procedures (C = clinician and P = PWA):
    (1) C sits opposite P and reads stimulus aloud to P.
    (2) C reads stimulus aloud to P, with C and P pointing to each word.
    (3) C and P read aloud together, with P continuing to point to each word; C adjusts rate and volume. The motor movement of pointing to each word may be a critical component.
    (4) Above step is repeated twice.
    (5) For each line or sentence, C states word for P to identify (e.g., "Show me 'big,'" "Show me 'on'").
    (6) For each line or sentence, C points to word for P to read, pointing to both content and functor words.
    (7) P reads stimulus aloud; C reads aloud with P as needed.

7. AphasiaScripts (Rehabilitation Institute of Chicago, 2007; Cherney & colleagues, 2008) is a computer program with an avatar "clinician" who assists the PWA to practice a personalized verbal conversational script that the "real" clinician has put into the program.
  a. In their research using AphasiaScripts, Cherney and colleagues have created at least three scripts for each PWA: one is a monologue telling a personal story and the other two are dialogues.
  b. Scripts were up to 20 conversational turns long and were audio recorded on a laptop by the SLP.
  c. Procedures for the PWA to learn the script include:
    (1) Sentence and conversation practice. Reading the script aloud with the following cues:
      (a) Visual verbal: Words are highlighted on the screen.
      (b) Visual motor: Correct articulatory movements are seen on the avatar clinician's head.
      (c) Auditory: Words are heard.
    (2) Cues are removed in a step-by-step process in a fixed order.
    (3) The PWA practices the script at home, with the assistance of the virtual therapist if needed.
    (4) The PWA decides when to dispense the various types of cues and generally controls the pace of the script learning.

8. Other treatments for anomia.
  a. Lexical retrieval problems are difficult to treat because of the nature of the deficit, that is, access to words is generally inconsistent.
  b. It is not a question of simply relearning a new vocabulary item as in normal language acquisition in childhood.
  c. Two main approaches to anomia treatment are to facilitate naming via cueing or to compensate for word-finding impairments in other ways.
    (1) Facilitation of naming via cueing, using external cues from the clinician or, ideally, internal cues generated by PWA themselves.
      (a) External cueing hierarchies systematically provide cues from those most likely to elicit the response to those least likely to do so; over time, the cues are faded out.
      (b) Order of cues in the hierarchies will vary across individuals: what is helpful for one person may not be helpful for another.
      (c) Types of cues include phonemic cues, verbal descriptions, first-letter cues, automatic completions and repetition, among many others.
      (d) Internal (self) cueing procedures include reinforcing what the PWA already does to self-cue, such as gesture (e.g., write the first letter of a word in the air or on paper or give verbal descriptions).
      (e) Clinicians can experiment with various cloze techniques (e.g., provide a missing

word) and practice ones that may work; sometimes even a neutral frame such as "well, it's a____" will help elicit the word.
(2) Compensating for anomia by focusing on getting the idea across rather than finding a specific word.
 (a) Therapy may aim to improve the use of natural circumlocutions by having the PWA provide information in a structured format.
  • What does the thing look like?
  • What is it made of? What size is it?
  • What do you do with it? What does it do?
  • What category does it belong to?
  • What type of place might you get it?
 (b) Encourage the PWA to use nonverbal means to express the concept: gesture how it would be used; draw a picture of it; point to a representation of it in a communication notebook.
d. Some clinicians recommend avoiding "what's it called?" therapy approaches in which the therapist presents one picture at a time and asks the PWA to name it.
(1) This task requires the PWA repeatedly to do exactly the thing they have most difficulty with and it is often a recipe for failure and frustration.
(2) Instead, one suggestion is to use a more divergent approach, such as laying out a set of 4 or 6 cards and saying, "Tell me anything you can about any of these cards."
 (a) If the PWA is able to say something appropriate, take that card away and replace with a new card; then repeat.
 (b) Success rates over the same number of trials will be much higher than presenting one card at a time and requiring one specific target response at that specific time.
 (c) Avoid having to use leading cues like phonemic cues, which help retrieve the word but rarely generalize to improved independent retrieval.
e. Treatment for Aphasic Perseveration (TAP; Helm-Estabrooks & Albert, 2004) is an anomia treatment for people with significant verbal perseveration that focuses on increasing conscious awareness of perseverative behaviors so that PWA learn to inhibit perseverations.
(1) Focuses on assisting the PWA in consciously inhibiting perseverative verbal behavior and is premised on the notion that if perseveration can be blocked, then correct naming behavior may be released.
(2) Candidates for TAP are people who show significant verbal perseveration on naming tasks (usually recurrent perseveration).
(3) It is not appropriate for PWA who have too little verbal output and are unable to respond to any cues, or those in whom naming is not severely impaired, or those whose perseveration is only mild.
(4) The method uses a cueing hierarchy to stimulate production of the correct name if the PWA cannot produce it independently.
(5) Strategies for helping the PWA inhibit perseverations are the important feature of the TAP procedure.
 (a) Explain what perseveration is, then ask the PWA to overtly try to inhibit perseveration by saying, "Don't say that word again; either give me a different word or don't say anything at all."
 (b) Make a point of changing categories and switching sets of items overtly: "We're all done with colors; now we're moving to household objects."
 (c) Use visual representation of perseverative errors, such as writing the perseverated word on a piece of paper, tearing it up and leaving the torn paper in a pile on the table.
 (d) Implement silent intervals of at least 5 seconds between items, allowing time for memory traces to fade.
 (e) Use short-filled intervals of an unrelated activity between items, such as imitating simple arm or hand movements.
f. Verb Network Strengthening Treatment (VNeST; Edmonds & colleagues, 2008) is a treatment to improve lexical retrieval of content words in sentences, recognizing the key role of verbs and the fact that PWA often have trouble with verb retrieval.
(1) VNeST uses a notion of bidirectional priming: A verb primes its agents, patients and instruments (linguistic terms for subjects and objects) and vice versa.
(2) VNeST procedure:
 (a) Provide a written verb and have the PWA generate three "who's" and three "what's" that could be used with it. Write these words on cards.
 (b) Ask the PWA to arrange cards to generate agent-verb and verb-object pairs and then read word pairs aloud.
 (c) Answer wh-questions about these pairs and make semantic judgments of correct and incorrect sentences read aloud by SLP.
 (d) Generate phrases without cards.
(3) Research on treatment with VNeST has indicated significant improvements in spontaneous verbal output may result for people with moderate and severe aphasia.

Treatments for Other Language Modalities

1. General considerations for treatments of A/C impairments.
   a. Try to keep the treatment task pure; if auditory comprehension is the target of treatment, avoid tasks that are dependent on verbal expression, reading comprehension or writing.
   b. Sample approaches have included:
      (1) Working to improve auditory attention, e.g., in people with severe press of speech or in people with TBI.
         (a) Listening for a specific target in an array of spoken words.
      (2) Working to lessen the severity of the A/C impairment.
         (a) Listening to a word and pointing to a picture that matches it from an array.
         (b) Responding to yes/no questions.
         (c) Following commands of increasing complexity.
         (d) Using multi-modality stimulation: presenting a stimulus as both a spoken word and a written word, then fading out the written word as A/C starts to improve.
         (e) Using sentence-level comprehension tasks: matching a sentence to a picture.
         (f) Using paragraph-level comprehension tasks: answering yes/no questions about a story.
      (3) Educating the family about A/C deficits.
         (a) Family members often overestimate A/C ability and may not always recognize the extent of A/C impairment in the PWA.
         (b) Training family members to use multi-modality input by always supplementing what they say with gestures and written key words when conversing with the PWA is often useful.
2. Treatment of Wernicke's Aphasia (TWA) is a structured method designed to improve auditory comprehension in people with Wernicke's aphasia who have significant difficulty understanding spoken language (Helm-Estabrooks & Albert, 2004).
   a. TWA is based on the clinical observation that if people could repeat a word, they may be more likely to comprehend it.
   b. It uses a more intact modality (reading comprehension) to assist a less intact modality (auditory comprehension).
   c. TWA is also based on the notion of deblocking—correct auditory comprehension is primed by first participating in oral reading and repetition tasks.
   d. Good candidates.
      (1) Moderate to severe Wernicke's aphasia.
      (2) Relative preservation of reading comprehension of single words.
      (3) Poor verbal repetition (i.e., not appropriate for those with transcortical sensory aphasia).
   e. Procedures include these four steps per target item:
      (1) Reading comprehension: Match a printed word to a picture from an array (e.g., "Which of these four pictures goes with this word?") and then show the written word *lion*.
      (2) Oral reading, e.g., "Can you read the word out loud?"
      (3) Repetition, e.g., "Now say it after me. Lion."
      (4) Auditory comprehension, e.g., "Now, which of these pictures is a lion?"
   f. Incorrect verbal responses on the oral reading or repetition steps are noted and tried as stimuli in subsequent sessions.
   g. After about 100 or so words are mastered, pictures of minimal pair words are introduced and the same procedure is used.
3. Treatments for alexia and agraphia.
   a. Principles of treatment of aphasic alexias.
      (1) The first step in developing a treatment plan for aphasic reading disorders is to conduct a thorough assessment that provides a full understanding of which of the key language abilities required for reading are still preserved or impaired.
      (2) Acquired alexias associated with aphasia may be quite different from the developmental reading disorders seen in childhood because adults with aphasia had normally functioning language and typical vocabulary development prior to their stroke.
      (3) Many people with aphasia are no longer able to use phoneme-to-grapheme (PGC) or grapheme-to-phoneme (GPC) conversion rules that they had learned as children, because the neural networks most important to these functions may have been either partially or completely damaged.
      (4) Attempts to relearn these conversion rules may be futile, in which case compensatory means to read are preferred in treatment.
      (5) In other cases, some partial preservation of these "phonics"-related skills may be able to be harnessed within a treatment plan.
      (6) Nevertheless, some of the approaches that have proven useful for developmental reading difficulties, such as using a multisensory structured approach may be useful for PWA, depending on the nature of the alexia that is being addressed.
      (7) Often alexias and agraphias are treated together because many PWA will have similar problems with reading and writing.

b. Specific treatment approaches for aphasic alexia.
  (1) Multiple Oral Re-reading (Beeson & Hillis, 2008) is a method designed for LBL readers who have impaired access to words in the graphemic input lexicon.
    (a) Read aloud a short text passage many times.
    (b) Practice the same passage as homework.
    (c) The multiple trials of reading the same passage aloud facilitate a shift away from LBL reading to whole-word reading by taking advantage of sentence context and familiarity of text.
  (2) Use of visual supports is a common strategy for people with deep dyslexia and other forms of aphasic reading difficulty who do not have access to grapheme-phoneme conversion rules.
    (a) Pairing functor words with visual pictures (e.g., the letter "I" with an eye drawn on the top of it, then fading out the pictures over time) as the PWA masters some of these common functor words.
    (b) Similar visual supports can also be used with content words by embedding the letters in a word into a picture representing the meaning of the word and then fading out the picture supports as the PWA gains consistent recognition of the word.
  (3) For people with deep dyslexia, strategies involve using their partially preserved access to semantic knowledge to help further refine their ability to comprehend written language. Activities such as finding the best written synonym to match a given written word will force the PWA to carefully consider finer-grained semantic information in coming up with the best answer.
  (4) Drills involving matching single words or phrases to pictures, explaining the meanings of newspaper headlines, filling in blanks in written sentences, answering comprehension questions about a written paragraph, completing crossword puzzles and many more.
  (5) Compensatory approaches for aphasic alexia.
    (a) Using text-to-speech software that will read aloud highlighted text on a computer screen.
    (b) Using books on tape and other resources available for those with visually based reading impairments.
    (c) Reading "pens" that will read aloud text that the pen has scanned.
c. Principles of treatment of aphasic agraphias.
  (1) The primary reason writing is difficult is due to the language disorder and not to the motoric impediment of having to use the nondominant hand.
  (2) The first step in developing a treatment plan for aphasic writing disorders is to conduct a thorough assessment that provides a full understanding of which of the key language abilities required for writing are still preserved or impaired, including lexical retrieval, spelling and writing of letters.
  (3) As for alexias, PWA may not have access to phoneme-grapheme conversion rules and therefore may not be able to respond to drills requiring them to "write the letter that goes with the sound /b/," for example.
  (4) Whole-word, visually based approaches, learning to re-create the "configuration" of the word may, therefore, be more useful.
d. Specific treatment approaches for agraphia.
  (1) Anagram Copy and Recall Treatment (ACRT; Beeson & Hillis, 2008; Helm-Estabrooks & Albert, 2004) is a method for agraphia that aims to strengthen words in the graphemic output lexicon so that they can be used for functional writing.
    (a) Reinforces the visual and kinesthetic aspects of writing through drill.
    (b) PWA are given letter tiles and asked to arrange them to spell a target word correctly.
    (c) They write by copying the word three times.
    (d) The tiles are removed and they try to write the word from memory.
    (e) Words introduced are then given as homework and the task is to write them approximately five times each.
    (f) In research studies of ACRT, there has been minimal carryover to untrained words, so it is important to use functionally useful target words.
  (2) Other treatment approaches for writing involve fade sheets, where the PWA is given a sheet on which to fill in progressively more and more letters for a given target word; exercises requiring them to fill in words in blanks within a sentence; completion of crossword puzzles; practice using a keyboard and using a word processor; and many more.
  (3) Compensatory approaches for aphasic agraphia.
    (a) Speech-to-text software that will write words on a computer screen spoken by the PWA.
      • These programs are only useful for those with very mild aphasia or for those with "pure agraphia."
    (b) Assisted-writing software programs that will predict words based on the initial letters that a PWA has typed; only useful for those with fairly intact visual word recognition skills.

(c) Software programs that will write words associated with pictures that are selected; the PWA does not have to spell or think of the words, only select the pictures.
4. Alternative communication treatments are approaches focused on assisting the PWA in communicating via means other than verbal expression.
   a. Visual Action Therapy (VAT) is a method developed by Helm-Estabrooks, Fitzpatrick, and Barresi (1982) for people with severe aphasia as a means to treat limb apraxia so that manual gestural communication may be an option.
      (1) Candidates for VAT are people with global aphasia who may not be able to respond to verbal treatment and who have limb apraxia.
      (2) VAT is a highly structured multistep program that trains PWA to produce manual gestures that represent objects.
      (3) Instructions are all given via clinician demonstration, primarily in silence, so VAT is appropriate for people with severe auditory comprehension impairment.
      (4) VAT programs targeted at improving both limb and oral-facial apraxia have been developed.
      (5) Sample goal: PWA will produce clearly recognizable gesture to represent an object that is not in view in 7 to 8 trials.
   b. Amer-Ind Gestural Training was developed by Madge Skelly (1979) and is based on a system of manual gestures to communicate information from "Universal American Indian Hand Talk" (Rao, 1994).
      (1) Amer-Ind is a system of manual gestures to communicate concrete ideas for functional communication.
      (2) The gestures are generally transparent, which means that a conversational partner should understand the meaning without having to learn the system.
      (3) Most gestures are adaptable for one-handed production for those with hemiparesis.
      (4) Limitations to learning Amer-Ind for PWA include limb apraxia.
      (5) Training generally proceeds with recognition of gestures produced by the SLP, then imitation of gestures, then independent production of gestures in response to either a spoken or picture stimulus.
      (6) Later steps of Amer-Ind involve training combinations of gestures to produce 2- and 3-gesture combinations.
      (7) A rare PWA may be so proficient at gestural communication that he or she may be able to produce complex pantomimes, but this sort of individual is uncommon in clinical practice.

c. Computer-assisted communication for PWA includes devices and software programs that are examples of augmentative and alternative communication (AAC) approaches. See Chapter 17 on augmentative and alternative communication.
   (1) Because language is impaired in PWA, the software that is appropriate for AAC is usually a picture-based, rather than a text-based, system.
   (2) Most systems have a combination of preprogrammed phrases that PWA can select as well as individual pictured vocabulary items that can be selected to create multi-icon messages.
   (3) Careful organization of content is required in order to make navigation as easy as possible; the optimal organization system has not yet been determined.
   (4) Learning to use these systems effectively can take many months of intensive therapy, and not every person with severe aphasia is able to become an independent user.
   (5) Computer-assisted communication systems that have been used with PWA include (among others):
      (a) C-Speak Aphasia (Nicholas & Elliott, 1998; Nicholas & colleagues, 2011).
      (b) Dynavox (www.dynavoxtech.com).
      (c) Lingraphica (www.aphasia.com; Aftonomous & colleagues, 2001).
      (d) Proloquo2go (www.proloquo2go.com; AssistiveWare, 2009–2010).
      (e) SentenceShaper® (Psycholinguistic Technologies).
      (f) TouchSpeak (www.touchspeak.co.uk).
      (g) Visual Scene Displays (Hux & colleagues, 2010).
d. Communicative drawing approaches are appropriate for individuals with severe aphasia who show some ability to produce representational drawings to communicate information.
   (1) Several methods have been described, including Back to the Drawing Board (BDB; Morgan & Helm-Estabrooks, 1987) and Helm-Estabrooks' Communicative Drawing Program (CDP; Helm-Estabrooks & Albert, 2004).
   (2) Effective methods involve caregivers and family members so that the "conversation" using drawing is an interactive one with both parties contributing.
      (a) The BDB program trains drawing of people in action sequences rather than using object pictures. It uses uncaptioned cartoon stimuli with minimal extraneous details that are relatively simple to draw. For example, from a set of 5 one-panel cartoons, 5 two-panel cartoons and 5 three-panel cartoons,

the clinician begins training with one-panel cartoons.
- (b) Trial 1: The PWA is asked to look carefully at the picture, and then it is taken away and the PWA is asked to draw it from memory. If the drawing produced by the PWA is a good rendition with all important elements of the original, then the clinician goes on to the next picture.
- (c) Trial 2: If the drawing lacks clarity or enough detail, the deficiencies are discussed, how it could be drawn is demonstrated and the PWA copies the original or the PWA copies the clinician's model version.
- (d) Trial 3: The PWA is asked to try again from memory. If the drawing is now acceptable, the PWA moves to next item.
- (e) When 3 of 5 one-panel cartoons are acceptable from memory, the PWA moves on to the two-panel cartoons and repeats all steps.
- (f) When 3 of 5 two-panels are "good," the PWA moves on to three-panel cartoon stimuli and repeats all steps.

e. The 10 steps of the Communicative Drawing Program (CDP):
  (1) Basic semantic-conceptual knowledge: Circle the objects that go together.
  (2) Knowledge of object color properties: Color in items with correct colored markers.
  (3) Outlining pictures of objects with distinct shape properties.
  (4) Copying geometric shapes.
  (5) Completing drawings with missing external and internal features.
  (6) Drawing objects with characteristics shapes from memory.
  (7) Drawing objects to command from stored representations.
  (8) Drawing objects within superordinate categories.
  (9) Generative drawing: Animals and modes of transportation.
  (10) Drawing cartooned scenes.

f. Communication notebooks. Many SLPs create personalized communication notebooks for PWA who have limited ability to express themselves verbally.
  (1) Several communication notebooks are commercially available, but individualized homemade notebooks are preferred by PWA and are generally more functional.
  (2) The PWA points to pictures or words in the notebook to communicate needs or ideas.
  (3) Treatment to use a communication notebook successfully is usually required and includes much practice finding specific pages as well as vocabulary items in the therapy session and in real-life communication situations.
  (4) Tips for creating a communication notebook.
    (a) Use a standard personal organizer that already contains telephone, address and calendar pages.
    (b) Use pictures and words for each concept represented.
    (c) Keep it simple and include personally relevant concepts that PWA want to communicate about.
    (d) Provide some organizational tabs, but keep the organization as simple as possible.
    (e) Sample pages to include in a functional communication notebook are listed in Table 12-9.

5. Community-based treatment approaches for PWA have been gaining in popularity in recent years and represent a shift away from impairment-based treatment approaches towards the Life Participation Approach to Aphasia (LPAA) model (Chapey & colleagues, 2001).
  a. The focus of community-based approaches is on enhancing quality of life with aphasia, rather than on fixing the impairments associated with aphasia.
  b. The focus is on the PWA within their environment and not just on the aphasia itself.
  c. Many community-based treatment approaches are based on the five core values of the LPAA:
    (1) The explicit goal of intervention is enhancement of life participation.
    (2) All those affected by aphasia are entitled to service (includes family members and friends).

Table 12-9

Sample Pages to Include in a Personalized Communication Notebook for a PWA

1. First page: explanations for "I have aphasia…" and "Aphasia is…."
2. Emergency information including name, address, telephone numbers to call in case of an emergency.
3. Autobiographical information: family trees, family photos, personal history timelines
4. Occupation pages
5. Small versions of local, state, national, and world maps
6. Lists of local towns, favorite restaurants, frequented places (stores, etc.)—use logos for these if possible
7. Specialized pages depending on individual's needs and interests, e.g., a Red Sox page, a crafts page
8. Transportation page
9. Finances page
10. Sports page(s)
11. Pockets to keep mementos: ticket stubs, programs of events attended, etc.
12. Small pad of paper and a pen to draw
13. (Optional) Pages of object items in categories (e.g., food items, clothing items, personal care items)

(3) The measures of success of interventions must include documented life enhancement changes.
(4) Both personal and environmental factors are targets of intervention.
(5) Emphasis is on availability of services as needed at all stages of aphasia (i.e., acutely poststroke through chronic).

d. Many community group programs have been established through the United States and abroad that offer a variety of ways in which the environment is made to be "aphasia-friendly." Programs offered include:
(1) Book clubs designed especially for PWA.
(2) Music, singing and drama groups.
(3) Psychosocial support groups for PWA run by the members themselves.
(4) Psychosocial support groups for family members and friends of PWA.
(5) Supported conversation groups with community volunteers trained to interact with PWA.
(6) Computer use and Internet classes.

e. Supported Conversation for Adults with Aphasia (SCA; Kagan, 1998) is a training program for clinicians and community volunteers developed by Aura Kagan and colleagues at the Toronto Aphasia Institute.
(1) Based on the idea that communication with PWA could be greatly enhanced by educating their communication partners instead of focusing on fixing the communication impairment of the PWA.
(2) The supported conversation training program educates conversational partners (family members, clinicians and community volunteers) about the symptoms of aphasia and suggests various ways to interact conversationally with PWA that are likely to be successful.
(3) Sample SCA techniques are presented in Table 12-10.

6. Efficacy of treatment for aphasia has been demonstrated repeatedly in carefully controlled research studies that are too numerous to review here.

Table 12-10

Sample Techniques Used in Supported Conversation for Adults with Aphasia (SCA)

	SAMPLE SCA TECHNIQUES FROM HTTP://WWW.APHASIA.CA/SCATEXT.HTML
Acknowledging competence of the PWA	Use a natural and not patronizing tone of voice. Choose adult, complex topics to discuss. Integrate supports into natural talk. Say "I know that you know." Attribute communication breakdowns to your failure, not to the PWA. Be open if you need to talk to a partner to get additional information. Openly acknowledge frustration shared by both.
Revealing competence of the PWA: Getting your message in	Use short, simple sentences and expressive voice. As you are talking, use gestures, write down key words and supplement with drawing. Eliminate distractions. Observe the PWA carefully to assess their comprehension of your input.
Revealing competence of the PWA: Helping them to get the message out	Ask yes/no questions and make sure they have a clear way to respond. Ask yes/no questions in a logical sequence from general to more specific. Ask one thing at a time. Ask PWA to gesture, point to something or write down a word. Give sufficient time to respond. Use fixed-choice questions sometimes.
Revealing competence of the PWA: Verifying the message	Summarize clearly and slowly what you think the PWA is to communicate. Add a gesture or written key word to your summary. Reflect back what you think they are saying. Expand on what you think they are saying. Summarize—pull things together at the end of a longer discussion.
General	Use only as many techniques as necessary. Expect that there will be breakdowns. Do not overuse techniques to avoid communication breakdowns at all costs.
Helpful materials to have on hand	Plenty of blank paper for drawing, writing Markers and pencils Cut-out window to isolate attention to a specific section of written or drawn material Self-adhesive notes Flashcard-size pieces of paper

a. Various meta-analyses have been conducted from which principles have emerged related to treatment for PWA.
  (1) Treatment must be provided at least twice per week (1-hour sessions) in order to be effective; less than that is no better than no treatment at all.
  (2) Effect sizes (a measure of change with treatment) are usually greatest in the acute post-stroke period, but PWA also make significant changes with treatment in the chronic period.
  (3) Treatment should be tailored to the specific profile of strengths and weaknesses in each individual in order to maximize effectiveness. In other words, there is no "one-size-fits-all" treatment for aphasia.
  (4) Therefore, recent research on aphasia has seen increasing use of single-subject (SS) research designs.
    (a) The PWA is used as his or her own "control" so there is no need for an untreated control group.
    (b) SS designs include designs such as the ABA design and the multiple-baseline design.
      - ABA design = Baseline (A) phase, treatment (B) phase and withdrawal (A) phase.
      - Multiple-baseline design:
        – Measure behavior at baseline (pretreatment) across different behaviors.
        – Treat one behavior only while probing performance on both behaviors.
        – Hopefully, only the treated behavior improves while the other one remains stable.
        – This design is useful for measuring response to treatment within the period of spontaneous recovery.
    • See Chapter 4 for research and evidence-based practice (EBP).

Recovery from Aphasia

Individual Recovery Patterns

1. Recovery from aphasia is related to numerous factors, and the pattern of recovery is unique to each individual.
2. The period of the first 6 months post-onset is generally referred to as a period where spontaneous recovery is taking place; that is, even without intervention, functions usually show improvement.
3. The widespread notion of a plateau in recovery after 6 months to 1 year post onset is probably false; many PWA continue to improve with and without treatment for many years in the chronic phase.
4. Neurophysiological mechanisms of recovery are complex but neuroimaging studies of PWA have shown several patterns.
   a. Neural tissue within an incomplete lesion region recovers to some extent and resumes normal or near-normal functioning.
   b. Peri-lesional regions adjacent to the area of brain damage take over functions previously conducted within the affected areas of the brain.
   c. Homologous regions in the right hemisphere become involved in functions that had previously been controlled by the affected areas in the left hemisphere.
   d. A combination of all of these patterns can occur.
   e. The neurophysiological mechanisms responsible for observed recovery may change according to time post onset over the course of recovery.

Factors Related to Recovery Patterns

1. Lesion location, lesion size and aphasia severity.
   a. Lesion location, size and aphasia severity are integrally related.
   b. Lesion size on its own is much less important to recovery patterns than lesion location (i.e., extent of damage within the language zone).
     (1) Extent of lesion in Wernicke's area is correlated with extent of recovery of auditory comprehension.
     (2) Persistent nonfluency of speech (stereotypies or phrase lengths of less than one word) has been associated with damage to specific cortical and subcortical regions of the frontal lobe.
2. Etiology.
   a. People with traumatic aphasia sometimes show more recovery of the aphasia than those with aphasias caused by strokes.
   b. People with hemorrhagic strokes causing aphasia sometimes recover better than those with aphasia from ischemic blockage strokes, provided the individual survived the initial event.
   c. Aphasia from primary progressive aphasia or any neurodegenerative condition will not recover but will deteriorate over time.
3. Aphasia type and severity.
   a. People with global aphasia (the most severe aphasia) may show less recovery than other

syndromes, but this depends on what is measured to evaluate recovery (e.g., verbal expression vs. communicative effectiveness in other modalities).
  b. Common changes in aphasia syndromes over the course of recovery.
     (1) Wernicke's → conduction → mild anomic.
     (2) Global → mixed nonfluent → severe Broca's.
     (3) Global → mixed nonfluent.
     (4) Broca's → milder Broca's.
4. Age.
  a. Age itself is an insignificant factor in recovery from aphasia in adults.
  b. However, increased age is associated with other health conditions such as diabetes, dementia syndromes and cerebrovascular disease that may affect recovery in negative ways.
  c. Normal aging also affects language in selected areas, such as reduced lexical retrieval, that may interact with recovery from aphasia.
5. Gender.
  a. Some studies have suggested that women may show slightly better recovery from aphasia, but most do not support this notion and show no gender differences in recovery patterns.
6. Handedness.
  a. Left-handers may show better recovery if they are in the minority of left-handers who have right-hemisphere dominance or mixed dominance for language.
7. Education level.
  a. Education level likely has no direct effect on recovery from aphasia, but as a component of socioeconomic status (SES), education has been observed to be related to initial severity level of aphasia; lower SES has been associated with more severe aphasia initially.
  b. This may be due to the notion of cognitive reserve—people with greater cognitive reserve may have less severe aphasia.
8. Presence and severity of other cognitive deficits.
9. Presence of significant nonlinguistic deficits in the domains of executive functions, memory and visuospatial functions is likely to result in less recovery from aphasia and less ability to respond to treatment.
10. Premorbid personality and other psychosocial factors are likely important to recovery but there has been little research on this.
  a. Premorbid psychiatric disorders such as significant depression are likely to have a negative effect.
  b. People who are shy or easily embarrassed may appear to recover less or be less likely to use compensatory means of communication.
  c. Family and friends' support is likely to be a significant factor in recovery.

Communication Disorders Associated with Right-Hemisphere Brain Damage (RBD)

Effects on Language

1. Strokes in the right hemisphere affect language differently than left-hemisphere strokes due to the dominance of the left hemisphere for language.
2. Aphasia resulting from a right-hemisphere lesion in a right-handed person is so rare that it is given its own name: crossed aphasia.
3. Left-handed persons may develop aphasia from a right-hemisphere lesion if they are in the minority of left-handers who have anomalous dominance.
4. Speech may be similarly affected by a right-hemisphere lesion, leading to a dysarthria if the right motor/sensory strip is affected.

Cognitive and Communication Symptoms

1. Cognitive and communication symptoms seen with damage to the right hemisphere are variable depending on lesion location but in general may include one or more of these:
  a. Problems understanding the nonliteral or figurative meaning of language (e.g., interpreting proverbs and understanding metaphors).
  b. Poor "theory of mind," i.e., understanding what is or is not shared knowledge or what the beliefs may be of another person.
  c. Poor ability to carry a tune and sometimes to recognize melodies.
  d. Difficulty expressing emotional states via facial expression or vocal intonation.
  e. Difficulty recognizing emotional states in others' facial expressions or vocal intonations.
  f. Flat affect, sometimes inappropriate affect or inappropriate "gallows" humor.
  g. Left neglect of space or lesser degrees of left hemi-inattention.
     (1) The spatial neglect seen in RBD is usually more severe than the spatial neglect or inattention to the right visual field that is seen in people with left-hemisphere strokes.

(2) This may impact the ability of a person with RBD to read written words even though they may not be alexic.
h. Impaired visuoconstructive abilities: The drawings produced by a person with RBD are often fragmented and lack an outer configuration or gestalt.
i. General inattention and distractibility; worse than is seen in those with left-hemisphere lesions.
j. Characteristic style of perseveration seen in writing: repeated individual letters, overwriting and poor spatial organization.
k. Taken together, all these symptoms often result in a very different personality style than prestroke.
l. Anosognosia, denial or unawareness of illness or deficit, is sometimes seen, usually in the acute period post onset.
   (1) Anosognosia tends to be seen only early post onset in RBD.
   (2) Anosognosia is extremely rare in LBD.
   (3) Anosognosia implies that the intact right hemisphere is perhaps more important to self-awareness than is the left hemisphere.

Assessment and Treatment

1. Assessment of individuals with RBD may be conducted with any of the assessment tools for language and cognition mentioned in the section on aphasia. Some specialized assessment tools for people with RBD that are used by SLPs include:
   a. The Mini Inventory of Right Brain Injury, 2nd edition (MIRBI-2; Pimental & Knight, 2000).
   b. The Ross Information Processing Assessment, 2nd edition (RIPA-2; Ross-Swain, 1996).
2. Treatment of people with RBD.
   a. SLPs often work with people who have RBD in rehabilitation settings.
   b. The focus of treatment may be on any one or a multiple of the symptoms listed under Cognitive and Communication Symptoms. Multicultural considerations for assessment of RBD.
      (1) Left neglect of space or inattention to stimuli in the left visual field can be quite debilitating and is often a focus of intervention by multiple rehabilitation clinicians (PT/OT/SLP).
      (2) Lessening of the left neglect or left inattention may be required prior to attempting other interventions, particularly when working on communication modalities such as reading.
      (3) Deficits in the comprehension of figurative language are also often a focus of treatment.
      (4) Impaired comprehension and expression of emotional states via facial expression or vocal intonation also greatly affects interpersonal communication and relationships and is often a target of intervention.
      (5) Treatment may also focus on improving speech intelligibility if dysarthria is present. See Chapter 13 on motor speech disorders.

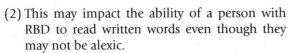

Neurodegenerative Syndromes Affecting Language and Cognition

Note: For information on neurodegenerative disorders such as amyotrophic lateral sclerosis (ALS) or multiple sclerosis (MS) that primarily affect motor speech and not language, see Chapter 13 on motor speech disorders.

Normal Aging

1. Awareness of the language and cognition changes seen in normal aging is important to the SLP as a basis for comparison when evaluating those who may have the beginnings of a dementia syndrome.
2. Because the range of performances expected in normal aging is somewhat broad, the boundary between what is considered "normal" and what is considered as possible dementia is somewhat fuzzy.
   a. In recent years, a category called mild cognitive impairment (MCI) has emerged that encompasses this fuzzy boundary area (see later section in this chapter on MCI).
3. Language and cognitive changes observed in normal aging are variable across individuals but include some common patterns relative to younger adults.
   a. Lexical retrieval ability on tests of naming and in conversation declines.
      (1) For example, for people in their mid-80s, Boston Naming Test (BNT) scores are 2.5 standard deviations below the mean scores of 30-year-olds.
      (2) Naming errors produced by elders are primarily categorized as circumlocutions; i.e., they are able to give appropriate semantic information but have difficulty retrieving the specific name.
      (3) This pattern has been described as the tip-of-the-tongue phenomenon, and people are able to say the target word when given phonemic cues.

(4) Proper noun retrieval (e.g., the names of people and cities) may also be particularly poor in normal aging.
b. Discourse production generally shows no impairment, with only subtle differences as people age.
c. Auditory comprehension of language shows some clear patterns of mild deficit, including increased difficulty with measures of inferencing, syntactic processing of certain embedded structures and semantic processing (e.g., of implausible sentences).
  (1) Most explanations of these patterns suggest that because working memory is vulnerable to aging, tasks that are dependent on WM will show deficits.
d. A discrepancy is seen in the Performance IQ (PIQ) vs. the Verbal IQ (VIQ) on the WAIS.
  (1) PIQ declines more steeply with increasing age than VIQ.
  (2) This reflects that visuoperceptual and visuoconstructional skills decline with increasing age on tasks such as block design, object assembly, drawing and copying tasks.
e. Memory functioning shows declines in working memory and free recall of word lists, but long-term memory is relatively resistant to aging.
f. On tasks of executive functioning, many skills remain unimpaired, but impairments are seen on tasks of divided attention.
4. Neuroanatomical changes seen in normal aging.
a. Decreased brain weight, gyral atrophy and loss of myelin.
b. Dilation of the cerebral ventricles.
c. Neuronal cell loss in hippocampus, amygdala, brainstem nuclei and cerebellum.
d. Neurofibrillary tangles, particularly in medial temporal lobe, and neuritic plaques in the frontal and parietal lobes.
e. Dopamine receptor density declines.
f. Auditory system changes peripherally and centrally.
  (1) Hearing and vision changes are common in normal aging and need to be considered when evaluating language and cognitive performance of people who are elderly.

Mild Cognitive Impairment

1. Mild cognitive impairment (MCI) is a term most commonly used to describe a subtle but measurable memory disorder.
2. A person with MCI has memory problems greater than normal for his or her age but does not show other symptoms of dementia, such as impaired judgment or reasoning.
3. The definition of MCI continues to evolve, and many people view it as a prodrome state (presyndrome) to Alzheimer's dementia or another form of dementia.

Dementia

1. A general broad definition of dementia states that it is a progressive neurological disorder affecting multiple cognitive domains, including memory, language, visuospatial skills, executive functions and behavior.
2. The Diagnostic and Statistical Manual (DSM-IV) definition for Alzheimer's dementia includes these four elements:
a. Memory must be impaired.
b. At least one of the other cognitive domains must also be impaired.
c. The disorder must impair work or social functioning.
d. The disorder must be progressive, showing a worsening of symptoms over time.
3. SLPs may be involved in the assessment and treatment of people with dementia seen in a variety of settings, including acute care, rehabilitation and long-term care hospitals; skilled nursing facilities; private practice clinics; and more.
4. Treatment provided by an SLP to a person with dementia often involves treating cognition and language in early and middle stages and swallowing in later stages. See Chapter 16 on dysphagia.
5. Assessment and intervention by an audiologist is also often required given the association of neurodegenerative syndromes with advancing age.

Assessment of Language and Cognition in People with Neurodegenerative Syndromes

1. The Mini-Mental State Exam (MMSE; Folstein, Folstein, & McHugh, 1975) is one of the most commonly used screening tests for cognitive dysfunction in adults.
a. It includes items to measure orientation to time and place, concentration, memory and language.
b. The maximum score on the MMSE is 30.
  (1) A score between 24 and 30 indicates "Uncertain Cognitive Impairment."
  (2) A score between 18 and 23 indicates "Mild to Moderate Cognitive Impairment."
  (3) A score between 0 and 17 indicates "Severe Cognitive Impairment."
  (4) Research studies on normal aging often use a score of ≥27 as a cutoff to insure their participants are not showing signs of dementia.

Table 12-11

The Subtests of the Arizona Battery for Communication Disorders of Dementia (ABCD)

Mental Status
Story Retelling—Immediate
Following Commands
Comparative Questions
Word Learning—Free Recall
Word Learning—Total Recall (free & cued)
Word Learning—Recognition
Repetition
Object Description
Reading Comprehension—Word
Reading Comprehension—Sentence
Generative Naming
Confrontation Naming
Concept Definition
Generative Drawing
Figure Copying
Story Retelling—Delayed

2. The Arizona Battery for Communication Disorders of Dementia (ABCD; Bayles & Tomoeda, 1993) is a comprehensive assessment tool specifically for people with dementia.
   a. See Table 12-11 for a listing of the subtests of the ABCD.
3. SLPs often use standardized language assessments such as the BDAE or the WAB or a similar comprehensive language battery with selected additional measures to evaluate nonverbal cognition.
   a. However, care should be taken when evaluating performance not to use the norms that are available for PWA when using these tests with people who have dementia.
   b. Norms for people with dementia are not available on the BDAE or the WAB.
4. The Cognitive Linguistic Quick Test (CLQT; Helm-Estabrooks, 2001) has both verbal and nonverbal subtests (clock drawing, mazes, trails, design memory, symbol cancellation and design generation) so it is an appropriate measure for people with suspected linguistic and nonlinguistic impairments.
5. There are several other dementia rating scales that have been developed for both clinical and research purposes, including the Clinical Dementia Rating Scale (CDR), the Dementia Rating Scale (DRS) and the Alzheimer's Disease Assessment Scale: Cognitive Subscale (ADAS-COG).

Characteristics of the Neurodegenerative Syndromes

1. Alzheimer's dementias (AD).
   a. AD is a common dementia syndrome named after researcher Alois Alzheimer. It is the leading cause of dementia in adults and approximately 2%–4% of people over age 65 have AD.
   b. Many people believe that AD is actually a family of neurodegenerative brain disorders, not a single disease entity.
      (1) AD may have variable presentations such as AD with visuospatial impairments (visuospatial subtype).
      (2) A familial variant of AD has been identified that has a strong genetic component, which generally presents at younger ages and has a more rapid course of deterioration.
   c. Onset of AD usually begins when people are in their late 60s or 70s and prevalence increases dramatically with increasing age, such that up to 50% of people over age 85 may have AD.
   d. More women than men are affected, primarily because women have longer life expectancies than men.
   e. There is a somewhat higher risk for AD in African Americans than in Caucasians.
   f. Behaviorally, it is diagnosed by physicians as "probable AD" by a history of a progressive memory impairment of insidious onset.
   g. AD also presents with language deficits and eventually a behavioral comportment problem, but at first, social graces are well preserved.
   h. Average duration from onset of the disorder to death is 8 to 15 years.
   i. AD as a neuropathological entity is diagnosed definitively only postmortem by examining brain tissue and seeing both neurofibrillary tangles within neurons and amyloid plaques outside the neurons.
   j. AD is known as a disorder of the protein tau (tauopathy).
   k. Changes in brain functioning in AD are thought to be the result of the amyloid cascade, in which amyloid-beta proteins are deposited in the brain that eventually lead to fibril and plaque formation, death of neurons and finally mental impairment.
      (1) These changes start many years prior to any apparent symptoms of mental impairment.
      (2) The neurophysiological mechanisms precipitating the start of the cascade are not fully understood but are believed to be a combination of genetic risk factors, general health, cerebrovascular factors and environmental factors.
         (a) The apolipoprotein E (apoE-4) genotype has been identified as an important risk factor for the development of AD.
         (b) Diabetes and insulin resistance have also been associated with increased risk of AD.
      (3) Neuropathological changes in AD are first seen in medial temporal lobe structures, including the hippocampus and entorhinal cortex,

Table 12-12
The 10 Warning Signs of AD from the Alzheimer's Association Website (www.alz.org)
1. Memory loss that disrupts daily life
2. Challenges in planning or solving problems
3. Difficulty completing familiar tasks at home, at work or at leisure
4. Confusion with time or place
5. Trouble understanding visual images or spatial relationships
6. New problems with words in speaking or writing
7. Misplacing things and losing the ability to retrace steps
8. Decreased or poor judgment
9. Withdrawal from work or social activities
10. Changes in mood or personality

explaining why memory impairments are usually the first sign.
(4) As AD progresses, neuropathological changes proceed in a lateral direction to include the frontal lobe, lateral temporal lobe and parietal cortex, explaining why language and other cognitive changes become more pronounced over time.
(5) Mild to moderate pronounced atrophy is seen on neuroimaging.
l. The 10 warning signs of AD published by the Alzheimer's Association (www.alz.org) are presented in Table 12-12.
m. Language and communication symptoms in AD change over the course of the disorder; many clinicians divide the progression into at least three stages:
(1) Mild or early AD.
 (a) Verbal output is fluent, well-articulated and grammatical but shows a mild word-finding problem and is slightly empty and circumlocutory.
 (b) BNT scores are slightly to moderately reduced over age-matched norms and more naming errors are due to misperceptions than are seen in normal aging.
 (c) Auditory comprehension problems may be seen in formal testing but may be secondary to reduced attention.
 (d) Oral reading is preserved but reading comprehension deficits are seen in formal testing.
 (e) Writing resembles verbal output, i.e., somewhat rambling, but often shows preservation of spelling and good syntax.
 (f) Awareness of the disorder may still be present.
(2) Moderate or mid-stage AD.
 (a) Language changes are more obviously different from normal elderly, as spontaneous speech becomes profoundly anomic, circumlocutory and tangential; however, syntactic aspects of language remain intact.
 (b) Paraphasias of many types, including neologisms, may be present.
 (c) There is marked perseveration of individual phrases as well as of ideas.
 (d) Auditory comprehension deficit is more obvious in conversation.
 (e) The memory impairment interacts with the linguistic disorder so that the individual frequently repeats questions and is unable to retain information in answers that were given.
 (f) Awareness of deficits is quite poor.
(3) Severe or late-stage AD.
 (a) All language abilities show severe impairment and it is nearly impossible to conduct neuropsychological assessment.
 (b) Eventually the person with dementia stops talking and becomes mute.
 (c) There may be some preservation of repetition skills seen in echolalia; the individual may echo words spoken by others without apparent comprehension.
2. Vascular dementia (VaD) is a syndrome with diagnostic criteria that are currently in flux, but it generally refers to a dementia syndrome in which the cause is cerebrovascular disease of sufficient severity that multiple cognitive domains become impaired.
 a. *Important:* It is not necessarily progressive.
 b. Some describe it as a subset of a larger syndrome called vascular cognitive impairment (VCI).
  (1) If cognitive impairment only affects one domain of cognition, the individual may be labeled as having aphasia, apraxia, amnesia, etc., depending on what is affected, rather than VaD.
  (2) VCI is important to recognize because cerebrovascular disease can be treated and thus prevent the development of VaD.
 c. VaD may be the second most common form of adult dementia.
 d. The typical onset is between age 60 and 75 and more men than women are affected.
 e. Life expectancy after diagnosis is not as long as AD due to vascular disease and its association with other medical conditions.
 f. Risk factors for VaD are similar to those for other dementia syndromes and include hypertension as the most important risk factor, diabetes and increased age.
 g. The DSM-IV criteria for VaD are similar to those for AD.
  (1) There must be memory impairment.
   (a) *Note:* This has been questioned as a necessary criterion because not all people with VaD will show memory impairment.

(2) One or more other cognitive domains must be impaired.
(3) There must be impairment of social or occupational functioning.
(4) Changes must represent significant decline of functioning over baseline.
(5) Additionally, there must be neurological signs or symptoms or laboratory evidence of cerebrovascular disease that is judged to be etiologically related to the disturbance.

h. Different etiologic subtypes of VaD have been recognized.
(1) Lacunar state results from multiple small infarcts primarily in subcortical regions of the basal ganglia, thalamus, midbrain or brain stem.
(2) Multiple cortical infarcts caused by a series of strokes affecting arteries feeding the cortex.
(3) Binswanger's disease is a rarer disorder in which there are multiple small infarcts in subcortical white matter, usually related to severe hypertension.
(4) Cerebral Autosomal Dominant Arteriopathy with Subcortical Infarcts and Leukoencephalopathy (CADASIL) is an inherited form of VaD.

i. Symptoms seen in VaD.
(1) Symptoms are highly variable because the exact symptoms depend on the region of the brain that is affected by the cerebrovascular disease.
(2) Reported symptoms include confusion, problems with recent memory, wandering or getting lost, loss of continence, pseudobulbar affect, difficulty following instructions and problems handling money.
(3) If cortical regions are damaged, there are likely to be cortical impairments such as aphasia, apraxia, dysarthria, agnosia, hemiparesis, hemisensory deficits, etc.
(4) If extensive subcortical regions of the brain stem or cerebellum are involved, dysphagia may be present.
(5) Many reports stress the common appearance of executive system impairments due to disruption of frontal-subcortical circuits.

j. Differentiating VaD from AD.
(1) Memory is always impaired in AD; only sometimes in VaD.
(2) The course of the disorder always shows an insidious progression in AD; only sometimes is it progressive in VaD.

k. Importance for SLP.
(1) VaD may be present in addition to other dementias (e.g., it is not uncommon for people to receive diagnoses of both AD and VaD).
(2) VaD may not always be recognized or labeled as VaD if focus is on the aphasia (i.e., some people with global aphasia could, by the criteria presented for VaD, be appropriately labeled as having VaD).
(3) Some people with VaD may be able to respond to treatment for their communication impairments if other cognitive domains are only mildly affected.
(4) The label of dementia may imply to family members that there will be relentless decline over time; SLPs may need to explain that VaD is not necessarily always progressive.

3. Frontotemporal dementias (FTD) are a group of neurodegenerative disorders that includes the primary progressive aphasias (PPA) and a nonaphasic "frontal" dementia syndrome.
a. FTD is a somewhat rarer type of dementia than AD and is the label currently given to a group of dementia syndromes including what used to be called Pick's disease and the Pick's complex of disorders.
b. Additional terms for dementias now included in this complex of disorders are circumscribed cerebral atrophy, lobar atrophy, progressive subcortical gliosis, corticodentatonigral degeneration, frontal lobe degeneration, semantic dementia, corticobasal degeneration, dementia lacking distinctive histopathology (DLDH), dementia with motor neuron disease (MND), primary progressive apraxia and others.
c. The onset for this group of disorders is typically younger than for AD (mean age approximately 55 years), and the progression is somewhat more rapid than in AD (between 6 and 8 years in FTD).
d. There is extensive brain atrophy visible in the frontal and temporal lobes in particular, which is the reason for the label FTD.
e. FTD is characterized by a significant decrease in brain weight and by a variety of other neuropathologies.
f. Most FTDs are known to be disorders of various proteins (tau, TDP-43), and a recent familial variant has been discovered that is related to a specific genetic mutation.
g. General symptoms of FTD and differentiation from AD.
(1) Decrease in spontaneous output and mutism earlier than in AD.
(2) Communication deficits more pronounced than memory deficits.
(3) Parietal lobe functions often preserved (visuospatial construction, R-L orientation, calculations).
(4) More common in men than in women.
(5) Approximately one-third of cases have a positive family history of FTD.

(6) A subset of individuals develops motor neuron disease (ALS) with weakness and muscle wasting.
h. Three major clinical variants of FTD have been recognized, including frontal dementia and two types of progressive aphasia: semantic and progressive nonfluent aphasia.
   (1) Frontal variant FTD is also known as the behavioral variant of FTD and does NOT include aphasia. It is characterized by disinhibition, poor impulse control, apathy and antisocial behavior.
   (2) Executive function deficits in planning and organization.
   (3) Memory is relatively spared.
   (4) Spontaneous conversation is reduced but language may be unimpaired on naming tests and other formal measures.
   (5) Stereotypical or ritualized behaviors—insisting on a routine.
   (6) Using a "catch phrase" or stereotypy.
   (7) Significant increase in food preference towards sweet things.
   (8) Elements of Kluver-Bucy syndrome late in course of FTD.
      (a) Increased sexual activity.
      (b) Hyperorality (oral exploration of objects).
      (c) Apathy and placidity.
i. Primary progressive aphasia (PPA): Semantic dementia and progressive nonfluent aphasia collectively are termed PPA because progressive language disturbance is the main clinical finding in the absence of a more global dementia.
   (1) To be diagnosed as having PPA, only language must be impaired and this must be the case for the past 2 years.
   (2) Other causes of the language disturbance such as acute CVA must have been ruled out.
   (3) Eventually, the majority of people diagnosed with PPA will develop a more global dementia syndrome within about 5 years of onset.
   (4) Semantic dementia is characterized by a loss of information in semantic memory that results in a variety of linguistic disturbances.
      (a) Anomia in discourse with frequent use of circumlocutions, indefinite terms and word-finding pauses in conversation.
      (b) Naming is impaired on formal testing and there is reduced ability to generate category exemplars on word list-generation tasks.
      (c) Both verbal and nonverbal semantic knowledge about things and words is impaired.
      (d) Auditory comprehension is impaired and there is sometimes alienation of word meaning (e.g., "I hear you saying 'cork' but I just can't recall what cork means").
      (e) Surface dyslexia and surface dysgraphia are seen with overreliance on phonetic rules in reading such that only the grapheme-phoneme route is used, not whole-word reading.
      (f) Grammar and phonological aspects of language remain intact.
      (g) Relatively preserved cognitive abilities include visuoperceptual and spatial skills, working memory, problem solving, day-to-day or episodic memory and autobiographical memory.
      (h) If temporal atrophy is bilateral, there may be prosopagnosia (difficulty recognizing faces), which gets progressively worse.
      (i) Behavioral changes only slight at first but may emerge over time as in the frontal variant.
      (j) The progression of the neuropathology in semantic dementia is the reverse of the pattern seen in AD.
         • It starts laterally in the temporal lobe and progresses to include medial temporal structures over time.
         • Symptoms mirror this progression: Language is impaired at first and, over time, memory becomes more impaired (this is the opposite of the pattern seen in AD).
   (5) Nonfluent progressive aphasia is characterized by significant nonfluency of verbal output as a presenting symptom.
      (a) People with nonfluent progressive aphasia may appear to have a syndrome similar to Broca's aphasia.
      (b) Nonfluency gets progressively worse over time and eventually spontaneous verbal output deteriorates to mutism.
      (c) Auditory comprehension is preserved initially and for a while, in contrast to semantic dementia.
   (6) Recently, a third PPA syndrome has been recognized, known as logopenic or phonological PPA (Ogar, 2010).
      (a) It is less well defined than the other variants and shares some features with both the nonfluent and fluent variants of PPA.
      (b) There is a significant difficulty in word retrieval, but grammar and motor speech are relatively intact.
      (c) There is an obvious deficit in repetition, and phonemic paraphasic errors are interpreted as due to a deficit in the function of the "phonological loop" component of verbal working memory.
      (d) Thus, this variant shares features with conduction aphasia.
   (7) See Table 12-13 for a summary of the three PPA syndromes (semantic dementia, nonfluent PPA and logopenic PPA).

Table 12-13
Characteristics of the PPA Syndromes

	NONFLUENT VERBAL EXPRESSION	FLUENT VERBAL EXPRESSION	AUDITORY COMPREHENSION	PHRASE LENGTH	GRAMMAR	ARTICULATION	READING	WRITING
Nonfluent PPA	+	−	+	1–4 words	−	−	+	+
Fluent PPA/Semantic Dementia	−	+	−	5+ words	+	+	−	−
Logopenic/Phonological PPA	−	+	−	5+ words	+	+	+	+

+ = relative strength, − = relative weakness.
Summarized from Helm-Estabrooks, Albert, & Nicholas (2013). *Manual of Aphasia and Aphasia Therapy* (3rd ed.). Houston, TX: ProEd.

(8) Primary progressive apraxia of speech (PPAOS) has also been recognized as a motor speech disorder that has a nonacute presentation and is progressive in nature. See Chapter 13 on motor speech disorders.

4. Parkinson's disease (PD) and dementia with Lewy Bodies (DLB) are disorders caused by dysfunctions in brain regions that produce the neurotransmitter dopamine and the brain networks that rely on it.
   a. Parkinson's disease (PD).
      (1) PD is characterized by a significant movement disorder, often including a motor speech disorder known as hypokinetic dysarthria, and not infrequently a dementia later in the course of the disease. See Chapter 13 on motor speech disorders.
      (2) PD is a neurodegenerative disorder of middle and late life. Average age of onset is typically over the age of 50 but early onset PD may be on the rise.
      (3) Idiopathic PD has no known cause, but it does have a well-defined anatomical site of dysfunction and a specific pattern of biochemical pathology.
         (a) Dopamine-producing cells in the substantia nigra of the brain stem and other cells in the pons, medulla and midbrain start to die off, resulting in less dopamine available to the projection sites of these cells in the basal ganglia.
         (b) Severe neuronal loss in these regions is seen in PD, but approximately 50%–75% of dopamine stores must be depleted before symptoms first appear.
         (c) Another major pathologic marker is Lewy body inclusions in subcortical brain regions.
            • In DLB, Lewy bodies are seen in both subcortical and cortical regions.
      (4) Slightly more men than women are affected.
      (5) The time course of progression is highly variable across individuals.
      (6) PD and DLB are synucleinopathies, i.e., disorders of the protein synuclein, in contrast to AD and FTD, which are tauopathies.
      (7) Motor symptoms at the typical onset of PD that people complain of:
         (a) Resting tremor in one hand.
         (b) Generalized slowing of movement, stiffness of muscles and fatigue with motor activity.
         (c) Shortened stride length when walking.
         (d) Micrographia or writing much smaller than premorbid writing.
      (8) Cardinal motor signs of PD are termed extrapyramidal signs, since they represent functions of the extrapyramidal motor system rather than the primary pyramidal motor system.
         (a) Resting tremor.
         (b) Cogwheel rigidity in motor tone.
         (c) Bradykinesia and akinesia, including "masked face," reduced arm swing and reduced eye blinking.
         (d) Postural instability, shuffling and freezing of motor function, often leading to falls.
      (9) Depression occurs in approximately half of the cases of people with PD.
      (10) Hypokinetic dysarthria that significantly affects speech intelligibility is common in PD and is characterized by low volume of speech (hypophonia), monopitch, reduced stress, monoloudness, imprecise consonants, inappropriate silences, short rushes of speech, sometimes a harsh voice quality and breathy voice quality. See Chapter 13 on motor speech disorders.
      (11) Significant dementia develops in up to one-third of cases of PD.
         (a) PD with dementia may differ from DLB only in terms of the time course of the onset of motor symptoms vs. cognitive symptoms.
         (b) The dementia syndrome in PD is characterized by bradyphrenia (slowness of cognitive

processing), executive system dysfunction, some naming problems and difficulty retrieving recently stored memories rather than encoding new memories.
  (c) The presence of these neuropsychological deficits may have a significant effect on response to treatment for the dysarthria associated with PD, and SLPs must consider this in designing treatment plans and making treatment decisions.

Treatment of Communication in People with Neurodegenerative Syndromes

1. Common pharmacological and medical treatments for people with dementia.
  a. Many people diagnosed with dementia will receive pharmacological treatment for their dementia and the SLP should be familiar will some of the more common medications that people may be receiving.
  b. Medications for people with AD.
    (1) Research is ongoing with many of these medications; in general, they have limited effects on cognition, and at most may delay progression of the disorder for up to, but usually not more than, 6 months.
    (2) Cholinesterase inhibitors may be prescribed.
      (a) These prevent the breakdown of acetylcholine, thus making it more available to neurons.
      (b) Common medications of this type include Donepezil (Aricept®), Rivastigmine (Exelon®) and Galantamine (Reminyl®).
    (3) Memantine (Namenda®) was approved for treatment of moderate and severe AD and works with the neurotransmitter glutamate.
  c. For people with VaD, treatment will involve medications for the underlying cerebral vascular disease in order to prevent any further infarcts from occurring.
    (1) Medications such as those that control hypertension or prevent the development of blood clots may be prescribed.
    (2) In some cases, if no further vascular events occur, the symptoms may improve or plateau, unlike in most other dementia syndromes.
    (3) If the underlying cerebral vascular disease is not well controlled or is impossible to control, then the disorder will progress and symptoms will worsen.
  d. For people with PD, Sinemet, which provides a form of dopamine (levodopa or l-Dopa), is the most widely prescribed medication.
  e. For people with one of the FTD syndromes, there is no evidence that cholinesterase inhibitors like those given to people with AD or that dopamine medications like those given to people with PD are useful; nevertheless, many people may be prescribed these medications.
  f. Deep brain stimulation (DBS) is a surgical approach that has had great success in treating the motor disorder associated with PD.
    (1) DBS involves implantation of electrodes in the subthalamic nucleus.
    (2) Implantations may be unilateral or bilateral.
    (3) Stimulation of the electrodes is turned on or off by a pacemaker-like device under the clavicle.
    (4) However, some studies have shown no improvement or worsening of dysarthria in people who have been treated with DBS; others have found psychiatric side effects and worsening of performance on neuropsychological measures post surgery.
    (5) DBS is considered as a treatment option usually after people with PD find that their prescribed medications are less effective in controlling symptoms.
  g. People with DLB are sensitive to neuroleptic medications (such as those used for people with agitation and psychoses) and may exhibit even more Parkinsonian symptoms if treated with them.
    (1) Prior to the current understanding of DLB, the hallmark symptom of visual hallucinations was interpreted as indicative of a psychosis and therefore treated with antipsychotic medications.
    (2) These medications deplete dopamine, resulting in worsening of Parkinsonian symptoms.
2. Cognitive-communicative interventions for people with dementia.
  a. For people with dementia syndromes, the same array of treatment options as in stroke-caused aphasia may be tried in early stages, but expectations will differ because symptoms will worsen, not improve, over time.
  b. Therefore, clinicians will change their focus over the course of working with individuals with dementia, from maintaining optimal function to compensating for deficits, for example, using alternative and augmentative communication (AAC) approaches.
  c. AAC approaches may be introduced early before they are needed, in a manner similar to the approach for working with the speech disorder associated with neurodegenerative disorders such as ALS.
    (1) AAC approaches may be particularly useful for those with PPA who have not yet developed a significant dementia affecting other cognitive functions besides language.

(2) However, in many cases, by the time the aphasic disorder of PPA has progressed to the point that AAC approaches are needed, symptoms of a more global dementia may be evident.
(3) Deficits in executive functioning and memory may thus interfere with the ability of the person with PPA to independently or functionally use the AAC strategy.
(4) Memory books are common compensatory aids used with people who have dementia.
   (a) These are often albums containing photos of family members, important familiar locations and other important information that the person with dementia, their family members and other caregivers may wish to converse about.
   (b) Photos and pictures are captioned with text and names so that the person with dementia may be able to use these words to aid in recall during the discussions.
d. Practice guidelines for treatment of people with cognitive-communicative disorders associated with dementia have been developed by the Academy of Neurologic Communication Disorders and Sciences (ANCDS); reports on seven different types of approaches are available on their website: www.ancds.org. Complete references for these are also at the end of the chapter.
e. The following are brief descriptions of these seven approaches that have been used successfully in people with dementia:
   (1) Simulated presence therapy consists of treatments in which clinicians attempt to reduce agitation and other negative behaviors by simulating the presence of loved ones via pretaped messages or phone calls played to the person with dementia.
      (a) A family member or friend records a one-person "conversation" about enjoyable past events they had experienced with the person with dementia.
      (b) The recording is played for the person with dementia when they are agitated or experiencing negative emotions.
      (c) Recordings may be played on an audiotape or accessed by dialing a telephone number to simulate an actual telephone call with a loved one.
      (d) Listening to the prerecorded tape of their loved one's voice may result in improvement of mood and lessening of agitation.
   (2) Group reminiscence therapy consists of treatments in which groups of people with dementia are involved in discussions facilitated by professional clinical staff on topics from their pasts that they are still able to reminisce about, such as high school graduation.
      (a) Reminiscence therapy activates cognitive and linguistic abilities to promote increased life participation and decrease social isolation.
      (b) It focuses on discussion of the types of memories that many people with dementia are still able to recall— autobiographical memories from one's youth, for example.
      (c) Visual and auditory props (e.g., popular songs from an earlier era) may be used in the discussions to help stimulate memories and positive emotions.
   (3) Spaced-Retrieval Training (SRT) is a treatment for those with memory dysfunction that attempts to introduce new memory associations via repeated stimulus-response trials over increasingly longer intervals.
      (a) Potential targets for SRT are face-name or object-name associations, associations between an external cue and a desired new behavior and instilling positive alternatives to problem behaviors.
         • For example, SRT might be used to help establish a memory for where an important item was located, such as a wallet.
         • If successful, the individual with dementia would not be repeatedly asking staff where the wallet was located.
      (b) When successful, SRT is hypothesized to rely on procedural memory systems rather than declarative memory systems, which are usually impaired in dementia.
   (4) Caregiver-Administered Active Cognitive Stimulation for individuals with AD is a series of treatments administered by the caregiver, usually in the home environment, that are designed to engage the person with dementia in cognitively stimulating activities, such as playing card games, completing puzzles and discussing films or events.
      (a) Research has indicated that these activities may be more beneficial to maintenance of cognitive function than such passive activities as simply watching television shows.
      (b) This approach may require some education and training for the caregivers as well as effort on their part to make sure cognitively stimulating activities are available on a regular basis.
   (5) Educating Caregivers on Alzheimer's Disease and Training Communication Strategies are treatments designed to improve the communication environment by educating caregivers about what is expected in AD as it progresses and about the types of communication strategies that are most successful.

(a) Research on this approach showed increases in success of conversational interchanges, improved quality of life for the person with dementia and reduced caregiver burden (in most cases).

(b) Examples of strategies include asking yes/no questions rather than open-ended questions that are too difficult for the person with dementia due to memory deficit, use of memory books and use of simultaneous nonverbal cues by the caregiver.

(6) Computer-Assisted Cognitive Interventions (CACIs) include treatments presented via computer that may assist people with dementia with their memory and problem-solving deficits.

(a) Examples include programs that provide a virtual representation of a person's home or the local area so that locations of objects or routes to area locations can be learned and practiced ahead of time on a computer.

(b) CACIs are appropriate for those with mild-moderate dementia who have preserved motor learning and procedural memory skills and who have prior exposure to using computers.

(7) Montessori-Based Interventions are treatments based on Maria Montessori's principles of education and are designed to result in improvements in behavior, cognitive function and mood.

(a) Montessori principles:
- Learning within the context of purposeful and meaningful activities.
- Breaking activities down into their component parts and training parts in a sequential, structured manner.
- Incorporating multisensory materials.
- Learning in stages from observation to recognition to recall and finally to demonstration to others.

(b) Research on this approach used with people with dementia found improvements in engagement levels, social interaction and on some cognitive measures.

Multicultural Considerations in Working with People with Dementia

Cultural Viewpoint and Clinical Decision-Making

1. In many cultures, dementia is viewed differently from the "Western medical model" that prevails in the United States and that has been presented in this chapter.
2. Some cultures do not view dementia as a "disease" but rather as a natural consequence of aging.
   a. A person with dementia may be cared for within the context of the family without ever being evaluated by physicians.
   b. A person with dementia who develops other medical problems for which no medical intervention is sought may not want assessment or treatment for the dementia condition.
3. Some cultures view those with dementia as being possessed by demons or suffering from a mental illness rather than suffering from a neurological disorder.
4. Caregiving, in terms of who the primary caregivers are as well as what is expected of caregivers, is also variable across cultures.
5. Therefore, SLPs should not assume that the person with dementia they may be treating or the person's family members possess the same beliefs they have about the causes of dementia or how best to treat and care for the person with dementia.
6. SLPs should remain open and sensitive to cultural differences that will affect their clinical decision-making when working with people with dementia and their families.

References Cited

Aftonomos, L.B., Steele, R.D., Appelbaum, J.S., & Harris, V.M. (2001). Relationships between impairment-level assessments and functional-level assessments in aphasia: Findings from LCC treatment programmes. *Aphasiology*, 15(10–11), 951–964.

Albert, M.L., Spark, R.W., & Helm, N. (1973). Melodic intonation therapy for aphasia. *Archives of Neurology*, 29, 130–131.

Bayles, K., & Tomoeda, C. (1993). *The Arizona Battery for Communication Disorders of Dementia (ABCD)*. Austin, TX: Pro-ed.

Beeson, P.M., & Hillis, A.E. (2008). "Comprehension and Production of Written Words," Chapter 25 in R. Chapey (Ed.), *Language Intervention Strategies in Aphasia and Related Neurogenic Communication Disorders*, 5th ed. Philadelphia: Lippincott, Williams, and Wilkins.

Chapey, R., Duchan, J. F., Elman, R. J., Garcia, L. J., Kagan, A., Lyon, J. G., & Simmons-Mackie, N. (2001). "Life Participation Approach to Aphasia: A Statement of Values for the Future," in R. Chapey (Ed.), *Language Intervention Strategies in Aphasia and Related Neurogenic Communication Disorders*, 4th ed. Philadelphia: Lippincott, Williams, and Wilkins.

Cherney, L.R. (1995). Efficacy of oral reading in the treatment of two patients with chronic Broca's aphasia. *Topics in Stroke Rehabilitation*, 2(1), 57–67.

Cherney, L.R., Babbitt, E.M., & Oldani, J. (2004). Cross-Modal Improvements During Choral Reading: Case Studies. Presented at the Clinical Aphasiology Conference, Park City, Utah, May, 2004.

Cherney, L.R., Babbitt, E., Oldani, J., & Semik, P. (2005). Efficacy of Repeated Choral Reading for Individuals with Chronic Nonfluent Aphasia. Paper presented at the Clinical Aphasiology Conference, Sanibel, FL, June, 2005.

Cherney, L.R., Halper, A.S., Holland, A.L., & Cole, R. (2008). Computerized script training for aphasia: Preliminary results. *American Journal of Speech-Language Pathology*, 17, 19–35.

Cherney, L.R., Patterson, J.P., Raymer, A., Frymark, T., & Schooling, T. (2008). Evidence-based systematic review: Effects of intensity of treatment and constraint-induced language therapy for individuals with stroke-induced aphasia. *Journal of Speech, Language, and Hearing Research*, 51, 1282–99.

Davis, G.A., & Wilcox, M.J. (1981). Incorporating parameters of natural conversation in aphasia treatment, in R. Chapey (Ed.), *Language Intervention Strategies in Adult Aphasia*. Baltimore, MD: Williams and Wilkins.

Edmonds, L.A., Nadeau, S., & Kiran, S. (2008). Effect of verb network strengthening treatment (VNeST) on lexical retrieval of content words in sentences in persons with aphasia. *Aphasiology*, 23(3), 402–424.

Folstein, M.F., Folstein, S.E, & McHugh, P.R. (1975). "Mini-mental state." A practical method for grading the cognitive state of patients for the clinician. *Journal of Psychiatric Research*, 12(3), 189–198.

Frattali, C., Holland, A., Thompson, C., Wohl, C., & Ferketic, M. (2003). *Functional Assessment of Communication Skills for Adults (ASHA FACS)*. Rockville, MD: American Speech-Language Hearing Association.

Goldstein, K. (1948). *Language and Language Disturbances: Aphasic Symptom Complexes and Their Significance for Medicine and Theory of Language*. New York: Grune & Stratton.

Goodglass, H., Kaplan, E., & Barresi, B. (2001). *Boston Diagnostic Aphasia Examination (BDAE)*, 3rd ed. Austin, TX: Pro-ed.

Goodglass, H., Kaplan, E., & Barresi, B. (2001). *The Assessment of Aphasia and Related Disorders*, 3rd ed. Chapter 6: "Interpretive Summary: The Major Aphasic Syndromes." Philadelphia, PA: Lippincott Williams & Wilkins.

Helm-Estabrooks, N. (1992). *Aphasia Diagnostic Profiles (ADP)*. Austin, TX: Pro-ed.

Helm-Estabrooks, N. (2001). Cognitive Linguistic Quick Test (CLQT). San Antonio, TX: Pearson.

Helm-Estabrooks, N., & Albert, M.L. (2004). *Manual of Aphasia and Aphasia Therapy*, 2nd ed. Austin, TX: Pro-ed.

Helm-Estabrooks, N., Fitzpatrick, P., & Barresi, B. (1982). Visual Action Therapy for global aphasia. *Journal of Speech and Hearing Disorders*, 44, 385–389.

Helm-Estabrooks, N., & Nicholas, M. (2000). *Sentence Production Program for Aphasia (SPPA)*. Austin, TX: Pro-ed.

Helm-Estabrooks, N., Nicholas, M., & Morgan, A. (1989). *Melodic Intonation Therapy*. Austin, TX: Pro-ed.

Helm-Estabrooks, N., Ramsberger, G., Morgan, A., & Nicholas, M. (1989). *Boston Assessment of Severe Aphasia (BASA)*. Austin, TX: Pro-ed.

Holland, A., Frattali, C., & Fromm, D. (1999). *Communication Activities of Daily Living*, 2nd ed. (CADL-2). Austin, TX: Pro-ed.

Hux, K., Buechter, M., Wallace, S., & Weissling, K. (2010). Using visual scene displays to create a shared communication space for a person with aphasia. *Aphasiology*, 24(5), 643–660.

Kagan, A. (1998). Supported conversation for adults with aphasia: Methods and resources for training conversational partners. *Aphasiology*, 12, 851–864.

Kearns, K.P. (1985). Response elaboration training for patient initiated utterances. In R.H. Brookshire (Ed.), *Clinical Aphasiology* (pp. 196–204). Minneapolis, MN: BRK Publishers.

Kearns, K., & Scher, G.P. (1989). The generalization of response elaboration training effects. *Clinical Aphasiology*, 18, 223–245.

Kertesz, A. (2006). Western Aphasia Battery–Revised (WAB-R). San Antonio, TX: Pearson.

Lingraphica [Computer software]. Available at http://www.aphasia.com/.

Lomas, J., Pickard, L., Bester, S., Elbard, H., Finlayson, A., & Zoghaib, C. (1989). The Communicative Effectiveness Index: Development and psychometric evaluation of a functional communication measure for adult aphasia. *Journal of Speech and Hearing Disorders*, 54, 113–124.

Luria, A.R. (1970). *Traumatic Aphasia*. The Hague, Netherlands: Mouton and Co.

McKelvey, M.L., Dietz, A.R., Hux, K., Weissling, K., & Beukelman, D.R. (2007). Performance of a person with chronic aphasia using personal and contextual pictures in a visual scene display prototype. *Journal of Medical Speech-Language Pathology*, 15(3), 305–317.

Morgan, A., & Helm-Estabrooks, N. (1987). Back to the Drawing Board: A Treatment Program for Nonverbal Aphasic Patients. In R. Brookshire (Ed.), *Clinical Aphasiology Conference Proceedings* (pp. 64–72). Minneapolis, MN: BRK Publishers.

Nicholas, M., & Elliott, S. (1998). C-Speak Aphasia: A communication system for adults with aphasia. Solana Beach, CA: Mayer-Johnson.

Nicholas, M., Sinotte, M.P., & Helm-Estabrooks, N. (2011). C-Speak Aphasia alternative communication program for people with severe aphasia: Importance of executive functioning and semantic knowledge. *Neuropsychological Rehabilitation*, 21(3), 322–366.

Ogar, J.M. (2010). Primary progressive aphasia and its three variants. *Perspectives on Neurophysiology and Neurogenic Speech and Language Disorders*, 20, 5–12.

Paradis, M. (Ed.) (2001). *Manifestations of Aphasia Symptoms in Different Languages*. Oxford, UK: Pergamon Press.

Paradis, M., et al. Bilingual Aphasia Test (BAT). Montreal: McGill University. Test versions in many languages are available online at http://www.mcgill.ca/linguistics/research/bat/.

Pimental, P.A., & Knight, J.A. (2000). *MIRBI-2: The Mini Inventory of Right Brain Injury*, 2nd Ed. Austin, TX: Pro-ed.

Porch, B. (1967). *Porch Index of Communicative Ability*. Palo Alto, CA: Consulting Psychologists Press.

Porch, B. (2001). *Porch Index of Communicative Abilities Revised (PICA-R)*. Albuquerque, NM: PICA Programs.

Psycholinguistic Technologies, *Sentence Shaper*. Available from http://www.sentenceshaper.com/index.html.

Rao, P.R. (1994). Use of Amer-Ind code by persons with aphasia. In R. Chapey (Ed.), *Language Intervention Strategies in Adult Aphasia*. Baltimore: Williams and Wilkins.

Raven, J., Raven, J.C., & Court, J.H. (2003, updated 2004). *Manual for Raven's Progressive Matrices and Vocabulary Scales*. San Antonio, TX: Harcourt Assessment.

Rehabilitation Institute of Chicago (2007). AphasiaScripts [Computer software]. Chicago: Author.

Robey, R.R. (1998). A meta-analysis of clinical outcomes in the treatment of aphasia. *Journal of Speech, Language, and Hearing Research*, 41, 172–187.

Rosen, W., Mohs, R., & Davis, K. (1984). A new rating scale for Alzheimer's disease. *American Journal of Psychiatry*, 14, 1356–1364. (Ref. for ADAS-COG).

Ross-Swain, D. (1996). *The Ross Information Processing Assessment*, 2nd ed. (RIPA-2) Austin, TX: Pro-ed.

Schuell, H. (1965). *Minnesota Test for the Differential Diagnosis of Aphasia (MTDDA)*. Minneapolis, MN: U. of Minnesota Press. (No longer in print.)

Sparks, R., Helm, N., & Albert, M. (1973). Aphasia rehabilitation resulting from melodic intonation therapy. *Cortex*, 10, 303–316.

Skelly, M. (1979). *Amer-Ind Gestural Code Based on Universal American Indian Hand Talk*. New York: Elsevier.

Thompson, C.K., Choy, J.J., Holland, A., & Cole, R. (2010). Sentactics®: Computer-automated treatment of underlying forms. *Aphasiology*, 24(10), 1242–66.

Thompson, C.K., & Shapiro, L. (2007). Treating agrammatic aphasia within a linguistic framework: Treatment of underlying forms. *Aphasiology*, 19 (10–11), 1021–36.

Wechsler, D. (2008). *Wechsler Adult Intelligence Scale*, 4th ed. (WAIS-IV). San Antonio, TX: Pearson.

Wechsler, D. (2009). *Wechsler Memory Scale*, 4th ed. (WMS-IV). San Antonio, TX: Pearson.

References from the ANCDS: Guidelines for Treatment of Cognitive-Communication Disorders of Dementia, www.ancds.org

Bayles, K., Kim, E., Chapman, S., Zientz, J., Rackley, A., Mahendra, N., Hopper, T., & Cleary, S. (2006). Evidence-based practice recommendations for working with individuals with dementia: Simulated presence therapy. *Journal of Medical Speech-Language Pathology*, 14(3), xiii–xxi.

Hopper, T., Mahendra, N., Kim, E., Azuma, T., Bayles, K., Cleary, S., & Tomoeda, C. (2005). Evidence-based practice recommendations for working with individuals with dementia: Spaced-retrieval training. *Journal of Medical Speech-Language Pathology*, 13(4), xxvii–xxxiv.

Kim, E., Cleary, S., Hopper, T., Bayles, K., Mahendra, N., Azuma, T., & Rackley, A. (2006). Evidence-based practice recommendations for working with individuals with dementia: Group reminiscence therapy. *Journal of Medical Speech-Language Pathology*, 14(3), xxiii–xxxiv.

Mahendra, N., Kim, E., Bayles, K., Hopper, T., & Azuma, T. (2006). Evidence-based practice recommendations for working with individuals with dementia: Computer-assisted cognitive interventions (CACIs). *Journal of Medical Speech-Language Pathology*, 13(4), xxxv–xliv.

Mahendra, N., Hopper, T., Bayles, K., Azuma, T., Cleary S., & Kim, E. (2006). Evidence-based practice recommendations for working with individuals with dementia: Montessori-based interventions. *Journal of Medical Speech-Language Pathology*, 14(1), xv–xxv.

Zientz, J., Rackley, A., Chapman, S., Hopper, T., Mahendra, N., & Cleary, S. (2007). Evidence-based practice recommendations: Caregiver-administered active cognitive stimulation for individuals with Alzheimer's disease. *Journal of Medical Speech-Language Pathology*, 15(3), xxvii–xxxiv.

Zientz, J., Rackley, A., Chapman, S., Hopper, T., Mahendra, N., Kim, E., & Cleary, S. (2007). Evidence-based practice recommendations: Educating caregivers on Alzheimer's disease and training communication strategies. *Journal of Medical Speech-Language Pathology*, 15(1), liii–lxiv.

13

Motor Speech Disorders

GREG TURNER, PhD

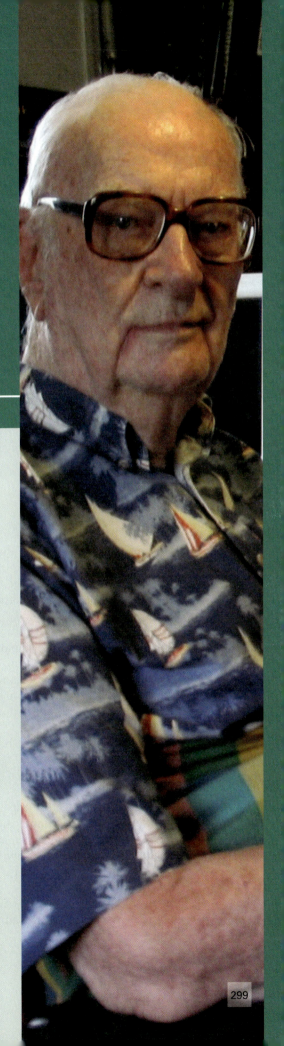

Chapter Outline

- Motor Speech Disorders, 300
- Assessment of Motor Speech Disorders, 303
- General Principles of Treatment of MSD, 310
- Treatment of Dysarthria, 311
- Treatment of Apraxia of Speech, 321
- References, 325

Motor Speech Disorders

Relevant Terms

1. The general label of "speaker" will refer to a speaker with a motor speech disorder, including a speaker with dysarthria or a speaker with apraxia of speech.
2. The acronym *MSD* is used to refer to the generic label *motor speech disorder*.
3. *Childhood motor speech disorders* is the term used to depict a MSD originating during childhood.
4. The acronym *AOS* is used to refer to the generic label *apraxia of speech*.
5. The acronym *CAS* is used to depict the onset of AOS during childhood.
6. *Developmental dysarthria*, or DD, is used when dysarthria occurs prior to acquisition of speech.
7. The term *childhood dysarthria* or the acronym CD is used to depict the onset of dysarthria during childhood, including both DD and acquired dysarthria after speech development is complete.

Dysarthrias

1. Definition.
   a. A group of speech disorders associated with an impairment to motor speech control and execution processes resulting from damage to the peripheral nervous system (PNS) and/or central nervous system (CNS).
   b. Anarthria or anarthric mutism is the inability to speak due to the severe impairment to motor speech control and execution processes as a result of damage to the PNS and/or CNS. Individuals exhibiting dysarthria are able to verbalize to speak, and for some individuals, to a limited extent.
2. General features of dysarthria for both children and adults.
   a. Onset: based on a developmental delay or acquired at any point across the lifespan.
   b. Neurological disease can impair the strength, speed, range, steadiness, tone, and/or accuracy of movements involving the respiratory, phonatory, resonatory and the articulatory components of speech production, resulting in both segmental and suprasegmental errors.
   c. A variety of different categories of disease influencing the nervous system can lead to dysarthria in adults (e.g., toxins, tumors, vascular disease and trauma).
   d. Cerebral palsy, muscular dystrophy and other childhood conditions influencing the nervous system may lead to dysarthria.
   e. Neurological disease influences not only speech but nonspeech activities such as feeding/swallowing and saliva management.
   f. Besides the presence of impairment, dysarthria leads to limitations in activity (e.g., reductions in speech intelligibility and naturalness) and restrictions in participation (i.e., social language use).
   g. Participation restrictions are not always related to speech activity limitations but also to cognitive, linguistic and physical (i.e., limited mobility) barriers associated with neurological disease.
   h. Various types of dysarthria exist as a result of differences in lesion location (e.g., hypokinetic dysarthria associated with a lesion to the basal ganglia).
   i. Presumed unique underlying pathophysiology associated with each type of dysarthria (e.g., weakness-flaccid; incoordination-ataxic).
   j. Each dysarthria type may be associated with common neurological signs.
   k. Each dysarthria type may be associated with a set of distinct perceptual features (refer to Table 13-1 for specific characteristics associated with each type of dysarthria).
   l. Congenital or an acquired onset of neurological disease prior to speech acquisition (i.e., developmental dysarthria) results in both developmental and neurologically based speech deficits.
   m. The acquired version of dysarthria occurring after speech acquisition has occurred is influenced largely by neurological disease; however, maturation of speech production does continue after a child obtains the ability to successfully produce the adult version of speech sound production.
   n. The character of the speech disorder may change as the child matures.
   o. The symptom complex associated with such conditions as cerebral palsy or Down syndrome can lead to a variety of other areas of concern (e.g., visual, attention, cognitive deficits).
   p. Language and literacy are concern for children with MSD, especially if neurological disease occurs prior to speech and language development.

Table 13-1
Perceptual Features Found in Dysarthria Types

DYSARTHRIA TYPE	PHONATORY DEFICITS	RESONATORY DEFICITS	RESPIRATORY DEFICITS	ARTICULATORY DEFICITS	PROSODIC DEFICITS
Flaccid Dysarthria	• Breathy vocal quality • Harsh vocal quality • Monopitch	• Hypernasality • Nasal emission	• Audible inspiration • Monoloudness • Short phrases	• Imprecise consonants	
Spastic Dysarthria	• Breathy vocal quality • Harsh vocal quality • Low pitch • Monopitch • Pitch breaks • Strained-strangled vocal quality	• Hypernasality	• Monoloudness • Short phrases	• Distorted vowels • Imprecise consonants • Slow rate of speech	• Excess and equal stress • Reduced stress
Ataxic Dysarthria	• Harsh vocal quality • Monopitch • Voice tremor		• Excess loudness variations • Monoloudness	• Distorted vowels • Irregular articulatory breakdowns • Prolonged phonemes • Slow rate of speech	• Excess and equal stress • Prolonged intervals
Hypokinetic Dysarthria	• Breathy vocal quality • Harsh vocal quality • Low pitch • Monopitch		• Monoloudness	• Imprecise consonants • Repeated phonemes • Short rushes of speech • Variable rate of speech	• Inappropriate silences • Overall increased rate of speech • Reduced stress
Hyperkinetic Dysarthria	• Harsh vocal quality • Monopitch • Strained-strangled vocal quality • Transient breathy vocal quality • Voice stoppages	• Hypernasality	• Excess loudness variations • Monoloudness • Short phrases • Sudden forced inspiration	• Distorted vowels • Imprecise consonants • Irregular articulatory breakdowns • Prolonged phonemes • Variable rate of speech	• Excess and equal stress • Inappropriate silences • Prolonged intervals • Reduced stress
Unilateral Upper Motor Neuron (UUMN) Dysarthria	• Harsh vocal quality • Hoarse vocal quality	• Hypernasality • Nasal emission	• Decreased loudness	• Imprecise consonants • Irregular articulatory breakdowns • Slow rate of speech	

Apraxia of Speech

1. Definition.
   a. Neurogenic speech disorder associated with impairment to motor planning and/or programming.
2. General features of acquired apraxia of speech in adults.
   a. Often the result of a lesion to the frontal or parietal lobe of the left cerebral hemisphere.
   b. Historical controversy between AOS being a language (phonological) or motoric (phonetic) disorder.
   c. Reflects a disruption in the process of the translation of correctly selected sounds to previously learned articulatory-kinematic parameters; parameters may be lost or an interruption in access may occur.
   d. Lack of neuromuscular impairment (e.g., paralysis, ataxia, involuntary movements).
   e. Difficulty with sequential movements for volitional speaking tasks.
   f. Often coexists with aphasia, and less often with dysarthria.
   g. Oral nonverbal apraxia frequently presents; limb apraxia may occur.
   h. Right lower face and right lingual weakness may occur but fails to account for limitations in speech activity.
   i. Exhibits deficits in articulation, rate and prosody.
   j. Severity ranges from a total inability to speak (severe AOS), to a few inconsistent articulation errors (mild AOS).
   k. Lack of agreement on standard diagnostic criteria for acquired AOS exists.
      (1) Natural variability of the disorder.
      (2) Difference in presentation of features across the severity continuum.
      (3) Co-occurring aphasia (and to a lesser extent dysarthria) makes it difficult isolate features unique to AOS.

Table 13-2

Examples of Clinical Characteristics Used to Diagnose Acquired Apraxia of Speech

SPEECH CHARACTERISTICS	SEQUENCING/RATE CHARACTERISTICS	OTHER CHARACTERISTICS
• Consonantal distortions • Vowel distortions • Lengthened speech segments • Speech sound substitutions • Articulatory groping behaviors • Initiation difficulties	• Slow rate of speech • Lengthened intersegmental durations • Increase errors with increased utterance length or complexity • Consistent errors in repeated utterances	• Abnormalities in prosody • Awareness of speech difficulties • Better automatic speech

Summarized from Waumbaugh, Duffy, McNeil, Robin, & Rogers (2006).

    (4) Possible existence of subtypes of AOS.
    (5) Variation in the degree of impairment across individuals.
    (6) Different methods clinical researchers have adopted to describe behaviors associated with AOS.
  l. Descriptive criteria.
    (1) Distinguishing the primary features unique to AOS.
    (2) Nondistinguishing or nondiscriminant features that can occur not only in AOS, but also in other disorders.
    (3) Features that cannot be used to discriminate AOS because they most likely occur as the result of another disorder (e.g., aphasia).
    (4) See Table 13-2.
3. Definition of childhood apraxia of speech.
  a. CAS is a controversial speech disorder.
  b. A recent report from the American Speech-Language-Hearing Association defined apraxia of speech in this way:
    (1) Childhood apraxia of speech (CAS) is a neurological childhood (pediatric) speech sound disorder in which the precision and consistency of movements underlying speech are impaired in the absence of neuromuscular deficits (e.g., abnormal reflexes, abnormal tone). CAS may occur as a result of known neurological impairment, in association with complex neurobehavioral disorders of known or unknown origin, or as an idiopathic neurogenic speech sound disorder. The core impairment in planning and/or programming spatiotemporal parameters of movement sequences results in errors in speech sound production and prosody.
4. Features of childhood apraxia of speech (CAS).
  a. Childhood speech disorder with neurological etiology.
  b. Viewed in some ways as a developmental counterpart to acquired AOS.
  c. Most often occurs as a congenital/development onset but can also be acquired (see definition above for three etiologic categories).
  d. There exists no universally accepted theory or model of the nature of CAS.
  e. Predominately viewed as a motorically based disorder (i.e., deficit in motor planning and programming); however, associated difficulties in expressive language have led some to hypothesize that a selection and sequencing deficit may extend to language processing.
  f. Deficit areas of CAS.
    (1) Nonspeech motor behaviors.
    (2) Motor speech behaviors.
    (3) Speech sounds and structure (i.e., words and syllable shapes).
    (4) Prosody.
    (5) Language.
    (6) Metalinguistic/phonemic awareness.
    (7) Literacy.
  g. Population estimates 1–2 children per 1000.
  h. Often co-occurs with a delay in language, less often with dysarthria.
  i. The disorder is often viewed as being resistant to change given the best therapeutic efforts.
  j. CAS associated with significant family histories of speech and language deficits, sex-linked (male) pattern of genetic transmission for some individuals, and the *FOXP2* gene appears to play a role in the disorder.
  k. Presently not associated with a specific site of lesion; however, some abnormalities located in cortical and subcortical areas of the nervous system.
  l. Difficulty with production of purposeful voluntary movements for speech in the absence of neuromuscular impairment.
  m. Presence of CAS will interact with phonological and literacy development, especially when apraxia is present prior to speech acquisition.
  n. Based on the *Childhood Apraxia of Speech: Technical Report* (AHSA, 2007), consensus indicated most

frequently occurring behavioral features of CAS include:
(1) Inconsistent errors on consonants and vowels in repeated productions of syllables and words.
(2) Lengthened and disrupted coarticulatory transitions between sounds and syllables.
(3) Inappropriate prosody, especially in the realization of lexical and phrasal stress.

o. The relevant number of identifying characteristics present in a child with CAS will depend on the severity of the motor planning and programming deficit, and the complex interaction between linguistic, motor development and motor planning and programming deficit.

Assessment of Motor Speech Disorders

Overview

1. Variety of possible reasons for assessment (see Table 13-3).
2. Reasons dependent on place of employment and phase of intervention.
3. One of the overall goals of assessment is clarifying the contributions of cognitive, linguistic, motor planning and programming, and motor execution impairment to the overall communication disorder.
4. Organization of the acquisition of assessment information for a speaker with MSD can occur within the International Classification of Functioning, Disability and Health Resources (ICF) framework. Information is obtained in the following areas: (1) description of impairment, (2) activity or functional limitations, (3) participation restrictions, and (4) environmental factors.
5. Typical clinical examination for MSD.
   a. History.
   b. Identifying coexisting disorders.
   c. Motor speech examination.
      (1) Dysarthria.
      (2) Apraxia.
   d. Evaluation of physical impairment.
   e. Differential diagnosis.
   f. Trial therapy.
   g. Development of long and short-term goals.

Obtain the Historical Information

1. Purpose: identify information to catalog in the areas of impairment, speech activity, participation and environment influencing communication.
2. Obtain history information (medical records, case history and speaker/caregiver interviews/questionnaires).
3. Identify and organize historical information associated with MSD.
   a. Nature (i.e., presence and location within the speech production system) and course of impairment.
   b. Type and frequency of functional limitations (e.g., naturalness, speech intelligibility).
   c. Perceived disabilities and restriction in participation.
      (1) Identify the communication needs.
      (2) Identify restrictions in meeting needs through self-report surveys.
4. Document observations during interactions with the speaker (e.g., perceptual observations of speech and language).
5. Identify and organize information identifying impairment in other areas (e.g., hearing, cognition, feeding/swallowing, language, literacy).

Table 13-3

Reasons for Assessment of Motor Speech Disorders (MSDs)

Screening
- Confirming presence or absence of motor speech disorder
- Refer for further assessment

Diagnostic Assessment
- Determine which motor speech disorder is present, including subtype (if applicable)
- Determine profile of patient strengths and weaknesses (i.e., treatment targets and scaffolds)
- Reevaluation for progress measurement

Adapted from McNeil & Kennedy (1984).

Identify the Presence of MSD and Other Associated Disorders

1. Based on the information from the History section, hypothesize about the type of non-MSD communication disorder(s) present.
2. Complete appropriate informal and formal testing to evaluate hypotheses (see appropriate chapters in this text for evaluating such areas as language, cognition, feeding/swallowing and literacy skills in both children and adults).
3. As testing proceeds for both children and adults, contributions of dysarthria and/or apraxia of speech, along with other cognitive/linguistic deficits (e.g., phonological disorders, aphasia, language delay, dementia), need to be thoroughly assessed to identify the correct direction for treatment.
4. Make referrals to other professionals as needed.
5. If either dysarthria (i.e., motor execution disorder) or apraxia of speech (i.e., motor planning and programming disorder) is suspected based on historical information, complete the motor speech examination.

Motor Speech Examination

1. Purpose: identify information to catalog in the area of speech activity/functional limitations.
2. Complete a detailed perceptual analysis.
   a. Obtain a speech sample, adopting methods that take into account the age of the speaker.
   b. For a speaker with dysarthria, utilize Mayo Clinic procedures for describing perceptual features of dysarthria. Based on Table 13-4, identify and/or rate speech dimensions associated with dysarthria.
   c. For speakers with apraxia of speech, perceptual features of the disorder are largely related to articulation and prosody.
   d. For CAS, the most frequently occurring features include:
      (1) Inconsistent errors on consonants and vowels in repeated productions of syllables and words.
      (2) Lengthened and disrupted coarticulatory transitions between sounds and syllables.
      (3) Inappropriate prosody, especially in the realization of lexical and phrasal stress.
3. Document speech activity/functional limitations.
   a. Naturalness.
      (1) Definition: overall adequacy of prosody.
      (2) Prosody is divided into:
         (a) Stress patterning.
         (b) Intonation.
         (c) Rate-rhythm.
      (3) Table 13-5 demonstrates prosodic features that are often disrupted in motor speech disorders.
      (4) Some options for documenting activity limitations in the area of naturalness.
         (a) Overall judgment via a Likert scale.
         (b) Identifying type and number of speech dimensions noted in Table 13-5.
         (c) Percentage of speech dimensions noted out of the total number of speech dimensions associated with naturalness in Table 13-5.
   b. Speech intelligibility.
      (1) Definition: extent of understanding of a speaker based on the acoustic signal.

Table 13-4

Mayo Clinic Speech Dimensions Summary

LABEL OF SPEECH CHARACTERISTIC

Respiratory Characteristics
- Audible inspiration; stridor
- Grunting on expiration

Vocal Characteristics
- Pitch: abnormally high or low; diplophonia; monopitch; pitch breaks
- Loudness: poor control, decay of loudness, voice too soft or too loud
- Quality: breathy; harsh; hoarse; strained/strangled
- Vocal tremor

Articulatory Characteristics
- Substitutions of sounds
- Distortions of consonants or vowels
- Imprecise production
- Specific weakness on pressure consonants (may be accompanied by nasal emission)

Sequencing/Rate Characteristics
- Difficulty with alternating movements of the articulators
- Errors increase with complexity of utterance or with increased rate
- Speech is too fast or too slow

Resonance Characteristics
- Hypernasality
- Hyponasality
- Nasal emission

Prosodic Characteristics
- Excess or equal stress on syllables
- Inappropriate silences (pausing)

Other Characteristics
- Coprolalia
- Palilalia
- Vocal tics

Adapted from the work of Darley, Aronson and Brown (1975) and Duffy (2013).

Table 13-5

Prosodic Impairments of Motor Speech Disorders

- Alternating pitch levels
- Alternating vocal loudness
- Excess and equal stress patterning
- Inappropriate silences (pauses)
- Increased intersegmental durations
- Increased rate of speech
- Monoloudness
- Monopitch
- Prolonged intervals during connected speech
- Reduced stress patterning
- Short rushes of speech
- Shortened phrase length
- Vocal loudness decay
- Vocal loudness variation

Adapted from Yorkston, Beukelman, Strand & Hakel (2010). *Management of motor speech disorders in children and adults*, 3rd ed. Austin: ProEd.

---

   (2) Used often as a measure of severity; however, comprehensibility and efficiency can also be measured.
   (3) Methods of evaluation.
    (a) Word intelligibility measures may include such measures as the Phonetic Contrast Test or the Test of Children's Speech (TOCS+) Intelligibility Measures (2–7 years of age).
    (b) Sentence intelligibility measures such as the Sentence Intelligibility Test and the TOCS+ Intelligibility Measures.
    (c) Subjective measures of speech intelligibility through equal-appearing interval scales, magnitude estimation or visual analog scales.
   (4) The clinician needs to be cautious when evaluating speech intelligibility because it can be influenced by a number of factors (e.g., listener familiarity, close or open set, mode of listening—audio vs. visual plus auditory).
   (5) Another measure related to intelligibility is comprehensibility. Comprehensibility refers to a listener's understanding of the speech of a speaker based not only on the acoustic signal but also the acoustic signal plus other information available to the listener during the communication interaction (e.g., gestures, semantic and syntactic context, and props within the communication environment).
   (6) Standardized measures of comprehensibility do not exist, but informal measures may be adopted with caution.
  c. Speaking rate.
   (1) Definition: rate at which speech units are produced within a given period of time (e.g., syllables or words per minute).
   (2) Conversational speaking gradually increases from 116 to 163 syllables per minute at age 3 to 162 to 220 syllables per minute by the age of 12, which is the typical speaking rate for adults.
   (3) An objective measure of speaking rate is calculated by dividing the number words spoken by the duration of the speech sample. This measure can be calculated with and without pauses. The length of the sample must be of adequate length to provide the best representation of the speaker's rate. Reading, monologue and conversation can be used.
  d. Efficiency.
   (1) Definition: rate of conveyance of intelligible or comprehensible speech.
   (2) Also useful as a severity measure and with other severity measures and is often related to participation restrictions.
   (3) Efficiency rate (ER) is calculated by dividing the rate of intelligible words per minute (IWPM) by the mean rate of intelligible words per minute for a group of normal controls. Increased efficiency is associated with values closer to 1.
   (4) A subjective measure involving efficiency, *Intelligibility Rating Scale for Motor Speech Disorders*, is based on comprehensibility.
  e. Articulatory adequacy.
   (1) Definition: perceptual adequacy of consonant and vowel production.
   (2) Children with MSD.
    (a) Standardized sound inventory tests (e.g., Goldman-Fristoe Test of Articulation) provide valuable information but should be supplemented with a spontaneous speech sample to capture the influence of the segmental and prosodic complexity associated with connected speech.
    (b) Obtain a phonetic repertoire using stimuli within the language abilities of the child.
    (c) For young children obtain a spontaneous speech sample, have child name objects and pictures (imitative or spontaneous) and parent report of phonetic skills (e.g., inventory of speech sounds, syllable shapes).
    (d) For older children with a 200+ word vocabulary, obtain a 75- to 100-utterance sample and a single word task, sampling production of all vowels and consonants of a language (i.e., standardized sound inventory test), as well as both monosyllabic and multisyllabic words.
    (e) Analysis of phonology and articulatory adequacy for both age groups (use transcription as needed for better description).
     • Inventory of all sounds, classes of sounds, and syllable and word shapes.

- Inventory of errors based on sounds, classes of sounds and syllable and words shapes associated with errors relative the adult form.
- Measure of error consistency.
- Inventory of syllable shapes not in repertoire.
- Results of stimulability testing.

(3) Older children and adults with MSD.
  (a) Phoneme Intelligibility Test (PIT) (part of the word intelligibility measures within the SIT software).
    - A single word or phrase reading test containing target sounds.
    - Unfamiliar listener identifies each word within a forced choice format.
    - Overall percent accuracy, percent of accurate vowels and percent of accuracy of overall consonants is calculated along with breakdown charts of percent correct for consonant manner.
    - These results provide a direction for treatment.
  (b) Phonetic Contrast Test (PCT).
    - A speaker verbally reads isolated words.
    - Unfamiliar listener identifies each word within a forced choice format.
    - Foils are presented, containing contrast errors typically present in the speech of speakers with dysarthria.
    - Contrast errors provide an explanation for the reductions in word intelligibility and direction for treatment.

f. Methods for evaluation of motor planning and programming.
  (1) Several standardized and nonstandardized examinations for evaluating motor planning and programming exist for both adults and children.
  (2) Typical purposes of completing the examination.
    (a) Screening.
    (b) Diagnosis.
    (c) Treatment planning.
    (d) Documenting change over time.
  (3) Adult AOS.
    (a) Standardized measures.
      - Apraxia Battery for Adults-2 (ABA-2).
        – Differentiates performance between AOS, aphasia and dysarthria.
        – Offers guidance for designing treatment by identifying error patterns.
    (b) Interpreting assessment results for individuals with acquired AOS in adults.
      - No published diagnostic test leading to reliable identification of AOS in adults presently exists; however, a consensus list of speech characteristics unique to AOS in adults based on the research literature and expert opinion is still forthcoming.
      - Beyond the diagnosis, of central importance is the identification of facilitating or influencing factors (e.g., utterance length, cueing, speaking rate, phonetic and linguistic complexity).
  (4) CAS.
    (a) Principle standardized measures.
      - Kaufman Speech Praxis Test for Children (KSPT).
        – Aid in the diagnosis, treatment planning and reassessment for children between the ages of 2 and 6 years suspected of exhibited CAS.
        – Performance on different tasks compared to normative charts.
        – Diagnosis and severity based on a checklist and rating scale.
      - Screening Test for Developmental Apraxia of Speech (STDAS-2).
        – Screen for the presence of CAS in children between the ages of 4 and 12 years (not diagnose), provide guidance for treatment, use for reassessment and use as a research tool.
        – Considers receptive/expressive language discrepancy and normative data for three subtests to calculate a likelihood level of CAS.
      - Verbal Motor Production Assessment for Children (VMPAC).
        – Identify the presence of disruptions in the motor control system used for speech in children 3–12 years of age, identify the level of disruption, and identify modalities (i.e., visual, tactile and auditory) useful in the intervention process.
        – The test provides assistance in identifying the presence of developmental dysarthria or CAS.
        – Speaker motor control plots are compared to normative plots for comparison.
      - The Apraxia Profile.
        – Aid in the differential diagnosis of CAS in children between the ages of 3 and 13 years, diagnose the presence or nonverbal oral apraxia, document change, and provide guidance for planning intervention.
        – A separate form for preschool and school-aged children.

- Decision about presence of CAS based on 10 characteristics thought to be unique to CAS.
  (b) Nonstandardized measures.
  - Motor Speech Examination for Children.
    - Due to similarity in the procedures, refer to the description of Motor Speech Examination for Apraxia.
  - Assessment of Children with Developmental Apraxia of Speech.
    - Used to obtain information regarding the presence and character of speech motor planning and programming deficits to use for diagnosis and treatment planning.
    - Tasks involve spontaneous speech sample, elicited speech (phonetic repertoire) and nonspeech behaviors.
    - Evaluate the productive phonetic repertoire of the speaker through spontaneous production or imitation including isolated sounds, different monosyllable syllabic structure, multisyllabic words of differing length and motorically challenging words and utterances.
    - Note where breakdown in articulation occurs; also evaluate the benefit of using different levels of auditory, visual and tactile cueing when errors occur; evaluate the ability of the child to self-correct.
    - Evaluate the ability to sequence nonspeech, monosyllabic and multisyllabic sequences; evaluate the latency, completeness and accuracy of tasks along with benefit of cueing if needed.

Factors Affecting Speech Activity

1. Identify factors influencing speech intelligibility, naturalness, articulatory adequacy and speaking rate.
2. Within both standardized and nonstandardized measures of apraxia of speech in both adults and children, factors such as phonetic complexity and utterance length are evaluated to observe the influence on phonetic integrity (articulatory adequacy).
3. The same concept can apply to speakers with dysarthria.
4. Factors influencing speech activity.
   a. Reducing influence of the subsystem impairment.
   b. Compensatory treatment strategies (trial therapy).
5. Some examples of factors that may influence speech activity include:
   a. Occluding the nose and noting the influence on speech intelligibility and articulatory adequacy (resonatory impairment).
   b. Decreasing speaking rate and noting the change in speech intelligibility (compensatory treatment strategy).
6. Document the influence and willingness of the speaker to adopt the method. Facilitative effect is useful for treatment planning and/or the development of hypotheses regarding impairment aimed at further assessment.

Impairments and Speech Activity

1. Based on Historical and Motor Speech Exam information, develop hypotheses regarding the influence of impairment on speech activity (e.g., impairment in tongue movement accounts for imprecision in a number of lingual consonants; speech intelligibility deficits ensuing from reduced loudness is a result of respiratory impairment).
2. Evaluate hypotheses through the measurement of impairment based on speech and nonspeech methods (see section "Evaluate for Presence of Neuromuscular Impairment").

Evaluate for Presence of Neuromuscular Impairment

1. Identification of the presence/absence of neuromuscular impairment; may be explanatory of speech deficit and support neurologic evaluation (e.g., identify specific cranial nerve impairment).
2. A traditional model of treatment for dysarthria involves identifying the physical and aerodynamic deficits in the four valves of speech production responsible for reductions in speech activity and treating those deficits (i.e., reducing impairment).
3. Examination involves predominant use of nonspeech tasks (e.g., instructions to protrude the tongue).
4. Evaluate parameters of impairment (size, strength, symmetry, speed, range of movement, tone, steadiness, accuracy and coordination).
5. Parameters measured (1) at rest, (2) during sustained postures and (3) during movement.
6. If apraxia of speech suspected, evaluate presence of oral and limb apraxia, and rule out neuromuscular impairment across subsystems as accounting for deficit in speech activity.

Differential Diagnosis

1. Individuals who are nonverbal or who present with limited speech are more difficult to diagnose.
2. Differential diagnosis for adults.
   a. Dysarthria from apraxia of speech (AOS).
      (1) The predominant lesion for AOS occurs in the frontal lobe and insula of the hemisphere dominate for language.
      (2) Speakers with apraxia typically do not exhibit neuromuscular conditions noted in dysarthria (e.g., hypertonicity, incoordination, weakness).
      (3) Speakers with apraxia typically do not exhibit feeding/swallowing deficits frequently present in dysarthria.
      (4) Nonverbal oral apraxia often presents in AOS but is not seen in dysarthria.
      (5) Typically only articulation and prosody are impaired in AOS, while frequently all subsystems are impaired in dysarthria.
      (6) Inconsistent speech sound error productions for AOS.
      (7) Volitional phonation can be impaired at times in apraxia. For person's dysarthria, both volitional and reflexive behaviors are impaired.
      (8) Speech sound errors are influenced by context (i.e., utterance length and phonetic complexity) for speakers with AOS compared with speakers with dysarthria.
      (9) Well-practiced tasks will be easier to perform for speakers with AOS than less familiar tasks.
   b. Dysarthria from aphasia.
      (1) Speakers with dysarthria typically fail to exhibit language deficits.
      (2) Speech production subsystem functioning is typically impaired with speakers with dysarthria but not speakers with aphasia.
      (3) Speakers with aphasia exhibit a variety of speech sound errors compared to largely distortion errors for individuals with dysarthria.
      (4) Dysarthria results from subcortical, cerebellar and cortical (bilateral) lesions, while the lesions for aphasia occur in the cortical areas of the hemisphere dominant for language, often the left.
   c. AOS from aphasia.
      (1) A speaker with apraxia:
         (a) Exhibits more errors in prosody.
         (b) Exhibits sound distortions.
         (c) Has difficulty initiating speech.
         (d) Attempts to self-correct.
         (e) Gropes in search of articulatory configurations.
      (2) Literal paraphasias (aphasic error) can be distinguished from errors produced by speakers with apraxia.
         (a) Aphasic errors are less predictable than apraxic errors.
         (b) Literal paraphasias always involve real English sounds, where some errors produced by speakers with apraxia may sound like a non-English sound.
         (c) Aphasic errors are more often "off target" in terms of place and manner.
3. Differential diagnosis for children.
   a. General considerations.
      (1) Extreme caution must be taken when attempting to diagnose children with limited experience or a limited repertoire of speech behaviors.
      (2) The motor limitations associated with a childhood motor speech disorders (CMSD) can influence language development, including phonological development.
      (3) The character of speech sound errors for CMSD as well as articulation and phonological dis-

Table 13-6

Differentiation of Childhood Dysarthria, Articulation Disorders, and Phonological Disorders

CHILDHOOD DYSARTHRIA (CD)	ARTICULATION DISORDER (A)	PHONOLOGICAL DISORDER (PD)
Neurologic diagnosis or site of lesion for speaker	Absence of neurologic diagnosis or site of lesion	Absence of neurologic diagnosis or site of lesion
Presence of neuromuscular impairment	Absence of neuromuscular impairment	Absence of neuromuscular impairment
Distortion errors (related to neuromuscular condition)	Distortion errors	No distortion errors
No substitution errors	No substitution errors	Substitution errors
Omission errors (related to neuromuscular condition)	Omission errors	Omission errors
Impaired prosody	Prosody intact	Prosody intact

Table 13-7

Differentiation of Childhood Apraxia of Speech, Articulation Disorders, and Phonological Disorders

CHILDHOOD APRAXIA OF SPEECH (CAS)	ARTICULATION DISORDER (A)	PHONOLOGICAL DISORDER (PD)
Inconsistency of speech sound errors	Consistency of speech sound errors	Consistency of speech sound errors
Deficits in lexical and phrase stress	No deficits in lexical and phrase stress	No deficits in lexical and phrase stress
Difficulty transitioning between sounds	No difficulty transitioning between sounds	No difficulty transitioning between sounds
Unusual errors (additions, prolongations, repetition of syllables)	No unusual errors	No unusual errors
Greater number of omission errors	Omission errors	Omission errors
Vowel and diphthong errors	No vowel or diphthong errors	No vowel or diphthong errors
Difficulties with nasality and nasal emissions	No difficulties with nasality or nasal emissions	No difficulties with nasality or nasal emissions
Groping behaviors and silent postures	No groping behaviors or silent postures	No groping behaviors or silent postures

Table 13-8

Differentiation of Childhood Dysarthria and Childhood Apraxia of Speech

CHILDHOOD DYSARTHRIA (CD)	CHILDHOOD APRAXIA OF SPEECH (CAS)
Neuromuscular conditions (hypertonicity, incoordination, weakness)	No neuromuscular conditions present
Frequent feeding/swallowing deficits	Atypical feeding/swallowing deficits
Frequently exhibit impairments to all speech subsystems and prosody	Impairments to articulation and prosody only
Speech sound errors are not influenced by context	Speech sound errors are influenced by context (i.e., utterance length and phonetic complexity)
Distortions most frequent	Variety of errors
Consistency in errors	Inconsistency in errors
No groping behaviors or silent postures	Groping behaviors and silent postures

orders may be similar, suggesting applying extreme caution when applying such errors to the differential diagnosis process.
   (4) CMSD and articulation and phonological disorders can co-occur.
  b. Differentiating childhood dysarthria (CD) from an articulation (A) or phonological disorder (PD).
  c. Differentiating CAS from A and PD.
  d. Differentiating CD from CAS.
4. Differential diagnosis across the dysarthrias (all ages).
  a. Informal assessment.
    (1) The following information can be used to differentiate among speakers with dysarthria. The greater number of pieces of categorical information that are available, the more the valid the differential diagnosis.
      (a) Speaker complaints.
      (b) Speech dimension features.
      (c) Site of lesion.
      (d) Common neurological signs.
      (e) Movement deficits.
      (f) Common subsystem impairment.
      (g) Clusters of auditory-perceptual characteristics.

Developing the Direction of Therapy

1. At the completion of the assessment process, organize information based on the ICF.
  a. Impairment.
  b. Limitation in speech activity.
  c. Restrictions in participation.
  d. Environmental factors.
2. What type of MSD is present? Provide supporting evidence.
3. Decide on prognosis base on cognitive function, receptive language, motivation, willingness to participate, severity, etc.
4. What long-term and short-term goals and procedures should be targeted for treatment?

General Principles of Treatment of MSD

General Principles

1. Treatment planning must take into account not only the communication disorder but other associated conditions (e.g., cognitive impairment, depression).
2. Treatment should be personalized for each individual with a motor speech disorder.
3. Treatment planning for MSD is broken down into (1) developing goals and (2) deciding on the treatment approaches to use.
    a. Treatment approaches involve behavioral, medical or prosthetic management.
4. The overall goal of therapy is to improve the ability to communicate through restoring lost function or compensate by helping individuals adjust to the loss of normal speech.
    a. Treatment does not solely target the speaker with an MSD, but also targets the communication partners.
5. Goals are driven by the severity of the speech activity limitations and the restrictions to participation.

Neuroplasticity

1. Reorganization of nervous system through transfer of restored or new behavior to spared parts of system.
2. Change can be positive (adaptive) and/or negative (maladaptive), and can occur immediately or slowly over time.
3. Neuroplasticity is influenced by type of experience.
    a. Therapeutically enriched environments (i.e., targeting the needs of client inside and outside the therapy room) are more likely to enhance plasticity.
    b. Plasticity may be task-specific (e.g., neural change only associated with specific task- nonspeech may not target plasticity for speech task).
    c. Progressively demanding treatment goals may lead to greater plasticity.
    d. Relevant, intensive and extended training more likely to induce plasticity.
4. Neuroplasticity is influenced by timing of experience.
    a. Neural change more likely early in recovery, but amount of surviving brain tissue can limit this change.
    b. Older nervous systems less plastic than younger.

Motor Learning Principles

1. General principles.
    a. Need an initial facilitative environment that leads to successful acquisition of motor skills.
    b. Successful treatment involves initially reducing cognitive and linguistic processing to allow more attention to focus on speech motor control skill development.
    c. After acquisition is achieved, treatment should focus on more challenging tasks for maximizing retention and generalization of skill.
2. Specific principles.
    a. Precursors to learning.
        (1) Establish motivation for learning by describing goals and methods to achieve goals.
        (2) Clinician provides instruction, modeling and demonstration of treatment methods.
    b. Massed and distributed practice schedules.
        (1) Mass practice involves practice without rest between trials.
        (2) Distributed practice involves short periods of practice with rest between trials.
        (3) Distributed practice schedule suggested to be the most effective for generalization, while mass practice leads to enhanced acquisition.
    c. Type of feedback.
        (1) Knowledge of results (KR) is feedback targeting the degree of success in achieving a motor behavior following a practice trial (e.g., "The /sh/ needs to be more distinct").
        (2) Knowledge of performance (KP) consists of specific feedback provided following practice regarding the quality of the motor behavior (e.g., "You need to round your lips more during the production of the /sh/").
        (3) KP can lead to improved acquisition, while KR is associated with improved retention.
    d. Amount of feedback.
        (1) Excessive feedback (i.e., feedback after every trial) may be less effective compared to a reduced or variable feedback schedule (e.g., feedback after every five trials).
        (2) Excessive feedback may be especially detrimental to motor learning in children.
        (3) Delaying the presentation of feedback after a trial may also improve motor learning (e.g., 3–5 second delay before giving feedback).
    e. Implicit and explicit learning.
        (1) Implicit learning involves acquisition of abstract knowledge without being aware of learning.
            (a) Neural substrates include prefrontal and motor areas, basal ganglia, and the cerebellum.
        (2) Explicit learning involves learning for memory or facts.

(a) Neural substrates include parietal and temporal cortices, the hippocampus and the thalamus.
(3) Depending on the lesion site(s) noted for a given speaker, implicit or explicit learning will be more or less effective in the learning process.
f. Specificity of training.
(1) Practice should approximate the movement of the targeted skill and the environmental conditions under which the skill is intended to be produced.
g. Intensive practice.
(1) Motor learning occurs as a result of intensive practice.
(2) Training sessions should be frequent, more than twice a week.
(3) Shorter sessions (e.g., 30 minutes).
(4) Maximize the number of practice trials within a session.
(a) Avoiding reinforcements taking too much time to administer.
(b) Limiting clinician talking time.
(c) Assigning practice outside of therapy session.
(5) Children require a longer period of cumulative practice compared to adults because, in comparison to adults, children exhibit:
(a) Shorter attention spans.
(b) Reduced short-term memory.
h. Other considerations.
(1) Self-learning by a speaker to achieve a targeted goal in treatment may lead to enhanced retention and generalization.
(2) In choosing tasks, consider the performance level of a task (i.e., error rate) as it can influence motivation and success.
(3) Consider the ordering of tasks based on the difficulty level of each task when organizing a treatment session (e.g., beginning and ending a session with the successful completion of an easier task may benefit motor learning).
(4) Fatigue brought on by physical activity may adversely influence speaker performance within a therapy session.
(5) Always allow time for a speaker to practice communicating within a session.

Candidacy for Treatment

1. A number of factors should be considered when deciding if a speaker will benefit and therefore, should receive treatment.
   a. Motor, sensory or cognitive deficits.
   b. Motivation.
   c. Medical diagnosis and prognosis.
   d. Need to communicate.
   e. Presence and degree of disability or handicap.
   f. Limits of the health care system.
   g. Communication partners.
   h. Environment where communication occurs.

Approaches to Treatment

1. Differ based on the type of motor speech disorder (i.e., AOS vs. dysarthria).
2. Within dysarthria, different approaches exist based on the underlying pathophysiology associated with the different types of dysarthria.
3. A variety of approaches exist for treating AOS (e.g., articulatory, rate and rhythm, intersystemic facilitation and reorganization).
4. Similarities exist between treatment for children and adults; however, less systematic treatment research noted for children.
5. When natural speech alone does not meet communication needs, augmentative and alternative approaches to communication are adopted.
6. Counseling and family education.
   a. Provide information (e.g., nature of the disorder, assessment process, direction for treatment, resource information).
   b. Provide both speaker and family appropriate counseling for psychological and emotional adjustment to communication disorder/neurological condition.
   c. Refer to mental health care professional as needed.

Treatment of Dysarthria

Principles of Treatment of Dysarthria in Children and Adults

1. General comments.
   a. Individualized treatment plan due to heterogeneity of the disorder.
   b. Focus of treatment based on severity.
      (1) Mild: maintain intelligibility while maximizing efficiency and naturalness.
      (2) Moderate: improve speech intelligibility.
      (3) Severe: supplement distorted speech and adopt a functional communication system.
   c. Organization of treatment strategies.
      (1) Speaker-oriented strategies.

(a) Maximize physiological functioning of subsystems (i.e., reduce impairment of subsystems responsible for limitations in speech intelligibility and naturalness) or between subsystems (i.e., improve valving of the velopharyngeal subsystem to improve function of other subsystems).
(b) Compensate in the continued presence of impairment (e.g., slow speaking rate to improve clarity of articulation and speech intelligibility).
(2) Communication-oriented or speech supplementation strategies (see section on strategies based on severity).
(a) Speaker approaches.
(b) Communication partner approaches.
(c) Combined speaker/communication partner approaches.
(3) Augmentative and alternative approaches.
d. Specific treatment technique adopted will depend on:
(1) Dysarthria type.
(2) Presence of linguistic and cognitive deficits.
(3) Potential for improvement of speech motor control.

Considerations for Children with Dysarthria

1. General considerations.
   a. Family members should be educated regarding the nature of the motor speech disorder, as well as effective ways to communicate with their child.
   b. Intervention should include targeting of both receptive and expressive language skills through the spoken and written language modalities.
2. Teaching communicative effectiveness.
   a. Communicative effectiveness and communicative repair strategies should be taught to the child as a means of enhancing their overall communicative effectiveness.
   b. Assist the child in appropriate word choice and sentence structure to aid in the comprehension of the listener.
   c. Communicative effectiveness and communicative repair strategies should be generalized to outside intervention sessions while increasing the child's confidence in their ability to use these strategies.
3. Speech ability and phonological knowledge.
   a. The child's phonological and phonetic repertoires and word and syllable shape repertoires should be expanded to the child's level of development.
   b. The child's length of utterance may be expanded through phonological training and multiple practice opportunities.
   c. Vocal loudness, vocal quality, and prosody may be targeted to increase the child's intelligibility.
   d. Phonological awareness and literacy skills should be targeted early in intervention.

Treatment of the Respiratory/Phonatory Subsystem

1. Improving respiratory support.
   a. Nonspeech treatment techniques.
      (1) Adopted for individuals not able to develop adequate subglottal pressure for phonation.
      (2) Behavioral techniques, examples of which are as follows:
         (a) Breathing against a resistive device (e.g., water manometer, resistive mask).
         (b) Pushing/pulling techniques.
         (c) Providing visual feedback on a computer screen of acoustic and aerodynamic measures.
         (d) Maximum inhalation and exhalation tasks.
   b. Postural adjustment treatment techniques.
      (1) Rationale.
         (a) Body position influences respiratory functioning; therefore, positioning an individual, especially someone wheelchair bound, can maximize respiratory support.
         (b) Training of speech breathing outside the typical upright position may not generalize.
      (2) Positioning techniques.
         (a) Upright position used with individuals with greater inspiratory than expiratory weakness, to assist the lowering of the abdominal content and the diaphragm via gravity (e.g., amyotrophic lateral sclerosis).
         (b) Supine position used with individuals exhibiting greater expiratory vs. inspiratory weakness as gravity and abdominal content move the diaphragm into the thoracic cavity (e.g., spinal cord injury).
   c. Prosthetic treatment techniques.
      (1) Rationale.
         (a) Less-frequently adopted techniques.
         (b) Important to consult with physical therapist prior to use.
         (c) Used to counter expiratory weakness and assist in creation of expiratory force for the generation of subglottal pressure during expiration.
         (d) Use on short-term basis until respiratory support improves or use on long-term basis

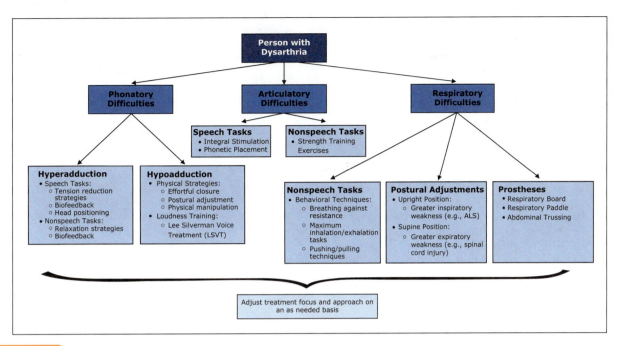

Figure 13-1 Flow Chart of Treatment Options for Impairments in Speakers with Dysarthria

Adapted from Spencer, Yorkston & Duffy (2003). Behavioral management of respiratory/phonatory dysfunction from dysarthria: A flowchart for guidance in clinical decision making. *Journal of Medical Speech-Language Pathology*, 11, xxxix-lxi.

if improvement of respiratory support does not occur.
  (2) Techniques.
    (a) Respiratory board or paddle.
    (b) Abdominal trussing.
  d. Speech treatment techniques.
    (1) Rationale.
      (a) Manipulation of breathing patterns involves instruction to achieve more normal respiratory function.
      (b) Biofeedback is based on the premise that change in the functioning of the respiratory system can occur when a speaker is provided with feedback of acoustic and/or physiologic measures of respiratory functioning; by receiving such feedback, the speaker can make adjustments to improve functioning.
    (2) Technique.
      (a) Manipulation of breathing patterns.
        • To increase and maintain subglottal pressure over a longer period of time, the speaker is instructed to inhale more deeply, exhale with greater muscular force, and/or use diaphragmatic (or abdominal) breathing.
      (b) Biofeedback.
        • Focuses on providing feedback to the speaker of aspects of respiratory functioning.

2. Improving coordination of respiration/phonation.
  a. Nonspeech treatment techniques.
    (1) Only use nonspeech tasks if speakers are unable to produce speech tasks and include speech stimuli as soon as possible.
    (2) Possible tasks.
      (a) Practicing speech-like breathing patterns (i.e., short inhalation followed by a long exhalation phase).
      (b) Practicing "inspiratory checking" without speaking by inhaling to about 50% of vital capacity and slowly exhaling via control of the chest wall and the abdomen, and not valving at the lips.
      (c) Support for use with individuals with cerebral palsy and traumatic brain injury, and also individuals with ataxic, spastic and mixed dysarthria.
  b. Speech treatment techniques.
    (1) Possible tasks.
      (a) Bring to speaker's awareness the speech breathing pattern (i.e., quick inhalation–long exhalation).
      (b) Apply different biofeedback methods for visualizing and/or sensing movement of the chest wall and abdomen while speaking (e.g., the clinician places his/her hands on the speaker's abdomen and has the speaker inhale to appropriate size for the speaking task).

(c) Identify optimal breath group (i.e., number of syllables produce comfortably in one breath) and target a gradual increase in the optimal breath group length.
3. Improving phonatory function.
   a. Treating hypoadduction.
      (1) Physical strategies.
         (a) Effortful closure.
            - Results in improved adduction and strength of vocal folds, increase loudness, and reduced breathy/hoarse voice quality (outcome measures).
         (b) Postural adjustments.
            - Involves turning head to left or right during phonation for individuals with paretic/paralyzed vocal folds.
            - Frequent use of strategy may be viewed as pragmatically undesirable; however, selective use in situations demanding increased loudness may be more palatable (compensatory strategy).
         (c) Physical manipulation.
            - Involves the clinician gently applying pressure to the thyroid lamina on the side of the paretic/paralyzed vocal fold while the speaker phonates.
            - If physical manipulation results in improvement of the voice in chronic conditions, surgical treatment (e.g., medialization) should be considered.
      (2) Lee Silverman Voice Treatment (LSVT).
         (a) Application of high-effort tasks to increase loudness and improve vocal fold function.
         (b) Originally targeted individuals with the hypokinetic dysarthria associated with idiopathic Parkinson disease (IPD) (however, applied to other neurological conditions such as multiple sclerosis, but greatest evidence for IPD).
         (c) Program.
            - Targets vocal loudness, breathiness, intonation and vocal stability.
            - Involves multiple repetitions of speech stimuli.
            - Adopts high-effort activities (e.g., maximum sustained phonation).
            - Intensive intervention schedule (four times a week for one month).
            - Heighten sensory awareness of increased loudness and effort through self-monitoring activities (i.e., recalibration).
            - Daily practice required.
         (d) Outcomes.
            - Improvement in a variety of perceptual, acoustic and physiologic measures of the voice (e.g., vocal quality, intensity, fundamental frequency variation, vocal fold adduction).
            - Improvements also noted in participation.
            - Shown to indirectly improve performance in other subsystems (i.e., articulation) and slowed speaking rate.
            - Maintenance of improvement out to 24 months.
         (e) Candidate criteria.
            - Exhibit hypoadduction of vocal folds, reduced loudness and vocal fatigue.
            - Poor respiratory support/effort.
            - Highly motivated to participate in intensive program (however, other forms of delivery continue to be evaluated).
            - Stimulable to cues to improve vocal performance.
            - Normal cognition, but benefit seen those with mild/moderate deficits.
   b. Treating hyperadduction.
      (1) Behavioral treatment of vocal quality resulting from hyperfunctioning in dysarthria is not typically undertaken due to lack of success (i.e., very limited evidence supporting success for any of the techniques discussed below).
      (2) Nonspeech treatment techniques.
         (a) Relaxation strategies.
            - Relaxation strategies result in inconsistent effects on hyperfunctioning.
         (b) Biofeedback of airflow or laryngeal muscle activity.
            - Biofeedback via Visipitch of nonvocal airflow.
            - Use of electromyography and videoendoscopic biofeedback for the control of laryngeal tension.
      (3) Speech treatment techniques.
         (a) Traditional tension-reducing strategies.
            - Based on the hypothesis that reduced laryngeal tension will be facilitated in the context of reflex-like or continuous phonation responses.
            - Initially the facilitating techniques are applied to isolated vowels and then extended to utterances of increasing length.
         (b) Biofeedback-enhanced relaxation.
            - Monitoring of physiologic and/or acoustic variables associated with phonation, typically through visual feedback, may allow a speaker to reduced hyperadduction.
            - Feedback variables include electromyographic, aerodynamic and videoendoscopic.

- (c) Head positioning and miscellaneous instruction.
  - Altering head positioning (e.g., forward-backward and/or side-to-side) during quiet, short duration phonations may lead to reduced hyperadduction for individuals with spastic cerebral palsy; inability to maintain reduced laryngeal tension may diminish as lung volume decreases as an utterance progresses; can become counterproductive.
- c. Improving phonatory coordination impairments.
  - (1) Phonatory coordination impairments lead to reduction or loss of distinctiveness of two specific phonetics contrasts (e.g., voice-voiceless).
  - (2) Apply contrastive production drills, a technique found in the section on treating the articulatory system to target phonatory coordination impairments.
- d. Augmentative and alternative communication (AAC).
  - (1) If significant reductions in speech activity and participation still exist after attempts to reduce impairment and/or adopt compensatory strategies, AAC technique must be considered.
  - (2) AAC devices targeting individuals with deficits in respiration/phonation.
    - (a) Vocal intensity controller.
      - Acts to monitor vocal intensity and inform the speaker if intensity falls below a targeted level.
    - (b) Portable amplifier.
      - Use with individuals with intact articulation skills but still indicate difficulty being heard in different speaking situation after implementation of behavior treatment aimed at improving loudness.
    - (c) Electrolarynx.
      - May be useful for speaker with aphonia or severe breathiness to enhance voicing.

Treatment of the Velopharyngeal Subsystem

1. Surgical management.
   a. Pharyngeal flap surgery (superiorly based flap).
   b. Injection of Teflon or surgical implants into the posterior pharyngeal wall.
2. Prosthetic management.
   a. Palatal lift.
      (1) General comments.
         (a) Viewed as an effective treatment for *selected* speakers with dysarthria who exhibit significant velopharyngeal weakness, most often those with flaccid dysarthria.
         (b) Results in a reduction in nasal airflow and an increase in intraoral pressure, leading to potential improvements in intelligibility and articulation, along with communication efficiency.
      (2) Design and function of the palatal lift.
         (a) A rigid acrylic appliance fabricated by a prosthodontist.
         (b) Consists of a retentive (palatal) portion covering the hard palate and a lift portion, which contacts the oral surface of the soft palate.
      (3) Construction/fitting of the palatal lift.
         (a) The prosthodontist and the speech-language pathologist collaborate during the construction/fitting process.
      (4) Candidacy criteria.
         (a) Different candidacy criteria depending on progressive vs. stable-recovering dysarthria exist (see Table 13-9 and 13-10).
         (b) Often the final decision to fit based on clinical judgment (i.e., weighing all clinical factors).
      (5) Minor devices.
         (a) Useful for some speakers who would benefit, but for various reasons (e.g., lack of acceptance, poor dentition, hyperactive gag reflex) cannot be fitted with a palatal lift.
         (b) Nose clip or pinching the nose.
            - Consider if nasal occlusion results in significant improvement in speech activity (e.g., speech intelligibility).
            - Typically pragmatically unacceptable; however, may be used on a temporary basis.
         (c) Nasal obturator.
            - A fabricated device placed in the nares for the purpose of impeding nasal airflow and allowing a speaker to increase intraoral air pressure.
            - For individuals who are poor candidates for a palatal lift.
3. Behavioral management.
   a. General comments.
      (1) Behavioral management techniques appropriate for those who can compensate or will have the ability to compensate as medical status of speaker improves.
      (2) Evaluating the ability to compensate is completed through stimulability testing.
      (3) For each condition, the clinician will provide instructions and evaluate if the speaker performed the instructions as specified and indicate if improvement in target speech outcome measure occurred.

Table 13-9

Characteristics of Good Candidates for Palatal Lift Fitting

- Able to inhibit gag reflex
- Adequate functioning of the speech subsystems (i.e., articulation, phonation, prosody, respiration, and resonance)
- Adequate or improving articulatory abilities for speech production
- Cognitive abilities are within functional limits, or mild deficits are noted
- Diagnosis of flaccid dysarthria (either recovering or progressive)
- Enough manual dexterity to independently operate palatal lift
- Pressure consonants are significantly more unintelligible than other consonant types
- Slow progression of symptoms (i.e., progressive dysarthria) or slow improvement of symptoms (i.e., recovering dysarthria)
- No presence of dysphagia
- Occlusion of the nares improves resonance
- Patient is motivated to maintain or improve speech abilities

Summarized from Yorkston, Spencer, Duffy, et al. (2001). Evidence-based practice guidelines for dysarthria: Management of velopharyngeal function. *Journal of Medical Speech-Language Pathology, 9*(4), 257–274.

Table 13-10

Characteristics of Poor Candidates for Palatal Lift Fitting

- Not able to inhibit gag reflex
- Poor functioning of the speech subsystems (i.e., articulation, phonation, prosody, respiration, and resonance)
- Declining articulatory abilities for speech production
- Moderate-to-severe cognitive deficits, particularly in executive functioning
- Diagnosis of spastic dysarthria (either recovering or progressive)
- Not enough manual dexterity to independently operate palatal lift
- All consonant types are equally unintelligible
- Rapid progression of symptoms (i.e., progressive dysarthria) or rapid improvement of symptoms (i.e., recovering dysarthria)
- Presence of dysphagia, or difficulty managing saliva
- Occlusion of the nares does not improve resonance
- Patient is unmotivated to maintain or improve speech abilities

Summarized from Yorkston, Spencer, Duffy, et al. (2001). Evidence-based practice guidelines for dysarthria: Management of velopharyngeal function. *Journal of Medical Speech-Language Pathology, 9*(4), 257–274.

(4) A clinically significant change in the outcome measure toward more normative values for a given condition would support compensation.
  b. Techniques.
    (1) Modifying speaking patterns.
      (a) Speak with increased effort.
      (b) Speak a slower than normal speaking rate.
      (c) Speak more precisely through the use of overarticulate speech.
    (2) Resistance treatment while speaking.
      (a) Involves speaking against airway resistance developed via a continuous positive airway pressure (CPAP) device.
    (3) Biofeedback.
      (a) Possible forms of feedback include visualization of nasal airflow or visualization of the pharyngeal walls.
    (4) Nonspeech techniques.
      (a) Evidence and expert opinion do not support effectiveness of nonspeech techniques (e.g., blowing bubbles, sensory inhibition tasks, etc.).

Treatment of the Articulatory Subsystem

1. General comments.
  a. Speech sound errors (i.e., vowel and consonant distortions) in dysarthria are not always related to neuromuscular impairment to the articulators (i.e., tongue, lips or jaw), but can be the result of impairment to other subsystems (e.g., velopharyngeal) or a combination of subsystem impairment.
  b. Treat subsystems in the order of the magnitude of their contributions to speech activity limitations and if multiple subsystems are impaired, typically the articulatory system is the last to be treated.
  c. Best practices suggest that the implementation of compensatory treatment techniques should not wait until the completion of treatment to reduce impairment.
2. Strategies for normalizing function (i.e., reduced impairment).
  a. Strengthening.
    (1) Assumes reductions in strength of articulatory structures (e.g., tongue), clearly contributes to deficits in articulation, but potentially also, to reductions in speech intelligibility and limitations in participation (i.e., disability).
    (2) Strength training can be completed with and without resistance and with and without biofeedback for a variety of movements of the tongue, lips and jaw.
    (3) Strengthening should lead to increased muscle tension, force and/or endurance and improve range of motion and speed of movement of the articulators.
    (4) Controversy regarding the use of oral-motor or nonspeech exercises to improve speech performance, including strengthening exercises.
      (a) Limited data regarding effectiveness of strength training.

(b) Weak correlations between measures of strength and speech deficits in speakers with dysarthria.
(5) Considerations.
(a) Most useful for speakers with flaccid dysarthria; however, some individuals with spastic, hypokinetic and unilateral upper motor neuron dysarthria may benefit.
(b) During speaking, individuals use only 10%–20% of the maximum force of the lips and tongue, so in general a speaker needs to be extremely weak for therapy to be considered.
(6) Organization of treatment.
(a) Treatment should involve multiple repetitions, sets and practice periods within and outside the therapy room.
b. Reducing muscle tone.
(1) Use of auditory or visual feedback of magnitude of muscle activity to reduce level of hypertonicity.
c. Traditional approaches.
(1) Integral stimulation.
(a) Clinician models production of utterance.
(b) The speaker is asked to watch and listen, and then say the target utterance after the clinician.
(2) Phonetic placement.
(a) Clinician describes and/or provides pictures of the articulator placement for targeted phoneme.
(b) Clinician physically positions or provides touch cues on where the articulator contact is in oral cavity.
(3) Phonetic derivation.
(a) Clinician using an intact nonspeech movement (e.g., whistling) as an initial movement from which to build or mold into the production of a target sound.
d. Surgical management.
(1) Neural anastomosis.
(a) Neural anastomosis involves surgically attaching a healthy functioning nerve to a damaged nerve.
(b) A side effect of hypoglossal-facial surgery may lead to impaired lingual articulation due to surgery-induced lingual weakness.
e. Pharmacologic management.
(1) Botulinum toxin injections.
(a) Botox has the potential as an effective treatment for a number of hyperkinesias.
(b) Emerging use of Botox in the treatment of speakers with spasticity.
3. Strategies for compensating for impairment.
a. Compensatory articulatory movements.
(1) Through self-exploration or training, a speaker can learn to make compensatory adjustments to achieve adequate production of erred phonemes.
(2) Type of compensatory strategy will be unique to the impairment profile of a speaker.
b. Minimal contrasts or contrastive production drills.
(1) Used for practice to make contrasting sounds perceptually distinct.
(2) The clinician instructs the speaker to make the two words as distinct as possible.
(3) The contrastive production drills can be applied to utterances beyond words (e.g., "The word is sent. The word is tent.").
c. Intelligibility drills.
(1) Speaker produces an unfamiliar utterance (e.g., words, phrases, sentences) to the clinician-listener for identification.
(2) If the listener identifies the correct utterance, then the speaker produces a new utterance; otherwise, the speaker is asked to produce the utterance a second time, making it more distinct.
(3) The drills.
(a) Promote self-discovery on how to make speech more intelligible, a primary goal of treatment.
(b) Provide both the speaker and listener experience with strategies to repair breakdowns in intelligibility.
d. Exaggeration of consonant production.
(1) Articulatory precision may be enhanced by instructing the speaker with dysarthria to speak with increased effort and at a slow rate.
e. Prosthetic management.
(1) Bite block.
(a) Consists of a small piece of acrylic or hard putty placed unilaterally between the lower and upper teeth laterally.
(b) When the speaker bites down on the block while speaking, abnormal jaw movement stabilized.
(c) May be helpful if jaw control is impaired to a greater extent than tongue or lower lip control and adversely influences their functioning due to anatomical connections.
(2) Other prosthetic devices influencing articulation.
(a) Prosthetic devices used to compensate for impairments in other parts of the speech production system can benefit articulation (i.e., palatal lift).
(b) Devices used to slow speaking rate (e.g., pacing and alphabet boards, delayed auditory feedback unit) can benefit precision of speech sound production and enhance speech intelligibility for some speakers with dysarthria.

Treatment of Prosody

1. General comments.
   a. Prosodic therapy focuses on naturalness for the mildly impaired speaker (i.e., intelligibility 90% or greater) and speech intelligibility for the speaker with moderate to severe dysarthria.
   b. The clinician must be aware of the trade-off between naturalness and speech intelligibility when planning treatment (e.g., therapy may target increased breath group flexibility in order to improve naturalness).
   c. Methods for improving prosody based on unique prosodic deficits in any of the three aspects of prosody (i.e., stress patterning, intonation and rate-rhythm).
   d. In treatment planning, improving respiratory support may lead to improvements in features of prosody.
   e. Treating prosody moves from highly structured tasks (e.g., contrastive stress tasks), to less structured tasks (e.g., marked and unmarked reading passages and conversational scripts), to spontaneous speech.
   f. Visual feedback of prosodic parameters (e.g., fundamental frequency, pause locations) can supplement and clarify perceptual judgments for both the clinician and speaker.
   g. Initiate self-monitoring activities early in the treatment process.
2. Treatment methods for use within breath groups.
   a. Techniques for treating reduced prosody.
      (1) Referential tasks.
         (a) Training material premarked for targeted prosodic feature (e.g., lexical stress, intonation).
         (b) The speaker is instructed to produce the targeted feature and the clinician/listener indicates feature they heard (e.g., syllable receiving lexical stress or intonation pattern).
         (c) If the speaker is less consistent at marking prosodic features, the clinician should increase times successful and train speaker to use method more consistently.
      (2) Contrastive stress tasks.
         (a) Classical application of a contrastive stress task involves a scripted response where the response utterances do not vary but the stress pattern does.
         (b) The stress pattern or prominence is placed on a specific syllable or word within the scripted response.
         (c) The clinician asks a series of questions for which the speaker is to respond using the core sentence with appropriate prosodic emphasis.
      (3) Modification of only one parameter to signal stress.
         (a) Targeting one prosodic feature (e.g., pitch, loudness, duration) compared to several can be more effective.
         (b) The feature of choice would be the feature the speaker appears to have most control over based on clinical observation; however, if this feature does not exist, duration should be targeted.
   b. Techniques for treating excessive prosody.
      (1) Reduce number of suprasegmental features signaling stress.
         (a) Speakers exhibiting excessive and equal stress or exaggerated signaling of stress (or another prosodic feature) may benefit using only one prosodic feature.
         (b) Altering duration to signal stress (i.e., insertion of a short pause) typically sounds more natural than alterations of fundamental frequency and intensity.
3. Treatment methods for use across breath groups.
   a. Limit breath group length and range.
      (1) If results from maximum phonation and/or counting tasks suggest a sufficient air supply for the production of longer breath groups, training should focus on increasing breath group lengths through the use of stimuli conducive to longer utterances.
      (2) If results from the two tasks suggest insufficient air supply, supportive of shorter breath groups, treatment should focus on factors leading to short breath groups (e.g., decreased respiratory support, poor valving of phonatory system).
      (3) If the flexibility of breath groups is not enhanced through treatment of other factors, then compensatory methods (e.g., better linking pauses to syntactic units) must be taught.
   b. Using both breath and nonbreath pauses.
      (1) Evaluate the number of words the speaker can produce on one breath.
      (2) If limited, work on increasing breath group length as noted previously.
      (3) If breath group length is adequate or became adequate after treatment, increase the use of nonbreath pauses.

Global Management Techniques

1. Global management techniques influence multiple speech production subsystems applied throughout the utterance and not to particular segments.

2. Techniques.
    a. Treatment of speaking rate.
        (1) Rationale.
            (a) Altering speaking rate (usually reducing rate) generally leads to improvement in sentence intelligibility and comprehensibility but not phoneme intelligibility.
            (b) Overall, slower rate may help to compensate for impairment across subsystems and also enhanced speech perception by communication partners.
        (2) Candidacy criteria.
            (a) Lack of specific candidacy criteria predicting who will benefit and to what extent, but typically used with individuals with reduced speech intelligibility.
        (3) Treatment strategies.
            (a) Rigid rate techniques.
                - Techniques.
                    – Alphabet supplementation.
                    – Hand and finger tapping or pacing board.
                    – Using a metronome to produce a syllable or a word in time with a beat.
                    – Delayed auditory feedback (DAF).
                - Advantages of rigid rate techniques.
                    – Slows speaking rate.
                    – Improves intelligibility for some speakers.
                    – Simple and inexpensive devices.
                    – Require minimal training.
                    – Allows for practice outside of therapy room.
                - Disadvantages of rigid rate techniques.
                    – Disrupt naturalness.
                    – Device cosmetically unacceptable by some speakers.
                    – Technique can be overlearned and lose effect.
            (b) Rate techniques that preserve prosody.
                - Rhythmic cueing.
                - "Backdoor" approaches.
                    – Phrasing and breath patterning.
                    – Pitch variation.
                    – Loudness control.
                    – Word and stress patterns.
                - Visual feedback.
                - Advantages of prosody preserving rate techniques.
                    – Slows speaking rate.
                    – Improves intelligibility for some speakers.
                    – Speech sounds more natural.
                    – Does not involve use of prosthetic device.
                - Disadvantages of prosody preserving rate techniques.
                    – Requires extensive training.
                    – Speaker must be highly motivated and physically capable of altering speaking rate in a relative natural fashion.
                    – Speaker less easily able to practice outside therapy initially.
    b. Treatment of loudness: use with speakers with reduced loudness and poor respiratory support; result in increased loudness and secondary benefits such precision of articulation; often used with hypokinetic dysarthria; however, can benefit other types.
        (1) Refer to section Treatment of the Respiratory/Phonatory Subsystem for details on Lee Silverman Voice Treatment (LSVT).
    c. Treatment of prosody: treatment of stress patterning, intonation and rate-rhythm includes functioning of a variety of subsystems; influences acoustic (e.g., F0 contours) and perceptual measures (e.g., precision of articulation, naturalness); often use with ataxic dysarthria but can benefit other dysarthria types.
        (1) Biofeedback (i.e., F0 or intensity contours).
        (2) Behavior instruction (training linguistic aspects of prosody, such as emphatic stress or pause usage).
    d. General instructions: influences clarity, intelligibility and precision in articulation; often used with mixed dysarthria, but can benefit other dysarthria types; in general, feedback about adequacy of productions results in greater improvement than instructions to talk clearly.
        (1) Provide instructions to produce clear speech.
        (2) Provide feedback about adequacy of production (i.e., feedback about clarity of an utterance or in repairing a misunderstood utterance).

Strategies to Enhance Participation

1. Intent of participation strategies is to improve communication in the presence of impairment; consists of environmental modifications, extra information (acoustic signal independent) to enhance understanding of distorted speech and improve comprehensibility, and repair strategies for communication breakdowns; strategies adopted dependent on the severity of dysarthria.
    a. Strategies adopted differ based on change of severity of dysarthria (i.e., from normal-sounding speech to limited natural speech).
    b. Speech sounds normal.
        (1) Treatment: counsel speaker on how to best compensate for barriers to communication. Organ-

ize communication interactions around times when he/she exhibits the least amount of fatigue or enhances/compensates for mobility limitation that causes a barrier to communication.
  c. Intelligible but unnatural sounding speech.
    (1) Treatment: identify communication barriers through use of communication diaries; analyze with the speaker factors associated with communication failures and successes; adjust communication style and environment to minimize communication breakdown and target communication success.
  d. Reduced intelligibility.
    (1) Treatment: enhance comprehensibility through adopting strategies aimed at providing extra or signal-independent information. Strategies are categorized into those used by the speaker with dysarthria, those used by the dysarthric speaker's communication partner (listener), and interaction strategies used together by both speaker and listener.
  e. Strategies used specifically by speakers with dysarthria.
    (1) Obtain listener attention and choose a communicative enhancing environment (i.e., well lit, quiet settings, minimal distractions, close approximation with communication partner).
    (2) Use semantic cues when initiating a topic or changing topic.
    (3) Enhancement of the message through use of complete, simple and predictable sentences.
    (4) Use gestures (i.e., eye gaze, pantomime, etc.) and props to initiate and maintain turn taking and for repairing of communication breakdowns.
    (5) Conserve energy for the most important communication exchanges to maximize comprehensibility.
    (6) Monitor communication partner comprehension through direct query and observation, and strive to maintain that comprehension.
  f. Strategies used specifically by the communication partners of speakers with dysarthria.
    (1) Maintain topic knowledge by monitoring message and querying to verify understanding; if communication breakdown occurs, immediately pursue repair strategies such as asking multiple questions, beginning from broad to more narrow topics.
    (2) Maximize the communication environment by communicating in a well-lit and quiet environment, devoid of distractions. Watch the speaker's face (maintain eye contact) and pay attention to nonverbal cues associated with communication of a message.
    (3) Combine clues to achieve comprehension.
    (4) Monitor and integrate all cues toward comprehension.
    (5) Maximize visual and hearing acuity: wear hearing aids and/or glasses/contacts.
  g. Interaction strategies used by both speakers of dysarthria and their communication partners.
    (1) Manage communication breakdown by adopting repair strategies; repair strategies are the responsibility of both speaker and listener.
    (2) Communication partners should develop agreed upon rules and cues used while communicating.
2. Limited natural intelligible speech.
  a. Treatment for speakers when natural speech alone is inadequate to meet communication needs and augmentative and alternative strategies are necessary; alphabet supplementation is one augmentative strategy used frequently. Refer to Chapter 17 in this text for application of other AAC methods.
    (1) Description of procedure.
      (a) Typically, speakers are trained to say each word of a message while simultaneously pointing to the first letter of the word located on the board (see Figure 13-2 for an example of an alphabet board).
        • Limits range of possible words spoken.
        • Adds short pause between words to enhance lexical segmentation during connected speech.
      (b) Slows the rate of production.
      (c) Used to repair communication breakdowns (e.g., spelling out words not understood).
    (2) Additional candidacy criteria beyond general requirements.
      (a) Consistent voluntary phonation.
      (b) Minimal literacy skills.
      (c) Reliable method for highlighting letters (typically touch letter with finger).

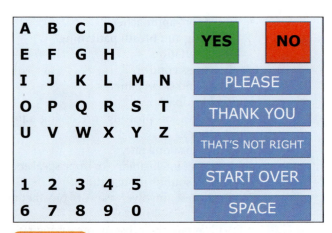

Figure 13-2 Alphabet Board

(d) Adequate cognitive and linguistic skills (e.g., pragmatic).
(3) Advantages.
    (a) Improves comprehensibility, and some speakers exhibit improved articulatory precision.
    (b) Faster than spelling out entire word.
    (c) Minimal cost.
    (d) Often minimal training involved.
(4) Disadvantages.
    (a) Slow rate adversely influences naturalness and communication efficiency.
    (b) For the most severe speakers, comprehensibility will fail to reach beyond 80%.
    (c) Possible future adaptation to technique (i.e., loose benefit).

Treatment of Apraxia of Speech

Treatment of Apraxia of Speech in Adults

1. Overview.
   a. Major goal to improve naturalness, effectiveness and efficiency, with a focus on articulation and prosody.
   b. Target reestablishing motor planning and programming or improving the ability to assemble, retrieve and execute planning and programming for speech.
   c. Based on the treatment literature on AOS, overall treatment can be successful, even with chronic cases; however, limited data exist for guiding decisions for deciding on a specific treatment for a specific speaker with AOS and predicting outcomes.
   d. Begin therapy with maximum cueing, with gradual fading of cues with success.
   e. Adopt principles of motor learning (see General Principles of Treatment for MSD above).
2. Treatment planning.
   a. Choose a motor or linguistic approach to treatment.
      (1) Decide on the separate contributions of AOS (i.e., motor planning and programming disorder) and any co-occurring aphasia (i.e., language disorder) to the communication deficit.
         (a) For some speakers, separating contributions is nearly impossible and combining motor and linguistic approaches of treatment must occur.
      (2) Significant contribution of AOS, use motor approach.
      (3) Significant contributions of aphasia, adopt melding of linguistic (i.e., target language deficits) and motor approaches.
   b. Considerations when choosing a specific motor approach.
      (1) Severity (e.g., articulatory kinematic methods used with more severely affected speakers).
      (2) Lack of prerequisite skills by speaker for specific motor approach (e.g., upper limb motor disabilities may rule out methods using hand tapping).
      (3) Training/experience of clinician.
   c. Selecting treatment targets.
      (1) Target meaningful sound combinations and not sound production.
      (2) Identify factors most adversely influencing communication.
         (a) Articulatory deviations, prosodic deviations and speech intelligibility.
         (b) Communication participation restrictions.
         (c) Environmental factors resulting in barriers to communication.
         (d) Counseling.
      (3) Refer to treatment information for reducing participation restriction and environment barriers in sections targeting individuals with dysarthria.
   d. Choosing speech stimuli.
      (1) General comments.
         (a) Use informal and formal testing to obtain:
            • An inventory of the nature of both accurate and inaccurate articulatory behaviors.
            • Factors influencing the articulatory behaviors (e.g., syllable shape, phonetic context, cueing effects).
         (b) Therapy success dependent on selection and ordering of stimuli.
         (c) Don't target individual phonemes unless for a very severe disorder.
      (2) Type of stimuli.
         (a) Choose functional stimuli with help of speaker and significant others (i.e., useful in meeting communication needs).
         (b) Initial stimuli should involve visible movements (i.e., anterior production) and movements that may benefit from tactile cueing.
         (c) The less severe the impairment, the greater length and articulatory and/or linguistic complexity of stimuli.

(d) Typically, speech stimuli are chosen; however, nonspeech targets (i.e., movements closely associated with speech sound positions) may be chosen for severe cases as initial building blocks to speech production.
(e) Often high-frequency, real words chosen over nonreal words and lower-frequency real words.
(f) Treating nonstimulable sounds and sounds with shared phonetic features may lead to better generalization.
(g) Speech sounds exhibiting low error rates should be targeted for more immediate success, but some support for improved generalization for targeting phonemes with high error percentages.
(h) Treatment typically targets more difficult end of the continuum (vowels, nasals, glides, plosives, fricatives, affricates, consonant clusters).
(i) Phonetic contrasts from least to most difficult.
- Oral/nasal.
- Voicing.
- Manner.
- Place.
(j) Stimuli may need to be chosen based on lack of certain sound contrast distinctions.
(k) Be cognizant of the influence prosody may have on articulation errors. If segmental distortion exists as a result of slow rate (i.e., exaggerated duration), need to target both prosodic and articulatory features. If place, manner or voicing errors are present, articulatory features should be targeted directly.

(3) Number of stimuli per session.
(a) Severity increases, set size decreases.
(b) Guiding factor: balance between mass and distributed practice.
(c) Target some stimuli for mass practice and others for distributed practice.
(d) As motor skills improve for certain stimuli, move those stimuli to distributed practice and add new stimuli, starting initially with mass practice.
(e) When stimuli receiving distributed practice meet accuracy criterion, shift to practice outside therapy room.
(f) Targeting more than one sound at a time can allow variable practice to occur (hypothesized to benefit generalization); however, may want to limit number of phonemes treated simultaneously (less than 3).

e. Intensity of treatment.
(1) Frequent sessions (e.g., four times per week).
(2) Length of session decreases with severity.

3. Motor approaches to treatment.
  a. Articulatory kinematic.
    (1) Key features.
      (a) Treatment focuses on improving spatial and temporal aspects of articulatory movement as a means to improve speech production.
      (b) Repeated, motoric practice of speech targets.
      (c) Facilitate articulatory accuracy through various forms of additional stimulation.
      (d) Provide movement information thought to be lacking or incorrect.
      (e) Involves conscious processing of various cues related to speech production.
      (f) Majority of evidence for more severe speakers with AOS.
    (2) Treatment targets.
      (a) Words (containing target sounds).
      (b) Short sentences or phrases.
    (3) Candidacy criteria.
      (a) Good auditory comprehension.
      (b) Aberrant speech sound production.
      (c) Motivated to improve speech.
      (d) Moderate to severe AOS.
    (4) Various techniques associated with the articulatory/kinematic category of treatment.
      (a) Modeling and repetition.
      (b) Integral stimulation.
      (c) Phonetic placement.
      (d) Phonetic derivation.
      (e) Key-word technique.
    (5) Overall results of articulatory kinematic treatment.
      (a) Improvement in the accuracy of trained sounds.
      (b) Training of an adequate number of exemplars for a given sound leads to accuracy improvements for untrained exemplars of the given sound.
      (c) Generalization to untrained sound typically does not occur.
  b. Rate and/or rhythm.
    (1) Key features.
      (a) Therapy techniques aimed to restore temporal control of speech production.
      (b) Assumes an underlying deficit in the timing of speech production (e.g., damaged central pattern generators) in individuals with AOS.
      (c) Rate and/or rhythm techniques focusing on slowing rate are hypothesized to benefit speech production by allowing additional

time for (1) planning and programming processes and (2) processing of feedback.
- (d) Other techniques (e.g., metronome or hand-tapping) may positively influence internal oscillatory mechanisms associated with speech production through entrainment or may refocus attention toward speech production processes.

(2) Treatment targets.
- (a) Varied types of targets.
- (b) Individual targets ranged from isolated vowels and vowel combinations to oral reading.
- (c) Targets often within a given treatment program involved a gradual increase in complexity with increasing treatment success.

(3) Candidacy criteria.
- (a) No specific restrictive criteria except for motivation to change behavior.

(4) Techniques.
- (a) Pacing via a metronome.
- (b) Hand tapping.
- (c) Utilization of a pacing board.

(5) Overall results for rate and/or rhythm treatment.
- (a) Improved articulation and fluency, a decrease in overall AOS symptoms, and reduced rate for trained material and mixed results for untrained material.

c. Alternative/augmentative communication (AAC).

(1) Key features.
- (a) AAC techniques aimed at substituting or supplementing verbal communication.
- (b) Verbal communication is viewed as less than adequate, and an alternate or supplemental form of communication is implemented.

(2) Treatment targets.
- (a) Range from skill training associated with the AAC system (e.g., acquisition of symbols) to application and acceptance by communication partners.

(3) Candidacy criteria.
- (a) Severe AOS.
- (b) Motivated to use AAC.
- (c) Adequate motor, visual, literacy and linguistic skills needed for the specific AAC system adopted.

(4) Techniques.
- (a) Comprehensive communication system.
- (b) Single systems involving pictures and symbols.
- (c) Voice output communication aid.

(5) AAC methods can be appropriate for some individuals with AOS who exhibit limited verbal output, but given the limited number of clinical research studies on this category of treatment, a prediction could not be made about success of treatment.

d. Intersystemic facilitation/reorganization.

(1) Key features.
- (a) Facilitate the function of an impaired system/modality (i.e., speaking) through a relatively intact system/modality (e.g., limb movement).
- (b) Hypothesized reasons for facilitating effects.
  - Provides additional sensory cues for speech production.
  - Use of limb gestures provide organizational framework for speech production.

(2) Treatment targets.
- (a) Words containing specific phonemes and sentences.
- (b) Accuracy of phonemes and word production and accuracy of gestures.

(3) Candidacy criteria.
- (a) Severe AOS.
- (b) Free of limb apraxia for use of meaningful gestures.
- (c) Ability to produce words, phrases or sentences for receiving nonmeaningful gestures.

(4) Techniques.
- (a) Gestural reorganization.
- (b) Singing.
- (c) Vibrotactile stimulation.

(5) Overall results for intersystemic facilitation/reorganization treatment.
- (a) Gestural reorganization.
  - Improvement in articulation and some improvement in gestures; however, uncertain about maintenance of gains.
  - Some generalization for gestures to untrained gestures.
- (b) Improvements for both vibrotactile stimulation and singing.
- (c) Improvements with intersystemic techniques.

Treatment of Childhood Apraxia of Speech

1. Overview.
   a. Treatment decision typically guided by understanding of disorder, but no universally accepted theory or model of CAS on which to base treatment.
   b. The predominant focus of therapy for CAS is to develop/improve motor planning and/or programming skills for speech sound production and prosody; however, other deficit areas may need attention (e.g., language, phonology, phonological awareness, literacy).

c. Consider other processing deficits (e.g., cognition, attention) in treatment planning.
d. A treatment plan should take into account ALL factors influencing communication (i.e., receptive/expressive language, phonological concerns, and literacy).

2. Basic principles of treatment.
   a. Goals.
      (1) Establish motor plans and programs for speaking.
      (2) Store the plans and program.
      (3) Habituate use of plans and programs to the level of automaticity.
   b. Treatment should incorporate motor learning principles (see General Principles of Treatment of MSD).
   c. Session characteristics.
      (1) Intensive and individualized treatment.
      (2) A clinician should maximize production practice during each practice session.
      (3) Adopt more frequent sessions (i.e., three to five per week) compared to traditional one to two sessions per week.
      (4) Length of session based on the attention/learning capabilities of child; however, 30-minute session appropriate for younger child.
   d. Practice stimuli.
      (1) Stimuli should typically include combinations of sounds.
      (2) Include a few words or phrases the child can use in daily communication (i.e., functional utterances).
      (3) In general, begin with less phonetically complex sounds and gradually increase in complexity as the child becomes more successful. For more severe speakers, may need to begin with nonmeaningful syllables in order to achieve building blocks of speech movement.
      (4) Choose stimuli the child can successfully imitate with cuing (i.e., auditory, visual and/or tactile) or through simultaneous repetition with clinician (integral stimulation procedures).
      (5) Build within the treatment hierarchy the gradual removal of forms of cueing (e.g., tactile, visual, auditory) or suprasegmental facilitator (e.g., slowing rate, stress) until achievement of spontaneous production of utterance.
      (6) Begin with smaller set of training words and increase in size with success; larger beginning set size with decreasing severity of the disorder.
      (7) After accomplishing correct production for a word in a set, begin practicing the word in a short sentence or phrase; add new word to original set.
   e. Use a multisensory approach to treatment (e.g., visual prompts, tactile cues, AAC).
   f. Teach the speaker to self-monitor.
   g. Auditory training typically not part of treatment program for CAS.
   h. Select some easily obtainable goals to ensure success and maintain motivation.
   i. May need to teach compensatory strategies (e.g., intrusive schwa for consonant clusters).
   j. Carryover and generalization of skills can be maximized through treating speakers within naturalistic environments.

3. Motor-based treatment methods.
   a. General comments.
      (1) A variety of different motor-based methods used to treat CAS.
      (2) Often methods are adoptions of techniques originally used with adults but take into account lack of experience with speaking in children.
      (3) Evidence supporting effectiveness is very limited for any one method of treatment.
   b. Factors to consider when choosing a specific motor-approach to treatment.
      (1) Severity (e.g., prosodic methods more appropriate for mild).
      (2) Presence of oral apraxia (may interfere with effective of cueing within some articulatory-based treatment methods).
      (3) Training/experience of clinician with method.
   c. Treatment methods.
      (1) Articulatory.
         (a) Key features.
            - Similar to the articulatory kinematic approach for adults with AOS.
            - The majority of articulatory treatment methods for CAS adopted features of integral stimulation (IS).
         (b) Specific methods.
            - Dynamic temporal and tactile cueing for speech motor learning.
              – Targets individual utterances within set of utterances chosen for client.
              – Utilizes motor learning principles such as mass and distributed practice and feedback schedules.
              – End result spontaneous productions with normal rate and prosody without cueing.
            - Nuffield Centre Dyspraxia Programme.
              – Based on a hierarchy, starting with core isolated sounds and consonant-vowel syllables, and gradually increasing the complexity of phonotactic structures and utterance length until reaching conversational speech.

- Controlling the phonotactic structure of utterances leads to the development of linguistic contrast.
- Visual materials supportive of literacy practice.
(2) Rhythm and/or rate.
  (a) Key features.
    - Provides speaker more time to evoke motor program and/or provide speaker with a longer time to process tactile and kinesthetic feedback information for positioning of articulators.
    - Hypothesized impaired prosody in CAS and rhythmic methods help to lay the groundwork for more improved speech rhythm, an important aspect of speech development.
    - Finally, the melody or intonation of speech along with hand tapping or signing can enhance speech production skills in speakers with a diagnosis of CAS.
  (b) Specific methods.
    - Different rhythm and/or rate methods.
    - Pairing movement of the body (e.g., foot or hand tapping for each syllable of a word) with speech production.
    - Melodic intonation therapy (MIT); refer to Chapter 12.
(3) Tactile/gestural.
  (a) Key features.
    - Provide multisensory input through both visual and kinesthetic cues.
    - Such cues thought to facilitate/enhance sequential speech movements.
  (b) Treatment methods.
    - Prompts for restructuring oral muscular phonetic targets.
      - Adoption of tactile cues to face and neck via hands to aid movement for syllable/word production.
      - Cues manner and place; presented in sequential order.
    - Targets meaningful utterances, moving to least to most motorically difficult.
    - Touch cues.
      - Utilized tactile cues on neck/face plus auditory and visual cues.
  (c) Stages of treatment.
    - Stage 1: nonsense syllable drills, learn cues, practice movement sequences, target self-monitoring.
    - Stage 2: move the movement sequences from stage 1 to nonsense and real monosyllabic and multisyllabic words; contrast through distinctive features.
    - Stage 3: continue sequencing skills to utterances of increasing length and eventually to conversational skills.
  (d) Adaptive cueing technique.
    - Gestural cueing (hand motion) for depiction of dynamic movement of articulators (tongue and jaw) in terms of place, manner and mandibular movement for consonants and vowels.
    - Hand gestures loosely based on manual sign alphabet.
    - Cues presented in synchrony with verbal production of an utterance by clinician for speech sequences (not individual phonemes).
(4) AAC.
  (a) Key features.
    - Adopted for speaker where communication needs are not being met through verbal means.
    - Can be supportive in language development.
    - Need to provide a rich, supportive environment where gains practice adopting AAC technique.
  (b) AAC methods.
    - Sign language.
    - Gesture.
    - Picture Exchange Communication System (PECS).

References

American Speech-Language-Hearing Association. (2007). Childhood apraxia of speech [Technical Report]. Available at: http://www.asha.org/policy/TR2007-00278/.

Ball, L. J., Beukelman, D. R., & Pattee, G. (2004). Communication effectiveness of individuals with amyotrophic lateral sclerosis. *Journal of Communication Disorders*, 37, 197–215.

Bashir, A. S., Grahamjones, F., & Bostwick, R. Y. (1984). "A Touch-Cue Method of Therapy for Developmental Verbal Apraxia" in W. H. Perkins & J. H. Northern (Eds.), *Seminars in Speech and Language*. New York: Thieme-Stratton, pp. 127–137.

Baylor, C. R., Yorkston, K. M., Eadie, T., Miller, R. M., & Amtmann, D. (2008). The levels of speech usage: A self-report scale for describing how people use speech. *Journal of Medical Speech-Language Pathology,* 16, 191–198.

Caruso, A. J., & Strand, E. (1999). *Clinical Management of Motor Speech Disorders in Children.* New York, NY: Thieme.

Clark, H. M. (2003). Neuromuscular treatments for speech and swallowing: A tutorial. *American Journal of Speech-Language Pathology,* 12, 400–415.

Crary, M. A. (1993). *Developmental Motor Speech Disorders.* San Diego, CA: Singular Publishing Group.

Darley, F. L., Aronson, A. E., & Brown, J. R. (1969a). Clusters of deviant speech dimensions in the dysarthrias. *Journal of Speech and Hearing Research,* 12, 462–496.

Darley, F. L., Aronson, A. E., & Brown, J. R. (1969b). Differential diagnostic patterns of dysarthrias. *Journal of Speech and Hearing Research,* 12, 246–269.

Darley, F. L., Aronson, A. E., & Brown, J. R. (1975). *Motor Speech Disorders.* Philadelphia, PA: W.B. Saunders.

Davis, B. L., &, Velleman, S. L. (2000). Differential diagnosis and treatment of developmental apraxia of speech in infants and toddlers. *Infant-Toddler Intervention,* 10, 177–192.

Duffy, J. R. (2005). *Motor Speech Disorders Substrates, Differential Diagnosis, and Management,* 2nd ed. St. Louis, MO: Mosby.

Duffy, J. R. (2007). "History, Current Practice, and Future Trends or Goals" in G. Weismer (Ed.), *Motor Speech Disorders: Essays for Ray Kent.* San Diego, CA: Plural Publishing Inc., pp. 7–56.

Duffy, J. R., & Abbs, J. (2003). Medical interventions for spasmodic dysphonia and some related conditions: A systematic review. *Journal of Medical Speech-Language Pathology,* 11, ix–lviii.

Dworkin, J. P. (1991). *Motor Speech Disorders: A Treatment Guide.* St. Louis, MO: Mosby.

Goldman-Eisler, F. (1968). *Psycholinguistics: Experiments in Spontaneous Speech.* New York, NY: Academic Press.

Hakel, M., Beukelman, D. R., Fager, S., Green, J., & Marshall, J. (2004). Nasal obturator for velopharyngeal dysfunction in dysarthria: Technical report on a one-way valve. *Journal of Medical Speech-Language Pathology,* 12, 155–159.

Hayden, D. A., & Square, P. A. (1994). Motor speech treatment hierarchy: A systems approach. *Clinics in Communication Disorders,* 4, 162–174.

Helfrich-Miller, K. E. (1994). Melodic intonation therapy for developmental apraxia. *Clinics in Communication Disorders,* 4, 175–182.

Hixon, T. J., & Hoit, J. D. (1998). Physical examination of the diaphragm by the speech-language pathologist. *American Journal of Speech-Language Pathology,* 7, 37–45.

Hixon, T. J., & Hoit, J. D. (1999). Physical examination of the abdominal wall by the speech-language pathologist. *American Journal of Speech-Language Pathology,* 8, 335–346.

Hixon, T. J., & Hoit, J. D. (2000). Physical examination of the rib cage by the speech-language pathologist. *American Journal of Speech-Language Pathology,* 9, 179–196.

Hodge, M. M. (2010). "Interventions for Children with Developmental Dysarthria" in A. L. Williams, S. McLeod, & R. McCauley (Eds.), *Interventions for Speech Sound Disorders in Children.* Baltimore, MD. Brookes Publishing Co., pp. 557–578.

Hodge, M. M., & Daniels, J. (2007). *Test of Children's Speech (TOC+) Intelligibility Measure* (Version 2.0) [Computer software]. Edmonton, AB: University of Alberta.

Hodge, M. M., & Hancock, H. R. (1994). Assessment of children with developmental apraxia of speech: A procedure. *Clinics in Communication Disorders,* 4, 102–118.

Kent, R. D., & Rosen, K. (2004). "Motor Control Perspectives on Motor Speech Disorders" in B. Maassen, R. D. Kent, H. F. M. Peters, P. H. H. M van Lieshout, & W. Hulstijn (Eds.), *Speech Motor Control in Normal and Disordered Speech.* Oxford, UK: University Press, pp. 285–311.

Kent, R. D., Weismer, G., Kent, J. F., & Rosenbek, J.C. (1989). Toward phonetic intelligibility testing in dysarthria. *Journal of Speech and Hearing Disorders,* 54, 482–499.

Klick, S. L. (1985). Adaptive cuing technique for use in treatment of dyspraxia. *Language, Speech and Hearing Services in Schools,* 16, 256–259.

Klick, S. L. (1994). Adapted cueing technique: Facilitating sequential phoneme production. *Clinical Communication Disorders,* 4, 183–189.

Love, R. J. (2000). *Childhood Motor Speech Disabilities,* 2nd ed. Boston, MA: Allyn and Bacon.

McCauley, R. J., & Strand, E. A. (2008). A review of standardized tests of nonverbal oral and speech motor performance in children. *American Journal of Speech-Language Pathology,* 17, 81–91.

McHenry, M. (2011). An exploration of listener variability in intelligibility judgments. *American Journal of Speech-Language Pathology,* 20, 119–123.

McNeil, M. R., Doyle, P. J., & Wambaugh, J. (2000). "Apraxia of Speech: A Treatable Disorder of Motor Planning and Programming" in S. E. Nadeau, L. J. Gonzalez Rothi, & B. Crosson (Eds.), *Aphasia and Language: Theory to Practice.* New York, NY: Guilford Press, pp. 221–266.

McNeil, M. R., & Kennedy, J. G. (1984). Measuring the effects of treatment for dysarthria: Knowing when to change or terminate. *Seminars in Speech and Language,* 4, 337–358.

McNeil, M. R., Robin, D. A., & Schmidt, R. A. (2009). "Apraxia of Speech: Definition and Differential Diagnosis" in *Clinical Management of Sensorimotor Speech Disorders,* 2nd ed. New York, NY: Thieme, pp. 249–258.

McNeil, M. R., Rosenbek, J. C., & Aronson, A. E. (1984). *The Dysarthrias: Physiology, Acoustics, Perception, Management.* San Diego, CA: College-Hill Press.

Morgan, A. T., & Vogel, A. P. (2008). Intervention for dysarthria associated with acquired brain injury in children and adolescents. *The Cochrane Database of Systematic Reviews,* 3. doi:10.1002/14651858.CD006279.pub2.

Morris, S. E. (1982). *Pre-Speech Scale: A Rating Scale for the Measurement of Pre-speech Behaviors from Birth Through Two Years.* Clifton, NJ: J.A. Preston.

Netsell, R. (1984). "Physiologic Studies of Dysarthria and Their Relevance to Treatment" in J. C. Rosenbek (Ed.), *Seminars in Speech and Language: Current Views of Dysarthria.* New York, NY: Thieme-Stratton.

Odell, D. H. (2002). Considerations in target selection in apraxia of speech treatment. *Seminars in Speech and Language,* 23, 309–323.

Pennington, L., Goldbart, J., & Marshall, J. (2003). Speech and language therapy to improve the communication skills of children with cerebral palsy. *The Cochrane Database of Systematic Reviews,* 3. doi:10.1002/14651858.CD003466.pub2.

Pindzola, R., Jenkins, M., & Lokken, F. (1989). Speaking rates of young children. *Language, Speech, and Hearing Services in the Schools*, 20, 133–138.

Ramig, L. O., Pawlas, A. A., & Countryman, S. (1995). *The Lee Silverman Voice Treatment.* Iowa City, IA: National Center for Voice and Speech.

Robbin, J., & Klee, T. (1987). Clinical assessment of oropharyngeal motor development in young children. *Journal of Speech and Hearing Disorders*, 52, 271–277.

Rosenbek, J. C. (1978). "Treating Apraxia of Speech" in D. F. Johns (Ed.), *Clinical Management of Neurogenic Communication Disorders.* Boston, MA: Little, Brown.

Rosenbek, J. C., & LaPointe, L. L. (1985). "The Dysarthrias: Description, Diagnosis, and Treatment" in D. F. Johns (Ed.), *Clinical Management of Neurogenic Communication Disorders*, 2nd ed. Boston: Little, Brown, pp. 97–152.

Rosenbek, J. C., Lemme, M. L., Ahern, M. R., Harris, E. H., & Wertz, R. T. (1973). A treatment for apraxia of speech in adults. *Journal of Speech and Hearing Disorders*, 38, 462–472.

Rosenbek, J. C., McNeil, M., & Aronson, A. E. (1984). *Apraxia of Speech: Physiology, Acoustics, Linguistics, Management.* San Diego, CA: College-Hill Press.

Shriberg, L. D. (1986). *Programs to Examine Phonetic and Phonologic Records in Children.* Madison, WI: University of Wisconsin.

Shriberg, L. D., Aram, D. M., & Kwiatkowski, J. (1997a). Developmental apraxia of speech: I. Descriptive and theoretical perspectives. *Journal of Speech, Language, and Hearing Research*, 40, 273–285.

Shriberg, L. D., Aram, D. M., & Kwiatkowski, J. (1997b). Development apraxia of speech. III. A subtype marked by inappropriate stress. *Journal of Speech, Language, and Hearing Research*, 40, 313–337.

Shriberg, L. D., & Kent, R. D. (2003). *Clinical Phonetics*, 3rd ed. Boston, MA: Allyn & Bacon.

Spencer, K. A., Yorkston, K. M. & Duffy, J. R. (2003). Behavioral management of respiratory/phonatory dysfunction from dysarthria: A flowchart for guidance in clinical decision making. *Journal of Medical Speech-Language Pathology*, 11, xxxix–lxi.

Square-Storer, P. A. (1989). *Acquired Apraxia of Speech in Aphasic Adults.* London: Taylor & Francis.

St. Louis, K. O., & Ruscello, D. (2000). *Oral Speech Mechanism Screening Examination,* 3rd ed. Austin, TX: Pro-Ed.

Strand, E. A. (1995). Treatment of motor speech disorders in children. *Seminars in Speech and Language*, 16, 126–139.

Strand, E. A., & Debertine, P. (2000). The efficacy of integral stimulation intervention with developmental apraxia of speech. *Journal of Medical Speech-Language Pathology*, 8, 295–300.

Strand, E. A., & McCauley, R. J. (1999). "Assessment Procedures for Treatment Planning in Children with Phonological and Motor Speech Disorders" in A. J. Caruso & E. A. Strand (Eds.), *Clinical Management of Motor Speech Disorders in Children.* New York, NY: Thieme, pp. 187–208.

Velleman, S. (2003). *Childhood Apraxia of Speech Resource Guide.* Clifton Park, NY: Delmar Learning.

Wambaugh, J. L., Duffy, J. R., McNeil, M. R., Robin, D. A., Rogers, M. A. (2006). Treatment guidelines for acquired apraxia of speech: Treatment descriptions and recommendations. *Journal of Medical Speech-Language Pathology*, 14, xxxv–lxvii.

Wambaugh, J., & Shuster, L. (2008). "The Nature and Management of Neuromotor Speech Disorders Accompanying Aphasia" in R. H. Chapey (Ed.), *Language Intervention Strategies in Aphasia and Related Neurogenic Communication Disorders*, 5th ed. Philadelphia, PA: Lippincott Williams & Wilkins, pp. 1009–1038.

Weismer, G. (2006). Philosophy of research in motor speech disorders. *Clinical Linguistics and Phonetics*, 20, 315–349.

Wertz, R. T., LaPointe, L. L., & Rosenbek, J. C. (1984). *Apraxia of Speech in Adults: The Disorder and Its Management.* New York, NY: Grune and Stratton.

Williams, P., & Stephens, H. (Eds.) (2004). *The Nuffield Centre Dyspraxia Programme*, 3rd ed. Windsor, UK: The Miracle Factory.

Williams, P., & Stephens, H. (2010). "The Nuffield Centre Dyspraxia Programme" in A.L. Williams, S. McLeod, & R. McCauley (Eds.), *Interventions for Speech Sound Disorders in Children.* Baltimore, MD. Brookes Publishing Co., pp. 159–178.

World Health Organization. (2001). *International Classification of Functioning, Disability and Health (ICF).* Geneva, Switzerland: Author.

Yorkston, K. M., Beukelman, D. R., & Bell, K. (1988). *Clinical Management of Dysarthric Speakers.* San Diego, CA: College-Hill Press.

Yorkston, K. M., Beukelman, D. R., Hakel, M., & Dorsey, M. (2007). *Speech Intelligibility Test for Windows.* Lincoln, NE: Institute for Rehabilitation Science and Engineering at Madonna Rehabilitation Hospital.

Yorkston, K. M., Beukelman, D. R., Strand, E. A., & Hakel, M. (2010). *Management of Motor Speech Disorders in Children and Adults*, 3rd ed. Austin, TX: ProEd.

Yorkston, K. M., Hakel, M., Beukelman, D. R., Fager, S. (2003). Evidence for effectiveness of treatment of loudness, rate, or prosody in dysarthria: A systematic review. *Journal of Medical Speech-Language Pathology*, 15, xi–xxxvi.

Yorkston, K. M., Spencer, K. A., & Duffy, J. R. (2003). Behavioral management of respiratory/phonatory dysfunction from dysarthria: A systematic review of the evidence. *Journal of Medical Speech-Language Pathology*, 11, xiii–xxxviii.

Yorkston, K. M., Spencer, K. A., Duffy, J. R., et al. (2001). Evidence-based practice guidelines for dysarthria: Management of velopharyngeal function. *Journal of Medical Speech-Language Pathology*, 9, 257–274.

Yoss, K. L. & Darley, F. L. (1974). Therapy in developmental apraxia of speech. *Language, Speech and Hearing Services in the Schools*, 5, 23–31.

SECTION IV

Structural Communication and Swallowing Disorders

Section Outline

- **Chapter 14:** Cleft Palate and Craniofacial Anomalies, 331
- **Chapter 15:** Voice Disorders in Children and Adults, 343
- **Chapter 16:** Dysphagia: Swallowing and Swallowing Disorders, 363

14

Cleft Palate and Craniofacial Anomalies

ANN W. KUMMER, PhD
AND MARGARET WILSON, MA

Chapter Outline

- Anatomy of the Face and Oropharyngeal Structures, 332
- Physiology of the Velopharyngeal Valve, 333
- Clefts, Craniofacial Anomalies and Syndromes, 335
- Resonance Disorders and Velopharyngeal Dysfunction, 338
- Evaluation and Treatment of Resonance and Velopharyngeal Function, 339
- References, 341

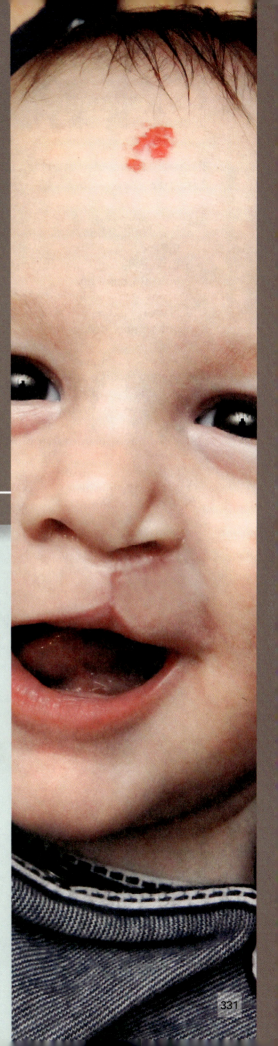

Anatomy of the Face and Oropharyngeal Structures

Nose, Nasal Cavity and Upper Lip

1. Outer nasal structures.
   a. Nasal bridge: bony structure that is located between the eyes.
   b. Columella: structure between the nostrils that supports the nasal tip.
   c. Ala nasi: the outside curved part around the nostril.
   d. Naris (plural nares): nostril.
2. Nasal septum: divides the nasal cavity into two sections.
   a. Vomer bone: trapezoidal-shaped bone in the nasal septum that is perpendicular to the palate.
   b. Perpendicular plate of the ethmoid.
   c. Quadrangular cartilage.
   d. Turbinates (also called conchae): long and narrow bony structures that protrude into the nasal cavity.
      (1) Superior turbinate.
      (2) Middle turbinate.
      (3) Inferior turbinate.
   e. Meatus (plural meatuses): passage in the nasal cavity that lies directly under a nasal turbinate.
      (1) Superior meatus.
      (2) Middle meatus.
      (3) Inferior meatus.
3. Upper lip.
   a. Philtrum: long dimple or indentation that courses from the columella down to the upper lip.
   b. Cupid's bow: the shape of the upper lip.
   c. Labial tubercle: prominent projection on the inferior border of the midsection of the upper lip.
   d. Vermillion: red tissue of the lips.

Oral Structures

1. Tongue.
   a. Dorsum of tongue (dorsal surface): top surface of tongue.
   b. Ventrum of tongue (ventral surface): under surface of tongue.
2. Faucial pillars and tonsils.
   a. Anterior and posterior faucial pillars: paired curtain-like structures in the back of the oral cavity on each side.
   b. Palatine tonsils: lymphoepithelial tissue found between the anterior and posterior faucial pillars on both sides.
   c. Lingual tonsils: masses of lymphoid tissue that are located at the base of the tongue and extend to the epiglottis.
3. Bones of the oral cavity (Figure 14-1).
   a. Alveolar ridge: outer surface of the hard palate that forms the bony support for the teeth.
   b. Incisive foramen: hole through the bone located in midline just behind the alveolar ridge of the maxillary arch.
   c. Premaxilla: triangular-shaped bone bordered on either side by the incisive suture lines and at the point by the incisive foramen.
   d. Hard palate: bony structure that separates the oral cavity from the nasal cavity.
   e. Pterygoid process of the sphenoid bone: provides attachments for velopharyngeal muscles. Contains:
      (1) Medial pterygoid plate.
      (2) Lateral pterygoid plate.
      (3) Pterygoid hamulus.
4. Velar structures (Figure 14-1).
   a. Velum (soft palate): soft, muscular structure, just posterior to the hard palate.
   b. Median palatine raphe: white suture line that can be seen coursing down the midline of the velum on the oral surface.
   c. Uvula: a teardrop-shaped structure that hangs freely from the posterior border of the velum.

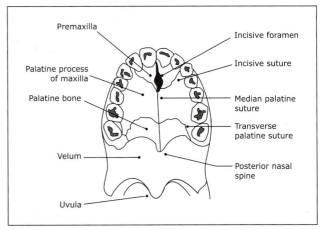

Figure 14-1 Structures of the Hard Palate and Velum

(From Kummer, A.W. 2008. *Cleft Palate and Craniofacial Anomalies: The Effects on Speech and Resonance*, 2nd ed. Clifton Park: Delmar Cengage, 2008, p. 9).

Pharyngeal Structures

1. Pharynx.
   a. Includes the throat area between the esophagus and the nasal cavity.
   b. Oropharynx: part of the pharynx that is at the level of the oral cavity or just posterior to the mouth.
   c. Nasopharynx: part of the pharynx that is above the oral cavity and velum and just posterior to the nasal cavity.
   d. Hypopharynx: part of the pharynx that is below the oral cavity and extends from the superior edge of the epiglottis inferiorly to the area of the esophagus and larynx.
   e. Posterior pharyngeal wall (PPW): back wall of the throat.
   f. Lateral pharyngeal walls (LPW): side walls of the throat.
2. Adenoids (also called "pharyngeal tonsils"): lymphoid tissue on the posterior pharyngeal wall of the nasopharynx, just behind the velum.
   a. Children often have velo-adenoidal closure during speech.
   b. Removal of the adenoids can affect velopharyngeal function.
3. Eustachian tube: membrane-lined tube that is lateral and slightly above the velum during phonation.
   a. Connects the middle ear with the pharynx on each side.
   b. Is responsible for middle ear function.

Physiology of the Velopharyngeal Valve

Velopharyngeal Function

1. Velar movement.
   a. During nasal breathing the velum rests against the base of the tongue, creating a patent airway (Figure 14-2).
   b. During speech the velum raises in a superior and posterior direction to contact the posterior pharyngeal wall or, in some cases, the lateral pharyngeal walls (Figure 14-3).
   c. "Knee action": the velum bends (like a knee) to provide maximum contact with the posterior pharyngeal wall over a large surface.
   d. "Velar dimple": indentation in the velum noted on the oral surface of the velum during phonation.

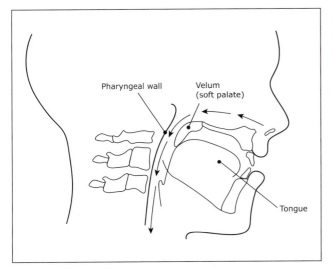

Figure 14-2 Lateral View of the Velum During Normal Nasal Breathing

(From Kummer, A.W. 2008. *Cleft Palate and Craniofacial Anomalies: The Effects on Speech and Resonance*, 2nd ed. Clifton Park: Delmar Cengage, 2008, p. 11).

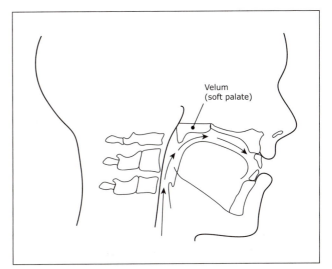

Figure 14-3 Lateral View of the Velum During Speech with Normal Velopharyngeal Closure

(From Kummer, A.W. 2008. *Cleft Palate and Craniofacial Anomalies: The Effects on Speech and Resonance*, 2nd ed. Clifton Park: Delmar Cengage, 2008, p. 11).

(1) Formed by the contraction of the levator muscles where they interdigitate.
(2) Usually located at a point that is about 80% of the distance from the hard palate to the end of the velum.
2. Lateral pharyngeal wall movement.
   a. Both walls move medially to close against the velum or, in some cases, to meet in midline behind the velum.
   b. There is variability as to the extent of movement in individuals.
   c. From oral cavity, walls may appear to bow outwards during movement for speech.
3. Posterior pharyngeal wall movement.
   a. Moves forward to assist in achieving contact against the velum, though this forward movement may be slight.
   b. Contributes less to closure.
4. Passavant's ridge.
   a. A shelf-like projection from the posterior pharyngeal wall that occurs inconsistently in some normal and abnormal individuals during velopharyngeal activities, such as speech, whistling and blowing.
   b. Not a permanent structure, but a dynamic structure that occurs during velopharyngeal movement and disappears when velopharyngeal activity ceases.
   c. Thought to be formed by contraction of the superior constrictor muscles.
   d. Usually occurs below velopharyngeal closure so it does not assist with closure.
   e. Does not indicate an abnormality and is not relevant when considering appropriate treatment.
5. Muscles of the velopharyngeal valve.
   a. All are paired muscles on each side of midline.
   b. Velopharyngeal sphincter requires the coordinated action of several different muscles.
      (1) Levator veli palatini: provide the main muscle mass of the velum.
         (a) Responsible for velar elevation in a 45-degree angle to close again the posterior pharyngeal wall.
         (b) Contraction is responsible for the "knee action" and also forms the velar dimple.
      (2) Superior constrictors: responsible for the medial displacement (constriction) of the lateral pharyngeal walls to narrow the velopharyngeal port to close around the velum.
      (3) Palatopharyngeus: associated with the medial movement of the lateral pharyngeal walls.
      (4) Palatoglossus: depresses the velum for production of nasal consonants in connected speech.
      (5) Salpingopharyngeus: have no significant role in achieving velopharyngeal closure.
      (6) Musculus uvulae: only intrinsic muscles of the velum.
         (a) Contracts during phonation to create a bulge on the superior and posterior part of the nasal surface of the velum.
         (b) Provides additional stiffness to the nasal side of the velum during velopharyngeal closure.
      (7) Tensor veli palatini: open the Eustachian tubes when the velum moves during swallowing or yawning; enhances middle ear aeration and drainage.
6. Motor and sensory innervation.
   a. Innervation arises from cranial nerves in the medulla.
   b. Motor and sensory innervation.
      (1) Pharyngeal plexus: a network of nerves that lies along the posterior wall of the pharynx.
      (2) Many cranial nerves provide motor and sensory innervation for the velopharyngeal complex.
         (a) Trigeminal (CN V).
         (b) Facial (CN VII).
         (c) Glossopharyngeal (CN IX).
         (d) Vagus (CN X).
         (e) Hypoglossal (CN XII).
7. Variations in velopharyngeal closure among speakers (normal and abnormal).
   a. Coronal.
      (1) Most common pattern.
      (2) Posterior movement of the soft palate closes against a broad area of the posterior pharyngeal wall.
      (3) There is little contribution from lateral pharyngeal walls.
      (4) When closure is complete, there is a coronal slit.
   b. Circular.
      (1) Second-most common pattern.
      (2) Soft palate moves posteriorly, the posterior pharyngeal wall moves anteriorly and the lateral pharyngeal walls move medially.
      (3) Closes like a true sphincter.
      (4) When closure is complete, there is a circular slit.
      (5) Passavant's ridge is commonly seen with this type of closure.
   c. Sagittal.
      (1) Least common pattern.
      (2) The lateral pharyngeal walls move medially to meet in midline behind the velum.
      (3) There is minimal posterior displacement of the soft palate for closure.
      (4) When closure is complete, there is a sagittal slit.
   d. The patient's basic pattern of closure can affect surgical treatment decisions for velopharyngeal insufficiency.
8. Variations with type of velopharyngeal activity.
   a. Nonpneumatic activities do not involve air pressure.

(1) Includes swallowing, gagging and vomiting.
(2) Velum rises very high in the pharynx and the lateral pharyngeal walls close tightly along their entire length.
(3) Closure appears to be exaggerated and is very firm.
  b. Pneumatic activities involve air pressure.
(1) Positive pressure activities such as blowing, whistling, singing and speech.
(2) Negative pressure activities: sucking and kissing.
(3) Closure occurs lower and is less exaggerated than with nonpneumatic activities.
  c. There is a different neurophysiological mechanism for different activities, which is why blowing and sucking exercises do not improve velopharyngeal function for speech.
  d. Other causes of variations in velopharyngeal closure.
(1) Phonemic content.
(2) Length of the utterance.
(3) Rate and fatigue.
(4) Changes with growth and age.
9. Physiologic subsystems for speech.
  a. Respiration.
  b. Phonation.
  c. Stress and intonation.
  d. Velopharyngeal function.
  e. Articulation.

Clefts, Craniofacial Anomalies and Syndromes

Cleft Lip and Palate

1. Primary palate structures.
   a. Located anterior to the incisive foramen.
   b. Includes lip and alveolar ridge.
   c. Develops at seven weeks' gestation.
   d. Embryological path from the incisive foramen to the lip.
2. Primary palate clefts.
   a. "Complete" clefts of the primary palate extend through the lip and alveolus to incisive foramen.
   b. Incomplete clefts do not extend all the way to the incisive foramen and can include:
      (1) A "forme fruste" or slight notch of the lip.
      (2) A cleft of the lip only.
      (3) A cleft of the lip and just part of the alveolus.
   c. Cleft location: unilateral or bilateral.
   d. Suture(s) affected: incisive sutures.
3. Secondary palate structures.
   a. Located posterior to incisive foramen.
   b. Includes hard palate, velum and uvula.
   c. Develops at nine weeks' gestation.
   d. Embryological path from the incisive foramen to the uvula.
4. Secondary palate clefts.
   a. "Complete" clefts of the secondary palate extend from the uvula to incisive foramen.
   b. Incomplete clefts do not extend all the way to the incisive foramen and can include:
      (1) A bifid uvula.
      (2) A cleft of velum only.
      (3) A cleft of the velum and just part of the hard palate.
   c. Cleft location: midline only.
   d. Suture affected: median palatine suture.
5. Effects of cleft lip and palate on speech.
   a. Dental and occlusal anomalies, particularly crossbites and Class III malocclusion.
   b. Hearing loss due to Eustachian tube malfunction.
   c. Velopharyngeal insufficiency (VPI). (See Syndromes Associated with Cleft Lip, Cleft Palate or VPI.)
6. Effects of cleft lip and palate on feeding.
   a. Cleft lip usually does not affect feeding.
   b. Cleft palate causes the inability to build up suction, due to the open cleft, and can also cause initial difficulties with compression of the nipple.
   c. Breastfeeding is usually not possible with cleft palate.
   d. With use of special nipples and bottles until the palate is repaired, most babies with clefts are able to feed well.

Sequence Associated with Cleft Palate

1. Pierre Robin sequence.
   a. Type of cleft: usually a wide, bell-shaped cleft palate.
   b. Craniofacial features: micrognathia (small mandible), glossoptosis (posterior tongue position).

c. Functional concerns.
   (1) Airway and feeding problems, particularly at birth, due to the micrognathia and glossoptosis.
   (2) Speech issues secondary to velopharyngeal insufficiency.

Syndromes Associated with Cleft Lip, Cleft Palate or VPI

1. Velocardiofacial syndrome (deletion 22q11.2 syndrome).
   a. Type of cleft: usually occult submucous cleft palate or velopharyngeal hypotonia.
   b. Craniofacial features.
      (1) *Velo*—often velopharyngeal dysfunction causing hypernasality.
      (2) *Cardio*—minor cardiac and vascular anomalies.
      (3) *Facial*.
         (a) Microcephaly, long face with vertical maxillary excess.
         (b) Micrognathia (small jaw) or retruded mandible, often with a Class II malocclusion.
         (c) Nasal anomalies including wide nasal bridge, narrow alar base and bulbous nasal tip.
         (d) Narrow palpebral fissures (slit-like eyes).
         (e) Malar flatness.
         (f) Thin upper lip.
         (g) Minor auricular anomalies.
         (h) Abundant scalp hair.
      (4) Other abnormalities: long, slender fingers; short stature.
      (5) Functional concerns: hypernasality and speech sound errors, language delay and learning problems and risk for psychiatric problems in adolescence.
2. Stickler syndrome.
   a. Type of cleft: cleft palate only.
   b. Craniofacial features.
      (1) Pierre Robin sequence with the characteristics of micrognathia, glossoptosis and wide bell-shaped cleft palate.
      (2) A wide, flat face with midface hypoplasia.
      (3) Epicanthal folds.
   c. Functional concerns.
      (1) Sensorineural hearing loss.
      (2) High myopia and risk for retinal detachments.
      (3) Risk for velopharyngeal insufficiency.
3. Fetal alcohol syndrome (FAS).
   a. Type of cleft: Pierre Robin sequence, cleft palate and cleft lip.
   b. Craniofacial features.
      (1) Short palpebral fissures.
      (2) Short nose, flat philtrum and thin upper lip.
      (3) Microcephaly.
   c. Functional concerns: developmental disabilities, behavior problems and speech and language disorders.
4. Trisomy 13.
   a. Type of cleft: cleft lip and palate; may have a midline cleft.
   b. Craniofacial features: holoprosencephaly, severe eye defects; midline facial deformities.
   c. Functional concerns: usually fatal before the first birthday.
5. Wolf-Hirschhorn syndrome.
   a. Type of cleft: cleft palate is common.
   b. Craniofacial features.
      (1) Distinctive facial appearance likened to a Greek helmet.
      (2) Hypertelorism.
      (3) Coloboma of the iris.
      (4) Prominent nasal bridge.
      (5) Microcephaly.
      (6) Micrognathia.
      (7) Short philtrum.
      (8) Dysplastic ears.
      (9) Pre-auricular tags.
   c. Functional concerns: developmental disabilities, speech and language disorders, occasional hearing loss.
6. Opitz G syndrome.
   a. Type of cleft: laryngeal cleft, cleft lip, cleft palate.
   b. Craniofacial features: hypertelorism, flat nasal bridge, thin upper lip and low-set ears.
   c. Functional concerns: voice and swallowing problems if there is a laryngeal cleft.
7. Van der Woude syndrome.
   a. Type of cleft: cleft lip and palate.
   b. Craniofacial features: bilateral lip pits on the lower lip; missing teeth.
   c. Functional concerns: speech disorders related to cleft lip and palate.
8. Orofaciodigital syndrome Type I (OFD I).
   a. Type of cleft: cleft lip, cleft palate, midline cleft lip.
   b. Craniofacial features.
      (1) Hypertelorism.
      (2) Lobulated tongue.
      (3) Multiple hyperplastic oral frenula.
      (4) Notching in alveolar ridge.
      (5) Broad nose.
      (6) Hydrocephalus.
      (7) Absence of corpus callosum.
   c. Functional concerns: developmental disabilities and speech and language disorders.

Craniosynostosis Syndromes

1. Saethre-Chotzen syndrome.
   a. Type of cleft: cleft palate or submucous cleft palate.
   b. Craniofacial features: oronasal synostosis, ptosis of the eyelids, midface hypoplasia, external ear anomalies.
   c. Functional concerns: risk for developmental disabilities.
2. Crouzon syndrome.
   a. Type of cleft: cleft palate; submucous cleft palate is occasionally seen.
   b. Craniofacial features: similar to Apert syndrome, including a broad forehead, flat occiput, exophthalmos, hypertelorism, antimongoloid slant, strabismus and midface hypoplasia/retrusion, Class III malocclusion, low-set ears.
   c. Functional concerns: risk for developmental disabilities and upper airway obstruction.
3. Apert syndrome.
   a. Type of cleft: cleft palate occurs infrequently.
   b. Craniofacial features: similar to Crouzon syndrome, including a prominent forehead with a flat occiput, exophthalmos, hypertelorism, antimongoloid slant, strabismus and midface hypoplasia/retrusion, Class III malocclusion, low-set ears.
   c. Functional concerns: developmental disabilities, speech and language disorders, upper airway obstruction.
4. Pfeiffer syndrome.
   a. Type of cleft: cleft palate is rare.
   b. Craniofacial features.
      (1) Coronal craniosynostosis.
      (2) Midface hypoplasia.
      (3) Shallow orbits with exophthalmos.
      (4) Hypertelorism.
      (5) Tracheal anomalies.
      (6) Upper airway stenosis.
   c. Functional concerns: hearing loss, developmental disabilities in Pfeiffer type 2 and type 3 and upper airway obstruction.

Other Syndromes

1. Hemifacial microsomia (oculoauriculovertebral dysplasia).
   a. Type of cleft: cleft lip and/or palate in about 15% of cases.
   b. Craniofacial features.
      (1) Facial asymmetry due to unilateral hypoplasia of the face, malar, maxillary and/or mandibular processes.
      (2) Cleft-like extension of corner of mouth.
      (3) Ear anomalies, including microtia or anotia and preauricular tags or pits.
      (4) Eye anomalies including colobomas of upper eyelid, epibulbar lipodermoids, microphthalmia.
      (5) Dysplasia or aplasia of temporomandibular joint, affecting the opening of the mouth and excursion of mandible.
   c. Functional concerns: hearing loss, occasional velopharyngeal insufficiency or incompetence due to unilateral velar paralysis or paresis.
2. CHARGE syndrome.
   a. Type of cleft: Pierre Robin sequence, cleft lip and palate.
   b. Primary features.
      (1) <u>C</u>oloboma.
      (2) <u>H</u>eart disease.
      (3) <u>A</u>tresia of the choanae.
      (4) <u>R</u>etarded growth and development.
      (5) <u>G</u>enital anomalies, cryptorchidism, micropenis, hypogonadism, delayed puberty.
      (6) <u>E</u>ar anomalies, hearing loss and deafness.
   c. Functional concerns: hearing loss or deafness, developmental disabilities, speech and language disorders.
3. Treacher Collins syndrome.
   a. Type of cleft: clefts occur infrequently, despite Pierre Robin sequence with pronounced micrognathia.
   b. Craniofacial features.
      (1) Downward slanting of the palpebral fissures.
      (2) Colobomas of the lower eyelids.
      (3) Microtia or middle ear anomalies.
      (4) Hypoplastic zygomatic arches and malar hypoplasia.
      (5) Macrostomia or microstomia.
      (6) Micrognathia.
      (7) Glossoptosis.
   c. Functional concerns: hearing loss.
4. Beckwith-Wiedemann syndrome.
   a. Type of cleft: none.
   b. Craniofacial features: hypertrophic facial features, macroglossia.
   c. Functional concerns: airway, feeding and speech disorders.

Resonance Disorders and Velopharyngeal Dysfunction

Normal Resonance and Velopharyngeal Function

1. Normal resonance.
   a. Determined by the function of the velopharyngeal valve.
   b. Affected by the size and shape of cavities of the vocal tract (pharynx, oral cavity, nasal cavity).
2. Velopharyngeal structures.
   a. Velum (soft palate).
   b. Lateral pharyngeal walls (LPW).
   c. Posterior pharyngeal walls (PPW).
   d. See anatomy section for more information.
3. Normal velopharyngeal function is dependent on:
   a. Normal anatomy (structure).
   b. Normal neurophysiology (function).
   c. Normal speech sound learning (articulation).

Velopharyngeal Dysfunction

1. Velopharyngeal insufficiency (VPI) (Figure 14-4).
   a. Associated anatomical defects.
      (1) History of cleft palate or submucous cleft (overt or occult).
      (2) Short velum.
      (3) Deep pharynx due to cervical spine or cranial base abnormalities.
      (4) Irregular adenoids.
      (5) Enlarged tonsils that intrude into nasopharynx and affect closure.
   b. Surgical or intervention causes.
      (1) Adenoidectomy.
      (2) Maxillary advancement (Le Fort I or distraction).
      (3) Treatment of nasopharyngeal tumors (surgical or radiation).
      (4) Cervical spine surgery through the mouth.
   c. Treatment: Always requires physical management (i.e., surgery or an obturator if surgery is not an option). Speech therapy is often required to change compensatory productions that developed as a result of the VPI.
2. Velopharyngeal incompetence (VPI) (Figure 14-5).
   a. Associated neurophysiological disorders.
      (1) Velar and/or pharyngeal hypotonia.
      (2) Velar paralysis or paresis due to brain stem or cranial nerve injury.
      (3) Neuromuscular disorders.
         (a) Myasthenia gravis.

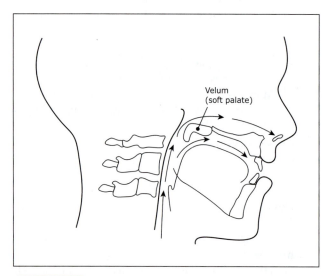

Figure 14-4 Velopharyngeal Insufficiency

Note the abnormality in structure in that the velum is too short for closure against the posterior pharyngeal wall during speech.

(From Kummer, A.W. 2008. *Cleft Palate and Craniofacial Anomalies: The Effects on Speech and Resonance*, 2nd ed. Clifton Park: Delmar Cengage, 2008, p. 179).

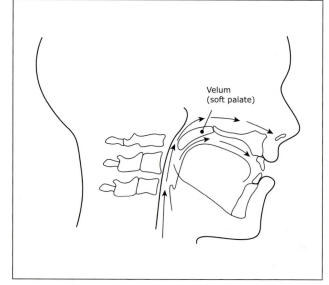

Figure 14-5 Velopharyngeal Incompetence

Note the poor movement of the velum during speech.

(From Kummer, A.W. 2008. *Cleft Palate and Craniofacial Anomalies: The Effects on Speech and Resonance*, 2nd ed. Clifton Park: Delmar Cengage, 2008, p. 179).

(b) Muscular dystrophy.
(c) Cerebral palsy.
(4) Dysarthria due to a central insult.
(5) Apraxia due to congenital or acquired neurological causes.
b. Treatment: With the exception of apraxia, usually requires physical management (i.e., palatal lift or even surgery in selected cases).
3. Velopharyngeal mislearning.
a. Caused by faulty articulation learning.
(1) Severe hearing loss or deafness causes abnormal resonance due to a lack of auditory feedback.
(2) Pharyngeal or nasal articulation of consonants results in phoneme-specific nasal emission.
(3) Pharyngeal or nasal articulation of vowels results in phoneme-specific hypernasality.
b. Treatment always requires speech therapy; never requires surgery.
4. Effects of velopharyngeal dysfunction on speech.
a. Hypernasality (see description under Resonance Disorders).
b. Nasal air emission resulting in:
(1) Weak or omitted consonants due to the lack of adequate air pressure.
(2) Short utterance length, due to the need to take frequent breaths to replenish the lost airflow through the nose.
(3) Dysphonia due to strain in the entire vocal tract in efforts to achieve velopharyngeal closure.
(4) Compensatory articulation productions: abnormal articulation placement in an attempt to compensate for the lack of air pressure in the oral cavity; usually produced in the pharynx where there is air pressure.
(5) Obligatory distortions: distortions due to abnormal structure (i.e., VPI), despite normal articulation placement.

Resonance Disorders

1. Hypernasality.
a. Too much sound resonating in the nasal cavity during speech.
b. Most perceptible on vowels (because vowels are voiced).
c. Voiced consonants may be nasalized (i.e., m / b, n / d).
d. Does not affect voiceless consonants, because resonance is the result of sound vibration.
e. Causes: VPI or a fistula (hole in the palate due to a palate repair breakdown); can even be caused by keeping the back of the tongue too high when articulating vowels.
2. Hyponasality.
a. Not enough sound resonating in the nasal cavity during speech.
b. Most perceptible on nasal consonants (/m/, /n/, /ŋ/).
c. Can also be noted on vowel sounds.
d. Cause: upper airway obstruction due to adenoid hypertrophy or nasal blockage.
3. Cul-de-sac resonance.
a. Occurs when the sound resonates in the pharynx or nasal cavity but is not released due to obstruction.
b. Commonly caused by enlarged tonsils, which block the entrance to the oral cavity, causing pharyngeal cul-de-sac resonance.
4. Mixed nasality.
a. Occurs when there is hypernasality and/or nasal air emission on oral consonants and hyponasality on nasal consonants.
b. Caused by apraxia or a combination of velopharyngeal dysfunction and upper airway obstruction.

Evaluation and Treatment of Resonance and Velopharyngeal Function

Evaluation of Resonance and Velopharyngeal Dysfunction

1. Perceptual evaluation.
a. Determine type of resonance (normal oral resonance, hypernasality, hyponasality, cul-de-sac resonance or mixed resonance).
b. Determine if there is nasal emission, and if so, whether it is consistent or phoneme-specific.
c. Determine if there are compensatory errors or obligatory distortions.
2. Oral examination.
a. Evaluate oral structures and function.
(1) Palatal arch and presence of fistula (if there is a history of cleft palate).
(2) Evidence of submucous cleft palate, including a bifid or hypoplastic uvula, an upside-down "V" shape of the velum during phonation or a zona pellucida (thin, bluish area in the soft palate). Occasionally you can palpate a notch in the hard palate.
(3) Position of uvula during phonation.

- (4) Size of tonsils.
- (5) Dental occlusion and teeth that may interfere with tongue tip movement.
- (6) Signs of oral-motor dysfunction.
- (7) Signs of upper airway obstruction.
  b. Can't evaluate velopharyngeal function because it is above the oral level.
3. Instrumental assessment.
   a. Nasometer.
      (1) Uses a headset to capture acoustic energy from the nasal cavity and oral cavity during the production of speech.
      (2) Gives a ratio of oral energy over total energy for a nasalance score, which can be compared to normative data.
   b. Aerodynamic instrumentation.
      (1) Uses catheters for the nose and mouth and pressure transducers.
      (2) Measures air pressure and airflow during production of a small speech segment.
      (3) Gives an estimate of velopharyngeal orifice size during speech production.
   c. Videofluoroscopy.
      (1) A multi-view, radiographic procedure of the velopharyngeal valve.
      (2) Requires multiple views, usually a lateral, frontal and base view, to assess velopharyngeal closure during speech.
   d. Nasopharyngoscopy.
      (1) An endoscope is passed through the nasal cavity to the nasopharyngeal port.
      (2) Allows the examiner to view the nasal surface of the velum and the entire velopharyngeal port during speech.

Treatment of Resonance and Velopharyngeal Dysfunction

1. Surgery for velopharyngeal insufficiency or incompetence (VPI).
   a. Velopharyngeal insufficiency or incompetence requires physical management, preferably surgical intervention.
   b. Speech therapy cannot correct hypernasality or nasal emission due to VPI.
   c. Common surgical procedures.
      (1) Pharyngeal augmentation: injection or implantation of a substance in the posterior pharyngeal wall or velum to fill in an opening.
      (2) Furlow Z-plasty: technique to repair the velum in an attempt to lengthen it.
      (3) Sphincter pharyngoplasty: the posterior faucial pillars (which include the palatopharyngeus muscles) are released at the base, rotated backward and overlapped on the posterior pharyngeal wall. This narrows the sides of the pharyngeal port but leaves the port open in midline.
      (4) Pharyngeal flap: a flap is elevated from the posterior pharyngeal wall and sutured into the velum to partially close the nasopharynx in midline.
         (a) Lateral ports are left on either side for nasal breathing and production of nasal sounds.
2. Prosthetic devices.
   a. Prosthetic devices are used either on a temporary basis or when surgery is not an option.
   b. Prosthetic device types.
      (1) Palatal lift: to raise the velum when velar mobility is poor.
      (2) Palatal obturator: to close or occlude an open cleft or fistula.
      (3) Speech bulb obturator: to occlude nasopharynx when velum is short.
3. Speech therapy.
   a. Speech therapy cannot correct hypernasality or nasal emission due to VPI.
   b. Speech therapy is appropriate after repair of the structure to address:
      (1) Compensatory articulation errors due to VPI.
         (a) Pharyngeal plosive.
         (b) Glottal stop (plosive).
         (c) Pharyngeal fricative/affricate.
         (d) Posterior nasal fricative.
      (2) Compensatory productions due to a fistula.
         (a) Velar fricatives.
         (b) Generalized backing.
      (3) Compensatory productions due to abnormal dental occlusion.
         (a) Palatal-dorsal productions.
      (4) Phoneme-specific nasal air emission, where nasal emission is due to faulty articulation. This occurs most commonly on sibilant sounds (/s/, /z/, /ʃ/, /ʒ/, /tʃ/, /dʒ/).
      (5) Variable resonance due to apraxia of speech.
      (6) Hypernasality or nasal emission following surgical correction.
         (a) Changing structure does not change function.
         (b) Patient needs to learn to use the corrected valve through auditory feedback.
   c. Techniques.
      (1) Auditory awareness and auditory feedback.
      (2) Articulation techniques to correct placement.
      (3) Drills and frequent practice (as is consistent with motor learning evidence).
      (4) Blowing exercises, sucking exercises, velar exercises or oral-motor exercises are NOT effective and are totally inappropriate.

d. Timeline for intervention and assessment for children with history of cleft lip and palate.
   (1) Birth to three years: should monitor language development and start language therapy, if needed.
   (2) Three years: should evaluate velopharyngeal function and start speech therapy, if needed.

References

American Cleft Palate–Craniofacial Association (ACPA). (2009). Parameters for evaluation and treatment of patients with cleft lip/ palate or other craniofacial anomalies. *Cleft Palate-Craniofacial Journal*, 30 (Suppl.), 1–16.

Kummer, A.W. (2009). "Assessment of Velopharyngeal Function." In J. E. Lossee & R. E. Kirschner (Eds.), *Comprehensive Cleft Care*. New York: McGraw-Hill.

Kummer, A.W. (2011). Disorders of resonance and airflow secondary to cleft palate and/or velopharyngeal dysfunction. *Seminars in Speech and Language*, 32(2), 141–149.

Kummer A.W. (2011). Perceptual assessment of resonance and velopharyngeal function. *Seminars in Speech and Language*, 32(2), 159–167.

Kummer, A.W. (2011). Speech therapy for errors secondary to cleft palate and velopharyngeal dysfunction. *Seminars in Speech and Language*, 32(2), 191–198.

Kummer, A.W. (2011). Types and causes of velopharyngeal dysfunction. *Seminars in Speech and Language*, 32(2), 150–158.

Kummer, A.W. (2014). *Cleft Palate and Craniofacial Anomalies: The Effects on Speech and Resonance*, 3rd ed. Clifton Park, NY: Cengage Learning.

Perry, J.L. (2011). Anatomy and physiology of the velopharyngeal mechanism. *Seminars in Speech and Language*, 32(2), 83–92.

Peterson-Falzone, S.J. (2011). Types of clefts and multianomaly craniofacial conditions. *Seminars in Speech and Language*, 32(2), 93–114.

Peterson-Falzone S.J., Hardin-Jones M.A., & Karnell, M.P. (2010). *Cleft Palate Speech*, 4th ed. St. Louis, MO: Elsevier.

Smith B.E., & Kuehn D.P. (2007). Speech evaluation of velopharyngeal dysfunction. *Journal of Craniofacial Surgery*, 18(2), 251–260.

15

Voice Disorders in Children and Adults

GAIL B. KEMPSTER, PhD

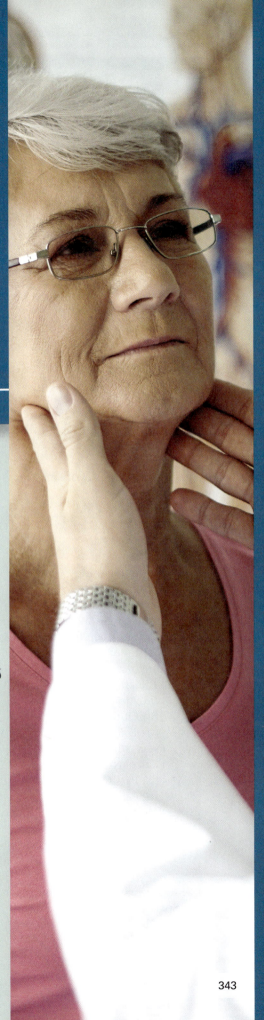

Chapter Outline

- Anatomy and Physiology of the Vocal Mechanism, 344
- Processes of Speech, 345
- Measures of Voice Production (Acoustic, Aerodynamic, Perceptual), 346
- Development of the Vocal Mechanism, 348
- Theories and Processes of Phonation, 348
- Etiologies and Characteristics of Vocal Pathologies, 349
- Pediatric Voice Problems, 354
- High-Risk and Special Needs Voice Populations, 355
- Voice Evaluation Protocol, 356
- Prevention of Voice Disorders and Promotion of Vocal Health, 358
- Evidence-Based Voice Treatment Approaches, 358
- Management Recommendations and Referrals, 358
- Management of Head and Neck Cancer, 359
- Anatomical and Physiologic Changes After Total Laryngectomy, 359
- Alaryngeal Voice Assessment Protocol, 360
- Alaryngeal Voice Treatment Approaches and Considerations, 360
- Other Head and Neck Cancer Effects on Speech, Voice and/or Swallowing, 360
- References, 361

Anatomy and Physiology of the Vocal Mechanism

Anatomy

1. Supportive framework comprised of bone and cartilages.
   a. Hyoid bone.
   b. Thyroid cartilage.
   c. Cricoid cartilage.
   d. Arytenoid cartilages.
   e. Epiglottis.
   f. Corniculate cartilages.
   g. Cuneiform cartilages.

Physiology

1. Extrinsic laryngeal and supplementary muscles.
   a. Suprahyoid muscles: move the larynx superiorly and anteriorly, or superiorly and posteriorly.
      (1) Mylohyoid.
      (2) Geniohyoid.
      (3) Anterior belly of digastric.
      (4) Hyoglossus.
      (5) Stylohyoid.
   b. Infrahyoid muscles: lower and stabilize the larynx.
      (1) Thyrohyoid.
      (2) Sternohyoid.
      (3) Sternothyroid.
      (4) Omohyoid.
      (5) Inferior constrictor.
2. Intrinsic laryngeal muscles.
   a. Abductors: open the vocal folds.
      (1) Posterior cricoarytenoids (PCA).
   b. Adductors: close the vocal folds.
      (1) Lateral cricoarytenoids (LCA).
      (2) Interarytenoids (IA).
         (a) Oblique interarytenoids.
         (b) Transverse interarytenoid.
   c. Tensors: stiffen or lengthen the vocal folds.
      (1) Cricoarytenoids (CT).
         (a) Pars recta.
         (b) Pars oblique.
      (2) Thyroarytenoids (TA): true vocal folds.
         (a) Medial/Internal (thyrovocalis).
         (b) Lateral/External (thyromuscularis).
         (c) TA may contribute as a vocal fold relaxer under some circumstances.
3. Associated anatomical features.
   a. Spaces.
      (1) Glottis: space between vocal folds.
      (2) Supraglottal area: space above vocal folds, below the base of the tongue.
      (3) Infraglottal area: space below true vocal folds.
      (4) Ventricle: space between true and false vocal folds.
      (5) Aditus: opening to the larynx.
      (6) Vestibule: region between false folds and aditus.
   b. Other muscles and tissues.
      (1) Ventricular folds: false vocal folds.
      (2) Quadrangular membrane: membrane lining the supraglottal region.
      (3) Conus elasticus: membrane lining the infraglottal region and connecting the thyroid, cricoid and arytenoid cartilages.
      (4) Vocal ligament: medial edges of the vocal folds, part of the conus elasticus, containing both elastic and collagenous fibers.
      (5) Macula flava: dense tissue connecting vocal folds to the cartilages at anterior and posterior ends.
      (6) Cricothyroid ligament: connects the cricoid and thyroid cartilages at the anterior midline; part of the conus elasticus.
      (7) Cricothyroid membrane: connects the cricoid and thyroid cartilages lateral to the cricothyroid ligament; part of the conus elasticus.
      (8) Aryepiglottic folds: connect the arytenoid cartilages and the epiglottis, contain the cuneiform cartilages, help in the closing/folding protective mechanism of the larynx.
4. Vocal fold histology.
   a. Layer structure of vocal folds.
      (1) Cover.
         (a) Squamous epithelium.
         (b) Superficial layer of the lamina propria.
      (2) Transition (form the vocal ligament).
         (a) Intermediate layer of the lamina propria.
         (b) Deep layer of the lamina propria.
      (3) Body.
         (a) Thyroarytenoid muscle.
   b. Important cellular elements in vocal fold tissue.
      (1) Interstitial proteins.
      (2) Elastin.
      (3) Collagen.
      (4) Basement membrane zone.
         (a) Complex layer of proteins.
         (b) Connects deepest layer of squamous cells to the superficial layer of the lamina propria.
      (5) Extracellular matrix.

(a) Substance of interstitial proteins, including hyaluronic acid, filling spaces between cells.
(b) Important in wound repair and regeneration of tissues.

Neuroanatomy of Phonation

1. Cranial nerve input to the larynx.
   a. Vagus nerve is cranial nerve X (CN X).
      (1) Cell body for motor neurons of CN X in nucleus ambiguus.
   b. Three branches of vagus go to the pharynx and larynx.
      (1) Pharyngeal nerve.
         (a) Innervates soft palate via pharyngeal plexus.
      (2) Superior laryngeal nerve (SLN).
         (a) Internal branch: sensory to glottal area and above.
         (b) External branch: motor to cricothyroid muscle.
      (3) Inferior laryngeal nerve (recurrent laryngeal nerve).
         (a) Sensory to glottal area and infraglottal area.
         (b) Motor to all intrinsic laryngeal muscles except cricothyroid.
         (c) Right and left branches differ in length. Left branch is longer because it wraps around the aorta before coursing upward. Right branch wraps around subclavian artery before entering larynx.
         (d) Enters larynx through the thyroid gland.

Processes of Speech

Breathing for Speech

1. Inhalation.
   a. Is an active process, resulting primarily from action of diaphragm and external intercostal muscles.
   b. When inhaling for speech, usually inhalation results in lung volumes above tidal breathing levels.
2. Exhalation.
   a. Is passive during quiet breathing.
      (1) Passive forces are those of gravity, elastic recoil and surface tension of the alveoli.
   b. Is active during breathing for speech.
      (1) Primary muscles include the internal intercostals (interosseous portions) and various other combinations of chest wall and abdominal wall muscles.
      (2) Pattern of exhalatory muscle activity (i.e., degree of chest vs. abdominal muscle contraction) varies from person to person and across activities.
3. Vital capacity.
   a. Amount of air available for use when lungs are inflated maximally.
4. Resting expiratory level (REL).
   a. The volume level in the lungs at the end of exhalation in tidal breathing, when no respiratory muscles are active.
   b. Volume level where the forces of contraction of the lungs are balanced by the forces of expansion of the chest wall.
5. Relaxation pressure.
   a. Pressure generated entirely by passive forces, pulling toward equilibrium at REL.
   b. Equals zero at resting expiratory level; increases when lung volume is above or below REL.
      (1) Relaxation pressure is positive above REL and negative below REL.
      (2) Expiratory pressure is positive.
      (3) Inspiratory pressure is negative.
6. Checking action.
   a. Activity of inhalatory muscles to control passive forces of exhalation in order to maintain steady subglottic pressure and airflow needed for speech production.
   b. These inhalatory muscles, primarily the external intercostals, stay activated until relaxation pressure equals subglottic pressure.
      (1) Average subglottic pressure during speech is 4–6 cm H_2O in conversational voice (increased for louder voices).
      (2) Relaxation pressure and subglottic pressure are equal at about 55% vital capacity. At this point, checking action ceases and muscles of exhalation gradually increase in activity to support the outflow of air.

Vocal Fold Vibration

1. Vocal fold opening.
   a. Vocal folds open for inhalation and to produce voiceless sounds due to action of the PCAs.

b. During voicing/vibration, vocal folds open due to the buildup of air below the vocal folds sufficient to overcome the resistance of the folds and push the tissue upward and apart. This results in the release of a puff of air into the supraglottal vocal tract.

2. Vocal fold closing.
   a. Vocal folds adduct due to action of the LCAs and IAs.
   b. However, during voicing/vibration, after the buildup of subglottal pressure pushes the vocal folds apart, closing the folds occurs due to elastic recoil force and the Bernoulli effect.
      (1) The Bernoulli effect occurs when a flow of air meets a constriction. This results in an increase in the airflow rate through the constriction balanced by an air pressure decrease at the point of the constriction. This decrease in air pressure at the point of the constriction creates a suction effect and pulls the vocal folds back toward one another.
      (2) The elastic recoil forces of the vocal fold tissues pull the folds back into their predetermined, closed position.

3. Vocal fold vibration.
   a. Occurs when the vocal folds are positioned in the adducted/closed position and airflow from the lungs causes repeated opening and closing.
   b. This repeated opening and closing is called "voicing" and occurs while airflow is continuous and the folds are held in a closed or nearly closed position at midline.

Phonation Type

1. Definition: the degree of vocal fold opening during speech production.
   a. Normal voice.
      (1) Regular bursts of air through the glottal opening.
      (2) Full opening and closing of vocal folds with vibration.
   b. Breathy.
      (1) Noise plus air burst.
      (2) Vocal folds partly open and partly closed; closed portion vibrates.
   c. Whisper.
      (1) Noisy friction airflow.
      (2) Narrow vocal fold opening, no vibration.
   d. Voiceless.
      (1) Noiseless airflow.
      (2) Vocal folds open, no vibration.
   e. Strained (creaky).
      (1) Irregular bursts of air through vibrating vocal folds.
      (2) Full vocal folds opening and closing with increased medial compression.
   f. Glottal fry (gravelly).
      (1) Low frequency, irregular air bursts.
      (2) Only a small portion of vocal fold margin opens and closes.
   g. Glottal stop.
      (1) No vibration at all; stoppage of airflow.
      (2) Folds fully shut with no vibration.

Registers

1. Definition of register.
   a. A series or range of consecutively phonated frequencies that can be produced with nearly identical voice quality and that ordinarily do not overlap.
   b. An individual's phonational range can be divided into three registers.
2. Pulse register.
   a. Lowest portion of one's phonational range.
   b. Vocal folds are relaxed and vibrate with minimal subglottic pressure.
   c. Frequency range is about 30–80 Hz.
   d. Closed phase is greatest portion of the glottal cycle.
   e. Sometimes heard as glottal fry.
3. Modal register.
   a. The largest portion of one's frequency range, comprising about 1.5 octaves.
   b. Voice quality has the greatest timbre and flexibility.
4. Loft register.
   a. Also known as falsetto, the highest portion of one's range.
   b. Vocal folds are stretched and tense/stiff, vibrating just at their medial edges. Airflow rate is increased.
   c. Transition from modal to loft occurs at about 300–350 Hz in both men and women.
      (1) Enters larynx through the thyroid gland.

Measures of Voice Production (Acoustic, Aerodynamic, Perceptual)

Normative values of many of the following measures are related to the age, gender and health status of the speaker and vary with the methodology used to elicit and extract them.

Acoustic Measures

1. Fundamental frequency.
   a. The number of times per second the vocal folds open and close during voicing.

b. Determined by vocal fold mass and stiffness.
c. Frequency is the inverse of period length. A glottal period is the time for the vocal folds to open and close one time, consisting of one glottal cycle.
2. Intensity.
   a. The sound pressure level generated by the acoustic shock wave traveling through the vocal tract.
   b. Intensity is determined by the subglottic pressure required to push the vocal folds open. This subglottic pressure is related to the degree of glottal resistance offered by the vocal folds.
   c. Relates to the amplitude of the acoustic waveform.
3. Jitter.
   a. The average cycle-to-cycle change in frequency from one cycle to the next.
   b. Jitter can be estimated using a variety of formulas, some of which use moving averages. Most often jitter is estimated taking the fundamental frequency (F_o) into account, with F_o serving as the denominator in the formula.
   c. Jitter is also known as pitch perturbation.
4. Shimmer.
   a. Is the average cycle-to-cycle change in amplitude (intensity) from one cycle to the next.
   b. Like jitter, can be estimated using a variety of formulas, some of which use moving averages. Shimmer is less dependent on average intensity, so can be calculated as absolute shimmer (without average intensity used in the denominator).
5. Noise measures.
   a. Spectral noise refers to elements of variability in the acoustic spectrum that create sound distortions.
   b. Can be measured by partitioning various sections of the acoustic spectrum. Noise throughout the acoustic spectrum is quite perceptible, while noise just in the high-frequency components of the spectrum is less noticeable.
   c. A variety of noise measurements provide information about the voiced signal, including:
      (1) Harmonics-to-noise ratio.
         (a) A measure that quantifies the amount of additive noise in the voice signal.
      (2) Long-term average spectrum.
         (a) A measure that describes the spectral characteristics of speech by averaging the contribution of individual speech sounds.
      (3) Cepstral measures.
      (4) Soft phonation index.
         (a) An acoustic analysis parameter that provides indication of vocal fold adduction and glottal closure during phonation.
      (5) Voice turbulence index.
         (a) A measurement that provides a quantitative index of breathiness.

Aerodynamic and Timing Measures

1. Airflow rate is the average rate of airflow through the vocal tract during phonation.
   a. Associated with the efficiency of phonation.
2. Subglottic pressure is pressure measured below the vocal folds, usually during vibration.
   a. Related to degree of medial compression of the closed vocal folds.
   b. Associated with the intensity of voice produced.
3. Glottal resistance is the ratio of subglottal pressure to airflow rate.
   a. Measured in cm H_2O/LPS.
   b. Associated with intensity at low and middle frequencies.
4. Maximum phonation time is the maximum time a subject can produce a vowel following a deep inhalation.
   a. May reflect phonation type in addition to characteristics of breath support for speech.
   b. Typically improves with practice and/or training.

Perceptual Measures

1. Quality of voice is that perceived by listeners as distinguished from pitch and loudness.
   a. Sometimes called timbre.
   b. Different aspects may be judged by listeners: severity, roughness, breathiness, strain, nasality.
      (1) Judgments of quality usually are less than reliable but may improve with training and standardized procedures.

Stroboscopic and Related Visual Measures

1. Symmetry refers to whether the left and right vocal folds move symmetrically during vibration. Are they mirror images of each other?
2. Amplitude is the extent of horizontal excursion of the vocal folds during vibration.
   a. Normal amplitude is about $\frac{1}{3}$ the width of the visible folds.
3. Periodicity is the regularity of (apparent) successive cycles of vibration.
4. Closed pattern refers to the position of the vocal folds and any space between them during the most closed phase of vibration.
   a. May be described as complete, incomplete, irregular, hour-glass-shaped, with an anterior or posterior chink.

5. Mucosal wave behavior corresponds to the movement of the superior surface, or cover, of the vocal fold laterally during vibration.
   a. Travels about half the width of the vocal folds at typical pitch and loudness.
6. Vocal fold edge can be described as smooth and even, irregular, with an excrescence, etc.
7. Appearance of the vocal folds is described, especially color, any supraglottal constriction, and presence of mucous.

Physiologic Measures

1. Force: a measure of collision force amplitudes in milliNewtons (mN), between the vibrating vocal folds; challenging to do in vivo.
2. Muscle activity: measured through electromyography whereby activation of single motor units and muscle fibers in general can be determined.

Development of the Vocal Mechanism

Growth and Development

1. Fetal development of the vocal mechanism.
   a. Larynx forms from branchial arches 4, 5 and 6.
   b. All structural elements are present by 3 months gestation.
2. From birth to puberty.
   a. At birth, the larynx is high in neck, contiguous with the hyoid bone.
   b. As growth occurs, larynx position moves downward, eventually opposite to C7.
   c. In infancy, tissues are very soft, prone to collapsing inward with increased airflow, especially when excess cellular fluid is present from an infection.
   d. Vocal ligament is present by age 2 and develops to about age 16.
3. Development during puberty.
   a. Laryngeal cartilages increase in size proportionally to each other.
      (1) Growth in males is 2–3 times that of females.
   b. Thyroid angle becomes more acute; also more obvious in males.
   c. Vocal fold length increases along with drop of modal pitch.
   d. Changes in related structures also occur, including lengthening of the neck and enlargement of thorax, increasing vital capacity.

Age-Related Changes

1. Changes in adulthood into old age.
   a. Gradual reduction in elastic fibers, increase in collagenous fibers, muscle atrophy in vocal folds themselves.
   b. Calcification of laryngeal cartilages begins after 20 years of age.
   c. Fundamental frequency decreases with age.
2. Other age-related changes.
   a. Weakening of muscles of breathing begins about age 40, with decreased elastic recoil of the chest wall.
   b. Vital capacity decreases, with proportional increase in residual volume.
   c. The conus elasticus, crico-arytenoid joint and mucous glands degenerate.
   d. More is known about age-related changes in men; some gender differences seem to be present, though data are limited.

Theories and Processes of Phonation

ADMET

1. ADMET is the aerodynamic myoelastic theory of phonation.
   a. Van den Berg proposed this theory to reflect what mechanisms are involved in one cycle of glottal vibration that results in vocal fold vibration.
      (1) The adductor muscles (LCAs and IAs) close the vocal folds to midline or near midline, while the tensors (CTs and TAs) stiffen the vocal folds to the desired fundamental frequency level.
      (2) With the vocal folds in a closed position, as the person begins to exhale, subglottal pressure builds beneath the vocal folds. Pressure builds until it is great enough to overcome the resistance of the vocal folds and push the vocal folds open.

(3) A noise burst of air, termed a "glottal pulse," is released, creating an acoustic shock wave traveling at the speed of sound through the vocal tract.
(4) Once the vocal folds have been blown open, forces of elastic recoil and the Bernoulli effect help to bring the folds back to their original position.
   (a) The Bernoulli effect indicates that at a point of constriction, airflow increases in rate and lateral pressure decreases. This has the effect of a vacuum, sucking the folds back toward one another.
   (b) As the vocal folds begin to be pulled closer and closer together, the Bernoulli effect increases since the constriction is becoming narrower and narrower.
(5) The opening and closing of the vocal folds during phonation is the result of the aerodynamic and muscular forces indicated above.
   (a) This implies that vocal fold vibration will continue as long as the vocal folds are in a closed or nearly closed position and air is flowing, building up sufficient pressure below the vocal folds to blow them apart.
   (b) The vocal folds do not open and close during voicing because of separate muscle contractions.

Cover-Body

1. Cover-body theory of vocal cord vibration.
   a. Proposed by Hirano and Kakita in 1985, this theory posits that the vocal fold cover moves independently of the body.
   b. The body of the vocal folds (i.e., the TA muscle) participates very little in vibratory movement.
   c. Movement of the vocal ligament, called the transition, falls in between the significant movement of the cover and the minimal movement of the body.
   d. This theory suggests that anything that interferes with the movement of the cover will affect the resulting voice quality.

Etiologies and Characteristics of Vocal Pathologies

Voice Problems

1. Phonotrauma etiology.
   a. Occupation.
   b. Personality and vocal "style."
   c. Activities involving frequent shouting.
2. Laryngopharyngeal reflex (LPR).
3. Allergies.
4. Family history/genetics.
5. Medications.

Voice Disorders

1. Common disorders associated with phonotrauma.
   a. Vocal nodules.
     (1) Etiology.
       (a) Nodules typically form from long periods of phonotrauma. Psychosocial stress may also contribute.
       (b) Traumatic vibratory behaviors result in an increase in intracellular fluid and a buildup of hyperkeratotic tissue with underlying fibrosis arising from the superficial layer of the lamina propria.
       (c) The resulting excrescence (i.e., an abnormal outgrowth) usually forms at the junction of the anterior one-third posterior two-thirds of the vocal folds (i.e., the middle of the membranous vocal folds).
     (2) Diagnostic characteristics.
       (a) Early nodules are often described as red, pinprick nodules that may develop into soft, fluid-filled lesions much like blisters, and ultimately may become harder and more callous-like.
       (b) Nodules are common in professional voice users, singers, aerobic instructors and the like. High-energy, prepubescent boys may also develop vocal nodules.
       (c) Voice quality ranges from mild to severely impaired and can be described variously as hoarse, breathy, harsh and/or raspy with phonation breaks and vocal effort. Quality usually worsens throughout the day.
       (d) Fundamental frequency may vary; maximum phonation time is reduced and jitter and shimmer are often increased.
     (3) Treatment.
       (a) Phonotraumatic behaviors should be reduced or eliminated to the extent possible.
       (b) Symptomatic voice treatment has been found effective using approaches such as

resonant voice therapy and confidential voice.
            (c) Nodules, particularly when hard and fibrotic, may be surgically removed, although non-surgical approaches are preferred by many physicians.
      b. Polyps.
         (1) Etiology.
            (a) Phonotrauma resulting in hyperfunctional vocal fold adduction results in wound formation arising in the superficial layer of the lamina propria.
            (b) Polyps may result from periods of phonotrauma or from a single traumatic incident.
         (2) Diagnostic characteristics.
            (a) Lesions may arise anywhere on the vocal fold cover, including the inferior surface of the vocal folds.
            (b) Polyps are unusually unilateral and may be pedunculated (attached by a stalk) or sessile (broad-based). Some may be hemorrhagic (filled with blood).
            (c) Voice quality may be minimally impaired or significantly changed. Pitch is typically lowered; jitter and shimmer are elevated.
            (d) Vocal fold closure may be affected, depending on the location of the polyp.
            (e) The patient may experience the sensation of something catching in the throat with heavy breathing or talking.
         (3) Treatment.
            (a) Short-term voice treatment focusing on improved vocal hygiene to reduce phonotrauma is thought to be helpful.
            (b) Many polyps require surgical removal to be eliminated.
      c. Polypoid degeneration (Reinke's edema).
         (1) Etiology.
            (a) Most often seen in women who are heavy smokers with chronic vocal abuse and perhaps gastroesophageal reflux disease (GERD).
            (b) The superficial layer of the lamina propria (Reinke's space) reacts to trauma by increasing fluid in the submucosal lining.
         (2) Diagnostic characteristics.
            (a) May be unilateral or bilateral and is typically asymmetrical.
            (b) The edema causes a loose, floppy appearance of the surface of the vocal fold, often pale in color. The cover of the vocal fold becomes less stiff.
            (c) Fundamental frequency is noticeably reduced with a reduced phonational range. Stroboscopic exam reveals decreased mucosal wave and decreased amplitude of vibration.
         (3) Treatment.
            (a) Phonosurgery combined with voice treatment focusing on vocal hygiene is standard.
            (b) The lesion will likely recur if the patient continues to smoke, so smoking cessation is considered key.
2. Other organic voice disorders.
   a. Cysts.
      (1) Etiology.
         (a) A cyst is a benign collection of material, such as fluid, surrounded by a membrane, typically arising from the superficial layer of the lamina propria.
         (b) Cysts may be congenital or form as a result of phonotrauma.
         (c) Two common types are mucous retention cysts, which result from a plugged mucous duct, and epidermoid cysts, where epithelial cells have become trapped and encapsulated in Reinke's space.
      (2) Characteristics.
         (a) Cysts vary in size and in location within Reinke's space of the vocal fold.
         (b) A cyst may be suspected whenever voice change does not resolve with conservative treatment and an adynamic portion of mucous wave on a vocal fold suggests increased stiffness of that fold.
         (c) Voice quality may vary depending on the size and location of the cyst and whether glottic closure is affected. Vocal fatigue may be reported along with some lowering of habitual pitch.
         (d) Sometimes cysts are seen to co-occur with other benign tissue changes in the vocal folds.
      (3) Treatment.
         (a) Voice therapy may help by improving vocal hygiene, reducing phonotrauma and promoting healing.
         (b) A vocal cyst will only be eliminated with careful surgical removal performed under a microscope.
   b. Human papilloma virus (HPV).
      (1) Etiology.
         (a) HPV infection in the larynx from types 6 and 11 results in recurrent respiratory papillomatosis.
         (b) Lesions may be found anywhere in the respiratory tract, although the vocal folds are the most common location.

(c) Childhood onset is linked to maternal genital infection; however, adult onset of the virus does occur.
(2) Characteristics.
  (a) Recurrent respiratory papillomatosis appears as masses of nonkeratinized stratified squamous epithelium that typically are white to pink or red in color. Single, multiple or clumps of lesions may be found.
  (b) A patient may exhibit a wide variety of changes in voice quality with frequent coughing or throat-clearing and may also experience some restriction in breathing with stridor.
(3) Treatment.
  (a) Although a variety of treatment approaches have been attempted (cryosurgery, antiviral injections), the current standard treatment involves repeated laser removal of the lesions with close monitoring.
  (b) Repeated removal of lesions from the vocal folds often results in the development of scar tissue, with a permanent disruption in voice quality as an outcome.
  (c) Children, especially, must be carefully monitored so that their breathing is not compromised. Many times, a tracheostomy tube is placed in these children until the vocal tract has grown and the recurrence of any lesions has been suspended.
c. Laryngitis (acute vs. chronic).
  (1) Etiology.
    (a) Acute laryngitis results in short-term loss of voice and/or impaired voice quality due to a bacterial or viral respiratory infection.
    (b) Chronic laryngitis can result from long-term vocal trauma, GERD and allergies, among other causes. Epithelial thickening and long-standing mucosal inflammation result that are not associated with an infection.
  (2) Diagnostic characteristics.
    (a) Voice quality is dysphonic and often described as rough, with increased spectral noise. Quality may decrease with increased talking.
    (b) Phonational range is reduced; jitter and shimmer are increased.
    (c) Patients may complain of dryness, and the laryngeal mucosa may appear dry, have areas of thickened secretions and show changes in color, such as increased redness.
    (d) Under stroboscopy the folds move asymmetrically and aperiodically.
    (e) Long-standing, negative effects of chronic laryngitis may result in permanent voice changes.
  (3) Treatment.
    (a) Reduce phonotrauma; control GERD; maintain adequate hydration.
3. Functional voice disorders.
  a. Muscle tension dysphonia (hyperfunctional dysphonia).
    (1) Etiology.
      (a) Chronic increased tension of the laryngeal musculature resulting in dysphonia that typically has multifactorial contributing etiologies.
      (b) This broad category designation is unclearly defined as a diagnostic entity.
    (2) Characteristics.
      (a) Vocal fold appearance is essentially normal, although hyper- or hypoadduction may be seen. Larynx may be held high in the neck with pain present on palpation.
      (b) Dysphonia can range from mild to severely dysphonic, often with a rough, strained quality. Voice breaks that are very short in duration may be seen using acoustic analysis programs.
      (c) Stroboscopy may reveal vibratory symmetry and abnormal glottal closure.
      (d) GERD may be a confounding finding.
    (3) Treatment.
      (a) Symptomatic voice therapy is the treatment of choice. Good evidence exists for benefit received from circumlaryngeal massage.
      (b) GERD should be managed and good vocal hygiene behaviors followed.
      (c) In some cases, Botox injections have been found to successfully break the cycle of chronic, unnecessary, excessive vocal tension.
  b. Psychogenic dysphonia/aphonia.
    (1) Etiology.
      (a) Voice change occurs associated with psychological causes, including anxiety or unconscious emotional distress; may be related to a single incident.
      (b) Is more common in women.
    (2) Diagnostic features.
      (a) Vocal folds tissue and movement are determined to be normal; however, during speech, the vocal folds are held in a partially abducted position, may hyperadduct or may appear bowed—all resulting in restricting normal vibration.
      (b) In some cases, voice may be produced sporadically or intermittently. Patients may complain of pain on talking.
      (c) Onset may occur after an upper respiratory infection.

(d) A normal cough is typically present, signaling an intact vocal mechanism despite the lack of normal volitional voice quality.
(3) Treatment.
  (a) Symptomatic voice treatment focusing on establishing and then extending a vocal tone is the treatment of choice.
  (b) Evidence supports the use of circumlaryngeal massage for this purpose.
  (c) Referral to a professional to help the patient understand and deal with underlying psychological issues can be appropriate.
  (d) Typically, once voice is reestablished and patients understand that they are in control of their voice, no further loss of voice occurs, or it is short-lived.

c. Puberphonia (mutational falsetto).
(1) Etiology.
  (a) Not clearly established. Is considered by most to be a functional voice disorder with possible psychological roots in some cases.
  (b) May be caused by the patient attempting to stabilize voicing during puberty when a "growth spurt" of the speech mechanism results in unstable pitch breaks.
(2) Characteristics.
  (a) Occurs more noticeably in males but can be found in females.
  (b) The larynx and other physical changes associated with puberty are normal.
  (c) Voice will be high in pitch with the larynx held in an elevated position, and neck tension may be evident.
  (d) Pitch breaks, phonation breaks, vocal fatigue and breathiness may also be present. Patient may not be able to shout with this voice.
(3) Treatment.
  (a) Voice therapy focusing on the production and then the establishment of a normal, lower pitch in a hierarchy from a single sound to conversation is the treatment of choice.
  (b) Treatment approaches may involve circumlaryngeal massage and/or hard, glottal attacks.
  (c) Initially, patients may have difficulty using the voice with family and friends and may not identify with the normal, lower voice as their own, but with continued use of the normal voice and with support, the transition to habitual use does occur.

d. Ventricular phonation (plica ventricularis).
(1) Etiology.
  (a) Adduction of the false vocal folds due to a psychological problem, a compensatory behavior, a component of a pattern of hyperfunction or as an unexplained phenomenon.
  (b) In rare cases, the false folds are used as a vibratory source of sound for individuals with nonfunctioning vocal folds.
(2) Characteristics.
  (a) The false vocal folds adduct and obscure the view of the underlying true vocal folds during voicing.
  (b) The true folds may remain in an open position or also close toward midline; the true folds do not appear to vibrate during attempts at phonation in most cases.
  (c) The resulting voice quality is low in pitch and loudness, monotone, rough/harsh, often diplophonic and has a significantly restricted pitch range.
(3) Treatment.
  (a) Symptomatic voice therapy is the treatment of choice when normal true vocal fold function is present.
  (b) Initial establishment of tone produced by the true folds is key, and if so produced, this tone is extended through a hierarchy of lengthening productions.

e. Vocal cord dysfunction (paradoxical vocal fold motion).
(1) Etiology.
  (a) Possible etiologies.
    • Upper airway sensitivity as a physiologic response to an irritant.
    • Psychogenic as a result of anxiety.
    • Laryngeal dystonia resulting from a neurological event or process.
(2) Characteristics.
  (a) A diamond-shaped posterior glottic chink can be seen endoscopically during inspiration and/or expiration.
  (b) The patient feels tightness in the neck and throat and may present with a cough or throat-clear just prior to an episode of difficulty breathing.
  (c) Some patients report distinct triggers, such as episodes associated with exercising or with strong odors (gasoline, perfume, coffee).
  (d) Asthma, allergies and GERD are comorbid factors in many patients.
  (e) Pulmonary function testing shows a reduced inspiratory flow volume.
  (f) Episodes of difficult breathing may vary from several episodes a day to only a few times a year. Patient's test results may be

entirely within normal limits when not experiencing an episode.
- (3) Treatment.
  - (a) Medical conditions such as GERD, allergies and asthma should be well controlled.
  - (b) Relaxed, open-throat breathing exercises are taught, often within an individually designed patient hierarchy of precipitating events.
  - (c) Recently, respiratory training exercises using resistance breathing devices have shown promise with this population.
4. Voice disorders of neurologic origin.
  a. Inferior (recurrent) laryngeal nerve paralysis.
   - (1) Etiology.
     - (a) The vagus nerve or its branches, either superior or inferior, may be damaged, leading to paresis or paralysis of the muscles of the larynx.
     - (b) Lesions may occur on one or both sides; a unilateral lesion is more common than bilateral lesions.
     - (c) Damage to the recurrent laryngeal nerve will affect all of the intrinsic laryngeal muscles except for the cricothyroid muscle.
     - (d) Common sources of damage include surgery (cardiac, thyroid or cervical spine), trauma, tumors, inflammatory processes or idiopathic, where no clear cause can be determined.
   - (2) Characteristics.
     - (a) Damage to the nerve results in the affected vocal fold typically resting in the paramedian position, just lateral to midline.
     - (b) The thyroarytenoid muscle fibers atrophy from lack of neurostimulation.
     - (c) The affected fold is unable to adduct to midline for normal vocal fold closure.
     - (d) Because of the paramedian position of the vocal fold and its flaccidity, the voice can be breathy/hoarse and soft, and patients typically have a weak cough.
     - (e) Maximum phonation time is decreased. Under stroboscopy, the vocal folds will vibrate asymmetrically and aperiodically. Greater than normal vibratory amplitudes and incomplete glottal closure are seen.
   - (3) Treatment.
     - (a) Unless the event precipitating the vocal paralysis is known and considered to be a permanent change, many physicians suggest patients wait for 6 months before electing for surgical management.
     - (b) A number of surgical options have been reported, including arytenoid adduction surgery, reinnervation techniques, use of injectable substances such as Teflon, fat, or collagen and vocal fold repositioning known as thyroplasty.
     - (c) Evidence indicates that thyroplasty results in superior vocal outcomes in comparison to some of the other treatment approaches.
     - (d) Voice therapy focusing on laryngeal adduction exercises or other kinematic approaches such as vocal function exercises may be helpful in maximizing voice quality.
  b. Superior laryngeal nerve (SLN) paralysis.
   - (1) Etiology.
     - (a) Damage to the superior laryngeal nerve may result from any of the events listed just above for the recurrent laryngeal nerve.
     - (b) However, usually the etiology of a superior laryngeal nerve paralysis is unknown, especially since the effects of a unilateral paralysis to only this nerve are quite subtle.
   - (2) Characteristics.
     - (a) If the internal branch of the SLN is affected, then sensation to the glottal and supraglottal regions is compromised.
     - (b) Unilateral damage to the external branch of the superior laryngeal nerve affects only the cricothyroid muscle. This causes an inability to lengthen the muscle on that side and results in altered pitch control and reduced pitch range.
     - (c) Patients may complain of vocal fatigue.
     - (d) Laryngoscopic/stroboscopic signs that may be present include a rotation or tilting of the larynx toward the normal side on phonation, slightly unequal levels of the folds at closure, reduced mucosal wave movement, incomplete glottal closure and reduced amplitude of vibration.
   - (3) Treatment.
     - (a) Surgical management may be recommended if the damage is bilateral.
     - (b) Voice therapy is helpful to maximize vocal quality and help minimize vocal fatigue and possible hyperfunction.
  c. Spasmodic dysphonia (SD).
   - (1) Etiology.
     - (a) Once thought to be psychogenic, spasmodic dysphonia is now considered a discrete vocal dystonia due to abnormalities in laryngeal motor control arising in the basal ganglia. However, the exact etiology remains unknown.
     - (b) Three types of SD are recognized: adductor SD, abductor SD and mixed SD.

- Of these, adductor SD is by far the most common and is found in approximately 90% of diagnosed cases.
            (c) SD is more common in women than in men.
            (d) Some patients with SD have other co-occurring neurologic abnormalities such as a vocal, head or hand tremor and blepharospasm.
        (2) Characteristics.
            (a) With adductor SD, patients experience irregular, uncontrolled, random closing spasms of the vocal folds during phonation. The resulting voice is often referred to as "strained-strangled."
            (b) Patients with abductor SD experience irregular, random, uncontrolled opening movements of the vocal folds, and the voice is heard as more breathy.
                - These spasms are most common in contexts with many voiced-voiceless transitions and are less noticeable or not present in a breath phrase with all voiced speech sounds.
            (c) Voice quality may be near normal during singing or when speaking in falsetto or for brief periods after laughing or crying.
            (d) Acoustic analysis research has shown that those with SD experience more than four voice breaks per production.
            (e) In some cases, SD may be difficult to differentially diagnose from muscle tension dysphonia, or patients may experience muscle tension dysphonia, which confounds the effects of the SD.
        (3) Treatment.
            (a) No cure exists for SD.
            (b) Behavioral treatment approaches used in voice therapy may be helpful, especially in incipient SD, but typically have limited effects.
            (c) Standard treatment now involves injection of botulinum toxin (Botox) into one or both vocal folds.
                - The effect of this treatment is to temporarily paralyze the vocal fold(s) such that the uncontrolled spasms cannot occur.
                - This effect wears off after 3 or more months, so management of vocal symptoms using Botox is long term, involving monitoring and regular repeated injections.
    d. Essential tremor of the voice (organic voice tremor).
        (1) Etiology.
            (a) Thought to result from a lesion in the extrapyramidal system of the central nervous system, voice tremor is also known to have a hereditary basis in some cases.
            (b) Voice tremor may be accompanied by a resting tremor of the face, head, hands or other muscles of the oral mechanism.
        (2) Characteristics.
            (a) Rhythmic oscillations of the larynx results in a voice often described as "quavering" and reminds listeners of aging.
            (b) The tremor is on the order of 4–12 cycles per second, which is slower than normal tremor and thus is obvious.
            (c) Essential tremor of the voice may begin in late adolescence or young adulthood but more commonly manifests in the fifth or sixth decade of life.
            (d) Vocal tremor worsens with fatigue or strong emotion.
            (e) The tremor may interfere with intelligibility, although complete voice breaks are not common.
        (3) Treatment.
            (a) Currently, no treatment has been found to be uniformly efficacious for patients with voice tremor.
            (b) Botox injections result in a slight reduction in the frequency and amplitude of the tremor, but the effect is only temporary.
            (c) Speech therapy to maximize intelligibility may be helpful. Strategies including shortening vowel durations, shortening phrase length and elevating pitch slightly have been suggested.

Pediatric Voice Problems

Congenital

1. Laryngomalacia.
    a. The most common congenital laryngeal disorder, diagnosed after birth due to the immature development of laryngeal cartilages.
    b. Pressure as air flows through the vocal tract results in the cartilages collapsing inward, causing stridor and respiratory distress.
    c. Sometimes surgery to protect the airway is performed until the problem resolves as the infant grows.

2. Subglottic stenosis.
   a. Also identified at birth due to respiratory distress. The condition is thought to be the result of failure in the development of vocal tract tissue, including tracheal cartilages.
   b. Reconstruction may be required, and these children may have long-term consequences affecting speech development.
   c. However, stenosis involving the soft tissues only may resolve as the child develops.
3. Laryngeal web.
   a. Congenital webs also manifest at birth with symptoms of stridor and difficulty breathing.
   b. Webs are common at the anterior commissure and are thought to result from a disruption in the normal development of the embryo. Webs can vary in thickness and length.
   c. Surgical removal is necessary to free the entire length of the vocal folds for vibration.

Acquired

1. The most common acquired voice problem in children is that of *bilateral vocal nodules.*
   a. This problem is thought to result from excessive voice use, including considerable yelling and effortful voice. GERD is also suspected to play a role in many cases.
   b. Many children with bilateral vocal nodules appear to "outgrow" them during puberty, but the exact reasons for this have not been determined.
   c. Other patients recall first noticing hoarseness and voice breaks associated with nodules during adolescence.
   d. Treatment commonly involves voice modification techniques and may include family counseling. Surgery for nodules is rarely recommended in children, although reflux management may be recommended.

High-Risk and Special Needs Voice Populations

Professional Voice Users

1. This population covers a wide range of professions and activities but can be grossly divided into two categories:
   a. Those individuals who need to talk a lot.
   b. Those individuals who need to talk loudly.
2. The following professions or activities have been associated with voice problems: actors, singers, cheerleaders, coaches, aerobic instructors, auctioneers, ministers, teachers, call center operators, salespeople.
3. Those whose occupations require hard and/or frequent voice use need careful laryngologic assessment and individualized treatment plans developed with specific patient needs in mind.
4. Most professional voice users need to take a long-term view of managing their voice problems in relation to their work and life needs.

Transgender Individuals

1. Some individuals work to be identified as a gender other than the one to which they were born. Their efforts to transgender may involve significant surgical and pharmacologic treatments. Voice therapy may be sought to improve the recognition of the intended gender.
2. A speech-language pathologist may assist in the therapy for elements related to gender identification, which include fundamental frequency, speaking rate, vocal intensity, aspects of quality and resonance, vocabulary and a variety of nonverbal behaviors.
3. Focusing on fundamental frequency is the most common, specific feature targeted in therapy, but the goal overall is to modify the overall image and identity projected by the patient.

Persons with Velopharyngeal Incompetency

1. The effect on the voice of velopharyngeal incompetency is primarily that of resonance. Research indicates that an opening in the velopharyngeal port greater than 20 cubic mm will typically result in the perception of hypernasality.
2. When velopharyngeal incompetence is consistent, patients will attempt to compensate for the poor closing of that valve by excessive closing of the laryngeal valve (i.e., the vocal folds). Repeated hyperfunction of this type may result, then, in formation of traumatic lesions on the vocal folds, such as vocal nodules, with those resulting vocal characteristics of hoarseness, voice breaks, lowered pitch and the like.

Persons with Hearing Loss

1. The voice quality of individuals with hearing loss may vary from that of normal, depending on the age of onset of the loss and the extent of the hearing deficit.
2. Hearing-impaired patients may have abnormal resonance characteristics and monotonous habitual pitch. Intonation patterns are likely to be disrupted, as well.

Voice Evaluation Protocol

Case History

1. Vocal history: questions involving the characteristics of the voice problem are of primary importance.
   a. These include a clear description of the onset and course of the problem, factors related to the variability over time and any changes associated with voice use in different situations.
2. Medical history: the patient should see the speech-language pathologist only after a medical diagnosis has been obtained.
   a. Other important elements of the patient's history are also of interest, including any medications the patient takes. The clinician needs to be informed of a patient's general health status and history with respect to surgeries, trauma, neurologic disease, allergies, asthma, reflux, other respiratory illnesses, smoking and other drug use and mental health.
   b. The medical history of other family members may be important.
3. Social history: voice problems are common in certain occupations and activities.
   a. How the individual uses the voice during a typical day is fundamental.
   b. How much and how effortfully the voice is used on a regular or occasional basis should also be determined.
   c. What is the patient's living situation?
   d. What stresses may be having an impact on the voice?

Functional Assessment: Assessing the Psychosocial Impact of Voice Disorders

1. International Classification of Functioning, Disability, and Health (ICF).
   a. Problems with human functioning are categorized into three inter-connected areas:
      (1) Impairments: problems in body function or alteration in body structure.
      (2) Activity limitations: difficulty in executing activities.
      (3) Participation restrictions: problems with involvement in any area of life.
   b. Disability refers to difficulties in any or all three areas of functioning.
      (1) Interaction of health conditions with personal and environmental factors.
   c. ICF covers all areas of human functioning and treats disability as a continuum.
2. Voice Handicap Index (VHI).
   a. A 30-item questionnaire with 10 questions in each of three domains (functional, physical, emotional).
   b. Uses a 0–4 ordinal scale with maximum score of 120.
   c. A change of greater than 18 points from one administration to another is considered significant.
   d. A modified version of the VHI, using only 10 questions, is also in use.
3. Voice-Related Quality of Life (VRQOL).
   a. A 10-item questionnaire with 6 questions in the physical domain and 4 questions in the social-emotional domain.
   b. Uses a scale from 1 (none) to 5 (as bad as it can be).
   c. Scores are put into a formula and converted to standard scores.
4. Functional Communication Measure (FCM).
   a. Developed by the American Speech-Language-Hearing Association for its National Outcomes Measurement project.
   b. Voice capability and quality is assessed on a 7-point scale reflecting functional capability.

Perceptual Assessment

1. GRBAS.
   a. Most common measurement tool used worldwide for estimating voice quality.
   b. Quality is judged on a 0–3 scale on the features: Grade, Rough, Breathy, Asthenic and Strained.

2. CAPE-V.
   a. Protocol with a form developed by authors associated with the Voice and Voice Disorders Special Interest Group of the American Speech-Language-Hearing Association.
   b. Clinicians rate voice quality features in three contexts (vowel, six specified sentences, conversation) on a 100 mm visual analog scale.
   c. Qualities judged are: Overall Severity, Roughness, Breathiness and Strained.
   d. Additional qualities may be assessed at the clinician's discretion.
3. Other perceptual quality instruments.
   a. Laver Voice Profiles (from Great Britain).
   b. Stockholm Voice Evaluation Approach.
   c. Buffalo Voice Profile.
   d. Perceptual Voice Profile (from Australia).

Acoustic Assessment

1. Common acoustic measures assessed during a voice evaluation.
   a. Modal fundamental frequency: the average habitual pitch of an individual in conversational speech and other speech tasks.
   b. Phonational range: the pitch range the patient can produce from low to high.
   c. Perturbation measures such as jitter and shimmer: instability measures reflecting variability in period and amplitude from cycle to cycle.
   d. Dysphonia severity index: a weighted combination of maximum phonation time, high and low frequency values and percent jitter to reflect perceived voice quality.
   e. Multidimensional voice profile: a computerized acoustic analysis program (KayPentax) that measures up to 19 different acoustic parameters from a segment of prolonged vowels and compares an individual's production to predetermined thresholds and norms.

Aerodynamic Assessment

1. Maximum phonation time: the maximum amount of time an individual can prolong a vowel on one breath of air.
2. Airflow rate: often measured along with pressure, airflow rate is an estimate of glottal valving efficiency.
3. Estimates of subglottic pressure: typically subglottic pressure estimates are made in reference to oral pressures determined just following release of the bilabial voiceless plosive /p/ using a mask integrated with special sensors, with air pressure, airflow and voice recorded simultaneously.
4. Laryngeal airway resistance: resistance is the ratio of air pressure to the flow of air through the glottis (pressure/flow) measured in units of cm of H_2O per cc per second.

Laryngologic/Stroboscopic Assessment

1. A speech-language pathologist may receive referrals for videolaryngoscopy/stroboscopy for the purpose of evaluating vocal fold vibratory characteristics. Besides documenting laryngeal appearance, the following features of vocal fold functioning are assessed:
   a. Glottal closure.
   b. Symmetry of movement.
   c. Periodicity.
   d. Amplitude of movement.
   e. Movement of the mucosal wave.

Hearing

1. A voice evaluation should include a hearing screening appropriate for the patient's age or otherwise note an impression of hearing ability from a functional perspective.

Common Additional Assessment Areas

1. Resonance.
   a. Most common perceptual features may include hyponasality, hypernasality, cul-de-sac resonance or observations of nasal emission.
2. Tremor.
   a. Voice tremor may be heard. Tremor of other structures of the speech mechanism or of the head or hands may be observed.
3. Motor speech production.
   a. Voice problems may co-occur as part of dysarthria symptoms. Should initial observations or the patient's history warrant, each speech subsystem should be assessed: respiration, phonation, articulation, resonance and prosody.
   b. A thorough oral-motor examination would begin this assessment.
4. Intelligibility.
   a. Should overall speech understandability be decreased, intelligibility should be assessed. This can be done by means of subjective judgments of how much is understood by a listener in known and unknown contexts, or better, by standardized testing such as the Sentence Intelligibility Test.

Prevention of Voice Disorders and Promotion of Vocal Health

Encouraging Voice Health

1. Phonotrauma:
   a. Sometimes referred to more generally as vocal abuse or vocal misuse, phonotrauma refers to those behaviors that are thought to contribute to the development of a voice problems.
2. Guidelines for good vocal health.
   a. Rare or minimal use of a loud, effortful voice or shouting.
   b. Attention to potential laryngo-pharyngeal reflux.
   c. Reducing unnecessary coughing and throat-clearing.
   d. Adequate hydration.
   e. Holistic elements: good nutrition, enough rest, regular physical exercise, good mental health.

Evidence-Based Voice Treatment Approaches

Management Approaches and Techniques with Good Evidence

1. *Resonant voice therapy* focuses on optimizing voice quality through a focus on maximizing oral-pharyngeal resonance and the degree of medial compression between the vocal folds.
2. *Botox* for injection into thyroarytenoid (usually) or other intrinsic muscles (less common) for treatment of spasmodic dysphonia and sometimes essential tremor of the voice.
3. *Vocal function exercises* have been shown to be useful in improving vocal range, stability, flexibility and resonance in a variety of normal and disordered populations.

Approaches and Techniques with Less Supporting Evidence

1. Boone has reported 25 facilitating approaches. Many of these are mentioned by other authors, though few have been studied with strong experimental controls.
2. A list of known techniques or approaches includes the Accent method, pushing, chewing, confidential voice, chanting, respiration training, and yawn-sigh, among many others.
3. Any technique used in treatment should be carefully chosen with specific patient characteristics and hypothesized physiological mechanisms in mind.

Management Recommendations and Referrals

Voice Therapy

1. When to recommend voice therapy.
   a. Evidence indicates voice therapy is effective for a particular problem.
   b. Voice does not give a positive image.
   c. Voice does not allow one to perform normal activities of daily living, including fulfilling one's job requirements.
2. Referrals to other professionals.
   a. Otolaryngology, neurology, psychology, singing teachers.

Management of Head and Neck Cancer

Surgery, Radiation and Chemotherapy

1. Strategies to cure the disease.
   a. Surgery alone.
   b. Radiotherapy alone.
   c. Surgery followed by radiation or chemoradiation.
   d. Chemotherapy followed by surgery, radiation or chemoradiation.
   e. Chemoradiation followed by surgery.
2. Effects related to surgery.
   a. Loss of function related to excised tissues, including effects on speech (speech distortions, voice and/or resonance changes) and swallowing (oral control, aspiration, residue issues).
3. Effects related to chemotherapy.
   a. Fatigue, nausea, loss of appetite, changes in taste and potentially hair loss.
4. Effects related to radiation.
   a. Inflammatory reactions, tissue fibrosis, loss of appetite, fatigue, xerostomia, necrosis, mucositis, pain.

Anatomical and Physiologic Changes After Total Laryngectomy

Total Laryngectomy Procedure

1. The entire larynx is removed in situ.
   a. Hyoid bone and intrinsic laryngeal cartilages down through first tracheal ring.
2. The respiratory tract is separated from the oral/digestive tract through creation of a permanent tracheostoma in the front of the neck.
3. If cancer has spread to the lymphatic system in the neck, the neck nodes and surrounding tissues are removed in a neck dissection.
   a. A radical neck dissection involves severing the spinal accessory nerve, which affects the ability to raise one's arm straight out to the side when neck tissue and lymph glands are removed.

Breathing, Speech, Voice and Swallowing Function After Total Laryngectomy

1. After a total laryngectomy, during respiration, air enters and leaves the pulmonary system through the open tracheostoma.
2. Following surgical healing, swallowing function typically returns to normal, unless affected by radiotherapy treatment to the neck.
3. Speech and voice production post larygngectomy surgery no longer can use the true vocal folds.
   a. Most common forms of alaryngeal voice production include the use of an electronic, artificial larynx or placement of a one-way valve (prosthesis) through a surgical puncture made between the trachea and the esophagus.
      (1) This latter form of voice production is called T-E voice, for "tracheoesophageal," and is produced via a TEP, or "tracheo-esophageal puncture."
      (2) T-E prostheses remain in place for months at a time.
      (3) When the tracheostoma is closed, either manually or by means of a two-way "speaking valve," air is shunted through the prosthesis into the upper esophagus. This airflow causes vibration of the upper esophageal and/or lower pharyngeal tissues. The voice produced is low in pitch and intensity with greater perturbation than normal voice.

Alaryngeal Voice Assessment Protocol

Applying the Protocol

1. Stimulability.
   a. Is the patient able to make sounds using the pharyngo-esophageal segment as a voicing source?
   b. Is spontaneous belching heard?
   c. Can a good placement for the head of an electro-larynx be found on the neck?
   d. Are the patient's articulation and rate of speech conducive to good posttreatment intelligibility?
2. Insufflation testing.
   a. Air is directed into the upper esophagus to see if the air can be released into the oral-pharynx and if vibration of upper esophageal tissues occurs.
   b. This testing is performed to see if after a total laryngectomy, vibration of the pharyngo-esophageal segment can be initiated and maintained for several seconds with relative ease.
3. Fitting of prosthesis.
   a. Most common type of prosthesis is a one-way, low-pressure valve inserted into the tissue space between the trachea and the esophagus at the back of the permanent stoma. The tissue space has been created by a surgical puncture at the time of surgery.
   b. Prostheses come in different lengths. Fit is determined by the SLP after referral from the otolaryngologist.
   c. The indwelling prosthesis typically stays in place for several months. Removal of an old prosthesis and insertion of a new one is accomplished in an office visit to the SLP or surgeon.
   d. A two-way breathing valve can be placed over the stoma opening to allow for hands-free voice production. If this valve does not work well for a particular patient, voicing is initiated by covering the stoma with a thumb to allow for the diversion of air.

Alaryngeal Voice Treatment Approaches and Considerations

TEP Voice Production and Troubleshooting

1. Improving TEP voice production.
   a. Once a prosthesis has been placed, patients must learn to coordinate breathing and voice for optimal speech production. This often involves attention to articulation, speech rate and phrasing.
   b. Optimal speech output is typically achieved after a small number of treatment sessions with motivated patients whose health status is stable.
   c. A significant decline in performance may signal recurrent disease, other health issues or problems with the prosthesis.
2. Troubleshooting prosthesis problems.
   a. Leakage may occur around or through a tracheoesophageal prosthesis, and these symptoms require different management strategies.
      (1) Leakage through a prosthesis often means the prosthesis needs to be changed.
      (2) Leakage around a prosthesis, on the other hand, suggests the need for a larger esophageal flange and/or a shorter prosthesis (but not a larger-diameter prosthesis).
   b. Patients using a TEP may be susceptible to fungal infections affecting the oral-pharynx, the tracheo-esophageal tract and/or the prosthesis itself.
      (1) Such infections require medical management, often with the use of antifungal medications.

Other Head and Neck Cancer Effects on Speech, Voice and/or Swallowing

Partial Laryngectomy

1. Partial laryngectomy is a general term referring to any surgery that involves removal of part (but not all) of the voice-producing mechanism.
2. Supra-glottic laryngectomy: the laryngeal structures and tissues above the level of the true vocal folds are surgically removed.
3. Hemi-laryngectomy: a vertical (sagittal) portion of laryngeal tissue is resected. This involves part or all of one vocal fold, sometimes including tissues above

the fold at the same time, and which sometimes may extend around the anterior commissure to include portions of the opposite vocal fold.
4. With partial laryngectomy surgery, voice, swallowing and sometimes resonance are often affected. The effects may be temporary or long term and are related to many factors, including how much tissue was surgically removed, other treatments the patient may have received and the patient's general health.

Total or Partial Glossectomy

1. Glossectomy refers to the surgical removal of tongue tissue. In most cases, this surgery results in some degree of swallowing difficulty due to oral stage changes and altered articulatory precision with subsequent reduced intelligibility.
2. In a total glossectomy, the entire tongue is removed. Speech intelligibility is dramatically affected due to limited articulatory ability. Swallowing, too, is difficult due to limited bolus control.
3. In a partial glossectomy, only a portion of tongue muscle is removed. In general, the proportion of tissue removed is directly related to the degree of the resulting speech and swallowing difficulty.

Other Surgical Treatments

1. Head and neck tumors may occur anywhere in the upper respiratory tract. Besides the larynx and tongue, other common sites include the floor of the mouth, tonsil and palate.
2. Treatment approaches are the same as for laryngeal cancers, involving surgery or radiotherapy alone or in combination, along with chemotherapy.

References

Boutsen, F., Cannito, M. P., Taylor, M., & Bender, B. (2002). Botox treatment in adductor spasmodic dysphonia: A meta-analysis. *Journal of Speech, Language and Hearing Research*, 45(3), 469.

Casper, J. K., Colton, R. H., & Gress, C. D. (1993). *Clinical Manual for Laryngectomy and Head/Neck Cancer Rehabilitation*. San Diego, CA: Singular Publishing Group, p. 197.

Colton, R. H., Casper, J. K., & Leonard, R. (2011). *Understanding Voice Problems: A Physiological Perspective for Diagnosis and Treatment*, 4th ed. Philadelphia, PA: Lippincott, Williams and Williams.

Daniloff, R., Schuckers, G., & Feth, L. (1980). *The Physiology of Speech and Hearing: An Introduction*. Englewood Cliffs, NJ: Prentice-Hall.

Hirano, M. (1981). *Clinical Examination of Voice. Disorders of Human Communication*. New York: Springer-Verlag.

Hirano, M., & Bless, D. M. (1993). *Videostroboscopic Examination of the Larynx*. San Diego, CA: Singular Publishing Group.

Hixon, T. J., Weismer, G., & Hoit, J. D. (2008). *Preclinical Speech Science: Anatomy, Physiology, Acoustics, and Perception*. San Diego, CA: Plural Publishing.

Hogikyan, N. D., & Sethuraman, G. (1999). Validation of an instrument to measure voice-related quality of life (V-RQOL). *Journal of Voice*, 13(4), 557–569.

Jacobson, B., Johnson, A., Grywalski, C., Silbergleit, A., Jacobson, G., Benninger, M., & Newman, C. (1997). The Voice Handicap Index (VHI): Development and validation. *American Journal of Speech Language Pathology*, 6(3), 66–70.

Kahane, J. (1982). Growth of the human prepubertal and pubertal larynx. *Journal of Speech and Hearing Research*, 25, 446–455.

Kent, R. D. (1994). *Reference Manual for Communicative Sciences and Disorders: Speech and Language*. Pro-ed.

Linville, S. E. (2001). *Vocal Aging*. San Diego, CA: Singular Thomson Learning.

Mathers-Schmidt, B. A. (2001). Paradoxical vocal fold motion: A tutorial on a complex disorder and the speech-language pathologist's role. *American Journal of Speech Language Pathology*, 10(2), 111–125.

Mathers-Schmidt, B. A., & Brilla, L. R. (2005). Inspiratory muscle training in exercise-induced paradoxical vocal fold motion. *Journal of Voice*, 19(4), 635–644.

Orlikoff, R. F., & Kahane, J. C. (1996). "Structure and Function of the Larynx" in *Principles of Experimental Phonetics*. Baltimore, MD: Mosby, pp. 112–181.

Roy, N., & Leeper, H. A. (1993). Effects of the manual laryngeal musculoskeletal tension reduction technique as a treatment for functional voice disorders: Perceptual and acoustic measures. *Journal of Voice*, 7(3), 242–249.

Roy, N., Weinrich, B., Gray, S. D., Tanner, K., Stemple, J. C., & Sapienza, C. M. (2 003). Three treatments for teachers with voice disorders: A randomized clinical trial. *Journal of Speech, Language and Hearing Research*, 46(3), 670–688.

Sapienza, C. M., & Ruddy, B. H. (2009). *Voice Disorders*. San Diego, CA: Plural Publishing Group.

Titze, I. R. (1994). *Principles of Voice Production*. Englewood Cliffs: Prentice Hall, pp. 279–306.

Ward, D. E. C., & van As-Brooks, C. J. (Eds.). (2007). *Head and Neck Cancer: Treatment, Rehabilitation, and Outcomes*. San Diego, CA: Plural Publishing Group.

Van den Berg, J. (1958). Myoelastic-aerodynamic theory of voice production. *Journal of Speech and Hearing Research*, 1(3), 227–244.

Zemlin, W. R. (1997). *Speech and Hearing Science, Anatomy and Physiology*, 4th ed. Upper Saddle River, NJ: Pearson Publishing.

16

Dysphagia: Swallowing and Swallowing Disorders

BARBARA C. SONIES, PhD

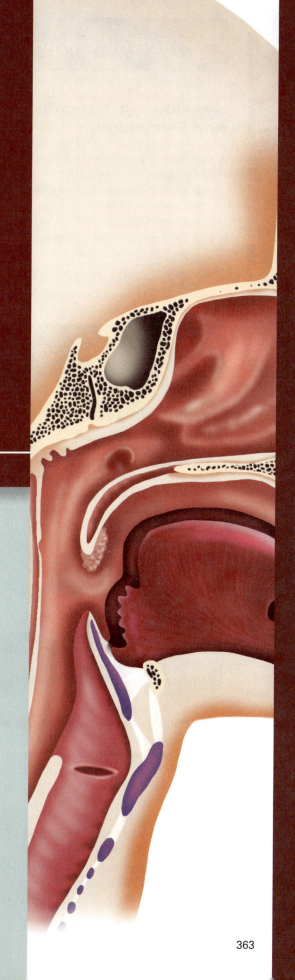

Chapter Outline

- Terminology, 364
- Normal Swallowing, 364
- Cranial Nerves and Cortical Control, 364
- Physiology of the Swallow, 366
- Dysphagia, 371
- Neuroplasticity and Swallowing, 375
- Head and Neck Cancer and Dysphagia, 375
- Aspiration and Penetration, 378
- Esophageal Disorders, 379
- Medications and Swallowing, 380
- Diagnostic Procedures, 380
- Instrumental Dysphagia Evaluation, 381
- Treatments, 384
- References, 387

Terminology

Swallowing, Feeding and Dysphagia

1. Swallowing is a patterned behavioral response that can be interrupted in its initial stages.
   a. It allows passage of a bolus from the oral cavity to the pharynx through the esophagus and into the stomach for further digestion.
   b. It encompasses the oral preparation of food, triggering of the swallow reflex, pharyngeal passage, airway protection and esophageal activity.
   c. Except for voluntary manipulation and preparation of food, swallowing is primarily involuntary.
2. Feeding refers to the oral manipulation of food prior to the initiation of the swallow. It involves the use of utensils to place food in the oral cavity.
3. Dysphagia is difficulty or abnormality in moving food from the mouth to the stomach.
   a. Dysphagia is a symptom of an underlying condition or disease and may result from a variety of neurologic, neuromotor, systemic, immunologic, developmental or iatrogenic conditions as well as infectious processes, surgery or trauma.

Normal Swallowing

Swallowing Anatomy

1. Anatomy of the swallow includes the structures of the upper aerodigestive tract (oral cavity, pharynx, larynx and the esophagus) and specific structures (lips, teeth, tongue, hard palate, soft palate, hyoid bone, mandible, floor of the mouth, faucial pillars, epiglottis) (Figure 16-1).
   a. Tongue.
      (1) Oral tongue (tip, blade, center, dorsum).
      (2) Pharyngeal tongue (base of the tongue, vallecular space).
   b. Pharynx: oropharynx, nasopharynx, hypopharynx and laryngopharynx.
      (1) The laryngopharynx contains the epiglottis, valleculae, pyriform sinuses and laryngeal aditus.
      (2) The pharyngeal musculature contains the superior, middle and inferior constrictor muscles.
      (3) Posterior and lateral pharyngeal walls.
   c. Esophagus.
      (1) Cricopharyngeal muscles compose the upper esophageal sphincter (UES).

Cranial Nerves and Cortical Control

Cranial Nerves and Swallowing

1. Six cranial nerves innervate the swallow and supply either motor or sensory input to the oropharynx and esophagus during the four overlapping phases of the swallow.
   a. Trigeminal (V)—sensory and motor.
      (1) Sensation in anterior two-thirds of tongue (hot and cold, oral pain).
      (2) Sensation to teeth, gums, and oral mucosa.
      (3) Salivary flow to major and minor glands.
      (4) Motor control of mouth opening, mandible motion and mastication.
      (5) Motor innervation to floor of mouth (FOM) muscles to elevate larynx and hyoid.
   b. Facial (VII)—sensory and motor.
      (1) Taste in anterior two-thirds of tongue.
      (2) Sensation to soft palate.
      (3) Salivation from all salivatory glands, except the parotid gland.
      (4) Motor control of lip motion and bilabial seal.
      (5) Motor control for the facial muscles, FOM muscles and cheeks.
      (6) Assists in elevation of hyoid and larynx to protect airway.
   c. Glossopharyngeal (IX)—sensory and motor.

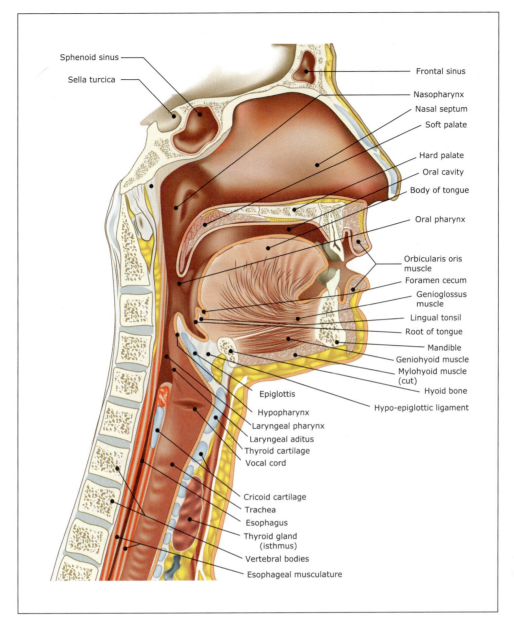

Figure 16-1 Anatomy of Swallowing

(1) Taste in posterior one-third of tongue.
(2) Sensation to faucial pillars and soft palate.
(3) Salivation from the parotid gland.
(4) Sensation to the pharynx and larynx.
(5) Motor velopharyngeal closure.
(6) Motor control of the upper pharyngeal constrictor muscle.
d. Vagus (X)—sensory and motor.
  (1) Controls sensory information for pharyngeal and esophageal phases.
    (a) Sensation for pharynx, larynx and trachea.
    (b) Visceral sensory for mucosa of the valleculae, pharynx, larynx, lungs, stomach and abdomen.
  (2) Motor innervation to the base of the tongue (BOT) and all pharyngeal muscles.
  (3) Major innervation to the larynx, diaphragm and lungs.
  (4) Pharyngeal contraction and esophageal peristalsis.
e. Spinal Accessory (XI)—motor only.
  (1) Partial innervation of soft palate and uvula.
    (a) Assists with velopharyngeal elevation.
  (2) Partial innervation of muscles of upper pharynx.
  (3) The primary function is to provide stability of shoulder and neck muscles during swallow and allow rotation of head and neck.

f. Hypoglossal (XII)—motor only.
      (1) Primary motor for all tongue muscles.
         (a) Seal oral cavity and prepare bolus.
      (2) Motor innervation of the pharynx.
         (a) Aids in hyolaryngeal elevation and airway protection.

Cortical and Subcortical Innervation

1. Cortical control of swallowing occurs in a widely distributed neural network.
2. The swallowing center (central pattern generator) is located in the medulla and pons.
3. MRI and PET studies indicate cortical activation in the sensorimotor cortex, insula, putamen, globus pallidus, thalamus, anterior cingulate gyrus, supplemental motor area (SMA), cerebellum and localized involvement of the basal ganglia.
4. Bilateral cortical activity occurs in the SMA.

Physiology of the Swallow

Overlapping and Sequential Phases

1. Oral preparatory phase.
   a. Entirely voluntary.
   b. Manipulate bolus to swallow-ready state.
   c. Food placed in oral cavity combines with saliva and is masticated to form a bolus. Requires mandible, teeth and lingual motion.
   d. Lip seal, saliva, oral sensation are important for recognition of food and for keeping food in the oral cavity.
      (1) Temperature, taste and smell.
      (2) Teeth, lips, tongue.
   e. Food preferences are important in voluntarily selecting what food will be consumed.
   f. Cultural and social components of social eating influence the process of eating.
   g. Can terminate swallow at will if undesirable.
   h. Anatomy of oral preparatory phase.
      (1) Main muscles: orbicularis oris, buccinator, tongue, masseter, medial and lateral pterygoids.
      (2) Cranial nerves: trigeminal (CN V), facial (CN VII), glossopharyngeal (CN IX), hypoglossal (CN XII).
2. Oral phase.
   a. Partially voluntary, because it requires some cortical control.
      (1) Can terminate swallow before food enters oropharynx.
      (2) Bolus is transferred to pharynx (duration from 1 to 1.5 seconds).
   b. The bolus is contained in a central groove on the tongue surface and moves posterior to the anterior faucial pillars (arches) where the swallow reflex is triggered to propel the bolus into the upper pharynx.
   c. The lips close, the tongue tip elevates to the alveolar ridge, the FOM muscles contract and the BOT approximates the posterior pharyngeal wall (PPW) to aid bolus flow.
   d. The hyoid bone moves anteriorly and superiorly as the tongue begins to move, bringing the larynx upward and forward to begin airway protection.
   e. The bolus passes the ramus of the mandible on fluoroscopic studies at the end of the oral phase and the start of the pharyngeal phase.
   f. The tongue dorsum and velum make contact to ensure that the bolus does not enter the nasopharynx.
   g. Bolus flow is horizontal in the oral cavity.
   h. Pressure changes within the oral cavity are caused by lip closure, tongue motion and lingual/velar/PPW contact and aid in bolus flow.
   i. Oropharyngeal component of a swallow is due to overlapping activity of muscles in hypopharynx and laryngopharynx.
   j. Muscles involved in oral phase and their cranial nerve innervations (Table 16-1A).
      (1) Orbicularis oris, mentalis, buccinator and risorius (CN VII).
      (2) Masseter, temporalis, pterygoids (CN V).
      (3) Tongue muscles (CN XII).
      (4) FOM muscles.
         (a) Mylohyoid (CN V).
         (b) Geniohyoid (CN XII).
         (c) Digastric (CNs V, XII).
      (5) Soft palate.
         (a) Levator veli palatini (CN X).

(b) Palatoglossus (anterior faucial pillars) (CNs IX, X, XI).
(c) Palatopharyngeus (posterior faucial pillars) (CNs X, XI).
k. Sensory components of the oral and oral preparatory phases.
(1) Trigeminal (CN V): anterior oral cavity.
(2) Facial (CN VII): sensation to anterior oral cavity.
(3) Glossopharyngeal (CN IX): sensation to posterior oral cavity.
3. Pharyngeal phase.
a. The bolus flows vertically through the pharynx to the esophagus, while the airway is protected from bolus entry.
(1) Combined with the oral phase, the duration is 1.5 seconds on average.
b. The tongue dorsum approximates the pharyngeal wall, and the velum remains elevated to create pressure for bolus flow.
c. The hyoid elevates, which lowers the epiglottis over the laryngeal aditus.
(1) Hyolaryngeal elevation is the fulcrum of a swallow.
d. Laryngeal elevation and partial vocal fold adduction occur to protect the airway.
(1) Hyolaryngeal elevation aids in opening the upper esophageal sphincter (UES).
e. Bolus flow through the pharynx is aided by pharyngeal constrictor muscle contractions, or stripping waves, that move the bolus.
(1) Superior pharyngeal constrictor muscle.
(2) Middle pharyngeal constrictor muscle.
(3) Inferior pharyngeal constrictor muscle is the cricopharyngeus muscle (part of UES).
f. Bolus flow bifurcates over the epiglottis, goes through the pyriform sinuses and combines in midline to enter the UES and the esophagus.
(1) The bolus clears immediately from the pharynx.
g. There is a brief period of apnea (.04 second) when the epiglottis is lowered, the lips are sealed and the velum is elevated.
h. Swallowing does not occur during respiration but is an expiratory pulse after a swallow.
i. Muscles of the pharynx propel the bolus, elevate the larynx and protect the airway.
4. Esophageal phase (Figure 16-2).
a. Totally involuntary, lasting 8–10 seconds, during which the bolus is moved into the stomach.
b. The esophagus is a collapsed, tube-like, muscular structure that lies posterior to the trachea.
c. The upper one-third is striated muscle connecting to pharynx. The lower two-thirds is smooth muscle connecting to stomach.
d. The UES relaxes and opens, allowing food/liquid to pass to the stomach by a series of peristaltic waves (contractions and relaxations).
(1) Primary, secondary and tertiary peristaltic waves.
e. Hyolaryngeal elevation, propulsion force of the bolus and density of the bolus aid in opening the UES.
f. The lower esophageal sphincter (LES) relaxes and the bolus enters stomach.
g. Innervation of the entire esophagus is by the vagus nerve (CN X).

Musculature of Swallowing, Function and CN Innervation

1. See Table 16-1A–G.

Swallowing and Normal Aging

1. Changes in oral and pharyngeal muscle function that occur with age cause delays in swallowing, but these must be differentiated from age-related diseases and conditions that cause dysphagia.
a. Common effects of aging on swallowing.
(1) Increased duration of swallow, delayed hyoid elevation, longer opening of UES, decline in pressure reserves, decreased lingual pressure and strength.
(2) Effects of sarcopenia (i.e., muscle wasting) affect tongue muscle and swallow functioning.
(3) Preference for softer foods due to poor dentition and decreased perception of viscosity.
(4) Reductions in smell and taste cause changing food preferences and need to enhance food with spices.
(5) Decreased muscle tone in pharynx and esophagus causes delayed passage of bolus, pooling in valleculae and slowed esophageal transport.
(6) Hiatal hernia and reflux are common, causing heartburn and gastroesophageal reflux disease (GERD).
(a) Many elderly have an inspiratory pattern of air intake during or just following a swallow. Normal pattern is expiratory.
(b) Causes laryngeal penetration and increased coughing during meals.
(7) Arthritis may reduce cricoarytenoid joint movement, laryngeal movement and airway protection.
(8) Oral mucosa may become thin and less elastic. This may affect denture wear. More common in smokers or those taking medications.

Table 16-1A

Muscles of Swallowing; CN Innervation and Function

MUSCLES OF NECK AND LARYNX: SUPRAHYOID		
MUSCLE	INNERVATION	FUNCTION
Digastric FOM	CN VII (anterior and posterior bellies from different branches)	Depresses mandible, elevates and steadies hyoid during swallowing
Stylohyoid	CN VII	Elevates and retracts hyoid and elongates FOM
Mylohyoid FOM	CN V (mandibular branch)	Elevates hyoid, FOM and tongue during swallowing
Geniohyoid FOM	Cervical 1 via CN XII	Pulls hyoid antero-superiorly, shortens FOM, widens pharynx
MUSCLES OF NECK AND LARYNX: INFRAHYOID		
MUSCLE	INNERVATION	FUNCTION
Omohyoid	Cervical 1–3 (branch of ansa Cervicalis), CN XII	Depresses, retracts, and steadies hyoid
Sternohyoid	Cervical 1–3 (branch of ansa Cervicalis), CN XII	Depresses hyoid following swallowing-related elevation
Sternothyroid	Cervical 2 & 3 (branch of ansa Cervicalis), CN XII	Depresses hyoid and larynx
Thyrohyoid	Cervical 1 via CN XII	Depresses hyoid and elevates larynx

Table 16-1B

Muscles of Swallowing; CN Innervation and Function

MUSCLES OF VELOPHARYNGEAL VALVE		
MUSCLE	INNERVATION	FUNCTION
Tensor veli palatini	CN V (medial pterygoid nerve of mandibular branch)	Tenses soft palate, opens tympanic tube during yawning and swallowing
Levator veli palatini	CN X (pharyngeal branch)	Elevates soft palate during yawning and swallowing
Palatoglossus	CN X (pharyngeal branch)	Elevates posterior tongue to create contact with soft palate
Palatopharyngeus	CN X (pharyngeal branch)	Contracts pharyngeal wall, tenses soft palate
Musculus uvulae	CN X (pharyngeal branch)	Shortens and pulls uvula superiorly

Table 16-1C

Muscles of Swallowing; CN Innervation and Function

PHARYNGEAL MUSCLES: INTERNAL LAYER		
MUSCLE	INNERVATION	FUNCTION
Palatopharyngeus	CN X (pharyngeal branch)	Elevates, shortens and widens the pharynx during swallowing and speaking
Salpingopharyngeus	CN X (pharyngeal branch)	Elevates, shortens and widens the pharynx during swallowing and speaking
Stylopharyngeus	CN IX	Elevates, shortens and widens the pharynx during swallowing and speaking
PHARYNGEAL MUSCLES: EXTERNAL LAYER		
MUSCLE	INNERVATION	FUNCTION
Superior constrictor	CN X (pharyngeal branch)	Constricts walls of the pharynx during swallowing
Middle constrictor	CN X (pharyngeal and laryngeal branches)	Constricts walls of the pharynx during swallowing
Inferior constrictor (including cricopharyngeus muscle)	CN X (pharyngeal and laryngeal branches)	Constricts walls of the pharynx during swallowing

Table 16-1D

Muscles of Swallowing; CN Innervation and Function

MUSCLES OF MASTICAION

MUSCLE	INNERVATION	FUNCTION
Temporal	CN V	Elevates mandible to close jaw
Masseter	CN V	Elevates mandible to close jaw, slightly protrudes jaw
Lateral pterygoid	CN V	Protracts mandible, depresses chin, contributes to lateral chewing movement
Medial pterygoid	CN V	Elevates mandible, protrudes mandible, contributes to smaller grinding movements

Table 16-1E

Muscles of Swallowing; CN Innervation and Function

INTRINSIC LARYNGEAL MUSCULATURE

MUSCLE	INNERVATION	FUNCTION
Cricothyroid	CN X (external laryngeal nerve)	Stretches and tenses vocal ligament
Thyroarytenoid	CN X (recurrent laryngeal nerve)	Relaxes vocal ligament
Posterior cricoarytenoid	CN X (recurrent laryngeal nerve)	Abducts vocal folds
Lateral cricoarytenoid	CN X (recurrent laryngeal nerve)	Adducts vocal folds
Interarytenoids (transverse and oblique)	CN X (recurrent laryngeal nerve)	Adducts arytenoid cartilages, closes glottis
Vocalis	CN X (recurrent laryngeal nerve)	Relaxes posterior vocal ligament while maintaining tension on anterior vocal ligament

Table 16-1F

Muscles of Swallowing; CN Innervation and Function

EXTRINSIC TONGUE MUSCLES

MUSCLE	INNERVATION	FUNCTION
Genioglossus	CN XII	Depresses tongue in mid-section, leading to tongue grooving
Hyoglossus	CN XII	Protrudes tongue, wags tongue to opposite side
Styloglossus	CN XII	Retracts and curls sides of tongue, contributing to tongue grooving
Palatoglossus	CN X	Elevates posterior tongue, depresses soft palate, constricts faucial pillars

INTRINSIC TONGUE MUSCLES

MUSCLE	INNERVATION	FUNCTION
Superior longitudinal	CN XII	Curls tongue longitudinally and up, elevates tongue apex, and retracts sides of tongue
Inferior longitudinal	CN XII	Curls tongue longitudinally and down, depresses tongue apex, retracts tongue
Transverse	CN XII	Narrows and elongates the tongue
Vertical	CN XII	Flattens and broadens the tongue

Table 16-1G

Muscles of Swallowing; CN Innervation and Function

MUSCLES OF THE LOWER FACE

MUSCLE	INNERVATION	FUNCTION
Orbicularis oris	CN VII	Adducts the lips, sealing off the oral cavity
Zygomaticus	CN VII	Draws the angle of the lips superiorly and posteriorly
Buccinator	CN VII	Draws lips against teeth
Risorius	CN VII	Retracts the angle of the lips posteriorly
Mentalis	CN VII	Raises the central portion of the lips
Platysma	CN VII	Depresses the jaw, draws the lower lip downward

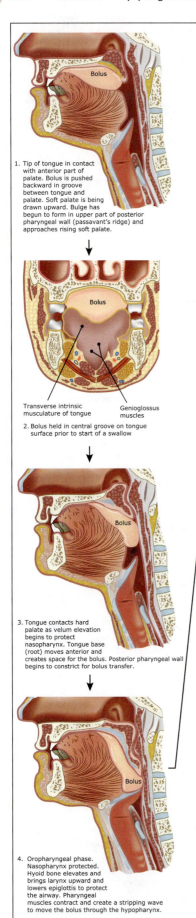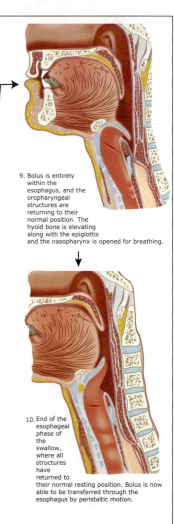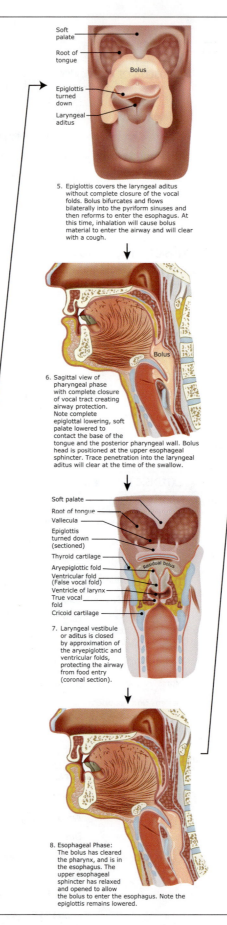

Figure 16-2 Anatomy of Bolus Flow in the Normal Swallow

(9) Salivary flow may lessen (xerostomia), causing dental decay and reduced lubrication needed for bolus flow through pharynx and esophagus. May also cause mineralization of teeth, neutralization of stomach acid and changes in oral sensation.
   (a) Pills can adhere to mucosa.
   (b) May be more common in postmenopausal females.
   (c) Reduced salivary flow common postradiation as glands susceptible to x-rays.
   (d) Reduced salivary flow also due to certain medications.
(10) Decrement in smell pervasive and is found to be important for oral preparation phase of swallow.
(11) Taste may or may not change significantly, but it is suggested that threshold for detection may increase, causing use of more tastants.
   (a) Tastant—any substance capable of eliciting gustatory excitation.

Dysphagia

Definition, Signs and Symptoms

1. From Greek *phaegin*, "to eat," plus *dys*, "disordered."
2. Difficulty moving food from the mouth to the stomach. Includes problems in oral manipulation, chewing, sucking and suckling (Figure 16-3).
3. Signs and symptoms (see Table 16-2).

Neurological Conditions

1. Stroke and Parkinson's disease are the most common neurological conditions that result in dysphagia.
   a. Other neurologic causes include amyotrophic lateral sclerosis (ALS), multiple sclerosis (MS), myasthenia gravis, muscular dystrophy, cerebral palsy,

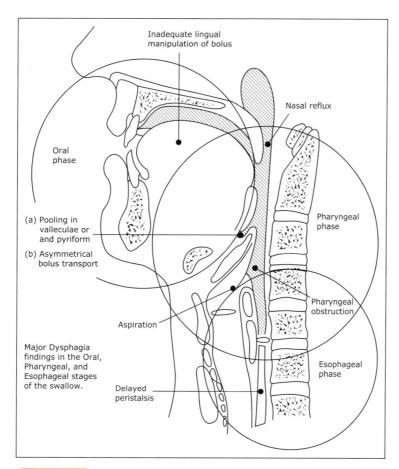

Figure 16-3 Signs and Symptoms of Dysphagia by Phase of Swallowing

Table 16-2

Signs and Symptoms of Oropharyngeal Dysphagia

GENERAL SIGNS AND SYMPTOMS

Patient reports feeling that something is stuck in his/her throat after eating
Excessive coughing during eating
Choking during eating
Excessive drooling
Wet, gurgling vocal quality after eating
Poor lung sounds-rasping
Dysphonia or loss of voice after meals
Pocketing of food in the mouth
Pills sticking in the throat
Shortness of breath after swallowing
Unexplained weight loss
Fever or sweating following meals
Pneumonia of unknown origin
Voice changes (e.g., hoarseness)
Heartburn or indigestion

Huntington's disease, postpolio, cortical tumors, polymyositis, trauma (head injury) and dementia.
  b. Any condition that impairs cortical function, cortical pathways, upper or lower motor neurons or subcortical function can impair swallowing.
2. Classification of these conditions includes, but is not limited to, the following categories:
  a. Vascular: stroke, transient ischemic attack (TIA).
  b. Infectious: meningitis, postpolio.
  c. Traumatic: brain injury, surgical.
  d. Autoimmune: polymyositis, MS, lupus, rheumatoid arthritis.
  e. Neoplastic: intracranial or cortical tumors.
  f. Degenerative: ALS, Huntington's disease, Parkinson's disease, multisystem atrophy (MSA), dementia.
  g. Neuropathies: cranial nerves.
  h. Congenital, structural: cleft palate.
  i. Neurodevelopmental: cerebral palsy, Down syndrome.
  j. Iatrogenic medication- or treatment-induced dysphagia (e.g., radiation, surgical).
3. Dysphagia symptoms.
  a. Tongue instability, incoordination, weakness and rocking motions during oral or oral preparatory phases.
  b. Impaired posterior or anterior tongue movements to prepare, form or transfer a bolus over the tongue surface to the pharynx.
  c. Impaired lip strength and movement and reduced lip seal needed to remove bolus from utensils.
  d. Abnormal chewing and impaired rotary jaw motions.
  e. Bolus residue in valleculae and/or pyriform sinuses.
    (1) Look for unilateral residue in pharynx.
  f. Nasal regurgitation and/or velopharyngeal incompetence.
  g. Residue on the lingual surface and posterior pharyngeal wall.
  h. Lack of epiglottal lowering.
  i. Impaired elevation of the hyolaryngeal complex.
  j. Laryngeal penetration or aspiration, back-up bolus from the pyriform sinuses or dripping from valleculae.
  k. Impaired opening of UES.
  l. Impaired esophageal peristalsis and reflux into the pharynx.
  m. Impaired oral sensation.
4. Stroke or cerebrovascular attack (CVA).
  a. Caused by vascular dysfunction (disruption of blood flow) leading to lack of oxygen to the brain and is the primary cause of dysphagia.
  b. Brain stem strokes can occur with damage in the medulla or pons.
  c. Bilateral damage to the pons and medulla may cause total dysphagia with poor prognosis.
    (1) Pontine (pons) stroke: Damage causes hypertonicity and delayed or absent swallow response.
      (a) Reduced laryngeal elevation.
      (b) Cricopharyngeal dysfunction.
      (c) Slow recovery.
    (2) Medullary stroke.
      (a) Nucleus tract solitarius or nucleus ambiguus lesions cause significant dysphagia.
      (b) Longer pharyngeal response times.
      (c) Increased duration for velar and laryngeal elevation.
      (d) Longer response time for cricopharyngeal sphincter (UES) opening.
      (e) If a unilateral stroke occurs, it results in a near-normal swallow with delayed triggering of pharyngeal swallow and pooling of residue in the valleculae and pyriform sinuses.
    (3) Wallenberg's syndrome is a form of brain stem stroke causing pharyngeal phase problems.
      (a) Due to lateral medullary infarct, caused by occlusion of the vertebral artery.
      (b) Although unilateral, it causes bilateral pharyngeal dysfunction, dysarthria, vertigo, ptosis, numbness and weakness of same side of the face.
  d. Subcortical strokes.
    (1) Milder symptoms, including mild oral and pharyngeal transit delays.
    (2) Greater pharyngeal phase findings, resulting in possible aspiration or laryngeal penetration.

(3) Therapy directed at triggering pharyngeal swallow and tongue base movement is often successful.
e. Cortical strokes.
  (1) Right hemisphere: more susceptible to pharyngeal problems, such as delayed pharyngeal stripping wave motion.
    (a) Mild oral delays, longer pharyngeal delays.
    (b) Aspiration before or during swallow due to incomplete laryngeal elevation.
  (2) Left hemisphere: difficulty in the oral phase of the swallow.
    (a) May have difficulty initiating a swallow (oral apraxia).
    (b) Mild delay in triggering pharyngeal phase, which may result in aspiration or laryngeal penetration before the swallow is triggered.
    (c) Better recovery of swallow function.
  (3) New evidence is emerging to indicate that there may be bilateral innervation from the right hemisphere to explain the increased severity of right-hemisphere strokes.
  (4) It is possible that the left hemisphere has more unilateral activation to the brain stem.
f. Persons with stroke usually respond well to dysphagia interventions, and since strokes often cause unilateral dysfunction including lingual weakness, function can be rehabilitated (see "Treatments" section).
g. Multiple strokes usually cause more swallowing dysfunction and poorer prognosis for recovery of swallowing ability.

5. Parkinson's disease.
  a. Dysphagia is found in approximately 50% of patients, especially those with disease progression.
  b. PD is a movement disorder caused by dopamine depletion in the substantia nigra in the subcortical region.
  c. Treated medically with levadopa and sinemet.
  d. Primary symptoms include resting tremor, rigidity, impaired postural reflexes and paucity of movement.
  e. Swallowing abnormalities include lingual rocking, pharyngeal dysmotility and pooling in the pharynx.
  f. Silent aspiration (being unaware of bolus entry into larynx without attempt to clear airway) subsequent to sensory dysfunction of oropharynx is a major finding.
  g. Tongue base sensory impairments may result in residue in the valleculae.
  h. Penetration and aspiration are also noted.
  i. Treatment focuses on sensory awareness and control of the oral swallow.
    (1) Expiratory muscle strength training (EMST) and Lee Silverman Voice Treatment (LSVT) treatment for voice may be helpful for treatment of oropharyngeal symptoms.

6. Progressive supranuclear palsy (PSP).
  a. A degenerative disorder of the CNS, caused by widespread neuronal degeneration in multiple systems in the brain stem and basal ganglia.
  b. PSP resembles PD but differs due to disturbed ocular motility and earlier signs of cognitive loss.
    (1) People with PSP are more aware of their dysphagia, and have more coughing and choking during eating.
  c. Patients are minimally responsive to dopamine.
  d. Swallowing rehabilitation is helpful.

7. Amyotrophic lateral sclerosis (ALS).
  a. A severe and rapid progressive degeneration of UMN and LMN tracts, causing severe motor dysfunction, dysarthria and dysphagia affecting all phases of swallow.
  b. Cognition is not impaired, and there is adequate retention of eye movement.
  c. Significant declines in respiratory function requiring total respiratory support.
  d. Patients develop severe dysphagia, leading to a need for nonoral feeding (usually percutaneous gastrostomy [PEG] tube).
  e. There is no known cure—dysphagia treatment is temporary and minimally successful.
  f. Family and patient counseling is essential in early stages.

8. Myasthenia gravis (MG).
  a. A LMN disorder in which conduction is impaired at the myoneural junction, due to a defect of acetylcholine release.
  b. Weakness that exacerbates with repeated effort is the primary symptom. Dysphagia occurs due to fatigue of the muscles of mastication.
    (1) Drooling, lingual holding of bolus.
    (2) Breathing difficulty, hoarseness.
    (3) Gagging and choking.
  c. Muscle strength evaluated by the Tensilon Test.
    (1) Tensilon (edrophonium) blocks the action of the enzyme that breaks down the transmitter.
    (2) Tensilon is an acetylcholine inhibitor.
    (3) May also use EMG to evaluate muscle strength.
  d. Medical treatments include removal of the thymus gland (thymectomy) and use of medication to help facilitate muscle movement.
  e. Behavioral treatment includes energy conservation.
    (1) Small meals, increased frequency.
    (2) Modify texture so less chewing effort needed for oral preparation.

9. Multiple sclerosis (MS).
  a. An immune-mediated demyelination of nerve fibers in the brain and spinal cord.
  b. Fluctuates and waxes and wanes in stages.
    (1) May be gradually progressive.
    (2) More common in white females.

(3) Slight risk of other autoimmune diseases.
c. Dysphagia occurs if corticobulbar tracts or brain stem pathways are affected.
d. General symptoms are delays in triggering a swallow, reduced tongue base retraction and pooling in the valleculae.
e. Medical treatment by high-dose intravenous corticosteroids and beta-interferon has been proven effective.

10. Huntington's disease.
    a. An autosomal-dominant, neurodegenerative disease that can be detected with blood tests.
    b. There is a progressive psychiatric disturbance.
    c. Dementia will become severe.
    d. Choreatic movements—involuntary movements.
    e. Respiratory failure may be terminal.
    f. Oropharyngeal dysphagia appears with disease progression.
        (1) Rapid, excessive rate of swallow, due to poor impulse control causing choking and gagging.
        (2) Buccal squirreling of bolus can occur, as well as premature swallowing of an unprepared bolus.
        (3) Holding the head in an extended position impairs the ability to swallow and causes airway compromise.
    g. Treatment for the patient's dysphagia is to feed them in an uncluttered space, with seating that provides head and trunk support.
        (1) Place food and drink directly into the mouth, using single, slowly paced bolus feedings.
        (2) The purpose is to control impulsivity and rapid feeding rate.

11. Postpolio syndrome.
    a. Viral-induced degeneration of the LMN and brain stem.
    b. The syndrome is due to degeneration of existing motor neuron endplates decades after an initial polio episode.
        (1) Bulbar or spinal classification of the disease, with bulbar classifications having initial signs of swallowing difficulty.
    c. Dysphagia occurs in almost all postpolio patients decades after the initial attack due to overuse of remaining motor neurons.
    d. Dysphagia symptoms are found in all phases of the swallow.
    e. Because of oropharyngeal muscle weakness, oral exercises are minimally effective, while postural and dietary treatments appear helpful.

12. Guillain-Barré syndrome.
    a. An autoimmune disorder affecting the peripheral nervous system, resulting in demyelination of cranial nerves.
    b. Causes weakness and sensory loss of the oral cavity, pharynx and larynx during the acute phase of the disease.
        (1) May require a feeding tube.
    c. Effects temporary and recovery is spontaneous.
    d. Plasmapheresis or intravenous immunoglobulin are highly effective cures.

13. Dystonias and dysphagia.
    a. Generalized dystonia.
        (1) Difficulty coordinating respiration and swallowing.
    b. Neck dystonia.
        (1) Cervical spasmodic torticollis causes delayed swallow initiation and vallecular residue.
    c. Laryngeal or spasmodic dystonia.
        (1) Swallowing preserved.
    d. Oromandibular dystonia (OMD-Meige syndrome).
        (1) Premature spillage of bolus into pharynx with vallecular residue, difficulty in oral preparation. Sometimes is progressive but responds to treatment.
    e. Lingual dystonia.
        (1) Biting of tongue, expel food from mouth.
    f. Treatments may include Botox injections or lesion surgery but effects remain inconclusive.

14. Dermatomyositis.
    a. An immune system disorder, which may appear in childhood.
    b. A serious condition in children, which appears as sun sensitivity.
    c. Begins as a skin rash of upper eyelids and periorbital region with scaly eruptions on knees, knuckles and elbows.
    d. Weakness, stiffness and pain in muscles in abdominal area.
    e. Dysphagia may appear and can be treated with medication such as steroids.
    f. Prednisone or corticosteroid treatment results in improvement in a majority of patients.

15. Traumatic brain injury (TBI).
    a. The leading cause of death and disability in the United States for persons 40 years and under.
        (1) Primary cause is motor vehicle accidents.
    b. Two types: closed head injury or penetrating head injury.
    c. Usually causes memory and other cognitive impairments.
    d. Dysphagia can also be present.
        (1) Secondary effects may be due to intubation and damage to pharyngeal anatomy.
        (2) Fractures of spinal column may affect recovery.
        (3) Cervical spinal cord injuries, spinal cord fusion surgery and effects of neck bracing may restrict swallowing.

(4) Problems in laryngeal elevation, airway closure and UES opening may result from trauma or surgery.
(5) May see abnormal oral reflexes if damage is to brain stem and may note many aspects of the complete range of possible deficits depending on the damage to the oropharyngeal structures and the nervous system.
  e. Prognosis ranges from good to unknown depending on location of injury.
16. Dementia.
  a. A cognitive impairment where dysphagia is not typical.
  b. Generally not associated with oral motor sensory deficits, except if there are findings of stroke, other brain injuries or a neurological condition in addition to the dementia.
  c. If there is dysphagia, it will appear in volitional eating, transporting food to the mouth, lack of awareness of food placed in the oral cavity and an inability to determine when to swallow.
    (1) Food agnosia: inability to recognize food.
    (2) Feeding apraxia: inability to remember how to swallow.
  d. Directed feeding and individual assistance during meals is often required.
  e. As cognition becomes more impaired, treatment may no longer be beneficial for swallowing or feeding.

Neuroplasticity and Swallowing

Central Nervous System and Dysphagia

1. Central nervous system.
  a. The central nervous system is known to have the ability to alter itself morphologically or functionally as a result of experience.
  b. This reorganization is an intrinsic property of the brain through which it is continually remodeled by experience.
    (1) Experience can take many forms, such as sensory stimulation, skill acquisition or repetition.
    (2) Adjacent undamaged areas of the cortex or undamaged tissue in other cortical areas on the intact hemisphere may take over functions that were lost.
2. Principles of neuroplasticity.
  a. Use it or lose it.
  b. Use it and improve it.
  c. Specificity.
  d. Repetition matters.
  e. Intensity matters.
  f. Time matters.
  g. Salience matters.
  h. Age matters.
  i. Transference.
  j. Inference.
3. Neuroplasticity and dysphagia.
  a. The evidence is beginning to accumulate that some of the motor tasks, especially lingual strengthening, may induce neuroplastic effects on swallowing due to cortical reorganization.
  b. This is one of the major new areas in treatment and offers encouraging promise of recovery.
  c. The various treatments we use may affect neuroplasticity and thus improve ability to swallow.

Head and Neck Cancer and Dysphagia

Characteristics, General Considerations and Prevalence

1. Most cancers that affect the oropharynx, larynx and/or esophagus will have a direct and negative impact on the ability to swallow.
  a. Due to the effects of surgical removal of tissue and fibrosis or necrosis of tissues after chemotherapy and/or radiation therapy.
2. The major posttreatment concern is swallowing and nutrition.
3. The prognosis is usually poor, with poor survival after five years.
  a. Most cases are smokers who consume alcohol and may not seek early medical care.
4. Risk factors for oropharyngeal cancer include:
  a. Sun exposure.
  b. Human papilloma virus (HPV).

c. Chronic acid reflux.
d. Inhalation and long-term exposure to airborne toxins.
5. Initial symptoms may include:
   a. Loose teeth.
   b. Red patches on mucosa or tongue.
   c. Bleeding.
   d. Oral candida or thrush.
   e. Ulcers.
   f. Ear pain.
   g. Feeling a mass.
6. Squamous cell cancers are the most prevalent.

Swallowing Recovery

1. In part associated with past behaviors, such as smoking and alcohol consumption, as well as the type and grade of tumor invasion, secondary metastasis and the amount of radiation used.
2. Surgery, radiation and chemotherapy treatments can all impair speech and swallowing.
3. Late radiation effects include:
   a. Tissue changes.
   b. Changes in oral bacteria due to lack of saliva.
4. Mucositis, or inflammation and infection of mucous membranes, causes pain and may be a severe limitation on the ability to swallow.
5. Tumors occur indiscriminately in nerves, muscles, bone and other tissues and can impair any and all aspects of swallowing.

Tumor Staging (TNM)

1. Relates to the size and location of the tumor(s)—larger numbers indicate greater severity and poorer prognosis.
   a. T1 (smallest) to T4 (largest) for tumor sizes.
   b. M relates to metastasis nodes.
      (1) M1 would mean that there was metastasis in one other area.
   c. N is the number of nodes in the tumor.
2. Surgical reconstruction ranges from wound closure in small lesions to a need for a tissue flap from another bodily area to close the surgical defect to microvascular grafts for blood flow.
3. The amount of remaining muscle, innervation, sensation and blood flow all relate to successful outcomes in dysphagia treatment.
4. Oral/dental prostheses are often important for swallowing rehabilitation.
5. Dysphagia evaluations should be conducted prior to surgery or medical intervention and after healing from acute effects postoperatively.
   a. Prior to surgery, the multidisciplinary evaluation should include a medical and drug history and a physical examination to determine if risks and symptoms of dysphagia occur.
   b. After surgery, the multidisciplinary evaluation should include determination of postsurgical effects, pain, swelling, radiation effects, xerostomia and mucous production.
6. Treatment for dysphagia should begin after major healing.
   a. Dental evaluation is required prior to radiotherapy.
   b. The evaluation and treatment must include a team including a physician, oncologist, dentist, nurse and social worker, in addition to the speech-language pathologist.
   c. Instrumental imaging techniques are used diagnostically to determine the site and size of the lesion.
      (1) CT scan of bone.
      (2) MRI of soft tissue.
      (3) Ultrasound of blood flow, soft tissue lesions and structural functioning.
   d. Different surgical procedures will have varying effects on swallowing and may require different treatment strategies.

Classification of Tumors

1. Some classifications are based on broad categories, such as oral, oropharyngeal and laryngeal.
2. Other classifications are more specific to the anatomy and can include the oropharynx, nasopharynx, hypopharynx, larynx, nasal cavity, salivary glands and esophagus.
3. Another classification system is specific to the organ itself.
4. Tongue tumors and glossectomy.
   a. Less than 50% of tissue removal typically results in only a temporary problem with a good prognosis.
   b. More than 50% of tissue removal will require more treatment.
   c. Treatments, including thermal tactile stimulation, lingual exercises, posterior bolus placement and backward head movement, are usually successful if the main problem targeted is oral transfer to pharynx.
   d. In a total glossectomy, deficits include:
      (1) Reduced BOT motion.
      (2) Difficulty with bolus propulsion.
      (3) Reduced hyolaryngeal elevation.
5. Tonsilar, FOM and pharyngeal tumors.
   a. Patients experience more difficulty swallowing as more structures can be involved.
   b. Anterior FOM may have adequate pharyngeal function.
      (1) If lingual suturing is used, the patient will have severe oral transfer problems and will require a method to transfer the bolus to the posterior lingual region.

(2) Methods may include:
  (a) Head movement.
  (b) Special utensils.
c. FOM, BOT and tonsilar resections will impair both oral and pharyngeal phases.
  (1) If the faucial arches are involved, the patient won't be able to trigger a swallow, resulting in residue in the valleculae.
  (2) Mendelsohn maneuver, sensory stimulation and prosthesis are methods that may be used.
  (3) Problems experienced may include:
    (a) Increased oral transit.
    (b) Pooling in the lateral sulcus.
    (c) Delayed swallow, with premature bolus spillage.
    (d) Reduced pharyngeal contraction.
    (e) Reduced hyolaryngeal elevation.
d. If treatment is radiation therapy, xerostomia and reduced range of motion will result.
  (1) Radiation effects can appear months after the treatment (late effects), which will impair the swallow.
  (2) Treatment should include exercises for range of motion of the jaw and tongue mobility.
    (a) The patient may be unable to chew, and will need to puree or thicken food.
    (b) Some cases will do best with liquids.
  (3) It is imperative to have the results of a modified barium swallow (MBS) for treatment planning.
6. Hypopharyngeal tumors.
  a. May present as a sore throat or a lack of symptoms until dysphagia appears.
7. Laryngeal tumors.
  a. Associated with a high risk of aspiration, due to reduced airway protection.
    (1) This will depend on where the tumor was located and how much of the structure was removed.
  b. Tumors can be categorized as indicated (reference is to above, at or below the glottis):
    (1) Supraglottic.
      (a) The epiglottis, aryepiglottic folds and false (ventricular) vocal folds may be resected.
      (b) 50%–70% of this population will aspirate and will benefit from supraglottic or safe swallow.
    (2) Glottic.
      (a) Treated wither with radiation or surgery and can range from a hemilaryngectomy to a total laryngectomy, where all cartilages and pyriform sinus may be resected.
      (b) Small tumors on the true vocal folds may respond to radiation, but if the tumor is larger, treatment may be combined with surgery.
      (c) Most laryngeal tumors are glottic.
    (3) Subglottic.
      (a) The structures below the glottis and above the inferior cricoid cartilage border.
      (b) May include muscles of the cricopharynx and can cause difficulty in bolus transfer to the esophagus.
      (c) Rare in the United States.

Surgical Procedures

1. Laryngectomy: surgical removal of all or part of the larynx.
  a. Partial laryngectomy (hemilaryngectomy).
    (1) Will spare portions of the laryngeal structure.
      (a) Organ preservation is the main focus.
    (2) Spares hyoid and epiglottis with good swallowing recovery.
    (3) Compensatory techniques include tilting the head forward and rotating it to the damaged side.
  b. Total laryngectomy.
    (1) Removes all of the laryngeal cartilages and separates the gastric and respiratory tracts.
    (2) Aspiration is not an issue, but this method may produce oropharyngeal swallowing problems.
  c. To achieve UES opening, one must generate force with the BOT against the PPW, producing a pumping motion of the tongue to compensate.
  d. Pseudoepiglottis is often constructed with a tissue fold at the BOT that can cause a problem and obstruct the pharynx or collect residue.
    (1) May need surgical intervention to correct this issue.
    (2) Scar tissue may form near the esophagus and further obstruct the area, requiring dilation for passage of material into the esophagus.
    (3) The patient may become a neck breather with an altered airway and reduced moisture, loss of taste and smell and an inability to blow the nose.
2. Any of these surgical procedures where tissue is removed and a flap is constructed from distal tissue may cause sensory and motor changes to the swallow.
  a. The effect may be backflow of a bolus into the oral cavity.
  b. Reassessment on an MBS in required to diagnose the effect.
  c. Tracheoesophageal puncture (TEP) is a placement of a small, flexible prosthesis into a tracheal stoma to prevent backflow and aspiration.
    (1) This device also serves as a voice prosthesis.
  d. Passy-Muir speaking valve has benefits for swallowing, as it helps restore sensation, taste and laryngeal closure.

3. Because of the great variability among patients with head and neck cancer, every period must be evaluated and individual treatment plans must be developed based on the extent of medical treatment, remaining structures, cognition and medical complications.

4. Specific treatment may use special feeding devices, intraoral prostheses and compensatory techniques implemented to increase the range of mandibular opening (e.g., using a device such as Therabite).

Aspiration and Penetration

Aspiration

1. Aspiration is the entry of food or liquid into the airway, below the true vocal folds, that eventually enters the lungs. It is best assessed on videofluoroscopy with an MBS.
2. Aspiration can occur before, during or after a swallow.
3. Healthy, normal people aspirate saliva during sleep, with no harmful effect. Aspiration is prevalent in bronchitis, asthma, GER, and in neurological conditions.
    a. Aspiration pneumonia will occur only if the material contains a respiratory pathogen (gram-negative bacteria).
        (1) Microaspiration of oropharyngeal secretions that have colonized with bacteria may occur.
        (2) Anaerobic bacteria: gram-negative, staphylococcus.
        (3) Artificial airways and intubation often cause problems due to bacterial growth on the plastic. Tube feeding may neutralize gastric acid, allowing bacteria to colonize.
4. Aspiration may occur with PEG placement, due to wicking effect, impaired sensation and collection of material on an inflated cuff when it is deflated.
5. Methods to detect aspiration may include use of blue dye or glucose monitors, which some believe are unreliable or unsafe compared to instrumental imaging techniques such as MBS and FEES (see section on instrumental assessment).
6. Suggestions to reduce the risk of aspiration in intubated or hospitalized patients include:
    a. Feeding in a semirecumbent position.
    b. Feeding with the cuff deflated.
    c. Aggressive suctioning.
    d. Supervised feeding.
    e. Not overfeeding.

Aspiration Pneumonia and Pneumonitis

1. Aspiration may lead to aspiration pneumonia (or aspiration pneumonitis) and increased health care costs. It is best assessed on videofluoroscopy with an MBS.
2. Oral hygiene is the most important predictor of aspiration pneumonia, and studies have shown that cleaning the teeth and reducing oral bacteria is especially important in nursing homes.
3. Aspiration pneumonitis (Mendelson's syndrome) is a "chemical injury caused by inhalation of sterile gastric contents . . . it differs from aspiration pneumonia, which is caused by inhalation of oropharyngeal secretions colonized by pathogenic bacteria."
    a. Occurs in patients who have disturbed consciousness, drug overdose, seizures, CVA or during anesthesia.
    b. Increases in severity as pH decreases (<2.5) or if food from the stomach is aspirated.

Penetration and Silent Aspiration

1. Penetration occurs when material enters the laryngeal aditus or laryngeal ventricle at some level above the vocal folds but does not pass into the airway.
2. In healthy older persons, penetration is often seen; however, material is ejected from the laryngeal aditus before the swallow.
    a. This is not considered a sign of dysphagia.
3. In silent aspiration, the individual is not aware of material entering the airway and, therefore, does not react. No effort is made to expel material from the airway (i.e., the patient does not cough).
    a. Usually occurs in individuals with impaired cognition, if there is a deficit in superior laryngeal nerve innervation to the larynx (causing sensory deficit) or if the vocal folds do not adduct protectively.

Aspiration-Penetration Scale

1. In combination with videofluoroscopic imaging, provides a quantitative method to express the occurrence of penetration or aspiration. Furthermore, it includes enough detail and is sensitive enough to describe additional aspects of swallowing events that are clinically relevant.

2. The Aspiration-Penetration Scale:
   a. Quantifies selected penetration and aspiration events during a videofluoroscopic swallow study.
   b. Does not quantify all events, such as amount and timing of penetration and aspiration.
   c. Can be included as a component of a total swallowing assessment battery.
   d. Is used to demonstrate functional change and the reduction of risk.
   e. Is the most commonly used rating scale for the MBS.
   f. Components.
      (1) Depth of bolus invasion into the airway.
      (2) Response of the client to the bolus.
         (a) Bolus material completely expelled, partially expelled or not expelled.
      (3) Severity.
         (a) Level of bolus entry.
         (b) Awareness of bolus and response to material.

The 8-Point Aspiration-Penetration Scale

1. Material does not enter the airway.
2. Material enters the airway, remains above the vocal folds and is ejected from the airway.
3. Material enters the airway, remains above the vocal folds and is NOT ejected from the airway.
4. Material enters the airway, contacts the vocal folds and is ejected from the airway.
5. Material enters the airway, contacts the vocal folds and is NOT ejected from the airway.
6. Material enters the airway, passes below the vocal folds and is ejected into the larynx or out of the airway.
7. Material enters the airway, passes below the vocal folds and is NOT ejected from the trachea, despite effort.
8. Material enters the airway, passes below the vocal folds and no effort is made to eject the material.

Esophageal Disorders

General Considerations for the SLP

1. Although the SLP does not treat esophageal disorders, which are the responsibility of the physician (gastroenterologist), they need to be familiar with the esophagus and know when to refer a patient for further study.
2. With the assistance of a radiologist, it is important to conduct a modified barium swallow and screen the esophagus for reflux, obstructions or other signs of abnormality. Since the problems in the oropharynx are often reflected by problems of the esophagus and vice versa, the SLP cannot ignore this structure.

Motility Disorders and GERD

1. Esophageal motility disorders are common in adults, especially in the elderly.
   a. Gastroesophageal reflux disease (GERD) is found in at least 2% of the population and 30% of those with oropharyngeal dysphagia.
2. One symptom of GERD is heartburn, which may occur after a meal, accompanied by acid reflux.
   a. Meals buffer gastric acid so that gastric pH rises above 5.
   b. There is a small area, the proximal cardiac/gastroesophageal junction, where acid does not get the effects of buffering.
3. Fatty meals give more buffering of the gastric acidity than a bland or spicy meal.
4. Rapid gastric emptying may cause higher postmeal gastric acidity and predispose one to reflux.
5. pH esophagogastric monitoring can determine if gastric emptying correlates with acid buffering.
6. Gastroesophageal reflux (GER) can result from inadequate relaxation of the lower esophageal sphincter, abnormal peristalsis and hiatal hernia.
   a. Common after meals (especially spicy or acidic foods) and when lying down.
   b. Risk factors include smoking, obesity, alcohol and medications for blood pressure.
7. Backflow: when stomach acid flows back upward into the esophagus, pharynx and oral cavity.
8. Laryngopharyngeal reflux (LPR) occurs when backflow rises to the level of the larynx, which can then accumulate in the pyriform sinuses and spill over into the larynx, causing aspiration and hoarseness.
   a. Other symptoms of GER include regurgitation, hoarseness and throat clearing, choking or gagging.
   b. Can be caused by inflammation or damage to mucosal lining of pharynx and larynx.
   c. GER is commonly treated with antireflux medications such as proton pump inhibitors.

(1) Medications may relax the LES and promote reflux.
(2) Tobacco, ethanol, dopamine, nitrates, morphine, diazepam, and calcium channel blockers.

Other Esophageal Abnormalities

1. Zenker's diverticulum: pocket or pouch that forms when the pharyngeal or esophageal muscles herniate.
    a. This usually occurs near the UES (Killian's triangle) and is seen when it fills with barium on fluoroscopy.
    b. If the diverticulum is filled, contents may drain out and spill over into the open airway after a swallow.
2. Pill-induced esophagitis: an inflammation of the wall of the esophagus produced by a pill or capsule that has lodged in the mucosa.
    a. This is often due to insufficient moisture to transfer a bolus and may become painful.
3. Obstructions in the esophagus will impair flow of the bolus and may cause pain.
4. Achalasia: absence of esophageal peristalsis and failure of the lower esophageal sphincter to relax.
    a. On barium study there is a "bird's beak" or narrowing at the LES. Regurgitation and weight loss are common.
5. Strictures and webs in the esophagus will obstruct bolus flow and can be diagnosed radiographically on a barium swallow of the esophagus performed by a radiologist.
    a. Strictures are treated with dilation.
6. Scleroderma: a motility disorder of the connective tissue that affects the smooth muscle region of the esophagus (lower two-thirds), weakening the LES. It is associated with increased GERD.
    a. Symptoms include heartburn and difficulty swallowing. Diagnosed by regular barium swallow study. Only symptoms can be treated, not the disease itself.
7. Tumors or neoplasms of the esophagus can form in the esophageal lining and obstruct bolus flow.
    a. May be more common in males with a history of drinking and smoking.
    b. Squamous cell carcinoma common in 90% of esophageal tumors.

Medications and Swallowing

Side Effects

1. Many clients with dysphagia are taking numerous medications that can affect the ability to swallow. This is especially true for the elderly and those with neurological conditions and disorders. The SLP needs to consider all medications when doing a swallowing evaluation to determine whether symptoms are medication-related.
2. Common result of medication is the reduction of salivary flow (xerostomia) to the oropharynx, which reduces the ability to mix a bolus and makes bolus transfer through the pharynx and esophagus difficult.
3. Medications can interfere with the oral voluntary phase of swallowing, as many have an impact on cognition or cause sedation, confusion and reduced alertness.
    a. Drugs include antianxiety drugs, antiepileptics, anticholinergics, antihistamines and antihypertensives.
4. Patients should be evaluated when their symptoms are controlled by medication or when they are "on."
5. Some medications cause muscle wasting or excessive muscle relaxation of the oropharyngeal muscles or the LES.
    a. Examples are antithyroid drugs, antacids, steroids, barbiturates, calcium channel blockers, dopaminergics and nitrates.
6. A complete drug history should be performed from chart review and in consultation with a pharmacist or nurse.

Diagnostic Procedures

Interview and Clinical Evaluation

1. An interview with the patient and caregiver is the first step in an evaluation.
    a. An assessment of function can occur at bedside or in an office setting.
    b. A complete evaluation of swallowing should include the interview, questionnaire of patient awareness of dysphagia, chart review, oral motor and feeding assessment and an instrumental swallowing study.

c. The purpose of the diagnostic evaluation process is to determine a treatment plan and a set of baseline performances upon which to compare change.
2. Clinical evaluation will serve as the basis for the instrumental evaluation. It will allow differentiation between normal and abnormal behavior, levels of severity, risks for aspiration and understanding of how a patient eats.
   a. Components include physical inspection of swallow mechanism, cranial nerve assessment, medical history, nutritional and respiratory status, cognition, oral sensation, secretion, taste and smell, lingual and labial strength and movement, velar sufficiency, phonation and oral reflexes.
   b. Observations of body tone, motor function, cough, chewing, rate of eating, mealtime discomfort, alertness and risks for dysphagia should be noted.
   c. 3-ounce water test may be used as a screening for aspiration.

Instrumental Dysphagia Evaluation

Definition and Purposes

1. The instrumental examination is the objective assessment of a patient's complaints that allows the clinician to plan treatment based on observed signs of dysphagia in the oropharyngeal, laryngeal and esophageal regions.
   a. The most commonly used instrumental procedure is the modified barium swallow (MBS) followed by fiberoptic nasoendoscopy, EMG, ultrasound, manometry and by less common research procedures such as scintigraphy or functional MRI.
2. Purposes of instrumental evaluation.
   a. Provide objective, visualized, dynamic, real-time documentation of anatomical and functional causes of swallowing impairment.
   b. Visualize bolus flow and control, swallowing timing, pharyngeal residue, response to bolus misdirection and airway protection.
   c. Determine aspiration risk, effect of modifications in body position, posture, treatment strategies and changes in bolus consistency on ability to swallow.
   d. Signs that require instrumental assessment include fever, pain, excessive effort, coughing, choking or difficulty breathing during or after swallowing.
      (1) Lack of cough or throat clearing with fever, pain or difficulty breathing may indicate silent aspiration and require assessment.
   e. Findings obtained from an instrumental evaluation include:
      (1) Oral and pharyngeal transit times.
      (2) Hyolaryngeal, epiglottic and lingual motion.
      (3) Aspiration, laryngeal penetration.
      (4) Movement of BOT, velum, pharyngeal walls.
      (5) Opening and relaxation of UES, esophageal motility, esophageal and pharyngeal reflux and pharyngeal backflow.
      (6) Vocal fold function, residue in pharynx.
      (7) Symmetry of structures and symmetry of bolus flow.
   f. Selection criteria for instrumental evaluation are intended to match the patient's clinical signs and symptoms with the most accurate, least invasive and safest technique.
      (1) Consider comfort, side effects, compliance, age and medical fragility and behavioral factors.
      (2) Aim for a technique that gives a complete, dynamic and pictorial image with the possibility of imaging from various positions.
      (3) MBS meets all of the above criteria but may not be advisable for an infant, someone with limited mobility or persons who have allergies to barium or who have a record of high doses of radiation exposure.

Modified Barium Swallow (MBS)

1. The modified barium swallow (MBS), also known as a videofluoroscopic swallowing study (VFS, VFSS), is the most complete method to assess oropharyngeal swallowing behavior for treatment planning purposes and follow-up.
2. Its major flaw is radiation exposure.
3. Small boluses are used in 3, 5 and 10 cc sizes for liquid barium while patient is upright. If patient presents with severe dysphagia, consider using 1 cc of liquid per trialed consistency.
   a. Most protocols use thin, nectar-thick and honey-thick barium and a cookie. Barium can be baked into cookies, mixed with pudding and impregnated into pills.
4. Scanning is done in both the lateral and anterior/posterior (AP) views.
   a. In the lateral view, the nasopharynx and entire oropharynx to the upper esophagus can be scanned to determine bolus transit and flow. The velum, tongue, BOT, epiglottis, FOM and hyoid bone are seen.

(1) Aspiration and penetration can be best viewed from the lateral view.
    b. In the AP view, one can image the bolus flow from the mouth, larynx and esophagus into the stomach.
        (1) AP view can identify asymmetries in bolus flow and unilateral residue in the pyriform sinus and valleculae.
        (2) In the AP view, barium can be detected in the laryngopharynx and trachea.
        (3) AP view is recommended for observing the esophagus from the UES to the LES.
    c. MBS is the best procedure to detect aspiration, penetration, swallow duration and pharyngeal and esophageal function.
5. Swallowing studies must be recorded on video or digital format for replay and frame-by-frame investigation of a swallow in real time.
6. Cautions and considerations in reviewing results include understanding that a MBS study is not a replica of a real meal and barium may cause a unique swallow pattern. Some caution should be used in interpretation of the study if aversion to the testing situation or lack of compliance is noted.
7. Clinician must wear protective lead aprons and remain out of the direct radiation field, especially females of child-bearing age.
8. The specific findings observed regarding swallowing physiology (function) in regard to bolus flow and observed signs and symptoms of dysphagia in relation to remedial postural techniques are seen in the following tables. These summary tables contain essential observations leading to remediation and follow-up of progress after dysphagia rehabilitation. The tabular information is derived from MBS studies (Tables 16-3 and 16-4).

Table 16-3

Swallowing Disturbances Observed on MBS

SWALLOWING DISTURBANCE	OBSERVABLE SYMPTOMS
Impaired epiglottic function	Laryngeal penetration or aspiration (MBS. FEES)
Laryngeal penetration or aspiration	Coughing, choking, wet/gurgly voice, harsh vocal quality related to meals
Silent aspiration	None on clinical exam but seen on instrumental study
Reduced laryngeal elevation	Penetration, aspiration, residue, effortful or incomplete swallows
Impairment in vocal fold adduction	Penetration due to reduced vocal fold closure, may cause aspiration
Mass or obstruction in pharynx	Pain when swallowing, bolus feels stuck in throat

Fiberoptic Endoscopic Evaluation of Swallowing (FEES)

1. Also known as nasoendoscopy, FEES uses a flexible fiberoptic naso-pharyngo-laryngoscope to observe the pharynx and larynx and vocal folds before and after a swallow.
2. During the swallow there is a "white out" and the view is obliterated. The oral and esophageal swallow are not able to be observed.
    a. The FEES is a procedure that allows one to see laryngeal penetration and pharyngeal residue using food coloring in a bolus such as applesauce.
3. There is no radiation and the equipment is portable. In some institutions, an otolaryngologist must insert the tube into the nares.
4. Although the effects are controversial, the use of a topical anesthetic (lidocaine) is common for insertion of the scope to avoid discomfort.
    a. Studies have not found any difference in outcome with and without anesthetic.
5. Special training is recommended for the SLP performing this procedure.
6. MBS is recommended for oral phase complaints or for initial examination of a client with dysphagia. FEES is used for bedridden or immobile patients and for a bedside evaluation or follow-up assessment of swallowing.
    a. FEES is often a component of a swallowing work station (e.g., Kay Elemetrics).
7. FEES provides a good assessment of laryngeal, velar and lingua-velar valving needed for a safe swallow.
8. FEES is unable to assess hyolaryngeal movement, bolus transfer and preparation and cannot visualize aspiration during a swallow. Unable to make measurements of swallowing duration and structures in motion.
    a. Copious secretions impair view of laryngopharynx, and microaspiration is not visible.
    b. Length of study must be monitored as it is often uncomfortable to swallow with a tube in the pharynx.
9. The study can be recorded for playback. Care must be taken to sterilize the scope and to use universal precautions, as oral secretions may contain bacterial or other infectious material.
10. May be a useful biofeedback technique and has value to determine food management without radiation.

Fiberoptic Endoscopic Evaluation of Swallowing with Sensory Testing (FEEST)

1. FEEST adds sensory testing of the larynx using air puffs to the laryngeal ventricle as a test of ability to swallow.

Table 16-4

A Postural Techniques Observed on VFS/MBS

PROBLEM OBSERVED ON MBS	POSTURE USED	RATIONALE
Reduced posterior propulsion of bolus over tongue	Slightly tilt head backward and then move head forward quickly	Gravity and oral pressure change helps clear oral cavity
Delay in triggering the pharyngeal swallow	Chin down in midline	Widens valleculae and narrows laryngeal aditus; may present bolus entry into airway
Reduced movement of the base of tongue	Chin down in midline or hawking and throat clearing	Pushes base of tongue closer to posterior pharyngeal wall
Aspiration during the swallow due to unilateral vocal fold impairment	Chin down with head rotated to close off the weakened side	Forces vocal fold closure on weaker side
Aspiration from oropharynx during the swallow	Chin lowered with a forceful swallow or hawking and throat clearing	May narrow laryngeal aditus and clear airway; may aid in vocal fold adduction and hyoid elevation
Residue in the valleculae or pyriform due to paresis/paralysis on one side of the pharynx	Rotate head toward the weaker side	Closes off the weaker side and permits bolus to flow down the stronger side
Slowed pharyngeal contractions	Side lying or forceful swallow	May help force bolus through the pharynx
Combination of unilateral oral and pharyngeal stasis (residue)	Head tilt and forceful swallow	Permits bolus to flow down the stronger side
Impaired laryngeal elevation and impaired UES opening	Mendelsohn maneuver	Manual manipulation raises the thyroid cartilage and may relax the UES

2. This is based on the theory that laryngeal or airway protection requires a cough response and that this technique is able to assess the reflexive cough.
3. It is postulated that persons with stroke or CN X problems may be silent aspirators without a cough, and this test may be able to predict that event.

Ultrasound Imaging (US)

1. A safe and noninvasive technique to view the oral and pharyngeal muscles and soft tissues.
2. Ultrasound is dynamic and can visualize real-time movements of the tongue, floor of the mouth, hyoid and larynx during swallowing using normal foods.
   a. Multiple planes can be seen and various postures and swallowing maneuvers can be imaged. Tumors and masses can be monitored during treatment.
3. US can be used as biofeedback during swallowing treatment, as ongoing images are digitized and can be played side-by-side with normal views for comparison purposes.
   a. Bolus preparation and bolus transfer can be seen along with specific movements of the tongue tip, blade and dorsum during oral preparation for the swallow and during the swallow.
4. Measurements of timing and duration of the swallow and movement of the tongue and hyoid bone can be made from digitized images.
   a. Hyolaryngeal elevation can be measured in conjunction with bolus transfer and lingual transport into the pharynx.
   b. Hyolaryngeal elevation, epiglottal lowering and airway protection are interrelated and can be measured objectively with US.
5. US is safe to use repeatedly and thus is advantageous for infants and children who are high risk or poor feeders.
6. It does not image bones and has a limited field of view depending on the scope of the transducer that is being used. Aspiration is not visible with submental imaging.
7. The larynx can be viewed and vocal fold adduction can be seen during phonation or swallowing.

Other Instrumental Procedures for Swallowing Research

1. Manometry is a medical procedure to view the pressure changes in the esophagus and pharynx during swallowing. It may be performed under sedation to view the gastric system or without sedation to view the pharynx and esophagus.
   a. Manometry has been paired with MBS, called manofluorography, to visualize and quantify the relationship between pressure changes and bolus flow.

2. Scintigraphy is a radiographic procedure that uses radioactive tracer T99 (technetium sulfur colloid) mixed into foods.
   a. The bolus flow and location is detected by a specialized gamma camera, or collimator, and the radiation emitted from the bolus is measured.
   b. Can detect bolus volume and quantify the amount of aspiration or bolus in the system well after a swallow.
   c. Does not display anatomy or the cause of abnormal bolus flow. It is an excellent, but rarely used, method to examine aspiration and gastric motility.
3. fMRI, or functional magnetic resonance imaging, is a sophisticated radiographic technique using alternating magnetic fields to delineate soft tissues and blood vessels.
   a. Gives excellent tissue resolution and will most likely become more prominent when the issue of movement artifact is better resolved. At present, rapid movement, such as in swallowing, impedes the image.
   b. Three-dimensional MRI images can be obtained and will prove invaluable in the next decade.
4. SEMG, or surface electromyography, requires the use of electrodes placed on the submental or neck region.
   a. The electrical signal generated by muscle contractions of the thyrohyoid muscle and FOM muscles during swallowing is produced.
   b. The signal begins at the onset of the swallow, with a peak rise and descending pattern at the end of the swallow. SEMG is often used as a biofeedback technique for swallowing.

Treatments

Direct or Indirect

1. Direct treatments use food, dietary modifications or postural changes and maneuvers during swallowing.
   a. The purpose of direct treatment is to modify the swallow by modifying food or feeding methods.
      (1) Modify posture, bolus size, texture, taste, smell and taste, tactile stimulation, focused on swallowing strategies.
      (2) Biofeedback with EMG or ultrasound.
      (3) Includes special swallowing techniques (e.g., supraglottic swallow, Mendelsohn maneuver, Shaker exercises).
2. Indirect, or rehabilitative, treatments do not use food during the actual exercises. More than one treatment technique is often required if a client has both oral and pharyngeal dysphagia. *Swallowing is the most effective exercise to retrain the swallow.*
   a. Treatment is undertaken to retrain the swallow phases, to prepare, collect and transfer a bolus over the tongue into the pharynx and into the esophagus.
   b. Purpose of indirect treatment is to modify the swallow mechanism and modify the patient without the use of food or liquid. Indirect treatments may involve oral exercises and those that simulate sucking, chewing, lip and lingual movement and a swallow.
      (1) Can include sensory stimulation of the swallowing mechanism, including use of cold or pressure.
      (2) Sour lemon bolus swallow—a frozen mixture may be used before a meal to stimulate oral or pharyngeal sensory awareness. Studies have indicated that a sour bolus will trigger a swallow.
      (3) Oral motor exercises, or neuromuscular treatments, are indirect treatments often used to strengthen and improve range of motion of the oral, facial, lingual, pharyngeal and laryngeal muscles as a precursor to swallowing.
         (a) Consensus appears to be that these exercises have to be targeted to the deficit and be intense and repeated to have a lasting effect.

Supraglottic Swallow

1. Initially for head and neck patients with cancer to protect airway in supraglottic laryngectomies; used commonly for many etiologies.
2. Hold breath, take sip, swallow, cough and clear the airway, swallow again.
3. To protect airway before the swallow and to clear the airway of penetrated material that has accumulated during or after the swallow.
4. Super supraglottic swallow is different only in the amount of effort used before the swallow in breath holding.
   a. May increase anterior laryngeal motion and tongue base movement while aiding in UES opening.
   b. Contraindicated for coronary artery disease or recent stroke.

Mendelsohn Maneuver

1. Mendelsohn maneuver is a direct technique used during a swallow to manually lift the larynx and sustain a swallow at the height of laryngeal elevation.
2. Designed for those with reduced opening of the UES and cricopharyngeal muscle dysfunction.
3. Is difficult to learn and requires intact cognition.
4. Has been demonstrated to be effective with intensive use.

Masako Maneuver

1. Masako maneuver is a tongue-holding maneuver where the tongue is held outside of the mouth. This is based on the observation that during a swallow the posterior pharyngeal wall bulges forward and at the same time contacts the base of the tongue, which creates pharyngeal pressure.
2. Assists bolus flow through the pharynx.
3. It is not recommended to be used with food and has not been thoroughly studied.

Thermal Tactile Stimulation

1. Thermal tactile stimulation is also called thermal application.
2. Purpose is to trigger a pharyngeal swallow with use of sensory stimulation (cold) and contact (tactile pressure) to the anterior faucial arches and surrounding tongue and posterior pharyngeal area.
3. Useful for stroke and in persons with delay in triggering of the pharyngeal swallow.
4. It is used without food to heighten sensitivity so that the swallow can be stimulated when food is introduced.
5. Uses a cold, size 00 laryngeal mirror dipped in ice, making circular motions.
6. Studies vary in results.

Geriatric Patients

1. Treatment for geriatric patients usually focuses on tasks that focus on bolus flow, posture and diet modifications.
2. Fatigue is a factor in treating the elderly, so rigorous exercises often are not feasible.
   a. A specific treatment for elderly patients is used to increase muscle strength in the tongue.
3. Use of specific isometric exercises that use resistance to retrain lingual muscles has had positive effects on swallowing in the elderly. This is a rehabilitative treatment.
   a. Lingual strength retraining using the IOPI (Iowa Oral Performance Instrument) reverses loss of muscle mass and can increase muscle strength.
      (1) Incorporates progressive resistance programs for lingual strengthening. New devices are being tested and appear to be useful for improving swallowing.
   b. Sarcopenia is the term for reduced muscle mass common in the elderly.
      (1) Often a major factor in causing oropharyngeal dysphagia in the elderly and in elderly stroke patients. The lingual strengthening devices can lessen the effects of sarcopenia.

Shaker Exercise

1. Shaker exercise (upper esophageal sphincter [UES] augmentation) is an isometric neck exercise that has improved anterior laryngeal excursion and the anterior-posterior diameter of UES opening.
2. Found to improve UES opening and bolus flow in elderly and younger adults with dysphagia.
3. Consists of repetitions of sustained head-raising in supine position.
4. Considered a rehabilitative strategy. Suprahyoid muscle strengthening exercise that can be used to treat UES opening abnormalities.
5. Not recommended if cervical spine problems or radical neck dissection.
6. May be contraindicated if coronary disease.

Effortful Swallow

1. Effortful swallow found that when subjects were able to use a hard swallow with the IOPI they were able to increase oral lingual pressure and to increase duration of maximum hyoid elevation and closure of the laryngeal vestibule. This was helpful in reducing aspiration risk.

Postural Changes

1. Postural changes are compensatory techniques that are used to improve patient's safety and ability to transfer a bolus safely into the pharynx.
2. The patient must be able to understand the postural change in order to use it independently.
3. Postural maneuvers involve the body or head.
   a. Fundamental posture: seated upright or close to 45 degrees with hips flexed to 90 degrees to achieve best bolus flow and benefit of gravity on bolus transit to the esophagus. Pillows or a wedge are used.

Elevate head of the bed or wheelchair (postural techniques summarized below).
b. Tilt chin downward: if there is residue in valleculae or delayed triggering of swallow. Widens valleculae and narrows entry into larynx.
c. Turn or tilt head: rotate head to damaged side (left or right) if there is unilateral paralysis or paresis. This allows bolus to flow down stronger side. Reduces pharyngeal residue and aspiration risk.
d. Turn head to damaged side and tuck chin: useful if there is unilateral paralysis or paresis and slowed triggering of the swallow. Allows bolus to flow down the undamaged or stronger side. May be the most effective posture.
e. Tilt head back: lingual transit insufficient to move bolus. Will allow gravity to assist in bolus motion. May be useful in early ALS.
f. Side lying: for oral cancer or if risk of aspiration is not severe. Head of bed should be tilted upward at least 30 degrees and pillows used for back support.

Diet Modifications

1. Diet modifications should be instituted only after an objective swallow study to determine which bolus types are safe. Modifications can range from NPO (nothing by mouth) to a mechanical soft consistency or use of thickeners or special foods.
   a. Thicker liquids may help provide sensory input needed to trigger a swallow if bolus is held in the oral cavity. Thickened liquids may be appropriate for those with poor tongue or lip control.
   b. Moist foods with sauces and gravy are more cohesive and easier to transfer into the pharynx. Patients/caregivers may be advised to mash table foods and add sauces, gravy, melted butter and mayonnaise to produce a single soft, homogeneous texture.
      (1) Make sure that foods are not lumpy. Should be without uneven bits or coarse, crispy, crusty surfaces or peelings that are difficult to swallow.
   c. Purees may decrease choking risk or aspiration in neurologically impaired who have most difficulty with liquids due to inability to contain a bolus on the lingual surface. Steam or boil fruits and vegetables and then puree them.
   d. Use natural thickeners, nectars, tomato juice, cream soups, gelatins, hot cereals, puddings and custards.
   e. Increase protein intake with custards, shakes and milk powder.
   f. Use high-energy or high-protein foods when minimal intake or low appetite. Dairy creams, whipping cream, sour cream, cream cheese, butter, ice cream, whole milk, milk powder, yogurt, tofu and legumes.
      (1) Make sure person is not lactose intolerant.
   g. Assess oral hygiene and brush teeth or clean oral cavity as needed.
   h. It is important that the person is adequately hydrated. Water is essential for normal metabolism.
   i. Work with nutritionist/dietician and possibly implement the National Dysphagia Diet (NDD), which has four levels of a dysphagia diet paired with levels of dysphagia difficulty.
      (1) Thin liquid, thick liquid (nectar thick, honey thick, spoon thick), pureed or mechanical soft.
      (2) Different facilities use differing scales, and different products can be used to thicken liquids.
   j. NPO for those who are critically ill, comatose, unable to swallow, aspirate over 10% of all food consistencies or whose swallow is delayed for more than 10 seconds per bite.
      (1) Feeding tubes will be needed for these individuals and require special nutritional evaluation.
   k. Functional Oral Intake Scale (a 7-point scale often used to determine level of feeding needed for each patient).
      (1) Nothing by mouth.
      (2) Tube dependent with minimal attempts at food or liquid.
      (3) Tube dependent with consistent oral intake of food.
      (4) Total oral diet of a single consistency.
      (5) Total oral diet with multiple consistencies, but requiring special preparations or compensations.
      (6) Total oral diet with multiple consistencies, without special preparation but with specific food limitations.
      (7) Total oral diet with no restrictions.
   l. Oral hygiene is one of the most important treatments for patients who are in hospitals or nursing facilities or who are infirm, elderly and unable to take proper care of themselves.
   m. Oral hygiene protocols need to be individualized to meet the specific requirements of each patient. This can be done through oral hygiene consultations with dentistry, nursing and pharmacy.
   n. Simple basic oral care is often better than complicated routines. A soft toothbrush can be used for most purposes. Patients with teeth need fluoride.
   o. Products containing alcohol are not recommended because of its drying effect. Products containing petroleum are not recommended.
   p. Water-soluble products are recommended for hydration.
   q. Product ingredients should match the pH balance of the mouth (5.0 to 7.0).

Neuromuscular Electrical Stimulation (NMES)

1. A controversial technique that requires the use of electrodes placed submentally to provide electrical stimulation to the muscles of the neck.
2. Numerous studies have found inconclusive results with use of this technique.
3. It does not have positive results in children, progressive neurological conditions or in damaged tissues such as those that are often the result of radiation.

McNeill Dysphagia Therapy Program

1. A "systematic exercise-based" program combined with traditional swallowing therapy and surface electromyography biofeedback.
2. Patients improved functionally and were clinically better when these combined strategies were used.

Mealtime Strategies

1. Mealtime strategies for nursing home residents and patients with dementia can enhance the feeding experience and compensate for some of the behavioral and cognitive impairments in persons with dysphagia.
   a. Visual cues, improved lighting, minimal distractions, written reminders, one-step directions, food placement, increasing visual contrasts on the plate, modified cups and utensils are all helpful.
   b. Direct feeding supervision; soft foods; small, bite-sized items; one item at a time; easily chewed foods; added smell and taste enhancement to bland or pureed foods, grouping by compatibility are all helpful.

Surgical Options

1. Surgical options exist to:
   a. Improve opening of the UES (dilatation, myotomy, botulinum toxin).
   b. Enhance airway protection (laryngeal stents, tracheostomy, feeding tubes).
   c. Improve glottal closure (injection of biomaterials in the VF).
   d. Close the glottis (a serious procedure called medialization thyroplasty) to all foreign material, terminating phonation.
2. These are used only if all previous dysphagia treatments have proven ineffective and the individual is in constant risk of aspiration pneumonia.

References

Bass, N.H. (1997). "The Neurology of Swallowing" in Groher, M.E. (Ed.), *Dysphagia Diagnosis and Management*, 3rd ed. Boston: Butterworth-Heinemann.

Belafsky, P.C., & Rees, C.J. (2008). "Esophageal Phase Dysphagia" in R. Leonard & K. Kendall (Eds.), *Dysphagia Assessment and Treatment Planning: A Team Approach*, 2nd ed. San Diego: Plural Pub.

Brown, B.P., & Sonies, B.C. (1997). "Diagnostic Methods to Evaluate Swallowing Other than Barium Contrast" in A. Perlman & K. Schulze-Delrieu (Eds.), *Deglutition and Its Disorders*. San Diego: Singular Publishing Group Inc.

Brush, J.A., & Calkins, M.P. Environmental interventions and dementia-enhancing mealtimes in group dining rooms. *ASHA Leader* (June 17, 2008).

Brush, J.A., Slominski T., & Boczko, F. Meal time enhancements. *ASHA Leader* (May 23, 2006).

Buchholz, D.W., & Robbins, J. (1997). "Neurologic Diseases Affecting Oropharyngeal Swallowing" in A. Perlman & K. Schulze-Delrieu (Eds.), *Deglutition and Its Disorders*. San Diego: Singular Publishing Group Inc.

Burkhead, L.M. (2009). Applications of exercise science in dysphagia rehabilitation. *Perspectives on Swallowing and Swallowing Disorders, ASHA Division 13*, 18(2), 43–48.

Carnaby-Mann, G.S., & Crary, M.S. (2010). McNeill dysphagia therapy program: A case-control study. *Arch Physical Medicine and Rehabilitation*, 91, 743–749.

Clark, H.M. (2003). Neuromuscular treatments for speech and swallowing: A tutorial. *American Journal of Speech-Language Pathology*, 12(4), 400–415.

Coyle, J.L. (2002). Critical appraisal of a treatment publication: Electrical stimulation for the treatment of dysphagia. *Perspectives on Swallowing and Swallowing Disorders*, 11, 12–15.

Crary, M.A., Carnaby-Mann, G.D., & Faunce, A. (2007). Electrical stimulation therapy for dysphagia: Descriptive results of two surveys. *Dysphagia*, 22(3), 165–1731.

Daniels, S.K., & Foundas, A.L. (1997). The role of the insular cortex in dysphagia. *Dysphagia*, 12, 146–156.

De Pippo, K., Holas, M., Reding, M. (1992). Validation of the 3-oz water test for aspiration following stroke. *Archives of Neurology*, 49(12), 1259–61.

Doeltgen, S.H., Macrae, P., & Huckabee, M.L. (2011). Pharyngeal pressure generation during tongue-hold swallows across age groups. *American Journal of Speech-Language Pathology*, 20, 124–130.

Ehlpen, E. (1997). Pulmonary aspiration in hospitalized adults. *Nutrition in Clinical Practice*, 12(5), 13.

Feinberg, M. (1997). "The Effects of Medications on Swallowing" in G. Sonies (Ed.), *Dysphagia: A Continuum of Care.* Gaithersburg, MD: Aspen Pubs.

Gallagher, L., & Naidoo, P. (2009). Prescription drugs and their effects on swallowing. *Dysphagia,* 24, 159–166.

Groher, M.E. (1997). *Dysphagia Diagnosis and Management,* 3rd ed. Boston: Butterworth-Heinemann.

Huckabee, M.L., Deecke, L. Cannito, M.P., Gould, H.J., & Mayr, W. (2003). Cortical control mechanisms in volitional swallowing: The bereitschaftspotential. *Brain Topography,* 16(1), 3–17.

Huckabee, M.L., & Steele, C.M. (2006). Analysis of lingual contribution to submental sEMG measures and pharyngeal biomechanics during effortful swallow. *Archives of Physical Medicine and Rehabilitation,* 87, 1067–1072.

Humbert, I.A., Poletto, C.J., Saxon, K.G., Kearney, P.R., Crujido, L., Wright-Harp, W., et al. (2006). The effect of surface electrical stimulation on hyolaryngeal movement in normal individuals at rest and during swallowing. *Journal of Applied Physiology,* 101, 1657–1663.

Kleim, J.A., & Jones, T.A. (2008). Principles of experience-dependent neuroplasticity: Implications for rehabilitation after brain damage. *Journal of Speech, Language, and Hearing Research,* 51(1), S225–239.

Langmore, S.E., Schatz, K., & Olsen, N. (1988). Fiberoptic endoscopic examination of swallowing safety: A new procedure. *Dysphagia,* 2(4), 216–219.

Langmore, S.E., Terpenning, S., Schork, A., Chen, Y., Murray, J.T., Lopatin, D., & Loesche, W.J. (1998). Predictors of aspiration pneumonia: How important is dysphagia? *Dysphagia,* 13, 69–81.

Leonard, R., & Kendall, K. (2008). *Dysphagia Assessment and Treatment Planning: A Team Approach,* 2nd ed. San Diego: Plural Pub.

Leopold, D.A., Bartoshuk, L., Doty, R.L., Jafek, B., Smith, D.V., & Snow, J.B. (1989). Aging of the upper airway and the senses of taste and smell. *Otolaryngology—Head and Neck Surgery,* 100(4), 287–289.

Leopold, N.A., & Kagel, M.C. (1985). Dysphagia in Huntington's disease. *Archives of Neurology,* 42, 5–63.

Leow, P., Beckert, L., Anderson, T., & Huckabee, M. (2012). Changes in chemosensitivity and mechanosensitivity in aging and Parkinson's disease. *Dysphagia,* 27, 106–114.

Logemann, J.A. (1998). *Evaluation and Treatment of Swallowing Disorders,* 2nd ed. Austin, TX: Pro-ed.

Ludlow, C.L., Humbert, I., Saxon, K., Poletto, C.J., Sonies, B., & Crujido, L. (2007). Effects of surface electrical stimulation both at rest and during swallowing in chronic pharyngeal dysphagia. *Dysphagia,* 22, 1–10.

Marik, P.E. (2001). Aspiration pneumonia and aspiration pneumonitis. *New England Journal of Medicine,* 344(9), 665–671.

Martin, R. (2009). Neuroplasticity and swallowing. *Dysphagia,* 24(2), 218–229.

Martin-Harris, B., Brodsky, M.B., Price, C.C., Michel, Y., & Walters, B. (2003). Temporal coordination of pharyngeal and laryngeal dynamics with breathing during swallowing: Single liquid swallows. *Journal of Applied Physiology,* 94, 1735–43.

McCulloch, T., Jaffe, D.M., & Hoffman, H.T. (1997). "Diseases and Operation of Head and Neck Structures Affecting Swallowing" in A. Perlman & K. Schulze-Delrieu (Eds.), *Deglutition and Its Disorders.* San Diego: Plural Pub.

Miller, J.L., & Sonies, B.C. (2008). "Dynamic Imaging of the Tongue, Larynx and Pharynx During Swallowing" in L. Orloff (Ed.), *Head and Neck Ultrasonography.* San Diego: Plural Pub.

Netter, F.H. (1953). *The CIBA Collection of Medical Illustrations: Nervous System.* New York: CIBA Pharmaceutical Company.

Nicosia, M.A., Hind, J.A., Roecker, E.B., Carnes, M., Doyle, J., Dengel, G.A., & Robbins, J.A. (2000). Age effects on temporal evolution of isometric and swallowing pressure. *Journal of Gerontology Series A—Biological Sciences, Medical Sciences,* 55(11), M634–640.

Pelletier, C.A. (2007). Chemosenses, aging, and oropharyngeal dysphagia. *Topics in Geriatric Rehabilitation,* 23(3), 249–268.

Perlman, A., & Christensen, J. (1997). "Topography and Functional Anatomy of the Swallowing Structures" in A. Perlman & K. Schulze-Delrieu (Eds.), *Deglutition and Its Disorders.* San Diego: Singular Publishing Group Inc.

Perlman, A.L. (1997). "Application of Instrumental Procedures to the Evaluation and Treatment of Dysphagia" in B.C. Sonies (Ed.), *Dysphagia: A Continuum of Care.* Gaithersburg, MD: Aspen Publishers.

Ramig, L., Fox, C., & Sapir, S. (2007). "Speech, Voice and Swallowing in Parkinson Disease" in W. Koller & E. Melamed (Eds.), *Handbook of Clinical Neurology: Parkinson's and Parkinsonian Disorders.* Elsevier: United Kingdom, pp. 385–399.

Redstone, F., & West, J. F. (2004). The importance of postural control for feeding. *Pediatric Nursing,* 30(2), 97–100.

Robbins, J., Butler, S.G., Daniels, S.K., Diez Gross, R., Langmore, S., Lazarus, C.L., et al. (2008). Swallowing and dysphagia rehabilitation: Translating principles of neural plasticity into clinically oriented evidence. *Journal of Speech, Language, and Hearing Research,* 51(1), S 276–300.

Robbins, J., Kays, S.A., Gangnon, R.E., Hind, J.A., Hewitt, L., Gentry, L.R., & Taylor, A.J., (2007). The effects of lingual exercise in stroke patients with dysphagia. *Archives of Physical Medicine and Rehabilitation,* 88, 150–158.

Robbins, J., Hamilton, J.W., Lof, G.L., & Kempster, G.B. (1992). Oropharyngeal swallowing in normal adults of different ages. *Gastroenterology,* 103, 823–829.

Robbins, J.A., & Levine, R.L. (1988). Swallowing after unilateral stroke of the cerebral cortex: Preliminary experience. *Dysphagia,* 3, 11–17.

Rosenbek, J.D., Robbins J.A, Roecker E.B., Coyle, J.C., & Wood J.L. (1996). A Penetration-aspiration scale. *Dysphagia,* 11, 93–96.

Sapienza, C.M., & Wheeler, K. (2006). Respiratory muscle strength training: Functional outcomes versus plasticity. *Seminars in Speech and Language,* 27(4), 236–244.

Seikel, J.A., King, D.W., & Drumwright, D.G. (2010). *Anatomy & Physiology for Speech, Language, and Hearing,* 4th ed. Australia: Delmar Cengage Learning.

Shaker, R., Easterling C., Kern. M., Nitschke, T., Massey, B., Daniels, S., et al. (2002). Rehabilitation of swallowing by exercise in tube-fed patients with pharyngeal dysphagia secondary to abnormal UES opening. *Gastroenterology,* 122, 1314–1321.

Shaw, D.W., Cook, I.J., Gabb, M., Holloway, R.H., Simula, M.E., Panagopoulous, V., & Dent, J. (1995). Influence of normal aging on oral-pharyngeal and upper esophageal sphincter function during swallowing. *American Journal of Physiology*, 268(31), G389–396.

Shawker, T., Sonies, B.C., Hall, T.E., & Baum B. (1984) Ultrasound analysis of tongue, hyoid and larynx activity during swallowing. *Investigative Radiology*, 19(2), 82–86.

Shawker, T., Sonies, B., Stone, M., & Baum, B., (1983). Real-time ultrasound visualizaton of tongue movement during swallowing. *Journal of Clinical Ultrasound*, 11, 485–489.

Sonies, B.C. (1991). "The Aging Oropharyngeal System" in D. Ripich (Ed.), *Handbook of Geriatric Communication Disorders*. Austin, TX: Pro-Ed.

Sonies, B.C. (1992). "Oropharyngeal Dysphagia in the Elderly" in B.J. Baum (Ed.), *Clinics in Geriatric Medicine*. Philadelphia: W.B. Saunders.

Sonies, B.C. (2006). "Disorders of Swallowing" in N.B. Anderson & G.H. Shames (Eds.), *Human Communication Disorders*, 7th ed. Boston: Pearson.

Sonies, B.C., & Dalakas, M.C. (1991). Dysphagia in patients with the post-polio syndrome. *New England Journal of Medicine*, 324, 1162–67.

Sonies, B.C., & Dalakas, M.C. (1995). Progression of oral-motor and swallowing symptoms in the post-polio syndrome. *Annals of the New York Academy of Sciences*, 753, 85–95.

Sonies, B.C., Parent, L.J., Morrish, K., & Baum, B.J. (1988). Durational aspects of the oral-pharyngeal phase of swallow in normal adults. *Dysphagia*, 3, 1–10.

Spechler, S. (1992). Epidemiology and natural history of gastroesophageal reflux disease. *Digestion*, 51(suppl. 1), 24–291.

Suiter, D.M., & Leder, S.B. (2008). Clinical utility of the 3-ounce water test. *Dysphagia*. 23(3), 244–250.

Suzuki, M., Asada, Y., Ito, J., et al. (2003). Activation of cerebellum and basal ganglia on volitional swallowing detected by functional magnetic resonance imaging. *Dysphagia*, 18, 71–77.

Watkin K.L., & Miller, J.L. (1997). "Instrumental Imaging Technologies and Procedures" in B.C. Sonies (Ed.), *Dysphagia: A Continuum of Care*. Gaithersburg, MD: Aspen Publishers.

Wheeler, K.M., Chiara, T., & Sapienza, C.M. (2007). Surface electromyographic activity of the submental muscles during swallow and expiratory pressure threshold training tasks. *Dysphagia*, 22, 108–116.

Yoshida, M., Yoneyama, T., Akagawa, Y. Nippon, R., & Igakkai, Z. (2001). Oral care reduces pneumonia of elderly patients in nursing homes, irrespective of dentate or edentate status. *Japanese Journal of Geriatrics*, 38(4), 48–103.

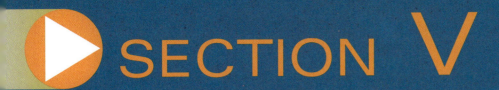

SECTION V

Special Considerations in Speech-Language Pathology Practice

Section Outline

- **Chapter 17:** Augmentative and Alternative Communication, 393
- **Chapter 18:** Audiology and Hearing Impairment, 409

17

Augmentative and Alternative Communication

MICHELLE L. GUTMANN, PhD

Chapter Outline

- Augmentative and Alternative Communication (AAC) and Related Terms, 394
- Communication Disorders Associated with Need for AAC, 394
- The Law and Access to AAC, 395
- Core Concepts in AAC, 395
- Assessment in AAC, 401
- Intervention in AAC, 403
- Anatomy of an AAC Device, 405
- Issues in AAC, 406
- Mobile Tablets and Apps, 406
- References, 407

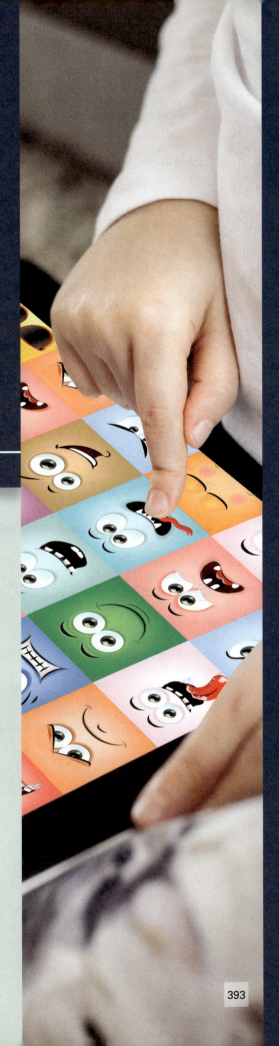

Augmentative and Alternative Communication (AAC) and Related Terms

Definition of AAC

1. Refers to forms of communication that either supplement and/or replace more conventional means of communication, typically referring to speech.
2. ASHA Position Statement on AAC.
   a. "Augmentative and alternative communication (AAC) refers to an area of research, clinical and educational practice. AAC involves attempts to study and, when necessary, compensate for temporary or permanent impairments, activity limitations and participation restriction of individuals with severe disorders of speech-language production and/or comprehension, including spoken and written modes of communication" (ASHA, 2005).
   b. AAC can be used to support receptive and expressive speech, language and/or communication disorders.

Candidacy for AAC

1. Anyone who cannot meet his/her daily written or spoken communication needs through speech or writing is a candidate for AAC.
2. People who need and/or use AAC, regardless of the type or severity of disability, are also referred to as people with complex communication needs (CCN).

Face-to-Face Communication (F2F)

1. Typically refers to spoken communication.

Written Communication

1. Typically refers to textual output.
2. May or not be printed as hard copy, and now includes sending text messages.

Communication Disorders Associated with Need for AAC

Developmental and Congenital Disorders

1. Autism spectrum disorders (ASD).
2. Cerebral palsy (CP).
3. Various syndromes (e.g., Down syndrome).
4. Severe and refractory phonological disorders.
5. Childhood apraxia of speech (CAS).
6. Intellectual disability.
7. Spina bifida.

Temporary vs. Permanent Need for AAC

1. Conditions that may necessitate temporary use of AAC.
   a. Intubation following surgery.
   b. Prescription of voice rest.
   c. Severe laryngitis.
2. Conditions that may necessitate permanent use of AAC.
   a. Total glossectomy and laryngectomy.
   b. Severe, chronic or progressive dysarthria.
   c. Severe and chronic aphasia.

Acquired Disorders

1. Brain tumor.
2. Stroke (cerebrovascular accident, or CVA).
3. Spinal cord injury (SCI).
4. Traumatic brain injury (TBI).
5. Multiple sclerosis (MS).
6. Guillain-Barré syndrome.
7. Huntington's disease (HD).
8. Head and neck cancers (HNCs) and other cancers that metastasize to the brain and affect speech, language and/or cognition.

AAC Across the Lifespan

1. AAC techniques, strategies and systems may be used across the lifespan to support both speech and language in development as well as in dissolution.
2. Although helpful, literacy skills are not necessary to use a variety of AAC options.
3. Recent research supports use of low-technology AAC options for people with a variety of disorders typically associated with aging, such as memory impairments, the dementias and progressive language disorders (e.g., primary progressive aphasia).

The Law and Access to AAC

Educational Settings

1. Free Appropriate Public Education (FAPE, 1975).
   a. Educational right of children with disabilities in the United States.
   b. Guaranteed by the Rehabilitation Act of 1973 and the Individuals with Disabilities Education Act (IDEA, 1990).
   c. Requires that children with disabilities receive support free of charge as is provided to nondisabled students.
   d. Provides access to general education services for children with disabilities by encouraging that support and related services be provided to children in their general education settings as much as possible.
   e. Does not entitle one to a mobile table or other specific type of device in school.
2. Individuals with Disabilities Education Act (IDEA, 1990).
   a. IDEA stipulates that assistive technology, of which AAC is part, must be provided if it is required as a part of a child's special education, related services or supplementary aids and services.
   b. The individual education plan (IEP) team must consider whether a child needs assistive technology devices and services to increase, maintain or improve functional capabilities.

Community Settings

1. Assistive Technology Act Amendments of 2004 (PL-108-364).
   a. Mandated assistive technology (AT) centers in each state and territory.
   b. Goal of each center to increase availability and utilization of AT services for individuals with disabilities.

Hospitals

1. Americans with Disabilities Act (ADA).
   a. Under the ADA, hospitals must provide effective means of communication for patients, family members and hospital visitors who are deaf or hard of hearing.
2. The Joint Commission's *Advancing Effective Communication, Cultural Competence, and Patient- and Family-Center Care: A Roadmap for Hospitals* (2010).
   a. A resource to help health care providers learn to communicate with patients so that each understands the other, regardless of cultural or linguistic differences, sensory impairments or limitations on ability to communicate via natural speech.
   b. The document addresses ways to improve overall patient-provider communication.
      (1) Develop language access services for patients (or providers) who speak languages other than English (including sign language) or who have limited health literacy.
      (2) Translate forms and instructional materials into other languages.
      (3) Address the needs of patients with disabilities, including those with speech, physical or cognitive impairments, blindness/low vision or hearing impairments.
      (4) Augmentative communication strategies and assistive technologies are requisite tools for many hospitalized patients.

Core Concepts in AAC

Unaided vs. Aided

1. Unaided AAC refers to the use of only the body to communicate, without external aids or equipment.
   a. Examples of unaided AAC include:
      (1) Gestures.
      (2) Manual signs.
      (3) Gaze.
      (4) Pantomime.
      (5) Head movements (e.g., nod/shake).
      (6) Vocalizations.
   b. Typically, unaided AAC uses the axis of the body.
2. Aided AAC refers to the use of external equipment to assist with communication.
   a. Examples of aided AAC.
      (1) Objects.
      (2) Pictures.
      (3) Line drawings.

(4) Labeled symbols.
(5) Speech output from some type of speech-generating device.
b. Typically, aided AAC extends beyond the body's axis.

Types of Aided AAC

1. No-tech refers to any type of AAC device/system that is nonelectronic (i.e., does not use a battery and cannot be plugged in).
   a. Examples of no tech AAC include:
      (1) Communication boards or displays.
      (2) Pencil and paper.
      (3) White-erase boards.
      (4) Use of symbol systems.
2. Low- to mid-tech refers to simple electronic devices on which a limited number of messages can be recorded and played back. These devices may not have rechargeable batteries.
   a. Examples of low- to mid-tech AAC.
      (1) Single or multiple message switches.
      (2) Very basic communication devices with a limited number of messages/cells.
3. High tech refers to more sophisticated electronic devices that support speech and/or written output. These devices may have rechargeable batteries.
   a. Examples of high-tech AAC.
      (1) Fully functional computers that run specialized software for communication.

Dedicated vs. Nondedicated Devices

1. All high-tech AAC devices and some mid-tech AAC options can be further classified as either dedicated or nondedicated (Figure 17-1).
2. Dedicated devices are devices whose sole purpose is to assist with communication, typically face-to-face communication, by providing speech output.
   a. Dedicated devices are referred to as speech-generating devices (SGDs).
3. Nondedicated devices are typically commercially available and support a range of functions in addition to speech output.
   a. Additional functions include, but are not limited to:
      (1) Access to the Internet.
      (2) Gaming.
      (3) Being an e-reader.
      (4) Word processing.
   b. Examples of nondedicated AAC.
      (1) Mobile tablets.
      (2) Laptop or notebook computers.
   c. Some nondedicated devices also support written output.

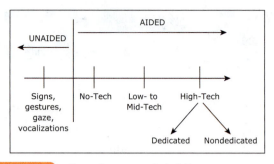

Figure 17-1 Continuum of AAC

Types of Aided AAC Symbols

1. All symbols represent some type of referent.
2. Symbols vary with respect to both complexity and the degree of transparency relative to the referent.
3. Iconicity is a characteristic of symbols.
   a. Iconicity refers to the association a person makes between a symbol and its referent.
4. Symbol transparency varies along an iconicity continuum, from:
   a. Opaque: symbol does not resemble referent (least transparent).
   b. Translucent: symbol bears some resemblance to referent (more transparent than opaque).
   c. Transparent: meaning of the symbol can be readily guessed in absence of referent (most transparent with respect to referent).
5. No tech AAC symbols.
   a. Real objects (e.g., a fork to represent "food/hungry").
   b. Partial objects (e.g., a drumstick to represent "drum/playing the drum").
   c. Miniature objects (e.g., a miniature dollhouse to represent "house/home").
6. No-, low- to mid- and high-tech AAC symbols.
   a. Photographs (e.g., black and white, colored).
   b. Line drawings (e.g., black on white background or white on black background).
   c. Text (i.e., orthography).
7. Depending on the individual's needs, an AAC system may comprise combinations of various aided AAC symbol types (e.g., photographs, line drawings and text).

Physical Characteristics of Aided AAC Systems

1. Aided AAC systems vary with respect to the following parameters:
   a. Number of symbols.
   b. Spacing between symbols.
   c. Size of symbols.
   d. Dimensions of display or device.
   e. Specifications of display or device (e.g., weight, height).

f. Type of display.
   (1) Static.
      (a) Display that doesn't change (e.g., low tech communication board).
   (2) Dynamic.
      (a) Screen changes following user input (e.g., ATM machines).
      (b) Input causes screen to change by branching to another page or another menu.

Additional Features of Aided AAC Systems

1. Portability.
   a. Whether or not the system is lightweight enough to be portable.
2. Adaptability.
   a. Whether or not the features on a device can be adjusted according to need. Often used with respect to whether the device supports alternate access.
3. Cosmesis.
   a. Aesthetic appeal of the device and whether it can be modified (e.g., addition of user-chosen colored panels or color choice of device).
4. Connectivity.
   a. Does the device support connection to the Internet, Bluetooth, etc.

Access

1. Physical access
   a. Direct selection: the user directly makes a choice on the system via touch, pointing, looking or speaking.
      (1) Touch via finger, hand, headstick, mouthstick, stylus. The medium comes into direct contact with AAC system screen.
      (2) Pointing via finger, hand or capacitive stylus. Medium does not come into direct contact with the screen of the AAC system, but is directed at specific target.
      (3) Looking via eye gaze or eye linking. The person using system makes selections via looking at targets.
         (a) Eye gaze systems typically require calibration.
      (4) Speaking using speech recognition software, the person using the system dictates what they wish to type.
   b. Alternate access: required when the user cannot directly make a choice on the system and must use alternate means to indicate desired target.
      (1) Scanning.
         (a) An indirect method of access. Choices are presented to the person using the AAC system, and the person indicates, via predetermined signal (typically using a switch) when the desired target is reached.
         (b) Scanning involves the selection set that is all of the messages, symbols and codes that are available at one time to the person using the AAC system.
      (2) Common scanning patterns.
         (a) Circular: device presents the selection set in a circle and scans them electronically, item by item, until a selection is made.
            • Simplest type of scanning.
         (b) Linear: device highlights each item in the first row of the selection set, followed by each item in the second row, etc., until a selection is made.
         (c) Row-column: scanning proceeds by highlighting each row until the user selects the row in which the target is located. Then scanning proceeds by highlighted each item or column until the desired target is reached.
         (d) Top-bottom: scanning proceeds such that the top half of the screen/display is highlighted followed by the bottom half of the screen/display. The user indicates where target is, and then that area (either top or bottom) is scanned using a row-column pattern.
         (e) Group item: scanning proceeds by group (e.g., color, semantically or thematically grouped items) until the user indicates which group target item is in. That group is then scanned using row-column scanning.
      (3) Selection control techniques (i.e., how a selection is made).
         (a) Directed (inverse) scanning: the cursor begins to move when the person activates and holds the switch. When the switch is released, a selection is made.
            • Useful for a person who can sustain activation and release in a timely manner.
         (b) Automatic (regular) scanning: the cursor moves automatically according to a preset pattern (e.g., row-column scanning), and when the person activates the switch, a selection is made.
            • Useful for a person who has difficulty sustaining and/or releasing the switch.
         (c) Step scanning: A 1:1 correspondence between cursor movement and switch activation. To select an item, the user stops activating the switch when the desired item is reached.
            • Useful for learning to scan but can be very fatiguing.

(4) Partner-assisted scanning (partner-dependent scanning).
   (a) Used when the person needing AAC cannot scan independently.
   (b) Communication partner presents choices to the AAC user.
   (c) The AAC user indicates when the desired target is met by a predetermined signal.
      • Typically, however, the person indicates "yes" and "no."
   (d) Requires training for communication partner(s).
   (e) Efficient when:
      • Both partners trained in system use.
      • System is organized to support this type of scanning.
(5) Auditory scanning.
   (a) Used when visual interaction with the device is not possible, due to visual problems (e.g., severe uncorrected vision problems, visual deficits postneurological insult, cortical visual impairment).
   (b) Choices are presented to the user auditorily, either out loud or privately via ear bud.
   (c) Person selects the message to be spoken via switch activation, and message is spoken publicly.
(6) Switches.
   (a) Scanning is accomplished using switches, which are pieces of hardware that open or close an electronic circuit.
   (b) Multitude of switches on the market.
   (c) Can use single-switch or multiple-switch scanning.
   (d) When two switches are used for scanning, one is used to navigate, the other to make a selection.
(7) Types of switches.
   (a) Mechanical: require activation pressure, some "travel" or excursion involved during activation.
   (b) Electrical: no pressure required, some travel required, provides less feedback.
   (c) Pneumatic: sip and puff, use inhalation and exhalation for activation.
   (d) Electronic: includes switches that work via infrared, sound, sensors or fiber optics.
   (e) Brain computer interface (BCI): still in development.
      • Does not require neuromuscular activation.
      • Captures changes in brain's electrical activity as intended activation.
      • Invasive electrodes are placed directly in the cortex.
      • Noninvasive recording sites at the scalp or via magnetic brain forces (e.g., MEG or MRI).
      • With noninvasive BCIs, must attenuate noise to enhance signal-to-noise ratio.

Switch Site Assessment

1. Most often conducted in conjunction with occupational and/or physical therapist to determine whether the patient has a consistent and nonfatiguing movement that can be used to activate a switch.
   a. Must consider the movement pattern.
      (1) Cannot be a movement that is difficult to perform or has the potential to create muscular or postural problems.
   b. Ideal switch site uses a small, isolated, volitional, controlled movement, with sustained pressure and controlled release.
   c. Switch site hierarchy.
      (1) Hands.
      (2) Head.
      (3) Mouth.
      (4) Feet.
      (5) Lower extremities.
      (6) Upper extremities.
      (7) Mind.
   d. Variety of rubrics for switch site assessment available.

Type of Communicator

1. Useful classification system for AAC users across both developmental and acquired disorders.
2. Emerging AAC communicator.
   a. Has extreme difficulty speaking, using symbols and responding to conversational input.
   b. May include apraxic component.
3. Contextual AAC communicator.
   a. More functional communicators than emerging communicators.
   b. Indicate basic needs by point; can recognize visual symbols (e.g., photographs, labels, signs, logos) and is aware of daily routines and schedules.
   c. Does not have the linguistic ability to independently initiate or add to a conversation.
   d. Can participate in conversation with assisted input to boost comprehension and with scaffolding for output.
4. Independent AAC communicator.
   a. Comprehends most of what he/she hears without contextual support.
   b. Can initiate intentional communication using a variety of strategies and modalities.
   c. Knows how to alternate among strategies and modalities to accomplish communicative goals.

Four Main Reasons for Communicative Interaction

1. Communication of needs and wants.
   a. To regulate the behavior of others to get needs and wants met.
   b. For example "I'm thirsty" tells the communication partner about a need for a drink.
2. Information transfer.
   a. To share information with others.
   b. Does not require action by communication partner.
3. Social closeness.
   a. To establish and maintain personal relationships.
   b. Interaction is of primary importance.
4. Social etiquette.
   a. To engage in brief interactions that conform to social conventions of politeness.
   b. For example, saying "good morning" as you pass a coworker in the hall, or saying "Hi, how are you?" without waiting for a response.

Communicative Competence for AAC Users

1. Four core competencies constitute communicative competence for an AAC user.
2. Model is foundational for guiding both assessment and intervention.
3. Communicative competence for AAC users includes:
   a. Linguistic competence.
      (1) Knowledge of the linguistic code used by one's AAC system (e.g., symbols, print, signs).
      (2) AAC user must also learn the language spoken/signed by members of the community so that they may receive messages.
   b. Operational competence.
      (1) The technical skills needed to operate the AAC system efficiently, which includes learning how to operate and maintain the system.
      (2) System maintenance (e.g., charging on a regular schedule) may be the responsibility of communication facilitators rather than the users themselves.
   c. Social competence.
      (1) Skills of social interaction, the pragmatics of communication.
      (2) These skills may be targeted directly in therapy to train the AAC user and may extend to training of facilitators how best to support the AAC user in social interactions.
   d. Strategic competence.
      (1) The ability of people who use AAC to invoke and use compensatory strategies to circumvent the functional limitations introduced by use of AAC systems.
         (a) Resolving communication breakdowns.
         (b) Using preprogrammed messages to indicate when a communication partner has misunderstood a message or when a communication partner should be patient while message composition is ongoing.
4. This model of communicative competence is applicable across the lifespan and cross-culturally.
5. Cultural views of disability, and particularly severe disability such as that often associated with CCN, may influence the acceptance of AAC and the extent to which a person with CCN may achieve these four competencies, regardless of true ability.

Rate Enhancement

1. Includes strategies and techniques used by AAC users to accelerate message formulation and transmission. Varying memory and learning requirements for each technique.
   a. Used to facilitate communication by attenuating the gap between speaking rate (typically 150–200 words per minute) and how quickly an AAC user can compose a message (approximately 15–25 times slower than the rate of spoken speech).
   b. Types of rate enhancement.
      (1) Prediction: used in smartphone technology. System uses various algorithms to predict word or message completion based on the portion of the word of message the AAC user has already formulated.
         (a) Single letter: the probability of a letter occurring based on the previous letters (e.g., in English, *q* is often followed by *u*).
         (b) Word-level: word prediction involves prediction of a constrained set of likely words, based on the word's frequency of use (e.g., in English, if the letters *q-u-i* are typed, the system may predict *quite, quiet, quill* in that order).
         (c) Linguistic prediction: prediction constrained and governed by the organizational patterns of the language (e.g., in English, if the user types *I* at the beginning of a sentence, the system presents only verbs that agree in tense with *I*, such as *I am, I go, I want*).
         (d) Phrase- or sentence-level: prediction based on units of language longer than a single word. Some high-level systems employ this type of prediction.
      (2) Coding: used to represent single words.
         (a) Alpha word codes: created by either truncation (i.e., using first few letters of a word, such as *comm* for *communication*) or contraction, which often involves deletion of some

of all of the vowels (e.g., *comnctn* for *communication*).
- (b) Alphanumeric word codes: use both numbers and letters to code for words or phrases.
  - Advantage is that the same letters can be used across words or phrases, the number differentiates them.
- (c) Letter-category word codes: the initial letter codes the superordinate category, and second letter is the first letter of the specific word.
  - For example, if *F* = *friends*, then *FA* could refer to Adam, while *FB* could refer to Brandon.
  - Similarly, if *B* = *beverages*, then *BC* could refer to coffee, and *BG* could refer to grape juice.
- (d) Numeric codes: arbitrary relation between number and word. Used when an AAC user has very limited motor abilities and needs many options represented in a small selection set.
  - The strength of this system is in the combinatorial power of words.
  - Requires extensive learning/memory or creation of a reference glossary.

(3) Message coding: used to encode messages.
- (a) Many of the same strategies used for words can be used for messages.
- (b) Alpha-letter encoding (i.e., salient letter encoding).
  - Capitalizes on knowledge of orthography and syntax.
  - The initial letters of salient content words are used to create the code.
  - For example, "hello, how are you?" could be coded *HHY* for the salient words of the message.
- (c) Abbreviation expansion (Abex).
  - Similar to alpha-letter encoding.
  - Uses the initial letters of core content words to formulate abbreviation.
  - Abbreviation cannot be a real word, otherwise when the word is typed, the system will insert the abbreviated message instead of the real word.
  - For example, "I am tired" should not be abbreviated *it*, as *it* is a real word. Rather, the phrase would need to be abbreviated as *ia* for *I am*....
- (d) Icon prediction.
  - Used with communication systems that use icons to code for words, phrases, sentences and longer units of text.
  - When an icon is selected, only those icons that can go with the original, either thematically or semantically, will be offered by the system.
  - Use of icon-based system required facility with words and multiple meanings.

(4) Color coding.
- (a) Fitzgerald key system: left-to-right, color-based, semantic-syntactic coding system.
  - Examples include nouns, verbs, modifiers, question words organized from left to right, with each syntactic category assigned a different color.

Organization and Layout of Communication Displays/ Devices

1. Goals associated with organization and layout.
   a. Maximize efficient communication.
   b. Minimize effort expended in communication.
   c. Promote language learning, as applicable.
2. Organization strategies.
   a. Grid displays.
      (1) Symbols, words and messages are arranged in a grid pattern.
      (2) Size of grid and number of symbols are determined during assessment.
      (3) Grid layout echoes linear pattern(s) of written syntax (e.g., subject-verb-object [SVO] sentences).
      (4) Examples of grid-type displays include, but are not limited to:
         (a) Fitzgerald key system (see above).
         (b) Schematic grid displays or topic boards.
            - Vocabulary is organized according to topic, event, routine or activity (e.g., going to school, circle time, work routines).
         (c) Pragmatic Organization Dynamic Display (PODD; Porter, 2007).
            - Developed to increase communicative efficiency across and within environments.
            - Pragmatic functions purposefully added to every page.
            - Words/phrases repeated as many times as necessary throughout the display.
            - Can be used by persons with CCN or via partner-assisted scanning.
   b. Visual scene displays (VSDs).
      (1) Image or picture that captures both environmental and action/interaction aspects of the context.
      (2) Used for people across levels of impairment, from children developing language to people with aphasia.
      (3) Involve hot spots where vocabulary/messages are programmed for use by the person with CCN.

(4) Some VSDs have navigational buttons around the main picture for ease of access to other pages/menus.
(5) When programmed thoughtfully, VSDs can be used for rate enhancement.
c. Alphabet displays.
(1) QWERTY or ABCD layout.
(2) Frequency of use layout.
(a) Letters that are more frequently used are laid out for easiest access.
(b) These layouts vary according to language.
(3) Vowels on the left, with consonants following.
(a) For example:
- A B C D
- E F G H
- I J K L M N
- O P Q R S T
- U V W X Y Z

Assessment in AAC

Candidacy for AAC

1. Anyone can be a candidate for AAC.
2. Do not need special skills already in place to be eligible for assessment.
3. Central to the entire assessment enterprise.
   a. Person with CCN.
   b. Significant others (e.g., family members, spouse, primary communication facilitator(s), etc.).

Importance of Team Assessment in AAC

1. Due to the multitude of skills needed for use of AAC, the input of professionals of differing backgrounds is necessary for thorough assessment.
2. Team composition will depend on the needs of the person with CCN.
3. The types of professionals involved in assessment for AAC include, but are not limited to:
   a. Speech-language pathologist (SLP).
   b. Physical therapist (PT).
   c. Occupational therapist (OT).
   d. Teacher.
   e. Special education teacher and/or resource person.
   f. Biomedical engineer.
   g. Vocational counselor.
   h. AT specialist.
4. All participants in the assessment process must share information regarding the findings of their assessments and recommendations as they relate to AAC.

Identification of Purpose for AAC

1. The purpose of AAC may be to support:
   a. Language development.
   b. Communication.
   c. Literacy acquisition.
   d. Employment.
2. Specify the priorities for what AAC will do for the person with CCN that he/she is not able to accomplish at present.

Skills/Status/Domains to Be Assessed

1. Cognition.
2. Language (receptive and expressive).
3. Speech intelligibility.
4. Sensory-perceptual status (e.g., vision and hearing).
5. Physical/health status.
6. Seating and mobility/motor abilities.
7. Literacy.

Phases of Assessment

1. Beukelman & Mirenda (2012) proposed a four-phase framework for assessment.
   a. Phase 1: referral for AAC assessment.
   b. Phase 2: initial assessment and intervention for today.
   c. Phase 3: detailed assessment for tomorrow.
   d. Phase 4: follow-up assessment.
2. This is an iterative process and is informed by the person with CCN's goals, needs, and medical diagnosis/diagnoses.

Models of Assessment

1. Participation Model (Beukelman & Mirenda, 2012).
   a. A systematic approach to assessment and intervention.

b. Based on participation requirements of routines, activities and interests of typically developing same-age peers of person with CCN.
c. Conduct a participation inventory or routines, activities and interests (e.g., home, school, work, recreation, religious, etc.).
d. Identify participation patterns of typically developing same-age peers of person with CCN (involves careful task analysis).
e. Assess how well a person with CCN is currently able to participate in desired task/routine/activity.
f. Identify participation barriers.
  (1) Opportunity barriers.
    (a) Imposed by forces external to the person with CCN.
    (b) Cannot be eliminated by provision of AAC.
    (c) Types of opportunity barriers.
      - Policy barriers: based on legislative decisions that govern various environments (e.g., restrictions on bringing AAC equipment into the ICU setting, person with CCN being placed in a nonmainstream class at school).
      - Practice barriers: procedures or conventions that have become commonplace in the environment (e.g., a school district barring a person with CCN from taking home AAC system home over the weekend and/or summer).
      - Knowledge barriers: caused by a lack of information on the part of the CCN's facilitator(s)/team members that results in decreased participation opportunities for the person with CCN (e.g., lack of familiarity with carry cases/second skins for AAC systems to protect from the elements, and so barring person with CCN from participating in outdoor activities with their AAC system).
      - Skill barriers: caused by facilitator difficulty implementing AAC technique or strategy (e.g., despite training, communication facilitator cannot adequately perform partner-assisted scanning).
      - Attitude barriers: caused by incorrect, outdated, outmoded and discriminatory attitudes regarding the abilities of people with CCN (e.g., a teacher who implicitly conveys lower expectations of a student with CCN than for other students in the class).
  (2) Access barriers.
    (a) Imposed by limitations of the individual with CCN and/or their current communication system.
    (b) Involve the capabilities, attitudes and resource limitations (perceived or otherwise) of the person with CCN vs. being externally imposed by society.
    (c) For example, a person with a neurodegenerative disease stops socializing due to changes in their ability to communicate. That person's friends want to maintain the friendship, but the person with CCN believes they can't participate in social activities given the changes in his/her functional status.

Assessment Tools

1. No standardized assessment batteries in AAC, due to the heterogeneity of populations that require AAC.
   a. No norm-referenced tests for the same reason.
2. Can administer standardized tests in nonstandardized ways (e.g., by varying response mode, altering instructions and time limitations, etc.) as long as it is reported that the test was administered and norms are not used.
3. Criterion referenced tests and inventories are commercially available.
4. Examples of inventories.
   a. *Social Networks: A Communication Inventory for Individuals with Complex Communication Needs and Their Communication Partners* (Blackstone & Hunt Berg, 2003).
      (1) Comprehensive inventory of communication-related behaviors and technology use as it relates to people with CCN and their communication partners.
      (2) Comes with a manual detailing how the inventory should be administered.
   b. *Augmentative & Alternative Communication Profile: A Continuum of Learning* (Kovach, 2009).
      (1) Based on Light's model of communicative competence.
      (2) Inventories to explore skill sets across all four competencies.
      (3) Provides mechanism for record-keeping across initial and follow-up assessments.
   c. Symbol Assessment (e.g., *Tangible Symbol Systems*, Rowland & Schweigert, 2000).
      (1) Provides a protocol for conducting a basic symbol assessment.
      (2) Symbol assessment is especially critical to AAC assessment for persons who are nonliterate.
      (3) Typically involves 10 items that are very familiar to the person with CCN.
      (4) Also involves colored photos, black and white photos, line drawings, line drawings that are color embellished and written words.

(5) Different-sized versions of all of the aforementioned types of representation are tried during a symbol assessment.
(6) Goals of symbol assessment are to determine:
   (a) Most abstract level of symbol/representation that person with CCN can reliably use.
   (b) Smallest size(s) of symbol/representation that person with CCN can reliably use.
(7) See Glennen & DeCoste (1997) or Beukelman & Mirenda (2012) references for full description of how to conduct symbol assessment.

Feature Matching

1. Process by which the skills and needs of the person with CCN are matched against the features of various AAC systems.
2. Iterative process while a system of best fit is found.
3. Can be used for both low- and high-tech AAC options, hardware and software.
   a. For example, a child with CP is seen for AAC assessment. After the team has conducted its assessment, it is determined that the child is not a direct selector, and so options that support scanning must be considered. Further, the child is not yet literate; however, that is an educational goal, so the AAC system must support both symbols and access to text/keyboard.
   b. For another example, an adult with amyotrophic lateral sclerosis (ALS) who is able to walk and use his/her hands wants a lightweight, portable AAC aid because his/her speech is severely dysarthric. After careful assessment across domains of function (e.g., cognition, sensory status, motor ability, speech and language), the team determines that this person is presently a direct selector and is literate. They proceed to identify options that meet the person's current needs (i.e., are portable, lightweight, allow direct selection and ready access to speech output and text), knowing that as the disorder runs its course, the feature match will likely change, which will necessitate changes in the AAC system.

System Selection

1. Culmination of feature-matching process, typically resulting in one or two options that will meet the person with CCN's needs.
2. When possible, arranging for a short-term loan of the recommended system(s) for the person with CCN to try in real (e.g., home, work, etc.) vs. clinic environments before a final decision is made.
3. If short-term loan or rental is not feasible, careful review of systems, components, training and supports necessary for system implementation can help guide decision-making.

Funding of AAC Systems

1. Some insurance policies cover AAC systems/SGDs as part of durable medical equipment (DME).
2. Insurance coverage is highly variable and is constantly changing.
3. Many SGDs that support connectivity (i.e., Internet) are currently not being funded.
4. Medicare is tending toward funding only dedicated AAC devices.
5. Check the website of the device vendor/manufacturer for updates on funding issues.

Intervention in AAC

Process of Intervention

1. Once assessment is complete, the team's focus shifts to the process of intervention, which may entail any or all of the following evidence-based techniques and steps.

Vocabulary Selection

1. Critical component of AAC intervention.
2. System usage often hinges on having age-, gender-, situational-appropriate and socially appropriate vocabulary.
3. Vocabulary (both expressive and receptive) information can be collected via informants who know the person with CCN across contexts (e.g., family, friends, teachers, clergy, coaches, friends, etc.).
4. Use vocabulary inventories to collect this information.
5. Typically, SLP will collate information from all sources.
6. Create vocabulary that will go on the person with CCN's system.
7. Two main types of vocabulary in AAC systems.
   a. Core: high-frequency words and phrases that are highly functional for the individual.

b. Fringe: words and phrases that are specific to a particular topic/activity/individual; often are content rich and not used that frequently.
8. Vocabulary must be updated regularly.
9. Additional types of vocabulary to consider.
   a. Developmental vocabulary: words/phrases that the person with CCN does not yet know but are included on the system to encourage vocabulary growth.
   b. Coverage vocabulary: those words/phrases that the person with CCN needs to communicate essential messages; typically relate to basic needs, and are context and age dependent.

Refinement of Symbol Selection and Placement on AAC System

1. Decisions regarding symbol placement.
   a. Location, with respect to the person with CCN's physical and visual access.
   b. Relative importance of symbol/vocabulary item.
      (1) High-frequency, high-priority items should be placed where the person with CCN can most readily access them.
      (2) Dimensions of system.
         (a) Low tech: Are there pages in a book or a lap-tray on a wheelchair?
         (b) High tech: Can the user navigate between pages/levels?

Training Person with CCN in System Use

1. Relates to operational competence.
2. Person with CCN should be trained on system usage and maintenance to the maximum of their capability.
3. Often a facilitator will perform maintenance, such as charging and cleaning a device.
4. Some operational features may not be introduced immediately, but will be introduced later.
5. Person with CCN's functional communication goals should guide prioritization of operational features to be taught.

Facilitator Training Requirements

1. Training each identified facilitator (e.g., parents, spouse, paraprofessional, siblings, etc.) in all aspects of operational competence.
2. Each new facilitator must be trained (e.g., even if system stays the same, but the paraprofessional changes, the new paraprofessional must be trained).
3. Training on how to update a system (e.g., add/delete vocabulary items as needed; download system updates from the Internet, if appropriate).
4. Demonstrating and training in AAC strategies and techniques to encourage system use.

Sample AAC Strategies and Techniques

1. Augmented input.
   a. Modeling how a system is used by providing input, in addition to speech, to the person with CCN so they receive input via AAC rather than via speech alone.
   b. Provides a powerful model of system use as a respected means of communication.
2. Expectant delay.
   a. Training facilitators to wait expectantly for a response.
   b. Count 1 to 5 slowly to themselves.
   c. Can even arch eyebrows to indicate that person is waiting for person with CCN to begin to respond.
3. Message co-construction.
   a. Training facilitators to encourage persons with CCN to supply the main content elements of their message.
   b. Communication partner confirms the content words.
   c. Communication partner then expands and elaborates these components.
   d. Resulting message is co-constructed.
4. Alphabet supplementation.
   a. For people with CCN who are literate and who have severely dysarthric speech.
   b. Use an alphabet display to point to the initial letter of each word as they say it.
   c. Combined effect of slowing speech rate and adding clarification for communication partner.
5. Topic supplementation.
   a. For people with CCN who have severely dysarthric speech and may/may not be literate.
   b. Use of communication boards that have lists (either written or pictorial) of commonly discussed topics.
   c. Person with CCN selects topic/context to cue the communication partner.
   d. Having the topic/context should theoretically facilitate:
      (1) The flow of relevant conversation.
      (2) Resolution of communication breakdown.

Anatomy of an AAC Device

Device Characteristics

1. Specifications and dimensions such as size, weight, screen size and number of keys/cells.
2. Location of the following features:
   a. Speaker(s).
   b. Message display.
   c. On/off keys.
   d. Adjusting volume.
   e. Speak key.
   f. Function keys (e.g., clear, backspace, delete).
3. Does the device support the use of a keyguard?
   a. Keyguard is a plastic or Plexiglass overlay that is made to help isolate each key/cell on the device to prevent the user from inadvertently activating keys/cells on the way to the target.
   b. Useful for people who use pointers and/or who have tremor.
4. Rate enhancement techniques supported.
   a. Word prediction.
   b. Icon prediction.
   c. Preprogrammed phrases.
5. Message display.
   a. Words, pictures or both.
   b. Speak each word/phrase.
   c. Speak on demand.
   d. Highlight each word as it speaks.
6. Message keys.
   a. Number and size of keys.
   b. Keys that can be reassigned at will.
7. Message feedback.
   a. Activation feedback: a specified signal that a key has been activated.
8. Key action.
   a. Does the device zoom/enlarge each message as selected?

Person Characteristics

1. Direct selector/alternate accessor.
2. Literate/nonliterate.
3. Ambulation.
4. Vision and hearing status.
5. Gross and fine motor skills.
6. Seating and mobility.
   a. Wheelchair (i.e., power, manual).
   b. If the person has a wheelchair, the device will need to be affixed to the chair using a mounting system (i.e., clamps, tubing and plates that allow the device to be attached to the chair so it can be used).

Commercially Available vs. Dedicated Device

1. Dedicated devices (SGDs).
   a. Sold by manufacturers.
   b. Insurance may require a physician's prescription and SLP report for purchase.
2. Commercially available.
   a. Mobile tablets.
   b. Laptop computers that can support special software.

Type of Screen

1. Static display.
2. Dynamic display.

Type of Input Supported

1. Text.
   a. Built-in or add-on keyboard.
   b. Onscreen keyboard.
2. Symbols.
3. Speech.
   a. Use of speech-to-text algorithm to convert speech to text.

Type of Speech Output

1. Synthesized speech.
   a. Computer-generated speech.
   b. May lack some prosodic contours.
   c. Text to speech (TTS).
      (1) Words or messages are retrieved from the device's memory or entered via text are converted to phonemes and allophones.
      (2) Device uses stored speech data to generate digital speech signals that correspond to phonetic representations of the text.
      (3) Device converts digital signals to analog speech waveforms that are spoken by the device.
      (4) Some devices do not store digital signals but use rule-based mathematical algorithms to generate speech sounds that correspond to phonetic representations entered by the system user.
      (5) Now available in male, female and child voices and in many different languages.

2. Digitized speech.
   a. Human speech that has been recorded, stored and reproduced.
   b. Stored as words and/or messages.
   c. Cannot be used to generate novel utterances because it is stored as words/messages.
3. Hybrid.
   a. Devices that support both synthesized and digitized speech.

Type of Message Formulation Supported

1. Single utterance/message units.
2. Sequence of words or phrases.
3. Spelling.

Type of Language Representation Supported

1. Phrase based.
2. VSDs.
3. Core words.
4. Semantic compaction (Minspeak).
   a. A branded set of icons used by a certain device company.
5. Orthography.

Type of Selection Methods Supported

1. Direct selection.
2. Alternate access: scanning (and what types of scanning).

Issues in AAC

Speech as Default System for Communication

1. Buy-in to AAC can be tough.
2. AAC may be viewed as a method of last resort by both clinicians and patients.
3. Reluctance to accept AAC.
4. May use speech long beyond the point it is viable.

AAC Impeding Speech Development

1. No research supports the claim that using AAC will impede speech development.
2. Research indicates that the use of AAC, both low and high tech, may promote increased communication (e.g., Blishchak, Lombardino, & Dyson, 2003; Millar, Light, & Schlosser, 2006).
3. Use of high-tech AAC options may provide repeated exposure to speech and language models that provide opportunity for imitation.

Financial Realities

1. Mobile tablets and apps are less expensive, nonstigmatizing and commercially available.
2. Dedicated devices (i.e., SGDs) are more expensive and not commercially available.
3. Insurance funding for SGDs is presently in flux.

Need for Ongoing Support for Persons with CCN and Their Facilitators

1. Who pays?
2. Who provides the service?
3. Who advocates for this support when the person with CCN either does not have an advocate and/or does not have consistent facilitators?

Mobile Tablets and Apps

Apps and AAC

1. Each app makes the tablet a qualitatively different device (Table 17-1).
2. Use feature matching to determine which app(s) best meet the person with CCN's needs.
3. Rubrics are available to assist with app feature matching.

Table 17-1

Pros and Cons of AAC Platforms

PLATFORM	PROS	CONS
Dedicated Devices (run Windows)	• Adaptable-support, direct selection and/or scanning • Warranty • Tech support • Built in switch ports, speakers and IR environmental controls	• Weight • Size • Cost • Fee to unlock features (e.g., access to Internet)
iDevices (run iOS)	• Weight • Size • Portability • Cosmesis • Connectivity • Many communication apps available • Cost	• Limited tech support for apps • Extra cost for speakers, protective cases and switch interface options • Apps designed for direct selection • Cost
Tablets (run Windows or Android)	• Weight • Size • Portability • Cosmesis • Connectivity • Some communication apps available • Cost	• Limited tech support for apps • Extra cost for speakers, protective cases and switch interface options • Apps designed for direct selection

Mobile Tablets (MTs) and AAC

1. Person with CCN must be able to touch, swipe and tap to use MT via direct selection.
2. More apps coming online for use via alternate access, but MTs are not designed for use via alternate access.
3. Funding for MTs and AAC apps is on a case-by-case basis.

Entertainment vs. Communication

1. Use of MT as AAC device may be sidelined by MT as an entertainment device.
2. Opinion differs with respect to needing separate MTs for communication and for entertainment.

References

American Speech-Language-Hearing Association. (2005). *Roles and Responsibilities of Speech-Language Pathologists with Respect to Augmentative and Alternative Communication: Position Statement.* Rockville, MD: ASHA. Available from www.asha.org/policy.

Beukelman, D. R., Garrett, K. L., & Yorkston, K. M. (2007). *Augmentative Communication Strategies for Adults with Acute or Chronic Medical Conditions.* Baltimore, MD: Paul H. Brookes Publishing Company.

Beukelman, D. R., & Mirenda, P. (2012). *Augmentative and Alternative Communication: Supporting Children and Adults with Complex Communication Needs,* 4th ed. Baltimore, MD: Paul H. Brookes Publishing Company.

Binger, C., & Kent-Walsh, J. (2010). *What Every Speech-Language Pathologist/Audiologist Should Know About Augmentative and Alternative Communication.* Boston, MA: Pearson Education, Inc.

Blackstone, S. W., & Hunt Berg, M. (2003). *Social Networks: A Communication Inventory for Individuals with Complex Communication Needs and Their Communication Partners.* Monterrey, CA: Augmentative Communication, Inc.

Blischak, D. M., Lombardino, L. J., & Dyson, A. T. (2003). Use of speech-generating devices: in support of natural speech. *Augmentative and Alternative Communication,* 19, 29–35.

Glennen, S. L., & DeCoste, D. C. (1997). *Handbook of Augmentative and Alternative Communication.* San Diego, CA: Singular Publishing Group, Inc.

Kovach, T. (2009). *Augmentative & Alternative Communication Profile: A Continuum of Learning.* East Moline, IL: LinguiSystems.

Lange, M. (2012). "Switch Mounting." Ablenet University. Recorded webinar. Available from http://www.ablenet.com.

Light, J. (1988). Interaction involving individuals using augmentative and alternative communication systems: State of the art and future directions for research. *Augmentative and Alternative Communication,* 4, 66–82.

Light, J. (1989). Toward a definition of communicative competence for individuals using augmentative and alternative communication system. *Augmentative and Alternative Communication*, 5 (2), 137–144.

Light, J., & McNaughton, D. (2014). Communicative competence for individuals who require augmentative and alternative communication: A new definition for a new era of communication? *Augmentative and Alternative Communication*, 30 (1), 1–18.

Millar, D. C., Light, J. C., & Schlosser, R. W. (2006). The impact of augmentative and alternative communication intervention on the speech production of individuals with developmental disabilities: A research review. *Journal of Speech, Language, and Hearing Research*, 49, 248–264.

Porter, G. (2007). Pragmatic Organisation Dynamic Display Communication Books. Victoria, Australia: Cerebral Palsy Education Centre.

Rowland, C., & Schweigert, P. (2000). *Tangible Symbol Systems Manual and DVD*. Portland, OR: Design to Learn. Available at http://www.designtolearn.com.

Soto, G., & Zangari, C. (2009). *Practically Speaking: Language, Literacy, & Academic Development for Students with AAC Needs*. Baltimore, MD: Paul H. Brookes Publishing Company.

The Joint Commission (2010). *Advancing Effective Communication, Cultural Competence, and Patient- and Family-Centered Care: A Roadmap for Hospitals*. Oakbrook Terrace, IL: Author. Retrieved Oct. 15, 2014 from http://www.jointcommission.org/Advancing_Effective_Communication_Cultural_Competence_and_Patient_and_Family_Centered_Care/.

18 Audiology and Hearing Impairment

CRAIG W. NEWMAN, PhD
SHARON A. SANDRIDGE, PhD
AND DONALD M. GOLDBERG, PhD

Chapter Outline

- Anatomy and Physiology of the Auditory System, 410
- Audiologic Evaluation, 415
- Hearing Disorders, 423
- Hearing Sensory Technology, 427
- Auditory Rehabilitation (Aural [Re]habilitation; Audiologic [Re]habilitation), 431
- References, 434
- Suggested Resources, 435

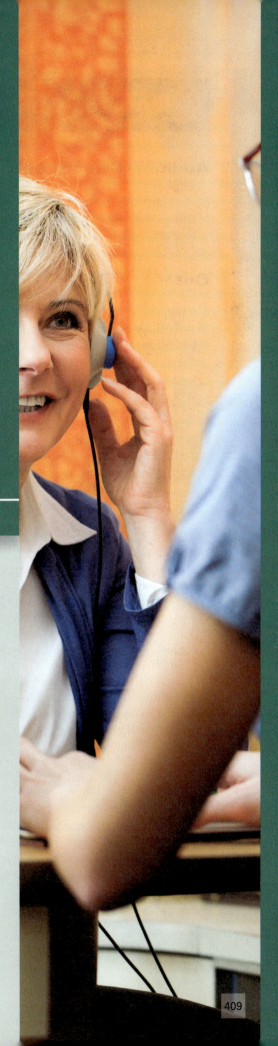

Anatomy and Physiology of the Auditory System

Auditory Structures

1. Anatomy of the auditory system consists of the structures of the outer ear, middle ear and inner ear (Figure 18-1).

Outer Ear (OE)

1. Pinna (auricle).
   a. Cartilage-framed appendage covered with skin.
   b. Appears around sixth week of gestation from the first and second branchial arches.
   c. Major structures of pinna (Figure 18-2).
      (1) Helix—folded outside edge of ear.
      (2) Antihelix—"y" shape upper part of ear.
      (3) Concha—bowl-shaped structure leading into the external auditory canal.
      (4) Tragus—triangular structure extension from face.
      (5) Antitragus—triangular structure arising from lower part of the lobe.
      (6) Lobe (lobule)—fatty and fibrous structure; can be attached or free.
   d. Attaches to cranium by skin, cartilage, three extrinsic muscles and extrinsic ligaments.
   e. Sensory innervation via trigeminal nerve (CN V).
2. External auditory meatus (EAM).
   a. S-shaped oval canal 25–35 mm in length opening at the pinna and terminating at the tympanic membrane.
   b. Outer (lateral) one-third of canal is cartilaginous and lined with skins, glands that produce cerumen and hair follicles (cilia) that move cerumen outward; medial two-thirds is osseous (bony).
   c. Innervated by trigeminal, facial and vagus nerves (CN V, VII and X).
3. Tympanic membrane (TM).
   a. Thin oval membrane that forms partition between the OE and the middle ear (ME).
   b. Layers.
      (1) Lateral epidermal layer continuous with the skin of the external auditory canal.
      (2) Intermediate fibrous layer consisting of radial and concentric fibers; provides structure to TM.
      (3) Medial mucosal layer continuous with the mucosa of the ME.
   c. The TM is a cone-shaped membrane with an area of 55 mm.
   d. The TM transduces sound—an acoustic vibration transformed into mechanical energy.

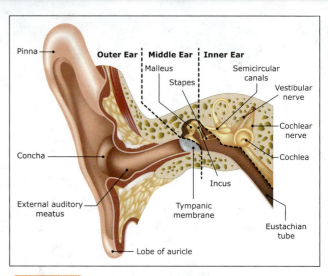

Figure 18-1 Cross-section of the peripheral auditory system illustrating the major anatomic structures within the outer, middle and inner ear.

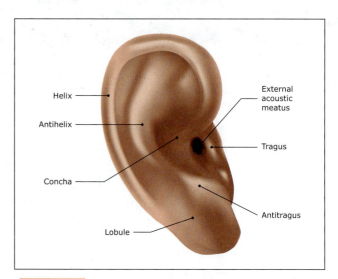

Figure 18-2 Illustration of the major structures of the pinna

4. Function.
   a. Auditory function—the OE collects sounds and channels it to the ME.
      (1) The pinna collects sound originating from in front of listener; reflects sounds (due to concave shape of pinna) coming from the back; this assists in front/back localization (especially for high-frequency sounds with short wavelengths).

(2) Serves as a natural filter enhancing or boosting higher frequency sounds approximately 10–12 dB.
(3) Natural resonance of the concha is approximately 5000 Hz.
(4) The EAM enhances sounds that have frequencies four times length of canal (1/4 wavelength theory); approximately 2500–2700 Hz (in adults).
b. Nonauditory function is protection.
(1) Cerumen is noxious to "intruders" such as insects and provides lubrication to the EAM.
(2) The S-shape prevents foreign objects, such as cotton swabs, from reaching TM and ME.

Middle Ear (ME)

1. Six-walled air-filled cavity within the petrous portion of the temporal bone.
   a. Roof (superior wall) is formed by thin plate of bone—tegmen tympani that separates ME from dura mater.
   b. Floor (inferior wall) separates ME from the internal jugular vein.
   c. Lateral wall is formed by the TM.
   d. Medial wall consists of the oval window, round window and the promontory (formed by first turn of cochlea).
   e. Posterior wall is the mastoid wall.
   f. Anterior wall is a small wall opening into the Eustachian tube.
2. Houses three ossicles (bones), five ligaments and two muscles (tendons).
   a. Ossicular chain—consists of three bones, which are the smallest in the human body, transferring the mechanical vibration from the tympanic membrane to the inner ear (IE).
      (1) Malleus—the most lateral (first) ossicle, consisting of a manubrium (handle), head, neck and lateral and anterior processes; attached to the TM (at the umbo) and the incus.
      (2) Incus—the middle and largest bone in the ossicular chain consisting of a body and a short, a long and a lenticular process.
      (3) Stapes—the most medial (third) and smallest ossicle consisting of a head, footplate and two crura. The footplate is held in the oval window by the annular ligament.
   b. Ligaments—five ligaments that suspend the ossicular chain in the ME.
      (1) Superior malleolar—attaches at head of malleus and the tegmen tympani.
      (2) Lateral malleolar—attaches to neck of malleus and bony wall.
      (3) Anterior malleolar—extends from anterior process of malleus to anterior wall.
      (4) Posterior incudal—attaches to short process of incus and posterior wall.
      (5) Annular ligament—attaches the stapes footplate to the oval window.
   c. Muscles—two muscles that serve to hold the ossicular chain in place and to reduce intensity reaching IE by pulling against each other to stiffen the system and reduce the efficiency of the ME. The ME muscles are muscles unique in their ability to exert the amount of force for their size.
      (1) Tensor tympani—a 2-cm-long muscle attaching to the head of the malleus; innervated by trigeminal nerve; pulls malleus medially.
      (2) Stapedius muscle—the smallest muscle in the body; attached to the neck of the stapes; innervated by the facial nerve; pulls stapes posteriorly and tilts footplate in oval window.
3. Eustachian tube—mucosal-lined pathway that ventilates the ME through the connection to the nasopharynx.
4. Function.
   a. The ME compensates for the impedance mismatch (loss of sound energy) between the acoustic signals from the OE and the cochlear fluids of the IE using two primary mechanisms; approximately 25–27 dB of the estimated 30-dB impedance mismatch is compensated by two primary effects.
      (1) Lever ratio.
         (a) The arm of the incus is shorter than the malleus, creating a lever effect that increases the force and decreases the velocity at the stapes; only accounts for gains of a few decibels.
         (b) Overall, approximately 25–27 dB of the estimated 30-dB impedance mismatch is compensated for by the areal ratio and lever ratio mechanism.
   b. ME muscles serve to increase the sensitivity of the auditory system for speech, especially in background noise, through stiffening of the ossicular chain (reducing low-frequency noise transmission) as well as serving as a protective process against intense sounds by attenuating or decreasing the intensity by 15 to 20 dB (frequency dependent).

Inner Ear (IE)

1. Complex structure residing within the petrous portion of the temporal bone; seen anatomically as one unit, however has two distinct functions—sense of hearing (cochlea) and sense of balance (semicircular canals and otolithic organs).
2. Osseous (bony) labyrinth is complex series of excavations in the bone containing a series of communicating membranous sacs and ducts (membranous labyrinth).
   a. Semicircular canals are responsible for angular movement; consists of three canals: lateral, posterior and superior.

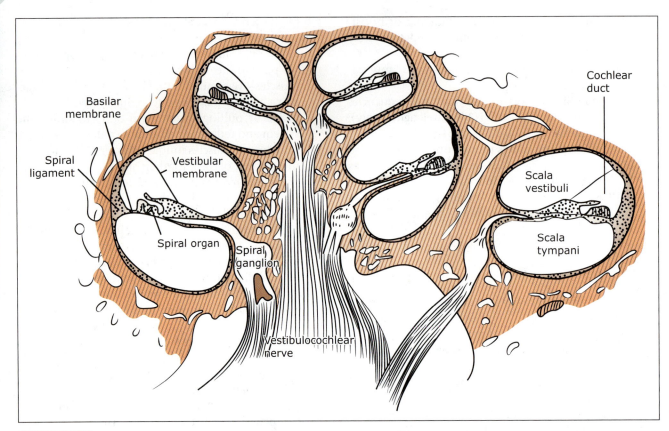

Figure 18-3 Cross-section of the cochlea illustrating the major anatomic structures within the scalae.

b. Vestibule is a 4-mm central chamber of the bony labyrinth housing the utricle and saccule, which are sensory organs responsible for detecting linear movement.
c. Cochlea—a snail-shaped structure containing the end-organ of hearing.

3. Cochlear structures (Figure 18-3).
   a. A bony canal surrounds a membranous tube, about 35 mm in length, and coils around a central core (modiolus) approximately 2¾ turns (in humans).
   b. The base of the cochlea, the largest turn, sits next to the vestibule; the apex, the smallest turn at the top of the cochlea, points anteriorly (toward the eye).
   c. The membranous labyrinth is divided into three canals.
      (1) Scala vestibuli—upper canal running from the oval window to the helicotrema (tip of cochlea); contains perilymph, a fluid similar to cerebrospinal fluid.
      (2) Scala tympani—lower canal running from the round window to the helicotrema (tip of cochlea); contains perilymph.
      (3) Scala media—middle canal divided from the scala vestibuli by Reissner's membrane and from the scala tympani by the basilar membrane; contains the organ of Corti, the end organ of hearing; contains endolymph.
   d. Organ of Corti consists of sensory hair cells, support cells, support membranes and ligaments (Figure 18-4).
      (1) Sensory hair cells—outer hair cells (OHC).
         (a) Approximately 13,500 per ear housed in three to four rows.
         (b) Test-tube-shaped; supported at base and apex only.
         (c) Three to five rows of stereocilia; W-shaped; graduated in length with the longest stereocilia in outside row.
         (d) Afferent and efferent nerve fibers synapse directing to the base of the hair cell; one afferent fiber synapses with as many as 10 OHC, providing convergent information.
         (e) Serve as a biologic modifier increasing or decreasing sensitivity to sounds by changing length of hair cells (as they lengthen, the tectorial membrane is moved further from the stereocilia of the inner hair cells, decreasing the sensitivity of the organ of Corti).

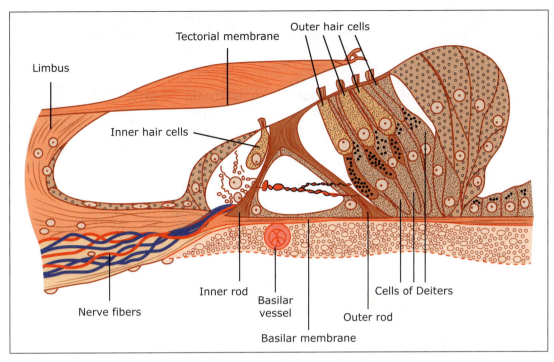

Figure 18-4 Cross-section of the organ of Corti within the cochlea.

(2) Sensory hair cells—inner hair cells (IHC).
  (a) Approximately 3500 per ear housed in one row.
  (b) Flask-shaped; completely surrounded by support cells.
  (c) Two to three rows of stereocilia; crescent-shaped; graduated in length, with the longest stereocilia in outside row.
  (d) Afferent nerve fibers synapse directing to hair cell; as many as 10 IHCs synapse to one afferent fiber, providing divergent information; efferent nerve fibers synapse on the afferent fibers.
  (e) Serve to process frequency, temporal (time) and intensity information to the auditory pathway.
(3) Support cells—serve as the core of the organ of Corti.
(4) Membranes.
  (a) Reissner's membrane—forms the roof of the scala media; may rupture with an active episode of Ménière's disease.
  (b) Basilar membrane—forms the floor of the scala media; the membrane becomes wider as it moves apically; as the width changes so does the mass and stiffness, yielding tonotopicity in which high frequencies are processed at the base (thinner and stiffer) and low frequencies at the apex (wider and more massive).
  (c) Tectorial membrane—a semitransparent, gelatinous structure that attaches medially to the spiral limbus and laterally to the top of the stereocilia of the OHCs; responsible for shearing the stereocilia of the hair cells.
4. Function.
  a. Changes the mechanical energy into hydromechanical energy and then into neural impulses.
    (1) Stapes acts like a piston, moving the fluid in the scala vestibule to create a wave—the traveling wave.
    (2) The fluid moves inward, pushing down on Reissner's membrane, which in turn creates a wave in the scala media.
    (3) The movement of the fluid causes the tectorial membrane and the basilar membrane to move, resulting in a shearing effect of the stereocilia.
    (4) The stereocilia movement causes calcium channels to open, exciting the hair cells; energy now becomes electrochemical.
    (5) The hair cells release neurotransmitter that binds with the nerve fibers, creating neural impulses.
    (6) The neural impulses travel via CN VIII (vestibulocochlear) through the internal auditory canal to the brain stem and synapse at the cochlear nucleus (the first nuclei in the central auditory nervous system).

b. Coding frequency.
  (1) Place theory—frequencies are encoded based on place along basilar membrane; responsible for frequency coding above 5000 Hz.
  (2) Temporal theory—auditory nerve is phase-locked to stimulus pattern and the brain encodes the timing pattern of the nerve firing.
  (3) Missing fundamental frequency—if the fundamental frequency is absent in a complex sound (e.g., 1000 Hz, 1200 Hz and 1400 Hz), the fundamental frequency (i.e., 200 Hz) will be heard even though it is not present in the sound.
c. Coding intensity.
  (1) As intensity increases, each nerve fiber fires more often; however, this is limited.
  (2) As intensity increases, a wider area of the basilar membrane is stimulated, resulting in greater number of nerve fibers activated.

Vestibulocochlear Nerve (CN VIII)

1. CN VIII is comprised of fibers from both the vestibular organs and the cochlea.
   a. Inferior vestibular nerve.
   b. Superior vestibular nerve.
   c. Cochlear nerve.
     (1) Consists of both Type I and II afferent fibers.

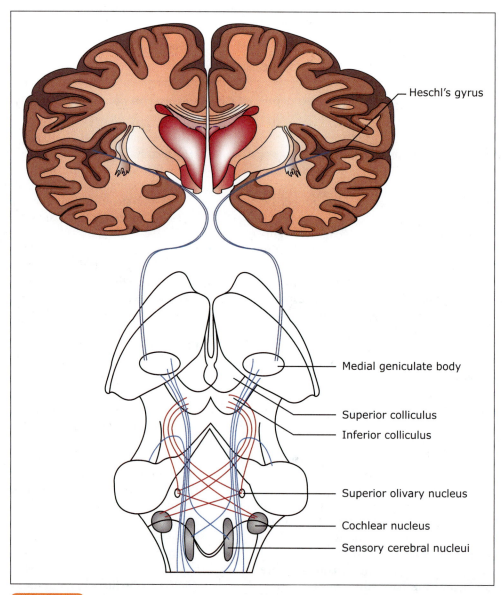

Figure 18-5 Schematic of the ascending central auditory nervous system pathways.

(2) Majority (95%) of Type I afferent fibers arise from the IHC; only 5% from OHC.
(3) Divergent pattern of nerve innervation for the IHC (1 hair cell to many nerve fibers); convergent pattern for OHC (many hair cells to 1 nerve fiber).
(4) Afferent fibers carry frequency, temporal and intensity information from the cochlea through the internal auditory canal to the ipsilateral cochlear nucleus (CN).

Brain Stem Pathways and Cortex (Figure 18-5)

1. All cochlear nerve fibers synapse at the ipsilateral anterior ventral cochlear nucleus (AVCN). Each nerve fiber bifurcates and either synapses at the posterior ventral cochlear nucleus (PVNC) or the dorsal cochlear nucleus (DCN).
2. From the CN, fiber tracts proceed to ipsilateral and contralateral superior olivary complex (SOC). The SOC is primarily responsible for localization and the acoustic reflex.
3. From the SOC, neural impulses travel up the lateral lemniscus, primarily a sensory fiber tract, to the inferior colliculus (IC).
4. From the IC, impulses travel via the brachium of the IC to the medial geniculate body (MGB), one of the nuclei of the thalamus.
5. From the MGB, the acoustic message is relayed to various areas for auditory processing. The primary area, AI, is located in the superior temporal gyrus or in Heschl's gyrus. Surrounding association areas are located in the temporal and insular lobes.

Audiologic Evaluation

Otoscopy

1. Otoscopy—a systematic visual inspection of the OE and surrounding tissue, EAM and TM.
2. Inspection components.
   a. External ear structures for anomalies such as skin tags or pits (sinuses), tenderness, redness or edema (swelling).
   b. EAM for obvious inflammation, growths, foreign objects, excessive cerumen, drainage.
   c. TM for presence of normal landmarks (e.g., cone of light, pearly-grey translucent color) or for any inflammation, perforation or any other obvious abnormalities in structure.
3. Pass criteria for visual inspection.
   a. Normal appearance of all structures.
   b. No complaints of pain when pinna or surrounding tissue is manipulated.
4. Referral for medical assessment.
   a. Reports of tenderness.
   b. Excessive or impacted cerumen.
   c. Sign of drainage or odor.
   d. Abnormal TM color (e.g., red/bulging).
   e. Growth/abnormality on canal wall.
   f. Foreign body.

Behavioral Assessment of Hearing

1. Psychoacoustic and measurement principles.
   a. Intensity—magnitude (amplitude) of a sound related to the perception of loudness.
      (1) Decibel (dB)—unit of measurement of intensity used in acoustics and audiometric testing; one-tenth of a Bel. dB is a relative unit; it is logarithmic, nonlinear and expressed in terms of various reference levels.
      (2) Sound pressure level (dB SPL)—intensity level based on an absolute *pressure* measurement; reference is 20 microPascals (20 µPa).
      (3) Hearing level (dB HL)—reference of normal human hearing thresholds for each audiometric frequency tested. Audiogram uses dB HL to plot thresholds (see definition below); audiometric zero (dB HL) is represented as a straight line on the audiogram but based on minimal audible curve in dB SPL.
      (4) Sensation level (SL)—any measurement that is made above an individual's threshold.
      (5) The y-axis (ordinate) on the audiogram is expressed in dB HL.

b. Frequency—cycles per second of the signal measured in hertz (Hz) related to the perception of pitch. For example, a 2000 Hz tone completes 2000 cycles in 1 second.
   (1) Period—amount of time it takes for one sine wave to complete one cycle; the reciprocal of frequency (period = 1/frequency).
   (2) Pure tone—a sound consisting of a single frequency.
   (3) Periodic sounds—variations of sound that are repetitive over time and that can be both simple (pure tone) and complex (voice).
   (4) Aperiodic sounds—complex sounds that are not repetitive over time.
   (5) The *x*-axis (abscissa) on the audiogram is expressed in Hz.
c. Sensitivity—capacity of sense organ to detect a stimulus.
   (1) Absolute sensitivity—ability to detect a faint sound.
   (2) Differential sensitivity (acuity)—ability to detect differences or changes; ability to detect differences between two frequencies or two different intensities.
   (3) Threshold—level at which a stimulus is perceived; clinical threshold defined as the lowest intensity to respond to the stimulus 50% of the time (e.g., two out of four trials using a bracketing approach).
   (4) Frequency range for hearing is 20 to 20,000 Hz at birth; intensity range is 0–140 dB.
2. Audiometer.
   a. Electronic instrument used to quantify hearing by producing sounds at calibrated intensities; sounds include pure tones, speech and noise.
   b. Sounds can be delivered by different transducers (device that changes energy from one form to another); options include headphones, insert phones, bone oscillator, sound field speakers.
   c. The attenuator controls the intensity of the signal, usually in 5 dB steps; however, some audiometers permit dB step sizes smaller than 5 dB (e.g., 2 dB steps).
   d. The duration of the signal is controlled by the interrupter switch.
      (1) The interrupter switch is turned *off* for the delivery of pure tone signal.
      (2) The interrupter switch is turned *on* when speech signals are presented.
   e. Can produce various sounds.
      (1) Pure tone signals are produced by the oscillator; octave and interactive frequencies are 125, 250, 500, 750, 1000, 1500, 2000, 3000, 4000, 6000 and 8000 Hz. Some audiometers can produce frequencies above 10,000 Hz.
      (2) Broadband signals (also known as white noise) are complex, aperiodic signals that contains all frequencies in the audible spectrum.
      (3) Narrowband noise is a white noise with frequencies above and below a center frequency filtered out.
      (4) Speech noise is a broadband noise containing frequencies between 300 and 3000 Hz and is used for masking during speech audiometry.
3. Pure tone audiometry.
   a. Pure tone audiometry serves several purposes.
      (1) Determines severity of hearing loss.
      (2) Provides information to help diagnose type of hearing loss (i.e., conductive, sensorineural or mixed).
      (3) Describes the configuration of hearing loss (i.e., pattern of pure tone thresholds from low to high frequencies).
      (4) Determines the intensity level at which other audiologic procedures will be performed.
      (5) Determines the need for further rehabilitative treatment, either hearing aid (HA) or cochlear implant (CI) candidacy.
   b. Air-conduction audiometry—stimulates the entire peripheral auditory system including both the *conductive* (OE and ME) and *sensorineural* portions (cochlea and CN VIII).
   c. Bone-conduction audiometry—bypasses the conductive mechanism; bone vibrator placed on mastoid to directly stimulate the IE.
   d. Audiogram—graph with frequency (measured in Hz) plotted on the *x*-axis and intensity (measured in dB HL) on the *y*-axis; denotes the assessed threshold as a function of frequency.
      (1) An audiogram is generated for each ear independently.
      (2) A standardized set of symbols is used to document air- and bone-conduction threshold results on the audiogram (Figure 18-6).
4. Audiogram interpretation.
   a. Degree of hearing loss—magnitude or severity of hearing loss.
      (1) Pure tone average (PTA)—average threshold value based on thresholds obtained at 500, 1000 and 2000 Hz.
      (2) Fletcher average—best *two* thresholds at 500, 1000 and 2000 Hz, which is often a better predictor of hearing for speech than the three-frequency PTA.
      (3) Classifications schemes have been developed to provide a metric of hearing loss ranging from normal hearing sensitivity to profound hearing loss (Table 18-1).

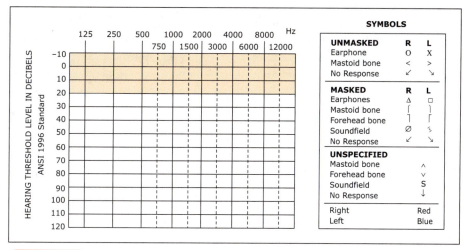

Figure 18-6 Example of an audiogram and associated audiometric symbols. Hz, Hertz.

Table 18-1

Hearing Loss Categories Based on Pure Tone Average (PTA; 500, 1000, 2000 Hz) and Associated Communication Impact

RANGE OF LOSS (IN dB HL)	DEGREE OF LOSS CATEGORY	POTENTIAL COMMUNICATION IMPACT
−10 to 15	Normal	No significant problem
16 to 25	Slight/minimal	Difficulty understanding faint speech especially in noise
26 to 40	Mild	Difficulty understanding faint or distant speech, even in quiet
41 to 55	Moderate	Hears conversational speech at a close range (approximately 3–5 feet)
56 to 70	Moderately severe	Hears loud conversational speech; significant difficulty in groups
71 to 90	Severe	Unable to hear conversational speech; able to distinguish vowels but not consonants
90+	Profound	May hear loud sounds; hearing is not primary communication mode

b. Types of hearing loss—determined by comparing air-conduction thresholds to bone-conduction thresholds for each ear independently (Figure 18-7)
  (1) Conductive hearing loss (CHL)—characterized by bone-conduction thresholds within normal range (0–20 dB HL) with air-conduction thresholds falling outside the normal limits for hearing; CHL results from problems associated with the OE and/or ME.
  (2) Sensorineural hearing loss (SNHL)—characterized by air-conduction and bone-conduction thresholds essentially equal (i.e., within 10 dB) and all thresholds outside normal range; SNHL results from disorders of the cochlea and/or CN VIII.
  (3) Mixed hearing loss—characterized by bone-conduction thresholds outside the normal hearing range with the air-conduction thresholds poorer than bone-conduction thresholds; combination of both CHL and SNHL. Difference between the air- and bone-conduction thresholds is known as the air-bone gap (ABG), reflecting the degree of conductive component contributing to the overall hearing loss.
c. Audiometric configurations.
  (1) Patterns that describe the relationship of low-frequency hearing to high-frequency hearing.
  (2) Example of mild gradually sloping to moderate SNHL means that hearing loss in the low frequencies is in the mild range with thresholds become gradually poorer (moderate range) in the higher frequencies.
d. Audiometric patterns that may reflect specific ear conditions (Figure 18-8).
  (1) A sensorineural notch at 3000 or 4000 Hz is consistent with noise exposure.
  (2) Rising conductive loss: reflects stiffness tilt associated with ME effusion (fluid in the ME space).
  (3) Sloping conductive loss: reflects mass tilt associated with a variety of conditions such as ossicular discontinuity, ME tumor and thickened TM.

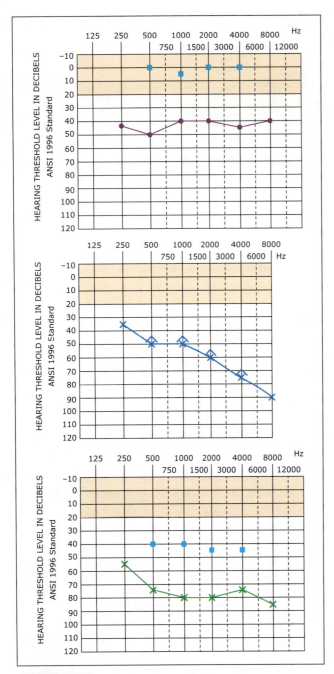

Figure 18-7 Audiometric results for (top) right conductive hearing loss; (middle) left sensorineural hearing loss; and (bottom) left mixed hearing loss.

(2) Quantifies suprathreshold speech recognition ability, which assists in determining site of lesion.
(3) Provides an estimate of communication function so that appropriate rehabilitative treatments options can be determined and outcomes monitored.
b. Speech recognition threshold (SRT).
 (1) The lowest hearing level at which one can correctly recognize speech stimuli, generally spondees, for each ear independently; reported in dB HL.
 (2) Spondee words—bisyllabic word with equal stress on each syllable (e.g., baseball, hotdog, airplane, northwest); most commonly used speech stimuli to assess the SRT.
 (3) SRT-PTA agreement—validates pure tone testing; SRT and PTA should each be within 6 dB; greater differences suggest erroneous hearing loss or equipment compromise.
c. Speech detection (awareness) threshold (SDT or SAT).
 (1) Lowest intensity level that speech can be detected; often established with young children; generally corresponds to the threshold of the best pure tone test frequency; reported in dB HL.
d. Speech/word recognition testing.
 (1) Estimate of one's ability to understand everyday speech.
 (2) Speech material presented at a suprathreshold level (see below).
 (3) Variety of speech materials.
  (a) Phonetically balanced (PB) words—monosyllable words that contain all the phonetic elements of connected discourse representative of everyday English speech; most commonly used:
   • Central Institute for the Deaf (CID) Auditory Test W-22.
   • Northwestern University Test No 6 (NU-6) word lists.
  (b) Other options include nonsense syllables, monosyllabic words, sentential approximations (nonsense sentences that are syntactically correct but meaningless) and sentences.
 (4) Response options.
  (a) Open response speech tests—test response is open and limited only by the patient's vocabulary.
  (b) Closed response speech tests—responses provided in a multiple-choice format.
 (5) Speech materials may be presented in a quiet or in a noise background (e.g., broadband noise, multitalker speech babble noise).

(4) Bone-conduction threshold at 2000 Hz is poorer than the other bone-conduction thresholds and appears like a SNHL at 2000 Hz; known as the Carhart notch, consistent with otosclerosis.
5. Speech audiometry.
 a. Speech audiometry serves several purposes.
  (1) Cross-checks validity of pure tone threshold results.

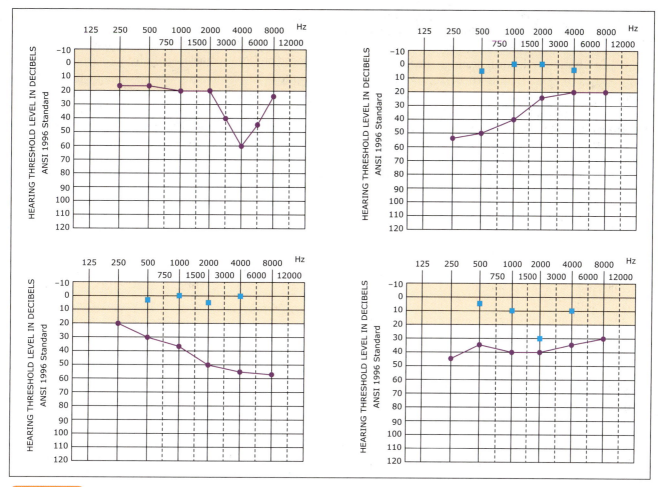

Figure 18-8 Examples of audiometric configurations: (top left) notch (sensorineural noise notch); (top right) stiffness tilt (rising conductive hearing loss); (bottom left) mass tilt (sloping conductive hearing loss); (bottom right) Carhart notch (otosclerosis).

(6) Presentation level of speech material—30 to 40 dB SL (i.e., above the SRT) or at the patient's most comfortable loudness (MCL) level.
(7) Presentation type—monitored live voice (MLV) or recorded; preferred method is recorded for comparison purposes.
(8) PB Max is the maximum word recognition score; may require completing a performance intensity (PI) function (assessing speech recognition at increasing intensities).
(9) Scoring—expressed as the percentage of words correct; Table 18-2 displays percent correct scores used in a classification scheme to estimate speech understanding ability. Presentation levels of word lists *must* be specified for correct score interpretation.

6. Clinical masking.
   a. Masking used to eliminate the participation of the nontest ear when evaluating the test ear to obtain valid thresholds.
      (1) Conducted by presenting a noise through an earphone to the nontest ear.
      (2) Narrowband noise is used as the masking signal for pure tone testing.
      (3) Speech noise is used as the masking signal for speech audiometry.
   b. Interaural attenuation (IA)—the amount of sound intensity needed before crossover (actual transmission of sound arriving at the nontest cochlea) occurs.

Table 18-2

Word Recognition Scores (in Percent Correct) for Monosyllabic Phonetically Balanced Words and Associated General Classification for Adults

SCORE	CATEGORY*
100 to 90	Excellent
88 to 80	Good
78 to 70	Fair
<68	Poor

*Maximum word recognition scores vary as a function of type and severity of hearing loss.

(1) For air-conduction testing, the minimum IA is approximately 40–50 dB for supraaural earphones and 60–70 dB for insert phones.
(2) For bone-conduction testing, the IA is 0 dB, suggesting that both cochleae are stimulated equally and simultaneously regardless of bone oscillator placement.
c. Undermasking—an insufficient amount of masking to produce the needed threshold shift.
d. Overmasking—occurs when the masking noise is so intense in the masked, nontest ear that the masking signal crosses over to the test cochlea, producing a false shift in threshold.
e. Shadow curve—observed when either no masking or an insufficient amount of masking is used and thresholds for the test ear "mimic" the responses from the cochlea of the nontest ear.
f. Masking dilemma—occurs when both ears have large ABGs and masking signal can only be presented at a level that results in overmasking.
g. Serious errors in diagnosing the type and severity of hearing loss can occur when masking is not used appropriately.
(1) A SNHL may be diagnosed as CHL.
(2) A profound hearing loss may be diagnosed as a moderate hearing loss.
7. Pediatric testing strategies—A variety of behavioral audiometric techniques have been adapted for testing children based on developmental age (see Table 18-3).
a. Behavioral observation audiometry (BOA).
(1) Conducted by presenting a stimulus via loudspeakers in a sound field and observing the infant's response.
(2) Response can be an eye blink (auro-palpebral reflex), a startle response in an awake infant or arousal response in a sleeping infant.
(3) Should be considered a screening, as it does not provide thresholds or ear-specific information.
b. Visual reinforcement audiometry (VRA).
(1) Child conditioned to look at a visual reinforcer when stimuli (speech, warbled tones or narrowband noise) are presented through loudspeakers or earphones.
(2) Information obtained represents minimal response levels versus true thresholds.
c. Conditioned play audiometry (CPA).
(1) Child is conditioned to perform a task (e.g., drop a block into a bucket) in response when stimuli (e.g., pure tones, narrowband noise, speech) are presented through loudspeakers or earphones.
(2) Responses may be minimal response levels or true thresholds.
8. Implication of audiometric test findings on auditory perception.
a. Relationship among speech sounds and the audiogram shown in Figure 18-9.

Table 18-3

Behavioral Audiometric Techniques Used with Children (Based on Developmental Age)

TECHNIQUE	APPROXIMATE AGE
Behavioral observation audiometry	< 7 months
Visual reinforcement audiometry	7 months to 2.5 years
Conditioned play audiometry	> 2.5 years

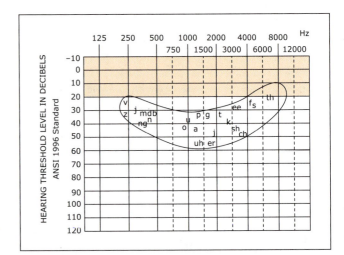

Figure 18-9 "Speech banana" illustrating the region which approximately represents phonemes as they fall on an audiogram.

b. Impact of hearing loss on communication depends on degree of sensitivity loss, audiometric configuration, type of hearing loss and degree and nature of speech perception deficits.
c. CHL (OE and/or ME).
(1) Attenuation of sound (reduction of volume of incoming signal).
(2) No difficulty understanding speech when loud enough.
(3) Occlusion effect—patient may speak softly because his or her own voice sounds loud.
(4) Paracusis willisii—ability to hear better in noisy environments.
(5) Some children with chronic fluctuating hearing loss during formative years may be at risk for delayed speech and language development, later academic and learning problems.
d. Sensory hearing loss (cochlear).
(1) Recruitment—rapid growth of loudness perception once threshold is crossed.
(2) Reduction in frequency resolution, which impacts speech understanding.
(3) Reduced dynamic range.
(4) Word recognition ability is reduced based on severity of hearing loss.

e. Neural hearing loss (CN VIII).
   (1) Word recognition ability is poorer than expected based on hearing loss severity.
   (2) Recognition in speech understanding declines with increases in intensity (rollover phenomenon).
   (3) Auditory adaptation occurs.
f. Brain stem disorder.
   (1) May have no effect on audiogram.
   (2) Difficulty hearing speech in noisy or complex listening situations.
g. Functional hearing loss (nonorganic, pseudohypacusis; malingering; psychogenic/hysterical hearing loss; erroneous)—intra- and intertest discrepancies that cannot be accounted for by known organic causes.
   (1) Poor SRT-PTA agreement (should not exceed 6 dB).
   (2) Patient repeats only half of the spondee (e.g., "hot" for "hotdog").
   (3) Absence of shadow curve (greater than 60 dB difference between right and left ears for unmasked air-conduction thresholds).
   (4) Bone-conduction thresholds poorer than air-conduction thresholds.

Physiologic Assessment of Auditory Function

1. Immittance measurement.
   a. Purposes of immittance testing.
      (1) Assesses ME function.
      (2) Differentiates cochlear from retrocochlear disorders (i.e., CN VIII and brain stem).
   b. Immittance is a generic measurement term for two reciprocal concepts.
      (1) Acoustic impedance—opposition to the transfer of acoustic energy.
      (2) Acoustic admittance—ease of sound flow through an acoustic system.
   c. Tympanometry.
      (1) Dynamic measure of energy flow through the TM and displayed on a tympanogram.
      (2) Tympanogram—graph plotting variation in air pressure and TM compliance.
         (a) y-axis plots acoustic immittance or TM compliance (how much sound passes through the TM or is bounced back into the EAM).
         (b) x-axis plots the change in pressure in deca-Pascals (daPa).
         (c) Largest peak on the tympanogram occurs when the pressure in the EAM is equal to the pressure in the ME.

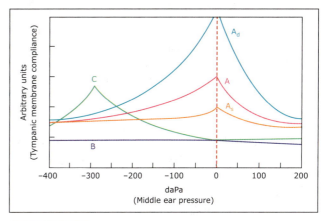

Figure 18-10 Schematic of five tympanogram types. Type A illustrates normal peak middle ear pressure (MEP) and tympanic membrane (TM) compliance (mobility); Type A_S illustrates normal peak MEP and reduced (shallow) TM compliance; Type A_D illustrates normal peak MEP and excessive (deep) TM compliance; Type B illustrates no peak pressure and flat shape; and Type C illustrates negative peak MEP and normal TM compliance.

Table 18-4

Tympanogram Type and Associated Disorders

TYPE (TYMPANOMETRIC SHAPE)	EXAMPLE DISORDER
A (normal pressure/normal compliance)	Normal middle ear function
A_S (normal pressure/reduced compliance)	Otosclerosis; ossicular fixation; moderate middle ear fluid
A_D (normal pressure/excessive compliance)	Disruption of ossicular chain; abnormal (hypermobile) tympanic membrane
B (flat configuration—no point of maximum compliance)	Middle ear effusion (e.g., otitis media); cerumen occlusion
C (negative pressure/normal compliance)	Eustachian tube disorder

(3) Tympanometric shapes—classified based on the height and location of the tympanometric peak (see Figure 18-10); shapes (i.e., Types A, A_S, A_D, B, C) are consistent with a variety of ME disorders (Table 18-4).
(4) Tympanometric gradient—width of the tympanogram (in daPa) measured at half of the height from the peak to the tail; abnormally wide tympanograms are consistent with ME dysfunction.
(5) Equivalent ear canal volume—an estimate of the volume of air between the probe tip in

the EAM and the TM; a large canal volume is consistent with a perforated TM or a patent (open) pressure-equalization (PE) tube.
  d. Acoustic reflex testing.
    (1) Measured by assessing change in acoustic admittance of the ear caused by a contraction of the stapedius muscle when a high intensity (i.e., typically, 70–100 dB HL) is presented.
    (2) Threshold is lowest intensity level at which ME immittance change can be detected in response to the acoustic stimuli.
    (3) Acoustic reflex is a bilateral phenomenon having ipsilateral (same side) and contralateral (opposite side) pathways involving peripheral and central structures.
    (4) Reflex decay measurement involves the suprathreshold analysis of the acoustic reflex to determine CN VIII function.
    (5) Provides differential diagnostic information.
      (a) Confirming ME disorders.
      (b) Distinguishing between sensory (cochlea) and neural (CN VIII) disease.
      (c) Identifying lower brain stem pathology.
      (d) Identifying facial nerve (CN VII) disorders.
2. Otoacoustic emissions (OAEs).
  a. OAEs—low-intensity sounds generated by the cochlea that travel back through the ME and are recorded in the EAM by a microphone.
  b. Present OAEs suggest normal or near-normal cochlear function in the presence of normal ME function; absent OAEs suggest some degree of hearing loss present in the presence of normal ME function.
  c. Multiple purposes for conducting OAEs.
    (1) Screening for hearing loss in newborns and infants.
    (2) Cross-checks for behavioral testing in difficult-to-test patients (e.g., a developmentally disabled child or adult; functional hearing loss).
    (3) Assists in the differential diagnosis of sensory (cochlear) and neural (CN VIII) hearing loss.
    (4) Monitoring for ototoxicity.
  d. Major categories of clinically useful OAEs.
    (1) Transient-evoked OAEs (TEOAEs)—testing uses a broadband signal (click) at 80–85 dB SPL to stimulate a wide range of frequencies in the cochlea; in general TEOAEs will be absent when cochlear hearing loss is greater than 30 dB HL (Figure 18-11).
    (2) Distortion-product OAEs (DP-OAEs)—testing using pair of tones (F1 and F2) presented at 65 and 55 dB; OHC create a distortion tone ($2f_1-f_2$), which is measured by microphone in EAM; reflects the nonlinear processes of the cochlea. DPOAEs will be absent when cochlear hearing loss is greater than 45 dB HL, in general (Figure 18-12).

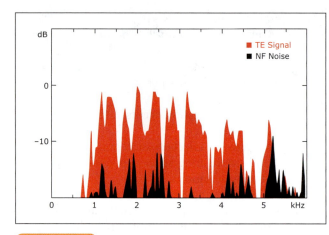

Figure 18-11 Example of a present Transient-Evoked Otoacoustic Emission (TE-OAE). The TE-OAE is shown in red with the background noise indicated by the black (NF-noise).

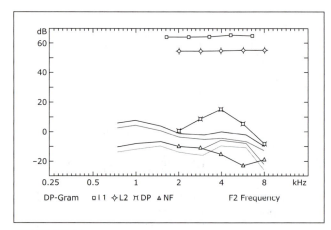

Figure 18-12 Example of a present Distortion-Product Otoacoustic Emission (DP-OAE). The top two sets of symbols of squares (L1) and triangles (L2) indicate the intensity of test signals (F1 and F2). The solid lines represent the 5th to 95th percentile range for established norms. The lower set of triangle symbols represents the noise floor; the squares represent the DP response.

3. Auditory-evoked potentials (AEPs).
  a. AEPs are a series of bioelectric responses (i.e., waveforms).
    (1) Recorded using surface electrodes (for most clinical applications) and computer-averaging techniques.
    (2) Waveform recordings consist of a series of peaks and troughs that can be measured in terms of their latency and amplitude.
    (3) Waveforms reflect neural synchrony and transmission of neural responses to acoustic stimuli along the auditory pathways.

b. Specific AEP tests.
  (1) Electrocochleography (ECochG).
    (a) Single biphasic response consisting of a summating potential (SP; response from the cochlea—primarily from basilar membrane and hair cell displacement) and compound action potential (AP; neural response from distal portion of CN VIII).
    (b) Compare amplitude of SP to the AP (SP/AP ratio) in diagnosis of Ménière's disease/endolymphatic hydrops.
    (c) Monitor latency of AP during surgical procedures involving auditory peripheral structures.
  (2) Auditory brain stem response (ABR).
    (a) Response occurs during the first 10 msec post onset of stimulus.
    (b) Waveform response is comprised of a series of waves. Waves I and II are generated by the distal and proximal portions of the CN VIII (respectively) and the remaining waves reflect neural function from multiple generator sites in the brain stem.
    (c) Clicks (broadband stimuli; corresponds to approximately 1000 to 4000 Hz region on the basilar membrane) or tone pips (filtered clicks more closely related to that frequency region on the basilar membrane) are used.
    (d) Latency-intensity function utilized to estimate hearing sensitivity in the difficult-to-test population; when behavioral audiometric testing cannot be completed (Figure 18-13).
      • ABR is NOT a true test of hearing, but is a reflection of neural activity in the auditory pathway that can be used to predict hearing sensitivity.
    (e) Monitor auditory nerve status during surgical procedures (e.g., removal of vestibular schwannoma or vestibular nerve section).
  (3) Auditory steady state response (ASSR). This technique uses a continuous frequency-specific signal that is frequency modulated, amplitude modulated or both. The presence/absence is determined by series of statistical algorithms that can be recorded within 10 dB of the behavioral thresholds.
  (4) Middle latency response (MLR).
    (a) Reflects activity of the auditory thalamocortical pathway.
    (b) Applications include estimation of low-frequency hearing thresholds, assessment of patients with CI/s and neurodiagnostic assessment of auditory pathway disease and central auditory processing disorders.
  (5) Auditory late responses.
    (a) Cortical responses; dependent upon one's state of arousal; has limited clinical application.
  (6) P3/P300.
    (a) Response requires active cognitive participation; response reflects multiple cortical generator sites.
    (b) Used to evaluate psychological events such as attention, alerting, arousal or memory.

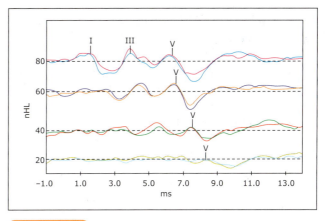

Figure 18-13 Example of an auditory brain stem response (ABR) latency-intensity function recorded from a normal hearing child. Note the increase in wave V latency and decrease in amplitude that occurs as stimulus intensity decreases. The lowest observable wave V represents the ABR threshold. nHL, normal hearing level; ms, milliseconds

Hearing Disorders

General Factors Causing Hearing Loss

1. Developmental deficits.
2. Infections.
3. Drugs.
4. Environmental toxins.
5. Trauma.
6. Vascular disorders.
7. Neural disorders.
8. Immune system disorders.
9. Bone disorders.
10. Aging processes.

OE and ME Disorders/Abnormalities

1. Primary disorders of the OE (the pinna, EAM or TM) and ME are presented in Tables 18-5 and 18-6 along with common treatments.
2. Disorders of the pinna and/or EAM typically do not result in hearing loss; cerumen in the EAM will cause hearing loss if it totally blocks the pathway.
3. Disorders of the ME typically cause a CHL; occurs whenever sound is blocked from reaching IE.
4. Maximum CHL is 60 dB (e.g., case of complete atresia).

IE (Cochlear) Disorders/Abnormalities

1. Primary disorders and treatments of the IE are presented in Table 18-7.
2. Abnormalities of the IE produce SNHL.
3. Audiometric configurations provides a gross estimation of the regions of the cochlea that are damaged by the pathology (e.g., high-frequency SNHL loss reflects damage to the basal end of the cochlea; a low-frequency SNHL reflects damage more to the apical portion of the cochlea).
4. Mild to moderate SNHL due primarily to damage of the OHC.
5. Severe to profound SNHL due to damage to both the OHC and IHC.

Table 18-5

Outer Ear Disorders

DISORDER	BRIEF DESCRIPTION
Anotia	Absent pinna
Microtia	Small pinna
Atresia	Absent or blocked external auditory meatus or canal
Stenosis	Narrowing of external auditory meatus
Foreign bodies	Miscellaneous objects in canal (e.g., bugs, peas)
Osteoma	Benign bony tumor
Exostosis	Benign bony tumor potentially due to swimming in cold water
Cerumen	Wax build-up, which may be impacted due to cotton swab use
Fungal/external otitis	"Swimmer's ear"
Tympanic Membrane (TM)	
TM perforation	Hole in TM (possibly due to trauma or infection)
Tympanosclerosis	Scarring of TM (often due to multiple perforations)

Table 18-6

Middle Ear Disorders

DISORDER	BRIEF DESCRIPTION
Otitis Media	Middle ear fluid, which may or may not be infectious (serous—noninfectious; mucoid; purulent); can be chronic or acute
Cholesteatoma	Nonmalignant growth, often following foreign body making its way into the ME space
Ossicular discontinuity	Trauma to any one or more of the ossicles—malleus, incus, stapes
Otosclerosis	"Stiffening" of the ossicles, due to bony growth, especially involving the stapes
Physical trauma/longitudinal fracture	Partial or total disarticulation of the ossicular chain
Barotrauma	Traumatic injury caused by rapid changes in atmospheric pressure (ascending/descending in airplane)
Glomus tumor	Neoplasm found in the middle ear that is a mass of cells with a vascular supply accompanied by pulsatile tinnitus
Tympanosclerosis	Formation of white plaques on the tympanic membrane

Table 18-7

Inner (Cochlear) Ear Disorders

DISORDER	BRIEF DESCRIPTION
Autoimmune hearing loss	Associated with autoimmune disorders; loss referring to abnormal immunologic responses where the body produces antibodies against its own tissue
Congenital pathologies	Hereditary or other hearing challenges identified at birth
Congenital infections	Most commonly associated with sensory hearing loss; includes cytomegalovirus (CMV), human immunodeficiency virus (HIV), rubella, syphilis, and toxoplasmosis
Noise-induced hearing loss	
Temporary threshold shift (TTS)	Short-term shift in hearing sensitivity due to acoustic trauma and/or noise
Permanent threshold shift (PTS)	Long-term shift in hearing sensitivity due to acoustic trauma and/or noise
Ototoxicity	Hearing loss caused by therapeutic agents (e.g., aminoglycosides; salicylates; loop diuretics; cisplatin) or other chemical substances (e.g., industrial solvents; carbon monoxide)
Ménière's disease	Results from overproduction of an inner ear fluid—endolymph (endolymphatic hydrops); triad of symptoms include: unilateral hearing loss; roaring tinnitus; vertigo (balance/nausea challenges) often accompanied by aural fullness
Presbycusis	Hearing loss related to aging process
Physical trauma/transverse fracture	Temporal bone fracture that causes damage to the membranous labyrinth of the cochlea

6. There are several perceptual consequences resulting from cochlear hearing loss.
   a. Loudness recruitment—an abnormally disproportionate increase in the sensation of loudness in response to auditory stimuli of normal volume.
   b. Dysacusis—difficulty understanding speech, which may result from a combination of frequency and harmonic distortion in the cochlea.
   c. Diplacusis—a difference in the perception of sound by the ears, either in time or in pitch, so that one sound is heard as two.
   d. Phonemic regression—significant difficulty in word recognition often associated with presbycusis.
7. Major management strategies for SNHL.
   a. Medical management of sudden SNHL is considered a medical emergency.
      (1) Corticosteroids may be delivered systemically or via intratympanic application.
      (2) Hyperbaric oxygen, currently not FDA approved for this indication, may be offered.
      (3) Patients with incomplete hearing recovery should be counseled regarding benefits/limitations of hearing aids (HA/s) and/or other hearing assistive technology.
   b. Ménière's disease—medical and surgical treatment.
      (1) Motion sickness medications [e.g., meclizine (Antivert) or diazepam (Valium)] to reduce vertigo symptoms and anti-nausea medications (e.g., promethazine) to control nausea and vomiting during episodes of vertigo; long-term use of diuretics to reduce fluid retention.
      (2) Medications injected into the ME and then absorbed into the IE may improve vertigo symptoms (gentamicin, steroids).
      (3) Surgery may be an option and include endolymphatic sac decompression, vestibular nerve section and labyrinthectomy.
      (4) Noninvasive procedures include vestibular rehabilitation therapy, HA/s, and use of Meniett device (application of positive pressure to the ME to improve fluid exchange).
      (5) Modification of diet including salt limitation and avoidance of monosodium glutamate (MSG) in prepared food.
   c. Noise-induced hearing loss (NIHL)—Table 18-8 displays damage-risk criteria for hearing loss.
      (1) Hearing loss prevention.
         (a) Use of hearing protection. There are different types of hearing protection such as foam earplugs, earmuffs and custom hearing protection devices; needed when in environment that is 85 dBA for more than 8 hours; if louder, need to reduce time by 50% for every 3 dB increase in intensity above 85 dBA.

Table 18-8

Damage-Risk Criteria (Based on NIOSH Criteria)

SOUND PRESSURE LEVEL	LENGTH OF EXPOSURE	EXAMPLES (IN dBA)
< 85	> 8 hours	Light traffic; dishwasher; blender
85 to 87	8 hours	Train; live show; snow blower
88 to 90	4 hours	Lawn mower; diesel truck; symphony concert
91 to 93	2 hours	Jazz concert; subway
94 to 96	1 hour	Personal stereo
97 to 99	30 minutes	Router; belt sander; drill; MRI machine
100 to 102	15 minutes	Nightclub/discotheque; snowmobile
103 to 105	7.5 minutes	Radial arm saw; chainsaw; rock concert
106 to 108	3.75 minutes	Circular saw; sporting event
109 to 111	1.87 minutes	Air raid siren; firecracker
111 to 113	< 1 minute	Revolver; automobile airbag

         (b) Turn volume down. Reduce volume and time when listening to personal music players or any other device that has a volume control. (Visit www.TurnItToTheLeft.com).
         (c) Walking away from the noise. Doubling the distance from the sound source decreases the intensity by 50%.
   d. HA/s (see complete section overview of HA/s).
   e. CI/s (see complete section overview of CI/s).

Retrocochlear (CN VIII, Brain Stem, Cortical) Disorders

1. Primary retrocochlear disorders are presented in Table 18-9.
2. There are several audiometric "red flags" associated with CN VIII disorders.
   a. Unilateral high-frequency SNHL.
   b. Unilateral tinnitus.
   c. Poorer word recognition scores that would be predicted based on pure tone audiometry.
   d. Dizziness.
   e. Normal tympanograms, elevated or absent acoustic reflexes and positive reflex decay.
   f. Abnormal ABR findings with prolongations of wave V.
3. Contrast-enhanced magnetic resonance imaging (MRI) is the gold standard for diagnosing vestibular schwannoma (VS).
   a. VS are slow growing and benign; treatment is recommended because growth may lead to

Table 18-9

Retrocochlear (CN VIII Nerve, Brain Stem, Cortex) Disorders

DISORDER	BRIEF DESCRIPTIONS
Brain stem infarct	Localized areas of ischemia produced by interruption of blood supply
Glioma	Tumor composed of neuroglia, or supporting cells of the brain that can affect auditory pathways
Presbycusis	Hearing loss related to aging process
Vestibular schwannoma	Often referred to as acoustic tumors (typically one-sided but can involve bilateral tumors; neurofibromatosis; NF-2)
Multiple sclerosis	Degenerative demyelinating disease, with auditory findings that may be detected during auditory evoked potential testing
Cerebrovascular accident	Stroke caused by interruption of blood supply to the brain due to an aneurysm, embolus or clot possibly resulting in language deficits and "cortical deafness"

multiple cranial neuropathies, brain stem compression, hydrocephalus and even death.
  b. A "watch-and-wait" approach may be taken when appropriate (e.g., elderly, medically fragile).
  c. Surgery options include different approaches (retrosigmoid, intralabyrinthine, middle fossa) each having their respective advantages and disadvantages.
  d. Stereotaxic radiosurgery (gamma-knife) is being increasingly used as an alternative to surgical removal of the tumor.
4. Intra-axial disorders (within the brain stem)—tests of central auditory function may show contralateral or bilateral effects, oftentimes with normal (or near normal) hearing sensitivity for pure tones.
5. Extra-axial disorders (outside the brain stem)—audiometric symptoms are on the same side as the disorder and patients may show a range (from mild to profound) of hearing sensitivity for pure tones.
6. Vascular accidents—disorders that interfere with blood supply to brain stem pathways and cortex.
  a. Thromboses—clots that form and remain in specific areas of the vessel.
  b. Embolisms—debris that circulates until it reaches a narrow vessel.
  c. Aneurysms—dilation of blood vessels causing the walls of vessels to stretch and dilate.
  d. Cerebrovascular accidents (CVA)—obstructions or ruptures of blood vessels within the brain causing a stroke.
  e. Atherosclerosis—hardening of the arteries.
7. (Central) auditory processing disorders (APD)—children or adults have difficulty interpreting auditory information (often exacerbated by background noise) even with normal peripheral hearing sensitivity.
  a. Intervention strategies include the enhancement of signal-to-noise ratio (SNR).
    (1) Using an FM system to increase teacher's voice over background classroom noise; could be personal or sound field.
    (2) Using environment treatments (e.g., curtains on windows, acoustic ceiling tiles, tennis balls on chair legs).
    (3) Providing written supplemental instructions/information.
    (4) Using preferential seating; this should be the last accommodation implemented.
  b. Children with APD may benefit from auditory training therapy and development of compensatory skills.

Auditory Neuropathy Spectrum Disorder (ANSD)

1. Previously known as auditory neuropathy/auditory dys-synchrony.
2. ANSD characterized by evidence of normal cochlear OHC (sensory) function and abnormal auditory nerve function.
3. Cause unknown; children born prematurely and having a stay in a neonatal intensive care unit (NICU) and/or hyperbilirubinemia are at increased risk.
4. Diagnostic criteria.
  a. Presence of normal or near-normal OAEs; although OAEs absent in approximately 30% of cases of ANSD.
  b. Presence of a cochlear microphonic (CM) assessed using ABR.
  c. Absent or markedly abnormal auditory brain stem response (ABR).
5. ABR is required as the screening method for newborns whenever there is a five-day or longer stay in the NICU.
6. Behavioral audiologic assessment.
  a. Audiogram—results may suggest any degree of hearing loss.
  b. Speech in quiet—results may not be consistent with audiometric findings.
  c. Speech in noise—results should show significant decrease in performance compared to testing in quiet.
  d. Immittance testing with acoustic reflexes—reflexes should be absent in presence of normal ME function.
  e. OAEs—should be present; although if absent does not rule out ANSD.
  f. ABR using both a condensation click and a rarefaction click to assess presence of a CM; a no-stimulus run should also be collected to verify that response is biologic, not electrical artifact from the headphones.

7. Responses to behavioral testing may be not consistent among tests; need to rely on parental report as well: "some days my child seems to hear—other days my child acts deaf."
8. Management options.
   a. HA/s—should be fit using standard pediatric fitting guidelines; however, if OAEs are present, HA/s should be fit to a mild hearing loss.
   b. CI/s considered when progress is limited; CI may bypass the dysfunctional area.
   c. Communication methodology—all options are available and presented to parents in an unbiased way to allow them to make an informed decision.

Hearing Sensory Technology

Hearing Aids (HA/s)

1. Components—All HA/s include several basic components (Figure 18-14).
   a. Microphone—transducer that converts acoustic sound into electrical signal.
      (1) Omnidirectional microphone—equally sensitive to sounds from all directions.
      (2) Directional microphone—more sensitive to sounds from specific angles.
      (3) Multi-microphones—combines more than one microphone.
   b. Amplifier—increases the gain (power) of the incoming signal.
      (1) Analog signal processing alters sounds via filters.
      (2) Digital signal processing alters sounds via conversion of sound into digital binary code (0, 1) and then by applying mathematical algorithms to the signal.
   c. Receiver—converts amplified electrical signal to an acoustic signal delivered to the ear.
   d. Battery—power source of HA.
   e. Other HA features:
      (1) Telecoil (t-coil)—coil of wire that creates an electromagnetic field when activated that communicates with the electromagnetic field from the telephone.
      (2) Channels—division of the frequency response of the HA into smaller units, permitting greater fitting precision.
      (3) Programs—separate fitting algorithms for specific listening situations (e.g., restaurants); selected either automatically or by push buttons on the devices or remote control.
2. Electroacoustic characteristics.
   a. Gain—amount or magnitude of amplification (in dB); quantified by the difference between the input into the HA and the HA output.
   b. Frequency response—amount of gain across the frequency range of the HA.
   c. Output sound pressure level (OSPL)—maximum output level of the HA.
   d. Linear sound processing—equal dB increase for all incoming sounds; i.e., soft, medium and loud input sounds amplified to the same degree.

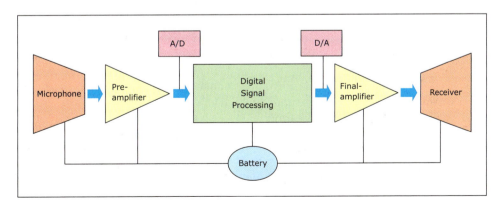

Figure 18-14 Block diagram of the basic components of a digital signal processing hearing aid. A/D, analog-to-digital converter; D/A, digital-to-analog converter.

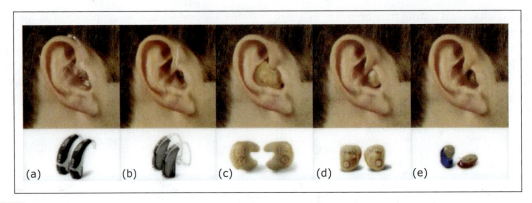

Figure 18-15 Photograph of major hearing aid styles: (A) behind-the-ear (BTE); (B) open fit micro BTE; (C) full shell in-the-ear (ITE); (D) half-shell ITE; (E) completely-in-the-canal (CIC).

Photographs are courtesy of Phonak.

    e. Nonlinear sound processing—amount of gain is dependent on the intensity of incoming sound; softer sounds are amplified more than louder sounds; most commonly used processing.
3. HA styles (see Figure 18-15):
    a. Behind the ear (BTE)—devices that sit on or behind the ear and are attached to a sound delivery system (e.g., tubing attached to earmold, slim tubing attached to small dome or receiver that sits in the EAM) to the ear canal.
       (1) RITE/RIC BTE—receiver-in-the-ear/receiver-in-canal BTE; used to create an open ear fit.
       (2) Open-fit BTE—EAM is not occluded with earmold; eliminates the occlusion effect (i.e., increased sound pressure level in the ear canal) that causes the HA user's voice to sound louder and hollow; increases physical comfort.
    b. Custom—family of in-the-ear (ITE) devices ranging in size from full shell (FS ITE), half shell (HS ITE), in the canal (ITC), to completely in the canal (CIC); all HA components housed within the shells.
       (1) Greater hearing loss requires larger-size device to prevent feedback (high-pitch ringing created by the HA) and provide sufficient gain, in general.
    c. Selection of a specific HA depends on a variety of factors, including the patient's ear canal and pinna anatomy, physical fit, degree of hearing loss, listening needs and patient preference.
    d. CROS HA/s—special HA fitting applications when conventional HA configurations may be inappropriate; provide bilateral (i.e., two-sided) hearing; not binaural (two-ear) hearing.
       (1) Contralateral routing of signal (CROS)—used to compensate for single-sided deafness (SSD; no aidable hearing in one ear with normal hearing in other ear); microphone worn on poorer ear; signal transmitted wirelessly to receiver worn on better ear.

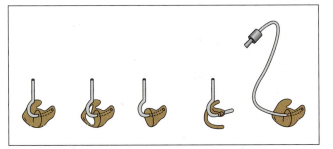

Figure 18-16 Examples of major earmold styles (left to right): full shell, skeleton, canal, free field/CROS, noncustom slim-tube.

       (2) Bilateral CROS (BiCROS)—used to compensate for asymmetric bilateral hearing loss; microphones worn on both ears; signal transmitted from poorer ear to better ear, which has a HA on/in it.
4. Earmolds (see Figure 18-16).
    a. Available in number of styles and materials, both of which can alter frequency response of the HA and affect the perceived quality of the patient's voice.
    b. Purpose of earmolds.
       (1) Attach traditional BTE to ear.
       (2) Deliver amplified sound to ear.
       (3) Modify the frequency response of the HA.
       (4) Prevents feedback.
    c. Earmold modifications.
       (1) Venting—channel that runs through the earmold; reduces feelings of fullness, prevents moisture in the ear canal and alters the low-frequency response characteristics.
       (2) Damping—acoustic filter/damper in the HA, tone hook or earmold that reduces the resonant peaks of the response (i.e., smoothes the frequency response, providing improved sound quality).

(3) Horn effect—use of "horn-shaped tubing" or "belled" bores in the earmold; provides enhancement of the high-frequency response.
5. HA fitting process.
   a. Multistep process to determine most appropriate devices to meet the needs of the patient.
      (1) Comprehensive audiologic evaluation.
         (a) Determines degree, type and configuration of hearing loss.
         (b) Determines need for medical treatment.
         (c) Assists in selecting specific amplification strategies (monaural versus binaural HA/s).
         (d) Assists in setting realistic expectations.
      (2) Hearing needs assessment and device selection.
         (a) Assessment of communication function and psychosocial consequences of hearing loss – use both objective calibrated speech materials (e.g., Quick Speech in Noise–QuickSIN test) and subjective self-report measures (e.g., Abbreviated Profile of Hearing Aid Benefit–APHAB; Hearing Handicap Inventory for the Elderly/Adult–HHIE/A).
         (b) Assessment of biopsychosocial variables such as visual status, manual dexterity, shape and dimension of pinna and ear canal, overall health, cognitive status, motivation, lifestyle, family support and financial factors.
         (c) Special considerations for children include tamper-resistant battery compartment, retention options for securing HA/s, t-coil/direct-audio input options.
      (3) HA fitting and orientation.
         (a) Verification that HA/earmolds are physically comfortable.
         (b) HA/s programmed to meet listening needs, focusing on naturalness of patient's voice, output within comfort level and without feedback.
         (c) Explanation of use and care of devices/earmolds.
         (d) Verification of ability to insert/remove HA/s, manipulate controls/ switches and change batteries.
         (e) Counseling of realistic expectations and effective communication strategies with the hearing devices.
      (4) Verification and validation of devices—processes to determine that the HA/s are performing appropriately and providing the expected benefit.
         (a) Verification—assesses adequacy of the HA; variety of strategies include:
            • Electroacoustic analysis (verifies frequency response characteristics, input/output functions of HA/s using calibrated signal in a specialized test box).
            • Real ear measurement (measures HA output at the TM using speech signals at different input levels).
            • Aided sound field testing using pure tones and speech signals (e.g., Hearing in Noise Test, Speech Perception in Noise test).
         (b) Validation—assesses one's perception of improvement in communication function following the HA fitting via:
            • Standardized questionnaires that are psychometrically robust (i.e., high test-retest reliability; e.g., International Outcome Inventory-Hearing Aids; HHIE/A administered in a pre-/postfitting paradigm).
6. Wireless connectivity options.
   a. Challenging listening situations/environments such as background noise, increased distance between sound source and listener and reverberation can be overcome with HA accessories using Bluetooth or FM wireless technology.
   b. Connect HA/s to telephones, televisions, personal music players via a device that streams directly to the HA/s.
   c. Wireless microphones can be worn on the talker's lapel, shirt or tie and stream directly to HA/s; other microphones can sit on table at restaurant or at a meeting and stream directly to HA/s.

Cochlear Implants (CI)

1. Components (Figure 18-17).
   a. Microphone—picks up sounds.
   b. External sound processor—filters and processes the sound; converts sound into digital signal; minicomputer inside the behind-the-ear piece (most common) or worn on the body (less common).
   c. Internal unit—converts digital signal into electrical signals via the internal receiver/stimulator that is attached to the electrode array.
   d. Electrode array—inserted surgically via an opening (cochleostomy) into the scala tympani in the area of the round window of the cochlea.
      (1) Electrical signals from the electrode array (bypassing the damaged hair cells in the IE) stimulate the CN VIII and auditory pathways to the brain for sound perception.
2. CI activation.
   a. Several weeks postsurgery, recipient returns to CI center where microphone and transmitting coil, speech or sound processor are activated.
   b. External sound processor uniquely programmed or MAPped (mapped) for each patient.

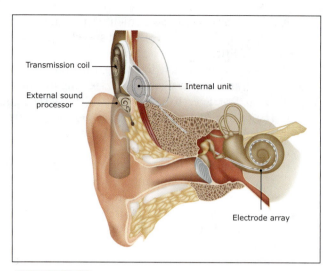

Figure 18-17 Major external and internal components of a cochlear implant system.

3. Current CI expectations.
   a. Helps to restore recipient's ability to detect and potentially understand sound information.
   b. May improve talking on the telephone, watching and listening to TV.
   c. May outperform many successful HA users with less severe hearing loss with today's technology.
   d. Length of deafness is predictor of performance; shorter length = better CI performance.
4. Pediatric candidacy criteria (established by the FDA).
   a. 12 to 24 months.
      (1) Profound SNHL in both ears.
      (2) No medical contraindications.
      (3) Lack of progress in the development of auditory skills.
      (4) High motivation and appropriate expectations from family.
   b. 2 years to 17 years, 11 months.
      (1) Severe-to-profound SNHL in both ears.
      (2) Lexical Neighborhood Test (LNT) scores of 30% or less in best-aided condition (for children 5 years to 17 years, 11 months).
      (3) Lack of progress in the development of auditory skills.
      (4) Multiple LNT (MLNT) scores of 30% or less in best-aided condition (for children, 25 months to 4 years, 11 months).
      (5) No medical contraindications.
      (6) High motivation and appropriate expectations (both child, when appropriate, and family).
5. Adult candidacy criteria—18 years and above; there is no upper age limit for CI surgery (established by the FDA).
   a. Moderate-to-profound SNHL in both ears.
   b. Preoperative Hearing In Noise Test (HINT) sentences recognition scores of 50% or less in the ear to be implanted and 60% or less in the opposite ear or binaurally.
   c. Prelinguistic or postlinguistic onset of severe-to-profound hearing loss.
   d. No medical contraindications.
   e. A desire to be part of the hearing world.
6. Candidacy evaluation.
   a. Candidacy is typically determined for pediatric and adult patients by a team of professionals.
   b. HA trial is usually required.
   c. Electrophysiologic testing (e.g., ABR with tone pips/bursts, ASSR) should be completed prior to the final candidacy decision.
   d. Radiographic studies (e.g., CT and/or MRI) are required to evaluate the patency (open) and overall structure of the cochlea, along with the visualization of auditory and vestibular landmarks.
   e. Aided audiogram reflecting auditory functioning with both HA/s (binaural amplification) and, ideally, testing with Left HA-ONLY and Right HA-ONLY, used to determine amplification benefit, if any.
   f. Some CI teams require that a developmental pediatrician see pediatric patients, and adult patients may need to be seen by a psychologist in order to determine that the patient and the family have realistic expectations about CI/s.
7. Terms related to CI use.
   a. Unilateral CI—one CI.
   b. Bilateral CI/s—two CI/s.
      (1) Simultaneous bilateral CI/s—CIs implanted during same surgical procedure.
      (2) Sequential bilateral CI/s—CI/s implanted at two separate surgeries, ranging from several months to multiple years apart.
8. Auditory brain stem implant (ABI).
   a. Currently only available for adult patients with damage to their auditory nerve (i.e., neurofibromatosis).

Bone-Anchored Auditory Implants (BAI)

1. Components.
   a. Microphone—picks up sound; part of externally worn sound processor.
   b. Externally worn processor—converts energy into a vibration.
   c. Surgically implanted titanium abutment and fixture—externally worn processor sits on abutment, which vibrates the skull when vibration received from processor; sound delivered to the IE via skull vibrations.
   d. Children younger than 5 years use a soft headband that holds the externally worn processor; not candidate for surgical implant until age 5 years.

2. Indications for use.
   a. CHL/mixed hearing loss—patients born with an incomplete, blocked or damaged OE, EAM (e.g., anotia, microtia, stenosis, atresia, among others) or ME, or with constantly draining ears due to chronic ear infections who may be unable to use standard HA/s.
   b. SSD—sound processor placed on the ear with the profound loss that stimulates contralateral (normal-hearing) ear via bone conduction.
3. Candidacy criteria.
   a. CHL or mixed hearing loss.
      (1) PTA bone conduction thresholds (500, 1000, 2000, 3000 Hz) for the indicated ear should be ≤45 to 65 dB HL, depending on the manufacturer and model of BAI.
      (2) Word recognition score >60%.
   b. SSD.
      (1) PTA air-conduction thresholds of the hearing ear (500, 1000, 2000, 3000 Hz) should be ≤20 dB HL.

Other Hearing-Assistive Technology

1. Frequency-modulated (FM) and infrared (IR) systems.
   a. User receives amplified signal directly from sound source using a wireless system; can increase the SNR; overcomes issues with background noise, distance and reverberation.
   b. Components.
      (1) Microphone—attached to sound source, such as a talker (e.g., parent, teacher, significant other, religious leader, actor on stage) or television.
      (2) Transmitter—sends signal to the receiver.
      (3) Receiver—receives signal from transmitter.
      (4) Transducers—headphones, loudspeakers, via neckloop or direct audio input (DAI) used with HA/s.
   c. FM signal—uses wireless radio wave; does not require line-of-site between the transmitter and receiver; may experience interference if another FM on same channel is in close proximity.
   d. IR signal—uses light waves; requires line-of-site transmission between transmitter and receiver; will not experience interference if another IR system in close proximity; signal may be compromised with direct sunlight.
2. Hearing-assistive technology (HAT).
   a. Alerting devices—include doorbells/door knockers, alarm clocks, telephone ringing, smoke detectors.
   b. Listening devices—include amplified telephones, television amplifiers.
   c. Text devices—text telephones (i.e., TTY, TT), captioned television.
3. Vibrotactile aid.
   a. Device that vibrates to transfer information about sounds.
   b. Assists in detecting and interpreting sounds through sense of touch.
   c. Vibrotactile aids provide awareness of sound and speech prosody; however, overall benefit is limited.

Auditory Rehabilitation (Aural [Re]habilitation; Audiologic [Re]habilitation)

World Health Organization (WHO) International Classification of Functioning, Disability and Health (ICF)

1. Provides model for understanding dimensions of health conditions and functioning under three domains; domains set the stage for developing auditory rehabilitation strategies.
   a. Impairment—measurable loss of hearing function (e.g., hair cell loss at the basal end of the cochlea causing a high-frequency hearing loss that can be measured using audiometry).
   b. Activity limitation (previously referred to as disability)—reflects the impact of hearing loss on the person's ability to communicate and understand environmental and speech signals (e.g., difficulty hearing in background noise or in reverberant environments).
   c. Participation restriction (previously referred to as handicap)—represents the nonauditory (e.g., social and emotional) problems faced by the patient with hearing loss in everyday situations (e.g., withdrawal and isolation from communication situations).

Definitions and Terminology

1. Terms used to describe the population of persons with hearing differences.
   a. Deaf and hard of hearing—currently used in U.S. federal legislation to describe children and adults with any degree of hearing sensitivity deficits/differences.
   b. Audiometrically deaf—refers to the most significant hearing sensitivity challenge based solely on audiologic testing (profound hearing loss).

c. Capital "D" Deaf—refers to persons who are culturally deaf, who would typically make use of American Sign Language (ASL), are proud to be deaf and may have been raised in Bi-Bi (bilingual-bicultural) environments, including schools for the Deaf.
2. Other terms used—often of varying accuracy and subject to rhetorical challenge or objections by some persons.
   a. Hearing loss—not all persons are born with hearing to lose.
   b. Hearing impaired or hearing impairment and hearing disabled or hearing disability—these terms have a negative connotation due to the words "impaired," "impairment," "disabled" and "disability."
   c. Hard of hearing—suggests minor hearing sensitivity deficit and, potentially, an ageist perception referring to the older adult.

Variables Associated with Hearing Differences

1. Age of onset.
   a. Congenital (at birth).
   b. Prelingual (birth to approximately 3 years of age).
   c. Postlingual (after speech and language have been developed).
   d. Acquired or adventitious hearing loss—refers to adults who develop hearing differences.
2. Age of identification.
3. Age and consistency of sensory technology use.
4. Family involvement and degree of stimulation/input to child.
5. Type of intervention services available.
6. Presence of other or multiple disabilities.

Communication Options, Opportunities and Modalities

1. Listening and spoken language.
   a. Auditory-verbal.
      (1) Method to facilitate optimal acquisition of spoken language through listening.
      (2) Parent-professional partnership is developed; professional teaches the parent/s or other caregivers how to teach their child to communicate using listening for spoken language development.
      (3) Previously referred to as unisensory and/or acoupedics.
   b. Auditory/oral.
      (1) Method to help children develop the spoken language and academic skills they need to be successful in a "regular" or "typical" classroom environment and to work and live in a predominantly hearing society.
      (2) Previously emphasized speechreading.
2. Manual communication.
   a. American Sign Language (ASL).
      (1) Visual-spatial language used by deaf/Deaf people in the United States and English-speaking parts of Canada.
      (2) ASL has its own grammar, syntax, idioms and vocabulary; uses space, direction and speed of movement and facial expression to mark grammar and convey meaning.
      (3) Has no spoken or written form.
   b. Bilingual-bicultural (Bi-Bi).
      (1) ASL is taught as the first language (bilingual).
      (2) Information about Deaf life and culture (bicultural) is addressed.
   c. Manually Coded English (MCE).
      (1) Uses some combination of ASL signs, special vocabulary, and English grammar (English word order) to visually communicate English.
      (2) Common forms include Seeing Essential English (SEE 1); Signed English; Signing Exact English (SEE 2).
3. Cued speech.
   a. System to clarify lipreading (speechreading) by using simple finger/hand movements or cues around the face to indicate pronunciation of any spoken word.
   b. Many spoken words look exactly alike on the mouth (e.g., the sounds /b,p,m/); these cues allow the user to distinguish the differences between the speech sounds in pronunciation.
4. Pidgin Sign English (PSE).
   a. Communication method that uses a combination of ASL, Signed English and fingerspelling (26 specific finger/hand positions that symbolize each of the 26 English alphabet letters).
   b. Often used in communication between deaf or hard of hearing signers.
5. Total communication (TC).
   a. Communication philosophy used to facilitate the development of language that considers the needs of the student or other user.
   b. May include use of sign, speech, gestures, mime, writing, pictures, fingerspelling, speechreading, and/or amplification (HA/s) or use of CI/s.

Auditory Rehabilitation Assessment Tools

1. Auditory.
   a. Ling Six Sound Test (Ling & Ling, 1978).
   b. Early Speech Perception (ESP) test battery (Moog & Geers, 1990).

c. Infant-Toddler Meaningful Auditory Integration Scale (IT-MAIS).
d. Meaningful Auditory Integration Scale (MAIS).
e. Parent's Evaluation of Aural/Oral Performance of Children (PEACH) (Ching & Hill, 2007).
f. Teacher's Evaluation of Aural/Oral Performance of Children (TEACH) (Ching & Hill, 2005).
g. Glendonald Auditory Screening Procedure (GASP!) (Erber, 1982).
h. The Listening Comprehension Test–2 (Bowers, Huisingh, & LoGiudice, 2006).
i. Test of Auditory Comprehension (TAC) (Foreworks, 1977).
j. Speech Perception Instructional Curriculum and Evaluation: For Children with Cochlear Implants and Hearing Aids (SPICE) (Moog, Biedenstein, & Davidson, 1995).

2. Speech.
a. Central Institute for the Deaf (CID) Picture SPeech INtelligibility Evaluation (SPINE) (Monsen, Moog, & Geers, 1988).
b. Phonetic Level Inventory/Phonologic Level Inventory (Ling, 2002).

3. Language.
a. Use of receptive and expressive language measures that are standardized on children with typical hearing.
b. In view of the increasing numbers of students who are deaf or hard of hearing who are mainstreamed, "typical" language measures are often recommended.
c. Attention to measures of both receptive and expressive language that thoroughly measure *form* (phonology, morphology and syntax/grammar), *content* (semantics) and *use* (pragmatics) are critical for comprehensive measurement (Bloom & Lahey, 1978).

Auditory Hierarchy of Listening

1. Detection.
a. The presence or absence of sound representing the foundation of the auditory hierarchy of listening.
b. A listener either hears or does not hear a stimulus and responds after sound is detected; for example, drops a block during Conditioned Play Audiometry or raises a hand when sound heard.
2. Discrimination.
a. Same versus different representing the next level of the hierarchy.
b. A discrimination task might include listening to "pa pa" and being asked to state if the syllables are the same or different; listening to "pa ba" and reporting if they are same or different.
3. Recognition and Identification.
a. Recognition—listener points to picture in response to an auditorily presented sound (e.g., NU-CHIPS or WIPI).
b. Identification—listener verbally repeats back the auditorily presented word (e.g., PB-K or NU-6 word lists).
4. Comprehension.
a. Listeners respond to linguistic information and provide a response that indicates they have "understood" what has been presented, representing the highest level of auditory functioning; for example, the listener responds correctly to the question, "What is your middle name?"

Educational Audiology Issues

1. Principles of school-age children hearing screening (5–18 years).
a. Risk factors.
(1) Parent/care provider, health care provider, teacher or other school personnel having concerns regarding hearing, speech, language or learning abilities.
(2) Family history of late or delayed onset hereditary hearing loss.
(3) Recurrent or persistent otitis media with effusion for at least 3 months.
(4) Craniofacial anomalies, including those with morphological abnormalities of the pinna and EAM.
(5) Stigmata or other findings associated with a syndrome know to include SNHL and/or CHL.
(6) Head trauma with loss of consciousness.
(7) Reported exposure to potentially damaging noise levels or ototoxic drugs.
b. Clinical procedures (audiologic criteria).
(1) Conduct screening under earphones/insert phones using 1000, 2000 and 4000 Hz tones at 20 dB HL.
(2) Must pass each frequency in each ear.
(3) If child does not pass any frequency in either ear, then reinstruct, reposition phones and rescreen within the same screening session in which the child fails.
(4) Pass children who pass the rescreening.
(5) Refer children who fail the rescreening or fail to condition to the screening task.
2. Classroom acoustics.
a. Noise—presence of unwanted sound that affects the SNR (i.e., intensity of signal strength relative to background noise). Sources of noise are:
(1) Internal—within the classroom, including other students, pencil sharpeners, shuffling chairs/tables and even the HVAC systems.

(2) External—outside of the classroom, including hallway noises, outside noise from the schoolyard, etc.

b. Reverberation—"bouncing of sound waves" or echoes often due to hard surfaces of the ceiling, floor and walls.

c. Distance—distance between the sound source and listener.

3. Classroom accommodations/modifications.

a. Use of FM or infrared systems.
(1) Use boom microphone or collar microphone versus lavaliere-type setup.
(a) Decreases clothing noise.
(b) Maintains consistent signal when head turned from side to side—moving closer or farther from microphone.
(2) Use pass-around microphone for the other students to talk into so that the student has access to each talker in the room.

b. Acoustic treatment.
(1) Low ceiling and acoustic tiles.
(2) Floor carpeting.
(3) Shades or curtains on windows or other hard surfaces.

c. Small class size.

d. Teachers who are accepting, welcoming and interested in having a child with a hearing loss in their classroom.

e. Provision of increased visual cues.
(1) Posting of written schedules, assignments and class content.
(2) Use of PowerPoint, black/chalk/SMART boards; CART, CAN; C-Print.

f. Annual in-services (minimally) for the full teaching faculty and support staff, including, for example, the cafeteria staff and the teachers and aides in the "specials" such as art, music, computer, etc.

g. Preferential seating—not considered sufficient, acceptable, or appropriate solution to students with hearing differences; idea of facing the "good ear" towards the teacher for students with unilateral hearing loss should be considered adequate.

References

Bilger, R. C., Nuetzel, J. M., & Rabinowitz, W. M. (1984). Standardization of a test of speech presented in noise. *Journal of Speech and Hearing Research*, 27, 32–48.

Bloom, L., & Lahey, M. (1978). *Language Developmen and Language Disorders*. New York: Wiley.

Bowers, L., Huisingh, R., & LoGiudice, C. (2006). *The Listening Comprehension Test—2*. East Moline, IL: LinguiSystems, Inc.

Ching, T. Y. C., & Hill, M. (2007). The Parent's Evaluation of Aural/Oral Performance in Children (PEACH) Scale: Normative data. *Journal of the American Academy of Audiology*, 18, 220–235.

Ching, T. Y. C., Hill, M., & Dillon, H. (2008). Effect of variations in hearing-aid frequency response on real-life functional performance of children with severe or profound hearing loss. *International Journal of Audiology*, 47, 461–475.

Cox, R. M., & Alexander, G. C. (2002). The International Outcome Inventory for Hearing aids (IOI-HA): Psychometric properties of the English version. *International Journal of Audiology*, 41, 30–35.

Cox, R. M., & Alexander, G. C. (1995). The Abbreviated Profile of Hearing Aid Benefit. *Ear and Hearing*, 16, 176–183.

Erber, N. (1982). *Auditory Training*. Washington, DC: AG Bell Association for the Deaf and Hard of Hearing.

Killion, M. C., Niquette, P. A., Gudmundson, G. I., Revit, L. J., & Banerjee, S. (2004). Development of a quick speech-in-noise test for measuring signal-to-noise ratio loss in normal-hearing and hearing-impaired listeners. *Journal of the Acoustic Society of America*, 116, 2395–2405.

Ling, D. (1994). *Speech and the Hearing-Impaired Child: Theory and Practice*, 2nd ed. Washington, DC: AG Bell Association for the Deaf and Hard of Hearing.

Ling, D., & Ling, A. (1978). *Aural Habilitation: Foundations of Verbal Learning in Hearing-Impaired Children*. Washington, DC: AG Bell Association.

Monsen, R., Moog, J., & Geers, A. (1988). *The CID Picture SPINE—Speech Intelligibility Evaluation*. St. Louis, MO: Central Institute for the Deaf.

Moog, J., & Geers, A. (1990). *The Early Speech Perception (ESP) Test*. St. Louis, MO: Central Institute for the Deaf.

Suggested Resources

Ching, T., & Hill, M. (2005). *Teacher's Evaluation of Aural/Oral Performance of Children (TEACH)*. New South Wales, Australia: Australian Hearing.

Clark, J. G., & English, K. (2004). *Counseling in Audiologic Practice: Helping Patients and Families Adjust to Hearing Loss.* Boston, MA: Pearson.

Estabrooks, W. (Ed.) (2012). *101 Frequently Asked Questions about Auditory-Verbal Practice.* Washington, DC: AG Bell Association for the Deaf and Hard of Hearing.

Hoversten, G.H. (1977). *Test of Auditory Comprehension (TAC) for Hearing Impaired Pupils—Reliability and Validity Study.* Los Angeles, CA: Los Angeles County Superintendent of Schools.

Johnson, C. (2012). *Introduction to Auditory Rehabilitation: A Contemporary Issues Approach.* Boston, MA: Pearson.

Ling, D. (2002). *Phonetic Level Inventory/Phonologic Level Inventory.* Washington, DC; Alexander Graham Bell Association for the Deaf.

Martin, F., & Clark, J. G. (2012). *Introduction to Audiology,* 12th ed. Boston, MA: Pearson.

Moog, B., Biedenstein, J., & Davidson, L.S. (1995). *Speech Perception Instructional Curriculum and Evaluation (SPICE).* St. Louis, MO;Central Institute for the Deaf.

Seikel, J. A., King, D. W., & Drumwright, D. G. (2005). *Anatomy & Physiology for Speech, Language, and Hearing,* 3rd ed. Clifton Park, NY: Thomson.

Welling, D., & Ukstins, C. (2013). *Fundamentals of Audiology for the Speech-Language Pathologist.* Burlington, MA: Jones & Bartlett Learning.

SECTION VI

Computer Simulated Examinations

Section Outline

- **Chapter 19:** Preparing for the Speech-Language Pathology Examination, 439
- **Chapter 20:** Computer Simulated Examinations, 455

19

Preparing for the Speech-Language Pathology Examination

ZACHARY M. SMITH, M.S.

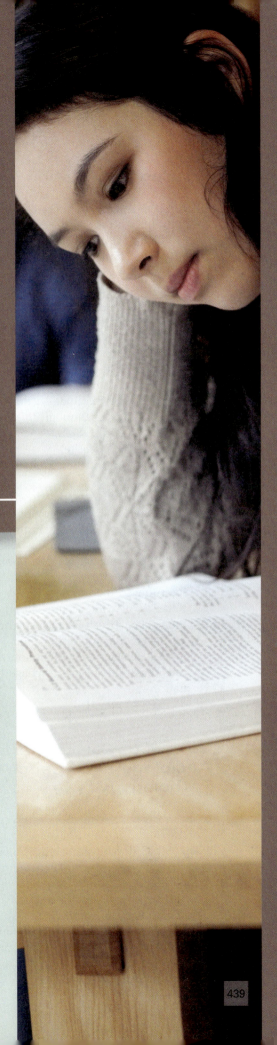

Chapter Outline

- Credentialing Agencies for Speech-Language Pathologists (SLPs), 440
- Speech-Language Pathology Examination Content and Format, 441
- Effective Examination Preparation, 442
- The Examination Day, 447
- Critical Thinking and Speech-Language Pathology Examination Performance, 449
- After the Examination, 452
- References, 454

Credentialing Agencies for Speech-Language Pathologists (SLPs)

American Speech-Language-Hearing Association (ASHA)

1. ASHA is the national professional organization for all SLPs in the United States.
   a. Holding ASHA certification, also known as the Certificate of Clinical Competence (CCC-SLP), means that the individual has met academic and professional standards and is prepared to begin practice in the field of speech-language pathology.
   b. ASHA also oversees the credentialing of audiologists and the registration of speech-language pathology assistants.
   c. SLPs may also hold ASHA membership, which entitles the individual access to large bodies of resources and information that can be helpful in clinical practice, although this is not necessary to become a certified SLP.
2. ASHA's official website (www.asha.org) posts the most current information about the certification process.
3. Additionally, ASHA works closely with Educational Testing Services (ETS) to develop and implement the Speech-Language Pathology Examination (ETS, 2014) as part of a catalog of examinations developed by ETS.
   a. The Speech-Language Pathology Examination is designed to assess graduating SLPs and those returning to the profession regarding their understanding of content and current practices within the field of speech-language pathology.
   b. To be eligible for certification (and licensure in most states), all individuals applying for their CCC must pass the Speech-Language Pathology Examination.

Council of Clinical Certification in Audiology and Speech-Language Pathology (CFCC)

1. The CFCC is the semiautonomous credentialing body of ASHA.
2. The CFCC develops and implements all policies of certification of speech-language pathologists and audiologists, including working with other agencies to develop the Speech-Language Pathology certification examination.
   a. The CFCC is charged with defining all standards related to clinical certification, granting certification to applying individuals and having sole authority to revoke certification on an as-needed basis.
   b. The CFCC grants individuals the CCC in speech-language pathology (the CCC-SLP) to those who have met all of the current standards for certification.
   c. The 2014 Standards of Certification is the most recent edition of standards that is required to be met by all individuals applying for the CCC-SLP.
      (1) Please visit http://www.asha.org/Certification/2014-Speech-Language-Pathology-Certification-Standards/ for the full 2014 Standards of Certification.

Educational Testing Services (ETS)

1. ETS is a nonprofit organization that works with ASHA to develop and implement the Speech-Language Pathology Examination.
2. ETS strives to provide fair and valid assessments in multiple areas of study, including speech-language pathology.
3. After developing the Speech-Language Pathology Examination, ETS works with the CFCC to establish an appropriate criterion score that must be reached in order to pass the exam.

State Licensure Boards

1. State licensure boards are agencies that are responsible for regulating professional activity of SLPs and for protecting the public interest. For most states, the demonstration of initial competency to enter practice is similar to the ASHA CCC-SLP requirements: graduate degree, passing Speech-Language Pathology Examination score, completion of 9-month fellowship.
2. It is important to note that some states do vary from ASHA standards. A list of current specific contacts for state licensing agencies can be found at www.asha.org/advocacy/state/.
   a. Once individuals have shown that they meet the state's standards, they are granted state licensure and are able to practice within their applying state.
3. Some states grant temporary licenses to those who are applying for permanent licensure and who hold permanent licensure from another state.
4. In many states, holders of the CCC-SLP are eligible for licensure and demonstration of other state requirements is unnecessary.

Speech-Language Pathology Examination Content and Format

Background

1. Speech-language pathology practice analysis.
   a. ASHA conducts a periodic SLP practice analysis (every 5–7 years), in order to determine "on the job" tasks for speech-language pathologists and to identify any emerging trends or other changes in the practice landscape.
   b. The analyses include large-scale surveys of practitioners, educators, clinical supervisors and clinic directors.
   c. The results of the surveys provide information on the knowledge, skills and abilities needed to be an independent practicing speech-language pathologist.
2. CFCC and practice analysis results.
   a. Based on the results of the SLP practice analysis, along with other information from within the field of speech-language pathology, the CFCC receives recommendations of change for the current standards of certification.
   b. The newly published standards of certification include information about requirements for the Speech-Language Pathology Examination.
3. Item development.
   a. The blueprint for the Speech-Language Pathology Examination is derived from the newly released standards for certification, which directly reflect the SLP practice analysis.
   b. Studies are periodically conducted to determine the validity of specific questions and their relevance to new clinicians.
      (1) These studies also determine the number of questions that a candidate must answer correctly, in order to achieve a passing score.
      (2) The CFCC uses the results of these studies to determine the final passing score criterion.
   c. From the results of all previously mentioned studies, ASHA proposes content areas for the Speech-Language Pathology Examination, and examination committees work with ETS to develop the examinations.
      (1) The examination committees are made up from ASHA-certified speech-language pathology members who work to develop questions.

Speech-Language Pathology Examination Content

1. Practice domains.
   a. The Speech-Language Pathology Examination comprises three domains of speech-language pathology practice, with each comprising a preset percentage of the exam. As of September 2014, these domains[1] are:
   (1) Foundations and Professional Practice, 44 questions.
      (a) Foundations.
         • Typical development and performance across the lifespan.
         • Factors that influence communication, feeding and swallowing.
      (b) Professional practice.
         • Wellness and prevention.
         • Culturally and linguistically appropriate service delivery.
         • Counseling, collaboration and teaming.
         • Documentation.
         • Ethics.
         • Legislation and client advocacy.
         • Research methodology and evidence-based practice.
   (2) Screening, Assessment, Evaluation and Diagnosis, 44 questions.
      (a) Screening.
         • Communication disorders.
         • Feeding and swallowing disorders.
      (b) Approaches to assessment and evaluation.
         • Developing case histories.
         • Selecting appropriate assessment instruments, procedures and materials.
         • Assessing factors that influence communication and swallowing disorders.
         • Assessment of anatomy and physiology.
         • Referrals.
      (c) Assessment procedures and assessment.
         • Speech sound production.
         • Fluency.
         • Voice, resonance and motor speech.
         • Receptive and expressive language.
         • Social aspects of communication, including pragmatics.
         • Cognitive aspects of communication.
         • Augmentative and alternative communication.
         • Hearing.
         • Feeding and swallowing.
      (d) Etiology.
         • Genetic.
         • Developmental.

---

[1] Information courtesy of American Speech-Language-Hearing Association (2014). Speech-Language Pathology Exam (5331) Content. Published online. Retrieved from: www.asha.org/Certification/praxis/Speech-Language-Pathology-Exam-5331-Content/.

- Disease processes.
- Auditory problems.
- Neurological.
- Structural and functional.
- Psychogenic.

(3) Planning, Implementation and Evaluation of Treatment, 44 questions.
  (a) Treatment planning.
   - Evaluating factors that can affect treatment.
   - Initiating and prioritizing treatment and developing goals.
   - Determining appropriate treatment details.
   - Generating a prognosis.
   - Communicating recommendations.
   - General treatment principles and procedures.
  (b) Treatment evaluation.
   - Establishing methods for monitoring treatment progress and outcomes to evaluate assessment and/or treatment plans.
   - Follow-up on posttreatment referrals and recommendations.
  (c) Treatment.
   - Speech sound production.
   - Fluency.
   - Voice, resonance and motor speech.
   - Receptive and expressive language.
   - Social aspects of communication, including pragmatics.
   - Communication impairments related to cognition.
   - Treatment involving augmentative and alternative communication.
   - Hearing and aural rehabilitation.
   - Swallowing and feeding.

Speech-Language Pathology Examination Format

1. According to the Speech-Language Pathology Examination Study Companion (ETS, 2014), the Speech-Language Pathology Examination consists of 132 selected response questions.
2. Selected response.
   a. Selected response questions require the test taker to select one or more choices from a field of given answers.
      (1) Multiple choice (MC) questions.
      (2) Checking more than one oval.
      (3) Clicking check boxes.
   b. Selected response questions often contain the phrase "which of the following" embedded somewhere in the question.
   c. There are selected response questions that include the words *not*, *least* and *except*.
      (1) When selected response contains one of these words, the examinee must select the answer that does not belong.
      (2) Reading these questions carefully is important to answering correctly.
   d. If a selected response includes graphs or images (i.e., audiograms, spectrograms, etc.), it is important to provide information pertinent only to the question being asked.

Effective Examination Preparation

Overview and General Guidelines

1. The Speech-Language Pathology Examination measures knowledge important for independent practice as a certified speech-language pathologist in a variety of different settings.
   a. There are four levels of objective examination questions, summarized in Table 19-1.
2. The ability to critically and clinically reason and evaluate questions is a skill necessary for success on the Speech-Language Pathology Examination.
   a. Table 19-2 summarizes types of critical reasoning to use during the Speech-Language Pathology Examination.

Psychological Outlook

1. Psychological outlook is an important factor for success when preparing and taking a professional examination.
   a. Positive outlook is a necessary foundation for effective studying and test taking, as it puts exam candidates in a mind-set for success.
      (1) Use previous successful academic and clinical experiences to bolster confidence in being prepared for the exam.
      (2) Discuss areas of strength and areas that might benefit from additional study time with professors, clinical supervisors and classmates. This feedback can provide a realistic picture that can build confidence.

Table 19-1

Levels of Examination Questions

QUESTION LEVEL AND DESCRIPTION	RELEVANCE TO SPEECH-LANGUAGE PATHOLOGY EXAMINATION	SPEECH-LANGUAGE PATHOLOGY EXAMINATION PREPARATION STRATEGY
1. **Knowledge** Recall of basic information.	A solid knowledge foundation of all information related to entry-level SLP practice is required to answer practice scenario items. It is highly likely that little to no items on the Speech-Language Pathology exam are solely at this level.	A strong commitment to studying is needed to remember all the information acquired during your SLP education. Fortunately, this text provides extensive information in an outline format to ease your review. Memorization of this information is required to be able to readily recall it during the 132 questions on the Speech-Language Pathology exam.
2. **Comprehension** Understanding of information to determine significance, consequences or implications.	The Speech-Language Pathology exam is not a matching column type of test; therefore, you cannot just recall information to be able to succeed on this exam. You must fully understand the content area to be able to understand the nuances of an exam item. A few items on the Speech-Language Pathology exam may be at this level.	When studying the text to review basic content and acquire your foundational knowledge, ask yourself how and why this fundamental information is important. Studying with a peer or a study group can provide you with additional insights about the relevance, significance, consequences and implications of the information. Do not enter the exam without strong comprehension of all major areas of SLP practice.
3. **Application** Use of information and application of rules, procedures, or theories to new situations.	The Speech-Language Pathology exam requires you to use your knowledge and comprehension as described above, along with the competencies you developed during your clinical placements, in a manner that best fits the specific practice scenario in an exam item. Many items from the Speech-Language Pathology exam are at this level, for a main goal of the exam is to assess your ability to respond competently to different situations.	Once you have acquired a solid knowledge base and good comprehension skills in all domains of SLP as put forth in this text, you should take practice Speech-Language Pathology exams. This type of exam requires you to apply your knowledge in a manner similar to the Speech-Language Pathology exam. Upon completion of these exams, you should analyze your performance, so that you can determine how well you are applying your knowledge.
4. **Analysis** Recognition of interrelationships between principles and interpretation or evaluation of data presented.	The Speech-Language Pathology exam assumes that you have mastered and comprehend entry-level knowledge, and that you can competently apply this information to diverse situations; therefore, it will ask you to analyze and respond to ambiguous, not "straight from the book" situations. Many items from the Speech-Language Pathology exam are also at this level, to determine your ability to be competent in complex practice situations.	Use the analyses of practice exams described above to reflect on your reasoning mistakes. Critically review the extensive rationales provided in this text for the correct exam answers. Reflecting with a peer or study group can be helpful in determining your gaps in analysis of exam items. Review the text's section on critical thinking skills and reflect on the questions provided in Table 1-5 to ascertain the actions you need to take to adequately prepare for the complexities of the Speech-Language Pathology exam.

Reference: Fleming-Castaldy, R.P. & Inda, K. (2014). "Effective *examination preparation*" in R. Fleming-Castaldy, National Occupational Therapy Certification Exam. *Review and Study Guide*, 7th ed. Evanston, IL: TherapyEd.

b. Doubt and negative outlook can be detrimental to performance on the Speech-Language Pathology Examination.
   (1) If developing a positive outlook may be difficult, be sure to access others who can be supportive and encouraging.
   (2) Keeping one's "eyes on the prize" of becoming a licensed and certified speech-language pathologist can help keep work and studying at the forefront and can help manage fear and anxiety.
c. If a previous attempt at taking the Speech-Language Pathology Examination was not successful, critique previous performance, including studying habits and methods, to evaluate the source of difficulty.
   (1) Knowing specific deficiencies in content or clinical reasoning/problem solving can be critical to improvement on the next test.
d. Table 19-3 summarizes psychological outlook and its relationship to success with the Speech-Language Pathology Examination.

Reviewing Professional Education

1. Establish current knowledge and skill level.
   a. The chapters of this review guide will help establish a plan of action for studying all pertinent aspects within the scope of SLP practice.
      (1) While proceeding through the chapters, make a "knowledge scale" consisting of: (1) know very well, (2) know adequately, (3) know little and (4) know nothing.

Table 19-2
Critical Reasoning Applied to Speech-Language Pathology Exam Items

TYPE OF REASONING	QUESTIONS TO CONSIDER	RELATIONSHIP TO EXAM SUCCESS
Procedural Reasoning Requires the systematic gathering and interpreting of data to identify problems, set goals, plan intervention and implement treatment strategies. It is the "doing" of practice.	What does the exam item tell/ask you about: Diagnosis? Symptoms? Prognosis? Assessment methods? Treatment protocols? Theories/practice frameworks to support procedures?	Correct answers on the Speech-Language Pathology exam will be consistent with the published evaluation standards and intervention protocols for a given clinical condition and congruent with established theories and relevant practice framework.
Interactive Reasoning Focuses on the client as a person and involves the therapeutic relationships between the practitioner, the individual, caregivers and significant others.	What does the exam item tell/ask you about: Rapport building? Family/caregiver involvement? Therapeutic use of self? Teaching/learning styles? Successful collaboration?	Correct answers on the Speech-Language Pathology exam will have the therapist engaging with the person, family, caregivers and others in an empathic, caring, respectful, collaborative and empowering manner.
Pragmatic Reasoning Considers the context(s) of service delivery, including the person's situation and the practice environment to identify the real possibilities for a person in a given setting.	What does the exam item tell/ask you about: Person's client factors? Practice setting characteristics? Reimbursement issues? Legal parameters? Referral options?	Correct answers on the Speech-Language Pathology exam will be realistic given the person's assets and limitations, his/her environmental supports and barriers and the practice setting's inherent opportunities or constraints.
Conditional Reasoning Represents an integration of procedural, interactive and pragmatic reasoning in the context of the client's narrative.[1] Focuses on past, current, and possible future social contexts.	What does the exam item tell/ask you about: The individual's unique roles, values, goals? Impact of illness on this person's function? How will the condition's course influence the person's future? Where the person will be able to live after discharge?	Correct answers on the Speech-Language Pathology exam will take into account all case information that is provided in the item scenario. Speech-Language Pathology exam items do not include extraneous details, so carefully reflect on the relevance of the information provided in each item scenario to determine the best answer.

Reference: Fleming-Castaldy, R.P., & Inda, K. (2014). "Effective examination preparation" In R. Fleming-Castaldy in R. Fleming-Castaldy, National Occupational Therapy Certification Exam. Review and Study Guide, 7th ed. Evanston, IL: TherapyEd.

[1] The application of narrative reasoning is not likely required during the Speech-Language Pathology exam, since this type of reasoning deals with the individual's speech-language story and uses critical imagination to help the person reach an imagined future. This important process is not readily measured by objective exam questions.

(a) Focus studying efforts on the content that falls toward the "know nothing" end of the scale to solidify knowledge in all content areas.

b. Using clinical reasoning skills gained during clinical placements will help navigate the questions posed on the Speech-Language Pathology Examination.
  (1) As of 2014, the Speech-Language Pathology Examination features changes in the format of questions, and the questions are structured to test clinical reasoning as well as a factual knowledge base.

c. Review coursework history in order to establish strengths and weaknesses.
  (1) Knowing which aspects of SLP practice that have been most challenging will determine a place to begin studying.

2. Establish a study plan of action.
  a. Items rated as "know little" or "know nothing" from the previously mentioned knowledge scale will become the most pertinent items for critical studying.
  b. Items rated as "know very well" or "know adequately" from the knowledge scale will become the items that require more review than critical study.
    (1) For example, if one has a strong knowledge base of assessment of the different disorders treated under the SLP's scope of practice, but has difficulty making goals or providing appropriate intervention approaches, one's studying may focus on intervention methods across disorders (i.e., treatment of speech sound disorders or adult acquired language disorders).
    (2) Finding trends throughout the chapters will help draw conclusions and provide an integrative learning experience that will prove to be invaluable in preparation for the exam.
  c. Remember that the Speech-Language Pathology Examination encompasses three distinct areas of practice equally, so be prepared to spend equal amounts of time studying each area.
    (1) Foundations and Professional Practice.
    (2) Screening, Assessment, Evaluation and Diagnosis.

Table 19-3
Psychological Outlook and the Speech-Language Pathology Exam

CONCEPT	PRINCIPLE	ACTIONS
Control	Only you can determine your future.	• Take charge; determine exactly what is needed to succeed. • Set goals to meet these needs. • Develop and implement concrete plans to succeed.
Self-Awareness	Knowing your innate capabilities enables you to build on strengths and effectively deal with limitations.	• Critically analyze test-taking errors and content knowledge gaps. • Be honest about your test-taking and content knowledge, strengths and limitations. • Avoid self-defeatist behavior.
Self-Confidence	Your past accomplishments provide a solid foundation for future success.	• Review exam content prior to completing practice exams. • Use a diversity of learning methods to achieve mastery. • Recognize and celebrate your successes and achievements.
Self-fulfilling Prophecy	Your self-expectancy will influence the outcomes of your efforts.	• Expect success. • Use positive self-talk throughout exam preparation. • Continue to think positively during the exam administration.
Self-Esteem	You are a person capable of excellence.	• Remember your personal and academic achievements. • SLP academic coursework and fieldwork are demanding; give yourself well-earned credit for your success.
Motivation	Your desire to succeed and a fear of failure can be channeled for success.	• Understand that the early stages of studying will have uncertain results. • Remind yourself of what initially motivated you to pursue a career as an SLP. • Harness fear and establish a doable study plan.
Courage	Taking responsibility for one's failures is key to success.	• Honestly critique precipitators/reasons for an exam failure. • Do not make excuses. • Do not strive for perfection.
Perseverance	You can only succeed if you persevere.	• Reestablish goals. • Seek support for goal attainment. • Utilize multiple resources to stay on track.
Freedom	You can freely choose your attitude.	• View test taking as an opportunity. • Keep your "eyes on the prize." • Exam success equates the achievement of your goal to become an SLP practitioner.

Reference: Fleming-Castaldy, R.P. & Inda, K. (2014). "Effective examination preparation" in R. Fleming-Castaldy, National Occupational Therapy Certification Exam. Review and Study Guide, 7th ed. Evanston, IL: TherapyEd.

---

      (3) Planning, Implementation and Evaluation of Treatment.
  d. Allow adequate time to prepare for the test, taking into account strengths and weaknesses as an exam taker.
      (1) Determine the appropriate time during graduate education to begin studying in order to achieve mastery of all material, including those that fall under the knowing nothing category.
      (2) Be aware of any constraints as a test taker (i.e., difficulty memorizing information, difficulty parsing out the important information to study, etc.) and make schedule adjustments accordingly.
  e. Assess study habits formed during professional program schooling and choose a route that is most effective.
  f. Create a strict study plan and follow through. Some study tips are as follows:
      (1) Study one major content area per session. This can include studying one of the comprehensive chapters in this book.
      (2) Limit any possible interruptions.
          (a) Turn off any electronics that are not essential to studying.
          (b) Parents/caregivers should make sure to arrange for help to allow ample opportunity to study without distraction.
          (c) Do not study by a computer or other devices, unless Internet restrictions for distracting websites can be enabled.
      (3) If something occurs that forces deviation from study schedules, immediately make an attempt to reschedule study time to make up for lost time.
3. Do not take any practice exams until adequate preparation has occurred, which entails following study plans and focusing on weak knowledge areas.
  a. Completing a practice exam before having adequately studied all areas of exam content will rein-

Table 19-4

Personalities of Test Takers

PERSONALITY TYPE	CHARACTERISTICS	ACTIONS
The Rusher	• Impatient. • Jumps to conclusions. • Skips key words. • Inadequate consideration of exam items.	• Take practice exams in a timed manner to establish a nondesperate pace and help realize that the time allotted for the exam is sufficient. • Use positive self-talk and relaxation techniques during the exam. • Employ the strategies provided in Tables 19-5 and 19-6 to slow your pace and not make the errors that are endemic to rushing.
The Turtle	• Overly slow and methodical. • Over attention to extraneous detail. • Reads and rereads exam items' details. • Misses the theme of exam items.	• Take practice exams in a timed manner to establish the pace of completing practice Speech-Language Pathology exams in 150 minutes, which is the amount of time given during the real examination. • Study in bullet format. • Use the strategies in Tables 19-5 and 19-6 to identify each item's focus and select the best answer, and then move on to the next item.
Squisher/Procrastinator	• Puts things off. • Does not reschedule missed study time. • Mastery of exam content is not attained and major knowledge gaps remain.	• Focus on developing a step-by-step plan. • Dig in and get started. • Adopt a "no excuses" attitude. • Join a study group or work with a study partner to stay on track.
Philosopher	• Is a thoughtful, talented, intelligent, and disciplined student. • Excels in essay questions. • Over analyzes and reads into exam items. • Wants to know everything and answer everything about the topic. • Overapplies clinical knowledge.	• Study in bullet, not paragraph, form. • Focus only on the exam item. • Look for simple, straightforward answers. • Remind yourself that your "job" on the exam is to select the best answer for the question posed, not to address all possible aspects of an item's scenario. • Apply the strategies provided in Table 1-5 and 1-6 to stay focused on answering each item as it is presented.
Lawyer	• Is a thoughtful, talented, intelligent, and disciplined student. • Picks out some bit of information and builds a case on that. • Reads into exam items to make a case for a preferred answer instead of determining what the question is asking.	• Focus on what the exam item is asking, and only what the exam item is asking. • Remind yourself that your "job" is to pass the Speech-Language Pathology exam, not to prove a point. • Remember that you can train to be a Speech-Language Pathology exam item writer and write "better" exam items after you pass the exam.

Second-Guesser	• Often a philosopher who reads into an item.
	• Frequently looks at the exam item from every angle.
	• Keeps changing answers, increasing anxiety, thinking less clearly and then changing answers more rapidly.
		• Apply a "lightbulb" strategy.
		  o Identify a good reason to reject your first answer (i.e., missing a key word).
		  o Identify a good reason to select a new answer (i.e., obtaining a solid hint from a subsequent exam item).
		• If you do not experience a lightbulb moment, do not change your answer.

Reference: Fleming-Castaldy, R.P. & Inda, K. (2014). "Effective examination preparation" in R. Fleming-Castaldy, National Occupational Therapy Certification Exam: Review & Study Guide, 7th ed. Evanston, IL: TherapyEd.

---

force feelings of fear and anxiety by demonstrating that continued gaps in knowledge exist.
  b. Completing a practice exam after having adequately studied the content areas will allow demonstration of the amount of knowledge gained while studying.
    (1) Taking practice exams at this point in studying will enforce feelings of confidence and self-esteem in knowledge of the material that a practicing SLP would encounter.
    (2) This will also give an opportunity to discover which areas of exam content may continue to be difficult and allow more time to focus on this material.

4. Using the practice exams that accompany this book can assist in determining a test-taking personality.
  a. Knowledge of test-taking personalities helps identify particular characteristics and strategies to aid in studying and test taking (Table 19-4).
5. It is important to take practice exams within the allotted time that would be given during the actual Speech-Language Pathology Examination Exam.
  a. This will allow practice with the visual, psychological and cognitive demands that come with taking an extended standardized test and becoming comfortable with them.

b. Practicing the test-taking strategies presented in this chapter during practice exams will help with generalization of skills to the real Speech-Language Pathology Examination.
6. Do not try to memorize any specific question that appears on any practice item used. Use questions to help assess knowledge.
   a. It is most important to review information and become comfortable with the structure of exam questions.

Key Preparation Resources

1. Effective preparation for the Speech-Language Pathology Examination requires understanding of two components to exam success: adequate content knowledge and effective test-taking skills.
2. This *Review and Study Guide* has been designed as a knowledge resource for individuals studying for the Speech-Language Pathology Examination and is a comprehensive compilation of information to help test takers succeed on the Speech-Language Pathology Examination and as a practicing SLP.
   a. The chapter authors are leading professionals in their respective areas of the field and draw from foundational textbooks and important research findings to form their chapters.
   b. Referring to the reference lists associated with each chapter may provide advanced knowledge of areas of SLP practice with which there may be weakness.
3. Reaching out to fellow students can prove to be a valuable resource.
   a. Forming study groups can help fill in gaps in knowledge for all members.
   b. Fellow students and friends can also serve as a psychological support, in the event that fear and anxiety surrounding the exam escalate.
4. Consulting academic and clinical resources, including professors and clinical supervisors, can help fill in gaps in knowledge from individuals who are experts in the field.
   a. Both professors and supervisors care about student clinicians' well-being and success within the field and have advanced knowledge of the content required for a successful career as an SLP.

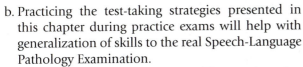

The Examination Day

Prepreparation and Planning

1. Be prepared physically and mentally.
   a. Get a good night's sleep prior to the Speech-Language Pathology Examination.
   b. Eat a well-balanced breakfast the morning of the Speech-Language Pathology Examination.
   c. Although coffee and tea may aid long nights of studying during professional programs, avoid too much caffeine prior to the test.
   d. Wear appropriate clothing for warm or cold testing centers, and make sure to wear layered clothing that can be changed easily (i.e., long sleeves that can easily be rolled up in the event that the temperature raises in the testing center).
      (1) Keep in mind that the time allotted for the test remains the same and is not paused for clothing adjustments.
   e. Make sure to use the restroom before entering the test room.
2. Be prepared emotionally.
   a. Before taking the exam, make sure to recall successes made throughout studying for the Speech-Language Pathology Examination.
      (1) This will enforce a positive mind-set before entering the testing center.
   b. Make sure to arrive early, to minimize any anxiety that could occur from potentially being late.
   c. Think about going to the testing center before the actual exam day, so routes are able to be mapped, including potential conflicts with public transportation, traffic, etc.
3. If something arises before the exam that requires cancellation of a test date, make sure to follow the procedures for cancellation outlined on the ETS website.

Test Center Procedures

1. Make sure to arrive at the test center at least 30 minutes prior to the start of the exam to allow ample time for check-in.
   a. Examination candidates that are late to the testing center may NOT be allowed into the exam and will have to forfeit any and all registration fees paid.
   b. Be aware that sometimes inclement weather or other conditions may cause a delay or cancellation of an exam time.

2. Before entering the testing center, the confidentiality agreement supplied by ETS must be signed.
   a. If the confidentiality agreement is not signed, entrance into the testing center will be denied and registration fees will not be refunded.
3. In order to sign in, a valid form of government-issued identification must be shown (see below for examples).
   a. The ID supplied must contain the examination candidate's name, picture and signature.
      (1) The name and signature used needs to match the name used when registering for the Speech-Language Pathology Examination.
         (a) Individuals who have a two-part last name or whose name has changed from the time they registered for the exam, will still need to provide a form of ID that matches the registration name.
         (b) If the form of ID does not contain a signature, it must be signed, or a supplemental form of ID must be produced as well.
   b. All documents and forms of identification used must be original and not expired.
      (1) No copies of any form of identification will be accepted by the testing center.
   c. If an acceptable form of ID is not brought, entrance to the testing center will be denied.
      (1) Acceptable forms of ID include:
         (a) Passport.
         (b) Valid, government-issued driver's license.
         (c) State or province ID provided by a motor vehicle registry.
         (d) National ID.
         (e) Military ID.
4. It is important to recognize that certain items are not allowed inside the testing center under any circumstance.
   a. Cell phones, smart phones, electronic watches, recording devices, scanning devices and photography equipment are not allowed, and if brought into the testing center, the examination candidate risks being released from the testing center with no refund of registration fee.
   b. Do not bring pencils, erasers or scrap paper, as these will be supplied at the testing center.
   c. The items that should be brought include:
      (1) An admissions ticket.
      (2) A valid form of ID.
      (3) Any health-related equipment needed.
         (a) Permission from respective testing centers needs to be received in order to bring such equipment.
   d. A locker will be supplied by the testing center to store personal items. Before entering the testing room, a search for banned personal items may be conducted.
      (1) Personal items may not be accessed at any point during the test or on any breaks.
5. Before starting the exam, a 30-minute practice time period will be given to allow examination candidates time to become familiar with the computer system.
   a. This practice period is designed to make sure that the exam moves smoothly.
   b. Scratch paper is not allowed during the practice time period.
6. During the exam, if any computer-related difficulties are experienced, testing center policy dictates that examination candidates raise their hand for a testing center employee's assistance.

Examination Time and Time Keeping

1. There are 150 minutes allotted to complete the Speech-Language Pathology Examination.
   a. There is an on-screen clock that will keep track of time as examination candidates continue through the exam.
   b. Although there is an on-screen clock, it is up to the examination candidates to keep their own pace.
      (1) The test is taken as a whole and is not broken into sections. As such, it is important to keep a steady pace throughout the exam.
      (2) If questions that are particularly difficult are encountered, it may be beneficial to move on to other questions in an attempt to answer as many questions as possible.
         (a) Remember, only questions that are answered correctly are counted toward the raw score, so the more questions that are answered, the more likely the raw score will grow.
   c. Allow a per question time limit, and stick to it, in order to continue to move through the exam at an appropriate pace.

Question Answering Strategies

1. Table 19-5 suggests general strategies for answering the questions that may be encountered while taking the Speech-Language Pathology Examination.
2. Table 19-6 suggests specific strategies for answering selected response questions on the Speech-Language Pathology Examination.
   a. These types of questions make up the bulk of the exam, so it is important to internalize these strategies!

Table 19-5

General Strategies for Answering Speech-Language Pathology Examination Questions

- Read the exam item carefully before selecting a response to the question posed.
- Employ relevant clinical experience.
  - Remember trends and consistent cases in your experience.
  - Do not call on unusual cases or atypical presentations.
- Read the exam item for key words that set a priority (e.g., pain, acute care, etc.).
- Apply clinical reasoning skills to determine the relevance of item info (i.e., diagnosis, setting, intervention and theoretical principles).
- Use your knowledge of medical terminology to decipher unknown terms by applying the meaning of known prefixes, suffixes, and root words.
- Select responses that most closely reflect the fundamental tenets of SLP (e.g., ethical actions, the use of functional communication).
- Choose client-centered, person-directed actions.
- Identify choices that focus on the emotional well-being of the person.
- Use your clinical judgment to support the best answer.
- Check your answer to see if it is:
  - Theoretically consistent with the exam scenario.
  - Diagnostically consistent with the exam scenario.
  - Developmentally consistent with the exam scenario.
- Eliminate choices that contain contraindications, as these must be incorrect.
- Consider eliminating options that state "always," "never," "all" or "only," as there are few absolutes in SLP practice.
- Eliminate unsafe options.
- Choose answers that reflect entry-level SLP practice.
- Remember the Speech-Language Pathology Examination is not a specialty certification exam.

Table 19-6

Specific Strategies for Answering Selected Response Questions

- Identify the theme of the selected response questions. Ask yourself, "What is the question posed REALLY asking?"
- Avoid "reading into" the selected response item. Read the question asked and nothing but the question.
- Identify choices that seem similar or equally plausible.
  - If two choices basically say the same thing, or use synonyms in their answers, both cannot be right; therefore, both can be eliminated.
- Carefully consider choices that are opposites of one another. If you cannot eliminate both opposites right away, one may be the correct answer.
- Determine the best answer using strategies identified in Table 19-5.
  - More than one answer may be "correct." Choose the one that is MOST correct.
- Select positive, active choices rather than passive, negative ones.
- Before changing an answer, make sure that you have a good reason to eliminate your original choice and a good reason to make your new choice.
  - Good reasons include realizing that you missed the theme or a key word (e.g., screening) of the exam item or you gained a clue from subsequent exam item (e.g., areas of the brain).
- Do not let second-guessing talk you out of the correct answer.

Critical Thinking and Speech-Language Pathology Examination Performance

Critical Thinking and the Speech-Language Pathology Examination

1. *Critical thinking* can be thought of as a process of evaluating and analyzing situations by drawing strengths from a person's knowledge, skills, experiences and objective logic in order to form reasonable conclusions.
   a. Critical thinking can be thought of as encompassing a variety of subskills, including:
      (1) Analysis.
      (2) Inference.
      (3) Evaluation.
      (4) Explanation.
      (5) Self-examination.
      (6) Self-correction.
2. Being able to think critically is a skill that is absolutely necessary for success on the Speech-Language Pathology Examination.
   a. The Speech-Language Pathology Examination does not simply test one's ability to reproduce information printed in a textbook or taught in lecture.
   b. Questions on the Speech-Language Pathology Examination require a strong knowledge foundation, but the ability to critically think, from the perspective

of a future speech and language clinician, can help examination candidates arrive at appropriate answers in an organized fashion.
   c. The Speech-Language Pathology Examination integrates the knowledge, skills and critical-thinking behaviors necessary for success as an entry-level SLP.
3. Because critical-thinking skills are employed on a daily basis as an SLP, it is important that these skills begin to be used long before taking the Speech-Language Pathology Examination.
   a. Most of the exam questions on the Speech-Language Pathology Examination are designed to be contextualized to the work an SLP would perform while in the field, which necessitates critical thinking in order to answer appropriately.
   b. Graduate academic and clinical work in speech-language pathology have started the foundation of critical-thinking skills, and it is important to draw from these experiences while studying for and during the Speech-Language Pathology Examination.

Analysis

1. *Analysis* is the ability to identify both the intended and actual relationships between concepts, facts, questions and descriptions of statements, beliefs, etc.
   a. This skill helps one examine concepts and the relationships between them.
2. Analysis is used in SLP practice through interpreting assessment results, reviewing case history information to retrieve important information (i.e., number of words spoken by a child, presenting medical illness for an adult) and to formulate a diagnosis for clients (i.e., Broca's aphasia, language disorder, etc.).
3. Analysis is required while answering many questions presented on the Speech-Language Pathology Examination.
   a. Information presented in graphs, charts or tables will mandate some form of analysis in order to correctly interpret information and determine its meaning.
4. Questions that tap an examination candidate's analysis skills can seem frustrating, due to potential lack of information. However, this closely simulates what a practicing SLP may encounter, as that SLP is rarely given a complete picture of the person(s) with whom they work.

Inference

1. *Inference* is the ability to identify and secure elements needed to draw reasonable conclusions, for hypotheses, consider relevant information and to form conclusions from data, statements, etc.
   a. This skill utilizes a specific knowledge base to make reasonable assumptions about new information.
2. Inference in used in SLP practice during assessment selection and when therapists infer potential client/patient symptoms based on limited information.
   a. For example, a note dictates that a new client does not make all of their sounds correctly, possibly necessitating the selection of an articulation/phonology assessment battery.
   b. As another example, while reviewing a patient's medical chart, the therapist notices "left MCA stroke," which leads them to infer the presence of aphasia.
3. Inference is also used in SLP practice in determining the best possible route of intervention for particular clients.
   a. Although all inferences should be based in some form of knowledge, they are not guaranteed to be 100% accurate. For example, when treating a child with a phonological disorder, the therapist cannot be certain that cycles approach would lead to the greatest gains for that child. For this reason, inference must utilize a clinician's knowledge and experience.
4. Because inference is regularly used in SLP practice and decision-making, it makes sense that this skill is important for success on the Speech-Language Pathology Examination.
   a. There are questions that prompt the examination candidate to determine likely presentations of disorders or appropriate approaches to treatment/intervention require inferential reasoning.
   b. Inference should be used cautiously when answering Speech-Language Pathology Examination questions because, if the information presented has not been considered appropriately or logically, an incorrect answer could be selected.
5. As inference is used frequently in daily SLP practice, it is not surprising that many of the Speech-Language Pathology Examination question require some level of inference.

Evaluation

1. *Evaluation* is the ability to assess the credibility of statements that represent a person's perceptions,

experience and judgment, as well as the ability to assess the logical strength of the relationship between statements, descriptions and questions.
   a. Evaluation aids in deciding whether or not a conclusion is valid, based on the facts presented.
2. Evaluation is used in SLP practice when difficult decisions need to be made, and there is no obvious answer or approach to use.
   a. In SLP practice, evaluation should be a conscious process to determine the trustworthiness of information used in generating a course of action.
      (1) Evaluation should be approached cautiously, as assigning too much value to information that has little relevance to a present case can lead to unintended consequences.
   b. Being able to assess the validity of research, in order to provide the best evidence-based practice (EBP) is something that requires keen evaluative skills.
   c. Situations that arise while in the field can be ambiguous and require a SLP to weigh sources of information for reliability, validity and applicability to the current situation in order to achieve the best result.
      (1) For example, while working with a patient who has a pulmonary disorder to improve swallowing endurance, the patient begins to experience shortness of breath. The clinician must evaluate whether or not to alert the patient's nurse.
3. Evaluation is required when answering questions on the Speech-Language Pathology Examination that deal with ethical dilemmas or when evaluating statements posed by research.
   a. In studying for the Speech-Language Pathology Examination, it helps to familiarize oneself with the evaluative process and practice evaluating statements made in research articles and case studies.

Explanation

1. An *explanation* states the results of the process of critical thinking in a way that justifies the reasoning used in reaching a conclusion.
   a. An explanation interprets results based on the information that was gathered to reach a conclusion.
2. Explanation is used in SLP practice when reaching a decision about a client's diagnosis using given information, when definitively explain why a particular treatment approach may prove to be beneficial and while advocating for the populations that SLPs serve.
   a. Explanation relies on solid foundational knowledge and skills, including knowledge of effects of diseases/deficits/disorders, the implications of treatment processes and the effect of communication and swallowing disorders on the quality of life affecting clients and patients.
3. Explanation on the Speech-Language Pathology Examination comes in the form of selecting the appropriate answer or answers for questions.
   a. Although there is no "check-box" in real situations, the check-box scenario found in the Speech-Language Pathology Examination directly assesses an examination candidate's explanation ability. By selecting the correct answers, a capacity for explanation has been shown.

Self-Examination

1. *Self-examination* is the ability to consciously reflect on previous occurrences in order to determine areas or acts of strengths in performance while also being able to interpret areas in which one could use improvement and why these could be improved.
2. Self-examination is typically used in SLP practice after assessment or treatment has been completed, in order to properly assess what behaviors have or have not been successful in that SLP's interactions with their clients.
   a. Engaging in self-examination after missteps in client interactions is important, because it allows the SLP to identify what behaviors caused the problem and how to effectively remedy these problems moving forward.
   b. Engaging in self-examination after successes is just as important for the therapist/client relationship, as it allows the SLP to determine what works well for particular clients in order to maximize their gains seen in treatment.
3. While the Speech-Language Pathology Examination may pose questions asking about changes to interaction style or therapy approach, it is likely that this skill is not going to feature prominently on the exam itself.
   a. The skill of self-examination is important during the study period for the Speech-Language Pathology Examination. If the amount of gains made during studying is not ideal, it is important to reflect on what is causing this, in order to make appropriate changes.
      (1) This is a continuing process throughout the time spent preparing for the Speech-Language Pathology Examination, as new problems may spring up farther down the road of studying.

Self-Correction

1. Using all of the other areas of critical thinking, self-correction allows a person to change his or her behavior for future occurrences that are similar in nature to a preceding event (i.e., future therapy session, future evaluations, etc.).
2. Self-correction is used in SLP practice after having engaged in self-examination so that one may move forward with appropriate changes.
   a. For example, perhaps an SLP's instructions or cueing was not effective during a particular session. After engaging in self-examination, that SLP can determine an appropriate correction in behavior in order to maximize the client's potential.
      (1) Invoking this change in behavior engages the SLP's self-correction abilities.
3. While self-correction can often be employed as a working SLP, this is a subskill of critical thinking that may not be employed as readily during the Speech-Language Pathology Examination.
   a. Because of the time limits during the administration of the Speech-Language Pathology Examination, it is important to work efficiently and to utilize self-correction only on an as-needed basis.

Developing Critical-Thinking Skills

1. Critical thinking entails a particular set of skills that are developed over an extended period of time and that continue to be refined over the course of one's career as an SLP.
   a. Time spent as a graduate student SLP clinician gives ample opportunity to begin forming these skills, but it is essential to continue to practice.
2. When studying for the Speech-Language Pathology Examination, take note of opportunities that arise for practice of any of the subskills of critical thinking, and capitalize on them.
3. Identifying any areas of potential weaknesses in critical thinking is a great way to practice critical-thinking skills.
   a. This identification establishes a foundation to analyze performance, make evaluations, engage in self-examination and make corrections in order to continue on the right path toward success.

After the Examination

Examination Scoring and Reporting

1. Equating Speech-Language Pathology Examination scores.
   a. The passing score for the Speech-Language Pathology Examination is established by ASHA and ETS, after statistical analysis of past test performance.
   b. Using performance of past exam candidates, ASHA and ETS are able to establish a criterion score that is fair and is reflective of passing performance.
2. Scoring procedures.
   a. Only questions answered correctly contribute to the final score, so it is better to answer questions that promote certainty, while moving on from difficult questions.
      (1) Remember, the more questions answered means more likely increases in the raw score.
      (2) Difficult questions are always able to be revisited after having gone through the remainder of the test.
   b. Each selected response question (i.e., multiple choice, multiple select, etc.) are worth one point toward the raw score.
      (1) These questions are automatically scored by computer.
   c. The raw score (number of questions answered correctly) is converted into a scaled score that adjusts for the difficulty of the test.
      (1) There are multiple versions of the Speech-Language Pathology Examination that are administered, and each contains different combinations of questions.
      (2) Using a scaled score ensures that all exam candidates have as fair a chance as possible to pass the Speech-Language Pathology Examination.
3. Scoring schedule and score reporting.
   a. Because the Speech-Language Pathology Examination is offered in specific testing windows, scores are available 10–11 days after each testing window is over.
      (1) Each testing window is approximately 11–12 days in length.

b. Exam candidates are encouraged to make an online ETS account, as score reports are available through the account.
   (1) Scores are available for exactly 1 year after their initial release, so exam candidates are also encouraged to save a copy of the score report to refer to later if needed.
c. In addition to exam candidates receiving their score, the score report is also sent to the candidate's graduate institute and to ASHA, for certification purposes.
   (1) The code to enter to ensure that ASHA receives Speech-Language Pathology Examination scores is R5031.
   (2) Codes for different graduate programs can be found at www.ets.org/s/praxis/pdf/aud_slp_attending_institution_recipient_codes.pdf.
   (3) As of 2014, passing Speech-Language Pathology Examination for ASHA certification is a scaled score of 162, on a 100- to 200-point scale.
d. Aggregate score reports are provided to the program directors for graduate programs in speech-language pathology for candidates who are graduates of the program.

Waiting For and Receiving Examination Results

1. The first step after completion of the exam is to accept that the exam is over and that there is a waiting period for receiving scores.
2. Focus on success and know that all questions were answered with the best reasoning possible.
3. Avoid focusing on any difficulties encountered during the exam, as this will increase feelings of fear and anxiety while waiting for scores.
4. Examination candidates should surround themselves with positivity, including friends, family members and other students.
5. Avoid discussions about the fairness of the exam and about the ability to pass the Speech-Language Pathology Examination.
6. After receiving score reports, if a passing score is achieved, look forward to beginning a clinical fellowship (CF) and to the start of a rewarding career as an SLP.
   a. If a passing score was not achieved, do not engage in feelings of sadness—know that there is always another attempt and that passing the Speech-Language Pathology Examination and becoming an SLP is still an attainable goal.

Retaking the Examination

1. Each Speech-Language Pathology Examination that is taken requires separate registration; however, the same online ETS account from the first attempt may be used repeatedly.
2. Eligibility to retake a Speech-Language Pathology Examination begins during the next available testing window.
   a. Testing windows for the Speech-Language Pathology Examination occur in the months of March, June, July, August, September and December.
   b. In the time spent waiting for the next selected testing window, there are several things to do:
      (1) Surrounding oneself with a supportive network of people may prove necessary in overcoming negative feelings of disappointment.
      (2) Review exam results and identify areas of strengths and weaknesses, in order to establish areas that should be reviewed while waiting.
      (3) Identify anything that may have caused the lack of success on the first attempt at passing the Speech-Language Pathology Examination. Reduce the chance of reoccurrence by minimizing these hindrances during a second attempt. These include behaviors such as:
         (a) Taking too long to answer certain questions.
         (b) Experiencing feelings of anxiety over questions that proved difficult or of those which promoted feelings of ambiguity.
         (c) Becoming distracted by how quickly other test takers are advancing through their tests.
         (d) Not arriving to the testing center with enough time to ease into the situation.
         (e) Either forgetting or forgoing assistance for the Speech-Language Pathology Examination if qualifications for disability assistance are met.
3. Be realistic about obstacles to success that can and cannot be changed. Evaluate those that can be changed, and come up with a solution that works.
4. Continue taking practice exams, in order to increase comfort with lengthy, computer-based standardized tests.
5. Know that having to retake the Speech-Language Pathology Examination will not prevent examination candidates from becoming well-rounded SLPs!

References

American Speech-Language-Hearing Association (2014). About the speech-language pathology Praxis exam. Retrieved from: http://www.asha.org/Certification/praxis/About-the-Speech-Language-Pathology-Praxis-Exam/.

American Speech-Language-Hearing Association (2014). Speech-language pathology exam (5331) content. Retrieved from: http://www.asha.org/Certification/praxis/Speech-Language-Pathology-Exam-5331-Content/.

American Speech-Language-Hearing Association (2014). Speech-language pathology practice analysis and curriculum study. Retrieved from: http://www.asha.org/Academic/accreditation/PracticeAnalysisSLP/.

American Speech-Language-Hearing Association (1997). Council for clinical certification in audiology and speech-language pathology. http://www.asha.org/About/governance/committees/CommitteeSmartForms/Council-for-Clinical-Certification-in-Audiology-and-Speech-Language-Pathology/.

Educational Testing Services (2014). On test day overview. Retrieved from: http://www.ets.org/praxis/test_day/.

Educational Testing Services (2014). Praxis scores overview. Retrieved from: http://www.ets.org/praxis/scores/.

Educational Testing Services (2014). Praxis II overview. Retrieved from: http://www.ets.org/praxis/about/praxisii/.

Educational Testing Services (2014). Praxis II test content and structure. Retrieved from: http://www.ets.org/praxis/about/praxisii/content/.

Educational Testing Services (2014). Registration, test centers, and dates. Published online. Retrieved from: http://www.ets.org/praxis/register/.

Educational Testing Services (2014). *The Praxis Study Companion: Speech-Language Pathology*. Ewing, NJ: Educational Testing Services. Retrieved from: http://www.ets.org/s/praxis/pdf/5331.pdf.

Facione, P. (1990). *Critical Thinking: A Statement of Expert Consensus for Purposes of Educational Assessment and Instruction. Research Findings and Recommendations*. Newark, DE: American Psychological Association.

Facione, P. (2006). *Critical Thinking: What It Is and Why It Counts*. Millbrae, CA: California Academic Press.

Facione, N. C., & Facione, P. A. (2006). *The Health Sciences Reasoning Test HSRT: Test Manual 2006 Edition*. Millbrae, CA: California Academic Press.

Fleming-Castaldy, R. P. (2014). *National Occupational Therapy Certification Exam: Review and Study Guide*, 7th ed. Evanston, IL: TherapyEd..

Much of the material in this chapter was used, with permission, from Rita Fleming-Castaldy's *National Occupational Therapy Certification Exam Review and Study Guide,* 7th edition (2014). Adaptations to fit the profession of speech-language pathology were made and new material was added.

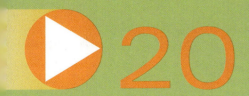

Computer Simulated Examinations

Examinations are on the flash drive. Follow the instructions. After completing each examination, your performance will be analyzed in terms of specific domains and categories. The questions that follow are the ones that constitute the software examinations. Separate TEACHING POINTS for each question contain explanations of the answer.

Domains of Knowledge

- Anatomy and Physiology of Communication and Swallowing
- Acoustics
- Language Acquisition
- Research, Evidence-Based Practice and Tests and Measurements
- The Practice of Speech-Language Pathology
- Speech Sound Disorders in Children
- Spoken Language Disorders in Children
- Written Language Disorders in the School-Age Population
- Autism Spectrum Disorders
- Stuttering and Other Fluency Disorders
- Acquired Language Disorders
- Motor Speech Disorders
- Cleft Palate and Other Craniofacial Anomalies
- Voice Disorders
- Dysphagia
- Augmentative and Alternative Communication (AAC)
- Audiology and Hearing Impairment

Categories

 Category 1—Foundations and Professional Practice

 Category 2—Screening, Assessment, Evaluation and Diagnosis

 Category 3—Planning, Implementation and Evaluation of Treatment

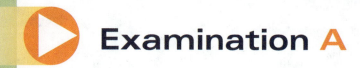

Examination A

A1

Augmentative and Alternative Communication (AAC)

A parent has brought a young child to an outpatient augmentative communication clinic for a full assessment. After reading the client's intake forms, the speech-language pathologist (SLP) believes the child is a candidate for augmentative and alternative communication (AAC) and is preparing tools for the assessment. Which approach to assessment should this SLP use?

Choices:
A. Select standardized assessment measures and vary response mode to see how the child best responds.
B. Select different subtests from multiple, standardized language assessments, to see to which kind of pictures the child best responds.
C. Select a standardized AAC inventory and administer according to direction, to see how the child's AAC skills compare to others in their age group.
D. Select multiple devices in order to determine the one to which the child best responds.

Teaching Points

Correct Answer: A

Currently, there are no standardized assessment batteries in AAC due to the heterogeneity of the populations that require AAC. An appropriate method of assessment in AAC is to administer standardized measures in nonstandardized ways in order to gather information about how the patient best communicates. Because there are no standardized assessment measures, there is no way to compare children with complex communication needs to one another. Additionally, it is more important to determine how the child best communicates rather than to which type of picture they respond, as their most effective communication may not depend on picture use. Finally, while it is important to determine a device the child responds well to, this is a step in the assessment process that comes after initial assessment.

A2

Acoustics

Compared to voiced stops, word-initial voiceless stops in English are expected to have a:

Choices:
A. Shorter voice onset time (VOT).
B. Longer VOT.
C. More compact spectrum.
D. More diffuse spectrum.

Teaching Points

Correct Answer: B

VOT duration distinguishes voiced and voiceless stops, with voiceless stops having longer VOTs, especially in word-initial position. A compact vs. diffuse spectrum distinguishes stop place of articulation, with bilabial stops having diffuse falling spectra, alveolar stops having diffuse rising spectra and velar stops having compact spectra.

A3

Dysphagia

A patient who has not been on the speech-language pathologist's (SLP's) caseload while at a long-term acute care setting begins complaining of gastroesophageal reflux-like (GERD-like) symptoms during and after every meal. The physician has asked the SLP to perform an evaluation, which comes back negative. After using instrumental assessment methods, it is discovered that the patient's lower esophageal sphincter (LES) is not functioning properly. Which of the following could potentially cause this patient's symptoms?

Choices:
A. Pharyngeal weakness, including muscle atrophy.
B. A change in medication, including addition of steroids.
C. Lingual weakness, including fibrillation.
D. Zenker's diverticulum, including residue.

Teaching Points

Correct Answer: B

When evaluating patients, it is important to keep in mind that medications are able to cause previously undiagnosed dysphagic problems. LES dysfunction has been attributed to medication, including steroids, antithyroid drugs and antacids, to name a few.

A4

Research, Evidence-Based Practice and Tests and Measurements

A speech scientist is analyzing data collected from a recently completed study. In order to properly analyze the data, she utilizes nonparametric statistical procedures. Which of the following scenarios **BEST** describes the scientist's data?

Choices:
A. There is not a normal distribution of the data.
B. There is a normal distribution of the data.
C. There is a small median for the data.
D. There is a small mode for the data.

Teaching Points

Correct Answer: A

Nonparametric statistical procedures are those that are not based on a normal curve model or are not normally distributed. Because the data collected from this speech scientist's study was analyzed using nonparametric statistical procedures, it is safe to say that there is not a normal distribution of the data. In contrast, if there was a normal distribution, the speech scientist would be able to implement the more powerful parametric statistical procedures of data analysis.

A5

Stuttering and Other Fluency Disorders

In evaluating a preschool child who stutters, it is important to observe the child interacting with the parent. The **PRIMARY** reason for this is:

Choices:
A. The most valid sample of communication and speech may be observed in the child's typical interaction with the parent.
B. Comfort with the parent is likely to reduce disfluency and make the child feel more comfortable.
C. There are a number of legal concerns that should be considered when separating the child from the parent.
D. The use of an informal speech sample reduces the need for any other standardized testing.

Teaching Points

Correct Answer: A

One of the biggest challenges in all speech and language assessment is obtaining a representative sample of an individual's "typical" communication in their own world. This is particularly challenging with very young children. By having the parent participate in a nondirected and noninterrupted conversation with the child, a more realistic and typical sample can usually be obtained.

A6

Acquired Language Disorders

A speech-language pathologist (SLP) working in a skilled nursing facility (SNF) has been assigned to design a treatment plan for a long-term resident. The patient was diagnosed with Alzheimer's dementia 5 years earlier and is considered to be in the mid-stage of the disorder. She has one daughter who is concerned about her, but who lives far across the country. The patient has been increasingly agitated and difficult for clinical staff to interact with. The intervention of **GREATEST BENEFIT** would be:

Choices:
A. A course of melodic intonation therapy (MIT) to increase phrase lengths and improve fluency of verbal output.
B. Using a simulated presence therapy technique, in which taped messages are played to the individual with dementia in times of agitation.
C. Using caregiver-administered active cognitive stimulation techniques, in which the SLP assists the family member in administering cognitive stimulating tasks such as playing card games and completing puzzles.
D. Training the patient on the use of a computerized augmentative communication system, such as Dynavox.

Teaching Points

Correct Answer: B

A person with Alzheimer's dementia that is in the mid-stage of the disorder and who has been increasingly agitated in the SNF is not a candidate for MIT, treatment to improve functional writing, or for using a computerized augmentative communication device. The patient is also not appropriate for caregiver-administered active cognitive stimulation techniques because the daughter lives across the country. Simulated presence therapy has been shown to calm agitation and improve social functioning in people with dementia.

A7

Audiology and Hearing Impairment

A person with hearing loss has complained that listening to conversational partners in noisy restaurants is very difficult. However, they still enjoy going out to eat with family and friends, regardless of this difficulty. Which level of the World Health Organization (WHO) International Classification of Functioning (ICF) **BEST** describes this person's hearing problem?

Choices:
A. Activity limitation.
B. Impairment.
C. Participation restriction.
D. Behavioral limitation.

Teaching Points

Correct Answer: A

An activity limitation reflects the impact of a hearing loss on the person's ability to communicate and understand environmental and speech signals. As this patient describes deficits with hearing in noisy environments, they are describing an activity limitation. In contrast, if this problem stopped this person from going into the community, this would be described as a participation restriction. An impairment refers to the measurable loss of hearing function (i.e., what is causing the hearing loss). Finally, there is no behavioral limitation as a part of the WHO ICF.

A8

Voice Disorders

A patient arrives at an acute rehabilitation hospital, following a hip replacement surgery. The physician has asked the speech-language pathologist (SLP) to perform a full evaluation of the patient, with suspicions of cognitive changes postsurgery. After performing the evaluation, the SLP documented a hoarse/rough vocal quality, which the patient reported was not there prior to the surgery. The SLP determines that the patient has not received adequate hydration and is consuming too much coffee during hospitalization. Which intervention should be utilized?

Choices:
A. Vocal hygiene information.
B. Medialization laryngoplasty.
C. Consultation with the physician for appropriate prescription drugs.
D. No treatment is necessary.

Teaching Points

Correct Answer: A

Adequate hydration is essential for normal laryngeal function. If the patient is not drinking enough water and is drinking excessive coffee (which acts as a drying agent), the person's vocal fold tissues may not be moving typically. Giving this patient vocal fold hygiene information, including the effects of water and drying agents on the vocal folds, may help the patient change behavior and restore normal vocal quality. Medialization laryngoplasty is a surgical intervention undertaken when there is unilateral vocal fold paralysis and is contraindicated otherwise. While prescription drugs may help reduce the swelling (i.e., nonsteroidal anti-inflammatory drugs), they may also cause other problems to arise (i.e., predisposition to vocal fold bleeding). As such, these should be attempted after vocal hygiene therapy has been ruled ineffective. Lastly, as the patient is presents with a complaint of change in perception, the SLP has an ethical obligation to help this patient to the best of his/her abilities.

A9

Speech Sound Disorders in Children

A child is brought into an outpatient speech and language clinic by her parents, with a chief complaint of "trouble speaking." After administration of a comprehensive speech sound evaluation, the speech-language pathologist (SLP) reveals the following speech sound errors: /rɪn/ for /rɪŋ/, /tæt/ for /kæt/ and /frɔd/ for /frɔg/. This child demonstrates difficulty producing sounds with which place of articulation?

Choices:
A. Alveolars.
B. Bilabials.
C. Velars.
D. Interdentals.

Teaching Points

Correct Answer: C

The speech errors that this child produces are errors for the following phonemes: /ŋ/, /g/ and /k/. These three speech sounds are produced when the back of the tongue comes into contact with the velum, and they are known are velar sounds. In contrast, alveolar sounds are produced when the tongue tip comes into contact with the alveolar ride, such as /t/ and /d/. Bilabial sounds are produced using both lips, such as /p/ and /b/. Finally, interdental sounds are produced when the tongue tip is placed between the two front teeth, such as /ð/ and /θ/.

A10

Anatomy and Physiology of Communication and Swallowing

Which muscle contributes to hyolaryngeal depression?

Choices:
A. Stylohyoid.
B. Geniohyoid.
C. Mylohyoid.
D. Sternohyoid.

Teaching Points

Correct Answer: D

The muscles most responsible for laryngeal depression are the infrahyoids, which include the sternohyoid, sternothyroid, omohyoid and thyrohyoid. The stylohyoid, geniohyoid and mylohyoid muscles are suprahyoid muscles and contribute to laryngeal elevation.

A11

Dysphagia

Following a car accident, a patient that is being treated by a speech-language pathologist (SLP) exhibits weakness in the orbicularis oris and buccinator muscles. Which of the following problems would be the **MOST LIKELY** presentation of this patient's dysphagia?

Choices:
A. Oral incontinence with anterior and lateral residue.
B. Pharyngeal delay with excessive residue.
C. Reduced opening of the upper esophageal sphincter.
D. Piecemeal deglutition with silent aspiration.

Teaching Points

Correct Answer: A

The orbicularis oris and buccinator are the muscles of the lips and cheeks, respectively. If these muscles are weak, the bolus may leak through the lips, or be left as residue in the anterior sulcus (i.e., the space between the bottom lip and the teeth) or the lateral sulci (i.e., the space between the cheeks and the teeth).

A12

Spoken Language Disorders in Children

Barbara is a young child with a severe cognitive deficit. Barbara's speech-language pathologist (SLP) is beginning to formulate a treatment plan for intervention and would like to focus on the MOST functional treatment targets during intervention. What should be targeted during Barbara's intervention sessions?

Choices:
A. Complex sentence structure.
B. Recreational vocabulary.
C. Phonological memory.
D. Joint attention skills.

Teaching Points

Correct Answer: B

Most children with cognitive deficits will learn some language, although normalization of language skills may not be the most appropriate expectation in these cases. For this population, functional language goals are the most appropriate treatment target, which may include focusing intervention on a limited language repertoire. For this child, as she is still relatively young, the most functional goal may be initially targeting vocabulary surrounding her favorite recreational activities as a means of improving their means of communication. Other functional tasks for this population include understanding of different syntactic structures and understanding useful vocabulary for the child's activities of daily living.

A13

Autism Spectrum Disorders

A child is brought to an outpatient clinic for a neuropsychological evaluation. Following the evaluation, the child is diagnosed with autism spectrum disorder; specifically with Level 2 severity in social communication. This child **MOST LIKELY** demonstrates:

Choices:
A. Difficulty initiating social interactions with peers.
B. Abnormal responses to social overtures.
C. Very limited social interaction.
D. Decreased interest in social interactions.

Teaching Points

Correct Answer: B

A Level 2 severity rating for social communication in autism spectrum disorder is characterized by marked deficits in verbal and nonverbal social communication that are apparent even with supports and reduced or abnormal responses to social overtures. In contrast to this, Level 1 severity ratings are characterized by noticeable deficits in social communication without supports, difficulty initiating and decreased interest in social interactions, and odd/unsuccessful attempts to make friends. Finally, Level 3 severity ratings are characterized by severe deficits in verbal and nonverbal social communication and very limited social interaction and response to social overtures.

A14

Speech Sound Disorders in Children

After performing a comprehensive speech evaluation on a pediatric client, a speech-language pathologist (SLP) has determined that the child demonstrates difficulty producing the /l/ phoneme, consistent with a phonetic error. Which method of intervention would be an appropriate selection for the SLP to utilize with this child?

Choices:
A. Minimal contrast method.
B. Distinctive feature approach.
C. Integral stimulation approach.
D. Cycles remediation approach.

Teaching Points

Correct Answer: C

The integral stimulation approach is an intervention method used for phonetic speech errors, in which emphasis on multiple input modes is used to help a child establish a speech sound into his/her repertoire. In contrast, the minimal contrast approach, distinctive features approach and cycles remediation approach are all intervention methods used for children with phonemic speech errors and would not be helpful in remediating this particular child's speech sound disorder as this child needs to learn the motor pattern to produce the /l/ phoneme.

A15

The Practice of Speech-Language Pathology

A patient in a hospital is being seen by multiple professionals, with each professional providing independent assessment and intervention. After each professional has completed initial assessment, each collaborates about the patient's treatment plan and shares information regarding the patient's status for each discipline. Which service delivery model is being utilized in the care of this patient?

Choices:
A. Unidisciplinary.
B. Transdisciplinary.
C. Multidisciplinary.
D. Interdisciplinary.

Teaching Points

Correct Answer: D

The interdisciplinary service delivery model dictates that the client is seen by multiple professionals who communicate regarding treatment and share information about overall status. However, independent assessment is completed by all involved disciplines, such as in this scenario. In contrast, multidisciplinary service delivery models dictate that the client is seen by multiple professionals with some communication between disciplines in regard to referral and follow-up, but with little cooperative service delivery. Transdisciplinary service delivery models dictate that professionals cooperate in service delivery and communicate frequently. Additionally, assessment and treatment are delivered by multiple professionals in a more natural environment. Unidisciplinary is not a service delivery model.

A16

Autism Spectrum Disorders

A speech-language pathologist (SLP) in the public school system has been working with a child with autism spectrum disorder. This child demonstrates severe deficits in social communication, and for this reason the SLP has decided to implement a peer mediation approach to intervention. Which of the following is an appropriate way for this SLP to implement this style of intervention?

Choices:
A. Have the child watch video clips of typically developing peers in order to model appropriate social communication.
B. Pair the child with an age-matched peer in order to model appropriate social communication.
C. Pair the child with an older peer in order to model later-occurring communication skills.
D. Have the child watch typically developing peers at recess in order to model appropriate play behaviors.

Teaching Points

Correct Answer: B

In the peer and play mediation method of intervention, children with autism spectrum disorder are encouraged to interact with their peers, as the peers provide a model for imitation. As the child with autism spectrum disorder gains social skills, opportunities for social interaction are increased. These social skills are learned in a developmental continuum, and the child is not expected to learn more age-advanced skills before reaching that developmental milestone. In addition, this method of intervention requires direct contact with peers to encourage maximum learning of social skills.

A17

Spoken Language Disorders in Children

A young child is brought into a speech and language clinic by his parents, with primary complaints of "little language use." Upon initial evaluation, the speech-language pathologist (SLP) determines that the child communicates appropriately through use of gestures for requests for actions and objects, but uses little verbal language. What would be of the **GREATEST BENEFIT** in the next step in this child's treatment?

Choices:
A. Expand the child's expressive syntax to include simple sentence structure.
B. Expand the child's expressive morphology to include plural markers.
C. Expand the child's receptive vocabulary to include more functional items.
D. Expand the child's repertoire to include vocalizations with gestures.

Teaching Points

Correct Answer: D

The child from this scenario demonstrates communicative intentions through his/her use of using gestures to request objects and actions. An appropriate next step for this would be to add vocalizations or words to the gestures, as a means of expanding expressive repertoire. This sets a foundational skill, on which later developing skills such as simple sentence structure and plural markers. As this child demonstrates the ability to request objects and actions successfully, he/she likely demonstrates age-appropriate receptive vocabulary skills and may not require intervention in this area.

A18

Acoustics

The speech-language pathologist (SLP) wants to use acoustic measurements of /r/ to document a child's progress in producing the sound. The **BEST** measurement to make is the amount of movement in:

Choices:
A. F0.
B. F1.
C. F2.
D. F3.

Teaching Points

Correct Answer: D
Correct articulation of English /r/ results in a clear drop in F3 frequency.

A19

Augmentative and Alternative Communication (AAC)

A speech-language pathologist (SLP) has been training a patient and his family in the use of a newly implemented augmentative and alternative communication (AAC) device. The SLP is targeting a strategy that allows the patient to supply the content elements of his message, after which the family members confirm these elements. The patient and family then expand on the message. Which strategy is the SLP utilizing with this family's approach to intervention?

Choices:
A. Alphabet supplementation.
B. Topic supplementation.
C. Augmented input.
D. Message co-construction.

Teaching Points

Correct Answer: D
The strategy of message co-construction requires the person with complex communication needs (CCNs) to supply the content elements of his/her message, which the communication partner then confirms. The partner then expands these components into a fully developed communicative message. As this closely matches

the strategy implemented by this SLP, it is likely a message coconstruction strategy is being used with this patient. In contrast to this, alphabet supplementation uses an alphabet display to point to the initial letter of each word when a patient says it to aid the intelligibility of the communication partner. Topic supplementation uses a communication board that has lists of commonly discussed topics. The person with CCN selects the topic to aid the intelligibility of the communication partner. Finally, augmented input is a strategy that employs modeling how a system is used to the person with CCN so they receive input via AAC rather than speech alone.

A20

Stuttering and Other Fluency Disorders

Secondary stuttering behaviors provide clinical significance in evaluation of the stuttering in children. Which of the following statement is **MOST ACCURATE** with regard to the significance of secondary behaviors?

Choices:
A. They indicate that the PWS is more likely to stutter as an adult.
B. They indicate that the PWS is exhibiting fear and embarrassment.
C. They indicate that the PWS is using escape and avoidance behaviors to deal with their stuttering.
D. They indicate that the PWS is familial.

Teaching Points

Correct Answer: C
Developmentally, when individuals who stutter begin to exhibit secondary behaviors, it serves as an important clinical signal. This indicates that the child has moved in the direction of attempting to control the core behaviors of prolongation and repetition, typically with motoric adjustments and blocks in voicing and airflow. The implications of the appearance of these behaviors may or not indicate any emotional reactions like fear or embarrassment.

A21

Acquired Language Disorders

Evaluation of a right-handed individual who had a left middle cerebral artery (MCA) stroke that affected only the anterior portion of the left MCA territory will demonstrate:

Choices:
A. Significant impairment of auditory comprehension and a right hemiparesis.
B. Visual agnosia and dysprosody.
C. Nonfluent aphasia with relative preservation of auditory comprehension and a right hemiparesis.
D. Severe dysphagia, but no aphasia.

Teaching Points

Correct Answer: C
Cerebrovascular accident in the anterior portion of the MCA territory is likely to affect portions of the language zone in the frontal lobe and the precentral gyrus (motor strip). Therefore the person is likely to have a nonfluent aphasia and a right hemiparesis. Since posterior language regions were not affected, the person will not have a fluent aphasia or a problem with auditory comprehension.

A22

Acoustics

The frequency of a periodic sound is increased by 100 hertz. What effect would this change in frequency have on the wavelength of the sound?

Choices:
A. There would be no change in wavelength.
B. There would be an increase in wavelength.
C. There would be a decrease in wavelength.
D. There would be a dampening of the sound.

Teaching Points

Correct Answer: C

Wavelength is the distance travelled by a sound during a single period. This measure has an inverse relationship with frequency. This means that higher frequency sounds would have a shorter wavelength whereas lower frequency sounds would have a longer wavelength. Therefore, if the frequency of a sound was increased, its wavelength would decrease accordingly.

A23

Written Language Disorders in the School-Age Population

A 7-year-old student on a speech-language pathologist's (SLP's) caseload at an elementary school shows strengths in rhyme awareness, phoneme blending and phoneme manipulation. Based on these strengths, the SLP would suspect that this student would have strengths in:

Choices:
A. Orthography skills.
B. Word attack skills.
C. Vocabulary skills.
D. Discourse processing abilities.

Teaching Points

Correct Answer: B

Word attack skills are dependent on skills in rhyme awareness and phonological awareness. Phonological awareness includes the ability to analyze and manipulate speech information, such as the blending and manipulation of phonemes that this student is able to do. Coupled with his/her strengths in rhyme awareness, this student would likely demonstrate strengths in the ability to recognize words based on phonological structure, structural analysis and morphological structure.

A24

The Practice of Speech-Language Pathology

A speech-language pathologist (SLP) has been asked to evaluate a new patient in an acute care hospital, after which point the SLP will provide treatment for this patient. The SLP currently has a full caseload, but was planning on discharging one of the patients the following day. How should this SLP proceed in order to better manage the caseload?

Choices:
A. Discharge the patient early, and send written notice.
B. Discuss discharge with their patient prior to terminating services.
C. Evaluate the new patient and begin providing intervention.
D. Have the department speech-language pathologist assistant (SLPA) proceed with the evaluation.

Teaching Points

Correct Answer: B

According to the ASHA Code of Ethics, Principle of Ethics I, Rule of Ethics R, "Individuals shall not discontinue service to those they are serving without providing reasonable notice." The SLP from this scenario is ethically bound to tell the current patient that he/she is nearing discharge (i.e., reaching all goals set) prior to termination of services. Because the SLP is working at a full caseload, it is not recommended to continue providing services to patients, as this may interfere with the quality of services rendered. Finally, SLPAs are not eligible to provide evaluation without assistance from the SLP.

A25

Augmentative and Alternative Communication (AAC)

John is a speech-language pathologist working with a patient in an outpatient augmentative communication center. John has been implementing an unaided augmentative and alternative communication (AAC) device for the patient to use in order to facilitate communication with family and friends. Which means of AAC would John **MOST LIKELY** utilize for the communicative purposes of this patient?

Choices:
A. Line drawings.
B. Speech-generating device.
C. Picture board.
D. Eye gaze.

Teaching Points

Correct Answer: D

Unaided AAC refers to the use of only the body to communicate, with no external aids or equipment. As eye gaze is a form of AAC that does not require equipment or aids to utilize, this would be the best choice for implementation with this patient. In contrast to this, line drawings, speech-generating devices and picture boards all require external equipment and would be in direct opposition to the needs of the patient from this scenario.

A26

Written Language Disorders in the School-Age Population

A 10-year-old girl with adequate vocabulary skills for her age reads one and two-syllable words accurately and with some fluency at the sentence level; however, she struggles with reading words of three or more syllable words. The **MOST** developmentally appropriate focus for improving her reading would be to teach:

Choices:
A. Grapheme-phoneme correspondence.
B. Structural analysis.
C. Story grammar components.
D. The six syllable types.

Teaching Points

Correct Answer: B

A student is likely to benefit from structural analysis instruction, or the instruction of reading and understanding the meaning behind different affixes, if they have the ability to read words with some degree of automaticity/fluency. Because this student demonstrates the ability to read one- to two-syllable words with sentence-level fluency, she most likely has an adequate understanding of grapheme-phoneme associations and the six syllable types. As story grammar instruction should be taught at a time when students are prepared for narrative reading, this student would not benefit from this type of intervention, as she is struggling with reading of three- and four-syllable words.

A27

Spoken Language Disorders in Children

A high school student presents with weaknesses in word recognition and spelling and has deficits in phonological and orthographic processing. The student shows relative strengths in underlying language skills, with typically average or above average abilities in the areas of vocabulary, morphology, syntax and discourse. This pattern of strengths and weaknesses is MOST TYPICALLY associated with a diagnosis of:

Choices:
A. Dyslexia.
B. Hyperlexia.
C. Language-learning disability.
D. Attention deficit disorder.

Teaching Points

Correct Answer: A

Students with language-learning disabilities and dyslexia demonstrate deficits in phonological processing, which includes their abilities with word recognition and spelling. The difference between these two diagnoses is that students with language-learning disability also demonstrate deficits in underlying language skills (i.e., vocabulary, morphology, syntax and discourse), whereas students with dyslexia have relative strengths in these areas.

A28

Spoken Language Disorders in Children

Mark is a child who demonstrates significant deficits in nonword repetition. An explanation for this may be that Mark:

Choices:
A. Has significant difficulty learning phonological structures.
B. Has unstable underlying phonological representations.
C. Has severe deficits in phonological awareness.
D. Has difficulty producing words with complex syllable structure.

Teaching Points

Correct Answer: B

Students who demonstrate difficulty repeating nonwords often have unstable phonological representations, which is suggestive of a language disorder. In contrast to this, students with poor phonological awareness often have difficulties with sound categorization, blending, segmentation, elision and deletion. Students with language disorders in general often have difficulty producing words containing complex syllable structures, but this does not strictly apply to nonword repetition. Finally, while difficulty learning phonological structures may be indicative of a language disorder, this too would not be strictly related to nonword repetition.

A29

Autism Spectrum Disorders

A speech and language scientist has focused her research efforts into proving that there are environmental causes for autism spectrum disorders. Which of the following would this scientist **MOST LIKELY** accept as a cause of autism spectrum disorders?

Choices:
A. Brain inflammation.
B. Chromosomal deficiencies.
C. Toxins.
D. Maternal blood supply.

Teaching Points

Correct Answer: C

Environmental theories of the cause of autism spectrum disorder often focus on environmental toxins (i.e., lead, chemicals, etc.) or vaccines as the cause of autism spectrum disorder. In contrast to this, chromosomal deficiencies as the cause of autism spectrum disorders fall under genetic research, whereas brain inflammation and maternal blood supply as the cause of autism spectrum disorders fall under neurochemical research.

A30

Cleft Palate and Other Craniofacial Anomalies

During a comprehensive speech evaluation, a speech-language pathologist (SLP) asks the child being evaluated to prolong the vowel /i/. The SLP asks the child to repeat the same vowel, but while pinching his/her nose closed. Upon completing this action, the SLP notices a change in the sound of the vowel. What type of resonance does this child **MOST LIKELY** demonstrate?

Choices:
A. Hypernasality.
B. Hyponasality.
C. Cul de sac resonance.
D. Mixed resonance.

Teaching Points

Correct Answer: A

Hypernasality would occur if excessive amounts of acoustic energy were released into the nasal cavities during speech. By occluding the nares, any energy in the nasal cavity would be forced into the oral cavity, and there would be no perception of hypernasality during these speech tasks. This type of evaluation would not reveal hyponasality, as this is a problem with normal nasal resonance. Additionally, cul de sac resonance would not be revealed, as this is a problem with sound already being obstructed in the pharyngeal or nasal cavities. Further obstruction would not make a change in perception.

A31
Acquired Language Disorders

Language assessment results for a person showed fluent verbal output with paraphasias and neologisms, as well as significant anomia. The individual also had great difficulty with comprehension. The person was able to repeat single words and sentences without error. Based on this scenario, the person would **MOST LIKELY** be diagnosed with:

Choices:
A. Wernicke's aphasia.
B. Transcortical motor aphasia.
C. Conduction aphasia.
D. Transcortical sensory aphasia.

Teaching Points

Correct Answer: D

The combination of fluent output, poor auditory comprehension and preserved verbal repetition is found in the syndrome of transcortical sensory aphasia. In contrast to this, a person with Wernicke's aphasia would demonstrate fluent verbal output, poor auditory comprehension and poor repetition of words. A person with transcortical motor aphasia would demonstrate nonfluent verbal output, good auditory comprehension and good repetition of words. Finally, a person with Conduction aphasia would demonstrate fluent verbal output, good auditory comprehension and poor repetition of words.

A32
Speech Sound Disorders in Children

A speech-language pathologist (SLP) is starting to work with a young child with a speech sound disorder. After reviewing the child's evaluation results, the SLP determines that the child is demonstrating errors in all word positions for the following phonemes: [l, t, g, ŋ, v, w]. The SLP would like to utilize a treatment method that will simultaneously target the child's speech sound errors. Which intervention would this SLP **MOST LIKELY** implement?

Choices:
A. Sensory-motor approach.
B. Integral stimulation.
C. Minimal pairs approach.
D. Multiple phoneme approach.

Teaching Points

Correct Answer: D

The multiple phoneme approach was developed for children with multiple phoneme errors, such as the child in this scenario. The child is given simultaneous instruction on errored phonemes, although the child may be at different phase of learning for each errored phoneme. In contrast to this, integral stimulation is an intervention method that helps establish a single phoneme at a time and concentrates on productions of that phoneme. The sensory-motor approach stresses the production of bi-syllable units and facilitative phonetic contexts to help in production of errored phonemes, but does not aid in simultaneous instruction of these phonemes. Finally, the minimal pairs method may be utilized when the child demonstrates homonymy in his/her speech, but does not focus on establishment of errored speech sounds.

A33

Research, Evidence-Based Practice and Tests and Measurements

A researcher is conducting a study comparing the performance of dyslexic versus nondyslexic participants during oral reading of written words presented rapidly versus slowly. This is an example of:

Choices:
A. Experimental research.
B. Descriptive research.
C. Mixed experimental-descriptive research.
D. Qualitative research.

Teaching Points

Correct Answer: C

For this scenario, it is best to separate out the experimental and descriptive portions of the study. The experimental portion comes from the manipulation of the independent variable (i.e., slow vs. rapid presentations of written words). The descriptive portion occurs because of the comparison between two groups based on subject attributes (i.e., dyslexic vs. nondyslexic readers). Because this study meets both of these conditions, it can be accurately called mixed experimental-descriptive research.

A34

Language Acquisition

A male child is brought to a speech and language clinic by his parents, who have told the speech-language pathologist (SLP) that the child refers to all round items as *ball*. This production includes describing words such as *moon*, *circle* and *orange*. Which of the following best describes this child's productions?

Choices:
A. Undergeneralization errors.
B. Phonological errors.
C. Overgeneralization errors.
D. Morphological errors.

A35

Audiology and Hearing Impairment

An audiologist has completed audiologic evaluation on a patient and has diagnosed the patient with a hearing loss localized to the middle ear. Which of the following structures could be experiencing a deficit?

Choices:
A. Cochlea.
B. Semicircular canals.
C. Ossicular chain.
D. Bony labyrinth.

Teaching Points

Correct Answer: C

The ossicular chain consists of the three bones or ossicles (malleus, incus and stapes) housed in the middle ear. As this patient is experiencing a middle ear disorder, the ossicular chain could be damaged. In contrast to this, the cochlea, semicircular canals and bony labyrinth are considered portions of the inner ear.

A36

Acoustics

The pitch contour for a vowel shows several abrupt changes that the speech-language pathologist (SLP) suspects may be inaccurate. The best way to objectively document accuracy or inaccuracy of the pitch contour is to:

Choices:
A. Listen to the vowel to see if abrupt changes in pitch can be detected.
B. Look at the waveform to see if it shows abrupt changes in pitch.
C. Look at an amplitude spectrum to see if the harmonics show abrupt changes in spacing.
D. Look at a narrowband spectrogram to see if the harmonic contours show abrupt changes.

Teaching Points

Correct Answer: D

A pitch contour should follow the same contour as the sound's harmonics. Harmonic contours are visible in a narrowband spectrogram. Listening to a vowel provides useful information, but not objective documentation. Pitch changes are more difficult to see in a waveform. Since an amplitude spectrum has no time access, it does not show pitch over time.

A37

The Practice of Speech-Language Pathology

A speech-language pathologist (SLP) has recently started working in an early intervention (EI) setting. The SLP has no prior experience in this setting and is curious about their specific role as an EI SLP. Which role does this SLP serve in their new setting?

Choices:
A. Providing Individual Education Plans (IEPs).
B. Providing a free and appropriate public education (FAPE).
C. Providing an Individualized Family Service Plan (IFSP).
D. Providing medical means of intervention for newborns.

Teaching Points

Correct Answer: C

SLPs that work in early intervention are responsible for providing and following an IFSP, which dictates goals and objectives for the child and family, including services to be provided, preservice levels, plan for intervention and evaluation of services/outcomes. SLPs that work in educational settings are responsible for providing IEPs and FAPEs. No SLP is eligible to provide medical means of intervention, for any client seen for services.

A38

Autism Spectrum Disorders

A child has been brought in to a physician's office for a comprehensive evaluation, with parent suspicions of autism spectrum disorder (ASD). Following the evaluation, the physician notes that the child demonstrates impairments in social interaction and restricted, repetitive behaviors, but demonstrates no delay in language or cognitive development. Which of the following disorders is this child **MOST LIKELY** demonstrating?

Choices:
A. Asperger's disorder.
B. Autism spectrum disorder.
C. Rhett's syndrome.
D. Pervasive developmental disorder not otherwise specified (PDD-NOS).

Teaching Points

Correct Answer: A

Asperger's disorder is a form of autism spectrum disorder, characterized by qualitative impairment in social interaction and restricted/repetitive behaviors, but with no significant delay in language or cognitive skills. In contrast to this, ASD involves deficits in language skills and may be accompanied by cognitive deficits as well. Rhett's syndrome is a form of ASD most common in girls and is associated with initially typical development followed by a decline in language and cognitive skills. PDD-NOS is a form of ASD that does not match the specific diagnostic criteria for other pervasive developmental disorders.

A39

Speech Sound Disorders in Children

Following a speech evaluation, a speech-language pathologist (SLP) has determined that the child he is working with demonstrates significant amounts of homonymy in his speech. For example, the child produces the word /bo/ for both /bot/ and /bo/. However, the child does produce the /t/ phoneme in other word positions. Which intervention approach would be of the GREATEST BENEFIT for the SLP to utilize in working with this particular child?

Choices:
A. Maximal contrast approach.
B. Integral stimulation.
C. Traditional approach.
D. Minimal pairs approach.

Teaching Points

Correct Answer: D

The goal of the minimal pairs method is to eliminate a child's creation of homonyms, or a singular production for multiple words. In this case, the child is producing /bo/ for both /bot/ and /bo/, which could be directly targeted utilizing this approach. In contrast, the maximal opposition method focuses on contrasting a target word with a maximally distinct sound (i.e., one that varies across a variety of features). However, in this method reduction of homonymy is indirectly addressed, unlike in the minimal pairs method. Both the traditional method and integral stimulation method are used to treat phonetic errors and are utilized to establish a sound that is not present in a child's repertoire. Because this child is able to produce /t/ in other word positions, these methods would not help alleviate the homonymy being experienced.

A40

Motor Speech Disorders

A speech-language pathologist (SLP) is developing a new assessment for acquired apraxia of speech. The SLP wishes to demonstrate the reliability of the assessment measure, as to better quantify the deficits in persons with apraxia. Which of the following should the SLP determine to prove the reliability of the assessment measure?

Choices:
A. Internal consistency, stability and equivalence of the measurement.
B. Content validity, criterion validity and construct validity of the measurement.
C. Interobserver agreement, standard deviation of scores and effect size of the measurement.
D. Sensitivity, specificity and average participant performance of the measurement.

Teaching Points

Correct Answer: A

In order for an assessment measurement to have good reliability, it needs to demonstrate stability (i.e., the same results upon multiple administrations), equivalence (i.e., comparison of participant results to results to an alternative form of the assessment), and internal consistency (i.e., results from one-half of the assessment to the other half from the same assessment). If all three of these conditions are met, the assessment has good reliability.

A41

Spoken Language Disorders in Children

Jordan is an elementary school student with a language disorder that is demonstrating significant difficulties in the classroom. After talking with his teacher, Jordan reveals that he has a hard time following classroom activities with specific deficits in content vocabulary. Given that Jordan has difficulty with content vocabulary, he would present with difficulty with:

Choices:
A. Vocabulary words that he has not yet learned.
B. Vocabulary words that are highly specific to his life.
C. Vocabulary words that allow him to follow classroom directions.
D. Vocabulary words specific to information in classroom assignments.

Teaching Points

Correct Answer: D
Content vocabulary consists of words that are specific to the information contained in instructional or curricular materials. In contrast to this, instructional vocabulary consists of words used in daily classroom instructions that students need to follow directions. Fringe vocabulary and developmental vocabulary are terms that refer to the type of vocabulary one may find on a person's augmentative communication device. Fringe vocabulary consists of words that are highly unique to the individual, whereas developmental vocabulary consists of words that the person does not know yet, but may learn through exposure.

A42

Voice Disorders

A patient arrives at an acute care hospital in order to have open heart surgery. After the surgery, the patient verbalizes complaints about a change in vocal quality, and a speech-language pathologist (SLP) is consulted. The SLP who performs the intake evaluation documents that the patient presents with an excessively high-pitched voice. Which of the following is a likely cause of this patient's change in vocal quality?

Choices:
A. Development of vocal fold nodules from screaming at the nurse.
B. A massive hemispheric stroke during the surgery.
C. Damage of the left recurrent laryngeal nerve during the surgery.
D. Persistence of anesthesia effects, resulting in a drug-induced change in vocal quality.

Teaching Points

Correct Answer: C
The recurrent laryngeal nerve innervates the thyroarytenoid muscle, which mediates normal tension in the vocal folds and controls lowering of pitch. This nerve also travels around the aortic arch on its way to innervate the intrinsic laryngeal musculature. If the recurrent laryngeal nerve is damaged (i.e., through open heart surgery complications), it may cause weakness in the thyroarytenoid muscle and reduce the patient's ability to lower pitch. However, the superior laryngeal nerve, which assists in pitch elevation, follows a different course than the recurrent laryngeal nerve and would not be damaged in open heart surgery. As this nerve would remain intact, the patient may experience higher-than-average pitch during oral communication. Although vocal fold nodules may arise from screaming at nurses, it would take prolonged periods of this phonotrauma to cause nodules to form, which would occur long postoperatively. A hallmark of upper motor neuron voice disorders, as would be seen in a hemispheric stroke, is a strained-strangled vocal quality, not a heightened pitch. Lastly, prolonged effects of medications may have a drying effect on the vocal folds and would cause a hoarse vocal quality but would not increase pitch.

A43

Anatomy and Physiology of Communication and Swallowing

A patient has recently sustained lower motor neuron damage to his/her trigeminal nerve (CN V) and is experiencing difficulty with mastication. Which of the following muscles could be experiencing deficits secondary to the nerve damage?

Choices:
A. Thyroarytenoid.
B. Masseter.
C. Hyoglossus.
D. Buccinator.

Teaching Points

Correct Answer: B

The masseter muscle is a large muscle that forms a sling around the ramus of the mandible. Upon contraction of this muscle, the jaw is raised to assist with mastication. The other muscles involved in mastication are the temporalis, external pterygoid and medial pterygoid.

A44

Voice Disorders

The principal of a local elementary school has come to an outpatient voice center in order to ask the speech-language pathologists (SLPs) to give a presentation to the high school teachers regarding vocal health. According to the principal's reports, a large number of teachers complain of difficulty voicing and require frequent sick days to recover. Which of the following options is NOT appropriate to use as a method to prevent voice disorders for this population of teachers?

Choices:
A. Using a sing-song voice to get students' attention.
B. Taking voice breaks in between classes.
C. Using a sticker chart for behavioral management.
D. Utilizing a seating chart for maximum vocal projection.

Teaching Points

Correct Answer: A

Teachers are part of a special population, known as professional voice users. Because teachers require use of their voice throughout the day, they are predisposed to phonotraumatic lesions. Effective strategies for teachers would require frequent voice rest, or nonvocal means of behavior intervention or gathering students' attention. If a teacher engages in a sing-song voice, they are prolonging their exposure to tissue vibration and continuing their chances of phonotraumatic lesions.

A45

Spoken Language Disorders in Children

A young child with a language disorder has recently been struggling with Tier 1 coursework for language arts. After consulting with the student's teacher, the speech-language pathologist (SLP) who works with this child has suggested the student may be a candidate for Tier 2 instruction. Which of the following is the **MOST APPROPRIATE** form of instruction for this child?

Choices:
A. The child receives in-class support from the SLP.
B. The teacher alters the coursework for the entire class.
C. The child receives one-on-one instruction from the SLP.
D. The teacher allows multiple resubmissions of all homework.

Teaching Points

Correct Answer: A

At Tier 2 in the Response to Intervention (RTI) model, a child will receive supportive or different forms of instruction as a means of helping them better grasp the material. If the child in this case was placed in RTI Level 2, they would most likely receive altered teaching from their classroom teacher or in-class supports (i.e., SLP intervention, paraprofessional, etc.). In contrast to this, if the child received one-on-one instruction for the material, this would fall under Level 3 of the RTI model, in which there is more intensive instruction and possible referral for special education services. The teacher altering the coursework for the entire classroom would not be a practical approach, as this may hinder the learning of other students. Finally, multiple resubmissions of homework assignments may not directly assist in the learning of the child from this scenario and would not be considered a part of the RTI model.

A46

Cleft Palate and Other Craniofacial Anomalies

A child is referred to a speech-language pathologist (SLP) by an otolaryngologist (ENT) with a presenting problem of "distorted speech." Following a comprehensive evaluation, the SLP determines that the child is experiencing significant nasal emission during speech. Based on this information, which of the following problems would this child **NOT** be experiencing?

Choices:
A. Short utterance length.
B. Compensatory errors.
C. Hypernasality.
D. Weak consonants.

Teaching Points

Correct Answer: C

Nasal emissions occur when there is air lost through the nasal cavity during speech production. As this air is required to maintain speech, the quicker loss of air that accompanies nasal emissions would cause short utterance length. Additionally, because this air is being released, there will be a lack of pressure buildup in the oral cavity, leading to weak consonants, which in turn would lead to compensatory productions. Nasal emissions on their own would not cause a change in a client's resonatory capabilities, therefore the client would not be perceived as hypernasal.

A47

Voice Disorders

A patient presents to the local voice clinic with complaints of difficulty producing voice, which is made worse during prolonged periods of vocal use. After receiving an initial evaluation by both the otolaryngologist (ENT) and the speech-language pathologist (SLP), the patient is diagnosed with muscle tension dysphonia, specifically with excess tension in the vocal fold adductor muscles. Which of the following treatment approaches is appropriate to utilize with this patient in an effort to alleviate these vocal problems?

Choices:
A. Lee Silverman Voice Treatment (LSVT).
B. Head turn maneuvers.
C. Straw phonation.
D. Circumlaryngeal massage.

Teaching Points

Correct Answer: D

Muscle tension dysphonia is a voice disorder characterized by chronic increased tension of the laryngeal musculature. The circumlaryngeal massage is a treatment method that can be utilized to effectively relax the laryngeal muscles and promote phonation in this population. The effects of the massage can last for extensive periods of time, and repeated massages may be utilized as possible. Head turn maneuvers and LSVT may be utilized in the hypofunctional vocal fold population, such as paralysis and Parkinson's disease. While straw phonation promotes easy onset of phonation, it does not reduce the increased tension in the laryngeal muscles found in muscle tension dysphonia.

A48

Spoken Language Disorders in Children

Speech and language researchers are attempting to determine the causes of language disorders in young children. They believe that specific biological feature differences in children are the root cause of language disorders. Which of the following would be the **MOST APPROPRIATE** hypothesis for these researchers?

Choices:
A. Language disorders are caused by brain asymmetry in children.
B. Language disorders are caused due to a lack of literacy opportunities in children.
C. Language disorders arise due to differences across language-learning environments in children.
D. Children with language disorders demonstrate limited processing capacity.

Teaching Points

Correct Answer: A

Potential causal factors for childhood language disorders may be broken down into biological, environmental and cognitive differences. Biological features that may account for childhood language disorders include brain asymmetry in children with language disorders and chromosomal differences. In contrast to this, limited processing capacity in children with language disorders are considered a cognitive deficit, and lack of literacy opportunities and limited language-learning environments are considered environmental differences.

A49

Autism Spectrum Disorders

A research team is currently investigating genetic theories to establish the cause of autism. The researchers have focused their research on children with autism spectrum disorder, who have faulty chromosome 11. Which of the following may be a hypothesis generated by these researchers?

Choices:
A. These children show lack of communication between neurons, causing their autism spectrum disorder.
B. These children show a lack of development of brain circuitry, causing their autism spectrum disorder.
C. These children show intellectual impairments, causing their autism spectrum disorder.
D. These children show faulting cell-to-cell signaling, causing their autism spectrum disorder.

Teaching Points

Correct Answer: A
Chromosome 11 consists of a group of genes involved in communication between neurons during brain development. If this research assumed chromosome 11 was implicated in autism spectrum disorder, they would most likely assume a lack of neuronal communication as the cause of the disorder. In contrast to this, chromosome 5 is responsible for development of brain circuitry, chromosome 15 is associated with intellectual impairment and chromosome 16 is responsible for cell-to-cell signaling and interaction.

A50

Autism Spectrum Disorders

Ruth is a speech-language pathologist (SLP) who is preparing to administer an assessment to a child suspected of having autism spectrum disorder in order to determine eligibility for intervention. Which of the following is an important consideration Ruth must factor in to her assessment of this child?

Choices:
A. The avoidance of criterion-referenced measurements in the assessment of autism spectrum disorders.
B. Informal observation of behaviors is a means of assessment not accepted by most school systems.
C. Form assessment measures are the most widely accepted method of determining eligibility.
D. The child must receive a diagnostic label following assessment in order to receive services.

Teaching Points

Correct Answer: A
When determining a child with autism spectrum disorder's eligibility for speech and language services, criterion referencing should be avoided. With this type of evaluation, cognitive and linguistic skills may be revealed as commensurate, which prompts many people to advocate against SLP intervention. In contrast to this, informal observations of behaviors exhibited by these children is critical in determining eligibility. Performance on a formal assessment may not be an accurate reflection of the child's abilities, and diagnostic labels may not be appropriate due to the heterogeneity of the autism spectrum disorder population.

A51

Dysphagia

After performing both bedside evaluation and instrumental assessment on a patient, consulting speech-language pathologists (SLPs) have determined the primary feature of their patient's dysphagia is characterized by a weak swallow. In order to improve the swallow, the SLPs have determined that the best treatment approach is to have the patient engage in swallowing-based exercises using boluses, with a minimum of three different swallowing exercises in each session. Which of the following principles of neuroplasticity is NOT explicitly targeted in the clinician's description?

Choices:
A. Use it or lose it.
B. Repetition matters.
C. Use it and improve it.
D. Age matters.

Teaching Points

Correct Answer: D
This SLP is using the approaches "use it or lose it" and "use it and improve it" simultaneously, because they are having the patient swallow boluses of real food in order to improve their swallowing. Additionally, because the SLP has chosen to have the patient engage in three swallows per bolus, they are engaging the principle of "repetition matters." While age would more than likely be a factor in deciding treatment approaches, the plan does not specifically address this in the approach.

A52

Stuttering and Other Fluency Disorders

Differentiating stuttering-like disfluencies from typical disfluencies is a clinical observation that:

Choices:
A. Always helps determine if someone is faking.
B. Helps determine the stage of stuttering in young children.
C. Is particularly important at more advanced stages of stuttering.
D. Is impossible to determine.

Teaching Points

Correct Answer: B
The differentiation of the type of disfluency being exhibited is a key feature in stuttering assessment and helps to determine whether treatment is indicated or not in these early years. In older children and adults (advanced stuttering), the type of stuttering has already been diagnosed, in most cases, and this distinction is of less importance.

A53

Motor Speech Disorders

A speech-language pathologist (SLP) has been working with an 8-year-old client for the last few weeks, in an effort to improve the client's intelligibility. The SLP decides that the child is an appropriate candidate for an integral stimulation approach to treatment. A key component of this methodology is a focus on:

Choices:
A. Articulation.
B. Rhythm and/or rate.
C. Tactile/gestural.
D. Augmentative and alternative communication.

Teaching Points

Correct Answer: A
The integral stimulation treatment approach follows when the speaker is asked to watch the clinician produce an utterance and then say the target after the clinician. Using this treatment approach focuses on the speaker's articulation of specific sounds/words and allows the speaker to compare his/her production with the production of typical speech from the clinician.

A54

Anatomy and Physiology of Communication and Swallowing

Inspiration during quiet breathing involves contraction of the diaphragm that:

Choices:
A. Increases the volume of the thoracic cavity and causes pressure in the lungs to increase.
B. Increases the volume to thoracic cavity and causes pressure in the lungs to decrease.
C. Decreases the volume of the thoracic cavity and causes pressure in the lungs to increase.
D. Decreases the volume of the thoracic cavity and causes pressure in the lungs to decrease.

Teaching Points

Correct Answer: B
When the diaphragm contracts, it pulls downward toward the abdominal cavity, increasing the volume of the thoracic cavity, where the lungs are housed. According to Boyle's law, as volume increases, pressure decreases. Thus, if the volume of the thoracic cavity increases, the pressure in the lungs decreases, which is the main drive behind inspiration.

A55

Speech Sound Disorders in Children

A child is brought into a local speech and language clinic for treatment of a speech sound disorder. When the speech-language pathologist (SLP) interviews the child's parents, they reveal that their child has severely hypernasal speech. On which of the following types of speech sound would this child's hypernasality be most audible?

Choices:
A. Nasals.
B. Velars.
C. Plosives.
D. Vowels.

Teaching Points

Correct Answer: D

Hypernasality occurs when too much sound is resonating in the nasal cavity during speech. This type of resonance disorder is most perceptible on vowels, because this type of sound class is always voiced and always produced with a completely occluded nasal cavity. Hypernasality may affect some types of voiced consonants, but voiceless consonants would remain unaffected, as hypernasality is the result of sound vibration that is not present during production of voiceless consonants.

A56

Audiology and Hearing Impairment

A patient has received comprehensive audiologic evaluation after complaints of hearing loss and was diagnosed with a vestibular schwannoma. What type of hearing loss, if any, would this patient be experiencing?

Choices:
A. Conductive hearing loss.
B. Mixed hearing loss.
C. Sensorineural hearing loss.
D. No hearing loss.

Teaching Points

Correct Answer: C

A sensorineural hearing loss is a type of hearing loss that results from disorders of the cochlea and/or CN VIII. Vestibular schwannomas are a type of acoustic tumor that affects the vestibulocochlear nerve (i.e., CN VIII). Because this is a disorder of a cranial nerve, it would lead to a sensorineural hearing loss. In contrast to this, a conductive hearing loss results from problems associated with the outer and/or middle ear. Lastly, mixed hearing loss includes problems congruent with both conductive and sensorineural hearing loss.

A57

Acoustics

The spectrum of a speaker's voice shows that H1 is 15 dB higher than H2 in amplitude. This **MOST LIKELY** indicates that the speaker has a:

Choices:
A. Breathy voice.
B. Modal voice.
C. Creaky voice.
D. High harmonic-to-noise ratio (HNR).

Teaching Points

Correct Answer: A

The relative amplitude of H1 and H2 provide an indicator of spectral tilt, which can differentiate voice quality changes between breathy, modal and creaky voice. Breathy voice is distinguished by an H1 that is higher in amplitude than H2. In modal voice, H1 and H2 are approximately equal in amplitude. In creaky voice, H1 is lower in amplitude than H2. HNR is a measure of overall harmonic-to-noise ratio rather than a comparison of H1-H2 amplitude.

A58

Motor Speech Disorders

The organizational framework of the treatment session can both positively and negatively influence success of therapy. A **UNIQUE** consideration when organizing treatment for children is:

Choices:
A. To avoid reinforcements that take too much time to administer.
B. The need for greater amounts of cumulative practice.
C. Clinician preparation.
D. The need for shorter treatment sessions.

Teaching Points

Correct Answer: B
When compared to adults, children exhibit shorter attention spans and reduced short-term memory. Because of these relative reductions when compared to adults, children will require greater amounts of cumulative practice in order to make the same amount of gains. Shorter treatment sessions, clinician preparation and an appropriate length of time prior to reinforcement are aspects of treatment that apply to both children and adults.

A59

Anatomy and Physiology of Communication and Swallowing

A person places a hand on a hot surface and experiences the sensation of heat. The feeling of heat is conveyed up to the primary somatosensory cortex in the parietal lobe. In order for this information to be received in this cortical area, it must first travel up the spinal column, via the:

Choices:
A. Lateral corticospinal tract.
B. Anterior corticospinal tract.
C. Anterolateral system.
D. Posterior column-lemniscal system.

Teaching Points

Correct Answer: C
If a person places a hand on a hot stove, this would cause pain and temperature sensation, which would be conveyed through the anterolateral system (pain, temperature and crude touch). The posterior column-medial lemniscus system is responsible for transmission of vibration, pressure and fine touch information. The lateral corticospinal tract and anterior corticospinal tract are both motor tracts, which control limb movement and girdle movement, respectively.

A60

Dysphagia

A speech-language pathologist (SLP) that works in a long-term acute care setting has received a physician request for a swallow evaluation. However, the only information that can be found in this patient's medical records regarding his/her swallowing status is that the patient was on a mechanical soft solid/thin liquid diet upon discharge from the acute care hospital. Which of the following consistencies is appropriate to bring into the bedside swallow evaluation?

Choices:
A. Pureed solids.
B. Mechanical soft solids.
C. Advanced soft solids.
D. All of the above.

Teaching Points

Correct Answer: D

It is appropriate to bring all of the textures mentioned to this patient's bedside swallow examination. Because the last note said that the patient was swallowing mechanical soft solids, the SLP should evaluate this consistency to check if the patient is safely and efficiently swallowing it. Pureed and advanced soft solids should also be tried to assess for an appropriate means of oral intake for the patient.

A61

Anatomy and Physiology of Communication and Swallowing

When forming the vowel /u/ in *boot*, which muscle **MOST LIKELY** contracts?

Choices:
A. Orbicularis oris.
B. Levator labii superioris.
C. Zygomatic major.
D. Risorius.

Teaching Points

Correct Answer: A

The orbicularis oris muscle is the sphincter-like muscle that surrounds the lips. Contraction of this muscle can lead to the lip-rounding associated with production of the /u/ phoneme in the word *boot*. In contrast to this, the levator labii superioris muscle contributes to elevation and everting of the upper lip. The zygomatic major contracts the corners of the mouth backward by simultaneously lifting and pulling the corners of the mouth sideways. Finally, the risorius muscle retracts the angle of the mouth upon contraction.

A62

Acoustics

The pitch contour of a vowel shows that the pitch begins at 200 hertz (Hz). If the pitch contour is accurate, the period at the beginning of the vowel will be:

Choices:
A. 0.005 sec.
B. 0.05 sec.
C. 0.005 Hz.
D. 0.05 Hz.

Teaching Points

Correct Answer: A

Frequency and period are in an inverse relationship. Period is a time measurement. If F0 = 200 Hz, the period will be 1/200 = 0.005 sec.

A63

Anatomy and Physiology of Communication and Swallowing

There are several parts of a neuron that are important in the transmission of neural signals throughout the body. Which of the following components is most important for receiving signals from other neurons?

Choices:
A. Soma.
B. Dendrite.
C. Axon.
D. Phospholipid bilayer.

Teaching Points

Correct Answer: B
Dendrites are the part of the neuron that are important in receiving action potentials from other neurons. The soma is the term for the cell body of the neuron, whereas the axon is the portion of the neuron that is important for propagation of action potentials to future neurons.

A64

Anatomy and Physiology of Communication and Swallowing

The spinal column is organized with respect to motor/sensory function, as well as upper and lower extremities. Cell bodies of lower motor neurons that control movement of the legs are generally found in:

Choices:
A. The precentral gyrus.
B. The postcentral gyrus.
C. The ventral horn of the spinal column.
D. The dorsal horn of the spinal column.

Teaching Points

Correct Answer: C
The ventral horns of the spinal column house the lower motor neurons responsible for movement, whereas the dorsal horns house neurons responsible for transmission of sensory information. The precentral and postcentral gyri are structures located in the cerebral hemispheres, which house the primary motor cortex and primary somatosensory cortices.

A65

Acquired Language Disorders

Language assessment results for a person showed: nonfluent verbal output with significant agrammatism, with a co-occurring apraxia of speech. The individual had relatively preserved auditory comprehension, but difficulty with repetition of even single words. Based on this scenario, the type of aphasia the person would **MOST LIKELY** be diagnosed with is:

Choices:
A. Global aphasia.
B. Transcortical motor aphasia.
C. Broca's aphasia.
D. Wernicke's aphasia.

Teaching Points

Correct Answer: C

A person with Broca's aphasia would present with nonfluent aphasia, significant agrammatism, intact auditory comprehension, deficits with repetition and a possibly co-occurring apraxia of speech. This is differentiated from global aphasia because of the spared auditory comprehension, transcortical motor aphasia because of the impaired repetition and Wernicke's aphasia because of the nonfluent verbal expression.

A66

Stuttering and Other Fluency Disorders

A speech-language pathologist (SLP) working in an elementary school is planning to enroll a kindergarten student in stuttering therapy after completing a careful diagnostic assessment. She discovers a policy that says children are not enrolled in fluency therapy in this particular school district until third grade. When she queries the rationale for the policy, she is told that "most students will grow out of stuttering and we don't want to waste resources." This is an example of :

Choices:
A. Unethical behavior.
B. Using school resources wisely.
C. Denial of the impact of developmental stuttering on a child's participation and benefit from the educational program.
D. Bad leadership.

Teaching Points

Correct Answer: D

While many school districts have had policies that delay treatment for children who stutter, there have been rulings that prohibit this practice. The argument has been made that stuttering is an impairment that can affect both educational performance and the participation of the child in the educational program. While many children will emerge as fluent speakers, the purpose of therapy for young children is to prevent the consequences of more advanced stuttering.

A67

Spoken Language Disorders in Children

A child and her mother are participating in a play evaluation with a speech-language pathologist. At one point in the evaluation, the mother asks her child, "Did Mary eat the cookie?" to which the child responds, "Yes, Mary ate the cookie." With which language structure does this child demonstrate difficulty?

Choices:
A. Narrative.
B. Ellipsis.
C. Dialect.
D. Acknowledgement.

Teaching Points

Correct Answer: B

Ellipsis refers to deleting already said information, even if it results in an ungrammatical sentence, and is a common structure in conversational language. As this child includes the information that "Mary ate the cookie," rather than "Yes, she did," she is demonstrating difficulty with ellipsis. Narrative refers to a decontextualized monologue that conveys a story, personal recount or retelling of a book or movie. Dialect refers to a style of speech related to ethnic, gender, region and generational differences. Finally, acknowledging is a form of communicative intention expressed by preschoolers.

A68
Research, Evidence-Based Practice and Tests and Measurements

A speech-language pathologist (SLP) is designing a study to research the effectiveness of a new treatment approach for aphasia, utilizing a time-series treatment design. He wants to be sure that the outcomes are valid, thus he wants to strengthen his treatment design as much as possible. Which of the following could this researcher include to maximize the strength of his study?

Choices:
A. Meta-analyses and systematic reviews.
B. Control groups and an analysis of variance (ANOVA).
C. Randomization and counterbalancing.
D. Multiple alternating treatments and baseline segments.

Teaching Points

Correct Answer: D

A time-series treatment design is a used for studying treatment efficacy. This specific type of design includes repeated baseline measures prior to treatment and includes systematic ongoing measurement of participant performance. The research performed using this type of design may be strengthened by including control subjects, a second baseline segment after treatment has begun, or multiple alternating treatment and baseline segments.

A69
Anatomy and Physiology of Communication and Swallowing

Dopamine is a neurotransmitter that plays an important role in neural signals involved in motor movement. Lack of dopamine in the substantia nigra has been associated with disease processes such as Parkinson's disease. What **BEST** describes the role of dopamine on basal ganglia circuits?

Choices:
A. Dopamine is excitatory to the direct and indirect pathways of the basal ganglia.
B. The net result of dopamine release to direct and indirect pathways of the basal ganglia is a facilitation of movement.
C. The net result of dopamine release to the direct pathway facilitates movement while release to the indirect pathway inhibits movement.
D. Dopamine is inhibitory to the direct and indirect pathways of the basal ganglia.

Teaching Points

Correct Answer: B

The net result of dopamine release into the basal ganglia control circuits is facilitation of movement, although the effect is different depending on which pathway is activated. Activation of the direct activation pathway assists with excitation of movement, whereas activation of the indirect activation pathway assists with inhibition of movement.

A70

Spoken Language Disorders in Children

Gus is a speech-language pathologist (SLP) working in an early childhood education setting. Recently, he has begun working with a child who has a significant language disorder. For this child, Gus has chosen to utilize induction teaching to facilitate the child's learning of language. Which of the following statements BEST describes this approach to intervention?

Choices:
A. Providing an enriched language-learning environment with no specific targets.
B. Targeting of specific forms and functions through repetition and modeling.
C. Increasing the rate at which a targeted form or function is learned.
D. Using a more explicit and systematic set of teaching steps.

Teaching Points

Correct Answer: D

Induction teaching refers to use a more explicit and systematic set of teaching steps, beyond modeling. When this form of instruction is utilized, it is not assumed the targeted form would have been learned without intervention or learned to the same degree. Use of induction teaching also leads to concomitant achievements in academic and/or social contexts. In contrast to this, facilitation refers to increasing the rate at which a targeted form or function is learned, focused stimulation refers to the targeting of specific forms and functions by the SLP through repetition or modeling, and general stimulation refers to a provision of an enriched language-learning environment with no specific target for learning.

A71

Augmentative and Alternative Communication (AAC)

Linda is an elderly woman who has recently sustained a large right middle cerebral artery infarction, resulting in a significant neglect and severe flaccid dysarthria. Linda's speech-language pathologist (SLP) has been implementing use of an augmentative and alternative communication (AAC) device to improve Linda's communicative effectiveness. The SLP has determined a list of high-frequency words for Linda to use in conversation and is determining the most appropriate placement of symbols on Linda's device. Which statement describes the MOST APPROPRIATE placement for Linda's symbols?

Choices:
A. On the right, so as to be more readily accessible.
B. In the middle, so as to encourage scanning.
C. On the left, so as to be more readily accessible.
D. On the border, so as to cancel effects of the neglect.

Teaching Points

Correct Answer: A

Placement of symbols should be informed by both the person with complex communication's physical and visual limitations to access. The most common form of neglect following a right hemisphere stroke is a left neglect, meaning the patient does not attend to (i.e., realize) there is stimuli on his/her left side. For this reason, the most appropriate placement of the user from this scenario's symbols is on the right, to maximize the chances that he/she will attend to and utilize the symbols for communication.

A72
Language Acquisition

Matthew is a 12-month-old boy whose pediatrician has referred him for assessment by the speech-language pathologist (SLP). The physician's referral message indicates that he is delayed in communication for his age. Which of the following is the **MOST LIKELY** behavior expected in children around 12 months?

Choices:
A. Single words or pointing.
B. Combinations of two words.
C. Grammatically complete sentences with minor phonological errors.
D. Vegetative sounds such as coughing, burping and some vocalizations.

Teaching Points

Correct Answer: A

Children are usually using single words or doing some pointing by about 12 months of age. Grammar emerges later in development. Vegetative sounds are nonlinguistic, and vocalizing comes much earlier in development.

A73
Voice Disorders

The voice team has been asked to evaluate a 3-month-old client presenting with parent-reported "weak cry." Following a comprehensive evaluation, which of the following findings would **NOT** be considered a typical laryngeal characteristic for this patient?

Choices:
A. A relatively small portion of vibrating vocal fold tissue.
B. Prominent arytenoid processes of the vocal folds.
C. Laryngeal positioning around cervical vertebra three.
D. The soft palate contacting the epiglottis at rest.

Teaching Points

Correct Answer: B

Differences between adult and infant larynges include shorter membranous vocal fold tissues, higher positioning of the larynx in the neck and the soft palate and epiglottis coming into contact with each other. Prominent arytenoid processes are associated with elderly vocal folds, as the vocal fold tissues begin to atrophy and reveal the arytenoid processes in this population. If there are prominent arytenoid processes seen during an infant's evaluation, this should be considered a red flag, and steps to treat this problem should be taken.

A74

Speech Sound Disorders in Children

Susie, a 5-year-old girl, is brought into a speech clinic for a full articulation and phonological evaluation, after being referred by her teacher. The speech-language pathologist (SLP) notices that she does not produce several "age-appropriate" phonemes. Which of the following is a phoneme that this child might have difficulty with producing, based on the given information?

Choices:
A. /s/.
B. /m/.
C. /r/.
D. /l/.

Teaching Points

Correct Answer: B

Of the phonemes listed, /m/ is a phoneme that is traditionally considered one of the earlier developing speech sounds, typically occurring by 3 years of age. The other phonemes listed are considered later developing sounds, typically occurring between the ages of 6 and 8 years. Therefore, if a 5-year-old client is demonstrating problems with production of age-appropriate phonemes, /m/ would be a phoneme that could prove difficult.

A75

Written Language Disorders in the School-Age Population

A speech-language pathologist (SLP) is asked to consult on a child in a first-grade classroom who is having difficulty with reading. When you arrive to perform the consult, the SLP discovers that the child comes from an unfamiliar cultural background. In order to better understand the case, what factors would **MOST LIKELY** influence learning to read?

Choices:
A. Language and literacy experiences in the home.
B. The child's reading preferences.
C. Parental reading and writing capabilities.
D. Family attitudes toward speech-language pathologists.

Teaching Points

Correct Answer: A

Attitudes toward language and literacy practices may vary greatly between cultures. By understanding the attitudes toward language and literacy within a particular student's home, an SLP may better be able to tailor assessment plans, which can lead to appropriate diagnosis. Additionally, the SLP may develop appropriate intervention plans to meet cultural expectations.

A76

The Practice of Speech-Language Pathology

A speech-language pathologist (SLP) in an outpatient speech and language clinic has been contacted by a patient interested in receiving cognitive therapy. The client claims to have been evaluated by another SLP and referred to this SLP for specific treatments for "attention and memory deficits." In this situation, the SLP should first:

Choices:
A. Administer his/her own assessment of the patient's cognitive abilities.
B. Accept the previous SLP's report and begin providing services.
C. Deny the patient services until contact with the previous SLP is established.
D. Begin intervention for this patient's cognitive deficit.

Teaching Points

Correct Answer: A

According to the ASHA Code of Ethics, Principle of Ethics IV, Rule of Ethics J, "Individuals shall not provide professional services without exercising independent professional judgment, regardless of referral source or prescription." Although the patient from this scenario may have been evaluated by a previous SLP, the patient did not divulge the date of the last evaluation, and much may have changed since that time. The SLP is fully within his/her own right as a professional to administer a cognitive-linguistic evaluation to this patient, and if results show that treatment is indicated, begin therapy. The SLP should always perform his/her own evaluation, to see if services are, indeed, required.

A77

Language Acquisition

Samantha is a 20-month-old toddler who has not met several of her early word-learning milestones. She demonstrates a small vocabulary and does not make two-word combinations. Using this information, which of the following BEST describes Samantha?

Choices:
A. She demonstrates an early language disorder.
B. She demonstrates an early language difference.
C. She is a typically developing toddler.
D. She demonstrates an early language delay.

Teaching Points

Correct Answer: D

Toddlers who do not meet early word-learning milestones in a timely manner, such as Samantha from this scenario, are referred to as late talkers. While most outgrow their early language delay, some will demonstrate language deficits that persist into preschool language disorders. Language differences refer to differing, but appropriate use of language. As Samantha has not reached several milestones, she is not a typically developing toddler.

A78

Motor Speech Disorders

The presence of development dysarthria has the potential to interfere with speech intelligibility as a result of impairment of motor skills. Therapy should focus on reduction of or compensation for the impairment. In addition to targeting motor development of the speech production system, what is the **MOST IMPORTANT** element to improve communication of the child with dysarthria?

Choices:
A. Treatment to reduce drooling.
B. Appropriate positioning of the child to maximize breathing for speech.
C. Development of repair strategies when communication breakdowns occur.
D. Targeting both receptive and expressive language skills.

Teaching Points

Correct Answer: D

Although dysarthria is a motor speech disorder, children with this type of speech difficulty are still in danger of lagging behind their peers in terms of receptive/expressive language development. Targeting receptive/expressive language within treatment sessions for children with dysarthria will promote age-appropriate development of language for these clients.

A79

Spoken Language Disorders in Children

Richard is a speech-language pathologist (SLP) in a preschool setting. Currently, he is working with a child who has specific deficits in morphological developments. Richard wants to establish that morphemes he has targeted in this child's intervention sessions are being used consistently. What level of use is appropriate for establishing acquisition of morphological structures?

Choices:
A. 85% of use in obligatory contexts.
B. 90% of use in obligatory contexts.
C. 95% of use in obligatory contexts.
D. 100% of use in obligatory contexts.

Teaching Points

Correct Answer: B

The consistency of morpheme use in obligatory contexts is the most appropriate measure for establishing the acquisition of a morpheme. This consistency can be calculated as the number of times the child correctly produced a specific morpheme (in obligatory context) divided by the total number of opportunities for that specific morpheme to have been produced in a spoken or written passage. Traditionally, the standard for establishing morpheme acquisition has been 90% of use in obligatory contexts.

A80
Speech Sound Disorders in Children

A speech-language pathologist (SLP) has been providing speech therapy to a child with a speech sound disorder. As this child demonstrates errors on multiple phonemes, the SLP has selected the cycles remediation approach for intervention with this child. What could the SLP do to utilize this treatment approach?

Choices:
A. Target a different phoneme each treatment session.
B. Provide multiple input modes to establish productions of phonemes.
C. Target different areas of language for generalization to phonological impairments.
D. Target word pairs that are contrasted by a single phoneme.

Teaching Points

Correct Answer: A

The cycles remediation approach targets a single errored phoneme per treatment session, and once all errored phonemes have been targeted a full "cycle" has been completed. A new cycle is then started, which builds off of the work completed in the previous cycle. This intervention method would be the best match to the SLP's wishes for intervention. In contrast, the integral stimulation approach utilizes multiple input modes to help a child learn the motor pattern for speech sound production. The maximal opposition approach utilizes sound pairs that are maximally different (i.e., by more than one feature) to help with errored speech sound production. Finally, the whole-language treatment approach targets multiple areas of language simultaneously to help build a child's phonological skills.

A81
Anatomy and Physiology of Communication and Swallowing

A person has a vital capacity of 5 liters and exchanges half a liter of air when typically breathing at rest. The person takes the biggest breath possible and inspires 3 liters of air. What is the expiratory reserve volume?

Choices:
A. 1.5 liters.
B. 2 liters.
C. 2.5 liters.
D. 3.5 liters.

Teaching Points

Correct Answer: A

A person's vital capacity is made of inspiratory reserve volume, expiratory reserve volume and tidal volume. In the presented scenario, the patient has a tidal volume of 0.5 liters (the amount of air exchanged passively) and an inspiratory reserve volume (found from the largest inspiration) of 3 liters. The remaining volume needed to reach the vital capacity of 5 liters is 1.5 liters of expiratory reserve volume.

A82

The Practice of Speech-Language Pathology

A speech-language pathologist (SLP) in an acute rehabilitation hospital has several patients on his/her caseload and has begun to feel highly overwhelmed by the amount of work that needs to be completed. However, the SLP is unsure of how to proceed in a way that reduces stress appropriately. Which of the following steps could the SLP take in order to better manage his/her caseload?

Choices:
A. Request a speech-language pathology assistant to perform all patient evaluations.
B. Request a fellow speech-language pathologist become lead clinician for some patients.
C. Discharge high-level patients from the caseload.
D. Continue working at the current pace with the current caseload.

Teaching Points

Correct Answer: B

According to the American Speech-Language-Hearing Association (ASHA) Code of Ethics, Principle of Ethics I, Rule of Ethics E, "Individuals who hold the Certificate of Clinical Competence shall not delegate tasks that require the unique skills, knowledge, and judgment that are within the scope of their profession to assistants, technicians, support personnel, or any nonprofessionals over whom they have supervisory responsibility." As this SLP is feeling significantly overwhelmed, he/she may not be able to appropriately deliver services to all patients on the SLP's caseload. The ASHA Code of Ethics prevents the SLP from delegating evaluations to an SLPA, and doing so would prove to be an unethical decision. In contrast to this, another SLP maintains the knowledge and skills to work with any patient, so relinquishing some patients would prove to be an ethical decision that may lead to better outcomes for all involved. Additionally, it is unethical to discharge patients simply for being "high level." A patient may be discharged from services when an SLP appropriately determines the patient has made maximum amounts of progress.

A83

Acoustics

In order to accurately measure voice onset time (VOT) in a series of stop consonants, the speech-language pathologist (SLP) should work from:

Choices:
A. Shorter VOT.
B. Longer VOT.
C. More compact spectrum.
D. More diffuse spectrum.

Teaching Points

Correct Answer: B

VOT is a time measurement. Time measurements should be made from broadband spectrograms or waveforms. Narrowband spectrograms have poor time resolution and should never be used for time measurements. Amplitude spectra have no time axis.

A84

Anatomy and Physiology of Communication and Swallowing

If a patient has denervation of the trigeminal nerve (CN V), which deficit would **MOST LIKELY** result?

Choices:
A. Reduced sensation of the trachea.
B. Reduced salivation from the parotid gland.
C. Reduced lingual control.
D. Reduced capacity for mastication.

Teaching Points

Correct Answer: D

CN V, the trigeminal nerve, controls sensation from the anterior two-thirds of the tongue and sensation of the teeth, gums and oral mucosa, controls salivary flow from the minor glands, and controls the muscles of mastication and helps with some muscles of laryngeal/hyoid elevation. The most likely presentation of a trigeminal nerve lesion would be a deficit with mastication, or chewing.

A85

Stuttering and Other Fluency Disorders

Mary is a speech-language pathologist (SLP) in a public school. She has received a referral from a classroom teacher for evaluation of a 10-year-old boy with a fast rate, history of language and learning problems and a high rate of disfluency that occurs in connected speech. The teacher indicates that the child doesn't seem too bothered by his problem. Mary completes her evaluation, which supports the teacher's assessment. This boy's fluency disorder is **MOST LIKELY** to be:

Choices:
A. Neurogenic fluency disorder.
B. Developmental stuttering.
C. Cluttering.
D. Psychogenic fluency disorder.

Teaching Points

Correct Answer: C

Cluttering is a fluency impairment that is seen in children and becomes prominent as they advance in school years. These children also usually show signs of learning difficulties and other motor problems. Excessive rate and lack of awareness are critical features that distinguish cluttering from other fluency disorders.

A86

The Practice of Speech-Language Pathology

A speech-language pathologist (SLP) at a skilled nursing facility currently has no patients on his/her caseload. After evaluating a newly admitted patient, the SLP determines the patient is functioning in the typical range, but on the border of a mild cognitive-linguistic disorder. The SLP is interested in working with this patient, but is unsure of what recommendations to make. How should the SLP proceed in the case of this patient?

Choices:
A. As the SLP needs to meet productivity standards, he/she should recommend services for the patient.
B. As the patient is on the border of a mild disorder, the SLP should recommend services.
C. As the patient is functioning in the typical range, the SLP should not recommend services.
D. As the SLP does not believe they have the skills to work with this patient, the SLP should not recommend services for the patient.

Teaching Points

Correct Answer: C

According to the ASHA Code of Ethics, Principle of Ethics III, Rule of Ethics C, "Individuals shall refer those served professionally solely on the basis of the interest of those being referred and not on any personal interest, financial or otherwise." As the patient is functioning in the typical range, it may not be in the patient's best interest to refer him/her for services. Although the SLP needs to meet productivity standards, the SLP may not ethically recommend the patient for services solely for this reason. Finally, if the SLP feels he/she does not have the skills to work with this patient, the SLP is still ethically bound to refer in the best interest of the patient and recommend that another SLP be the lead clinician.

A87

The Practice of Speech-Language Pathology

Allison is a speech-language pathologist (SLP) who has worked in the school system for the last 30 years. Recently, her friend's mother had a stroke, resulting in significant dysphagia. Allison's friend asks her if she could provide services, as Allison is the only SLP she knows. Allison has not given treatment to a patient with dysphagia since graduate school and has not attended any continuing education classes on the topic. What should Allison do in this situation?

Choices:
A. Refer her friend to a professional with more experience in the treatment of dysphagia.
B. Refer her friend to a colleague who works with clients with pediatric dysphagia.
C. Provide services to her friend's mother, as dysphagia falls within her scope of practice.
D. Provide recommendations for at-home exercises targeting improved functional swallowing abilities.

Teaching Points

Correct Answer: A

According to the ASHA Code of Ethics, Principle of Ethics II, Rule of Ethics B, "Individuals shall engage in only those aspects of the professions that are within the scope of their professional practice and competence, considering their level of education, training, and experience." As Allison has not provided intervention to adult clients with dysphagia in at least 30 years, her understanding of treatment, including at-home exercises, may be outdated. Therefore, she should make a referral to a professional with the most up-to-date knowledge, in order to provide the best services to her friend's mother. Additionally, a clinician working with the pediatric dysphagia population may not have a full understanding of how dysphagia affects the adult population and therefore should not be consulted.

A88

Dysphagia

An infant is brought into the emergency room, and the parents report that their child is continually vomiting after every meal and has not stopped crying for the past few days. After a full consult by speech-language pathologists (SLPs), nutritionists and gastrointestinal (GI) specialists, it is decided that the infant is suffering from pediatric gastroesophageal reflux disorder (GERD). Because infants are not yet mature enough to participate in treatment efforts on their own, which of the following is a treatment approach the SLP could share with the parents that is targeted at reducing the symptoms of pediatric GERD?

Choices:
A. Giving the child extremely acidic food, to counteract the stomach acid.
B. Positioning the infant on his/her back to allow gravity to counter the regurgitation.
C. Positioning the infant on the side, to avoid aspiration of regurgitated foods.
D. Positioning the infant upright, to reduce the regurgitation of food.

Teaching Points

Correct Answer: D
Pediatric GERD can be managed through postural techniques, nutritional approaches, medication, or surgical intervention. Because the infant needs immediate attention for the GERD symptoms, it is important to begin trying strategies as soon as the infant is medically stable. Positioning the infant in an upright position can help reduce the upflow of stomach contents, alleviating the infant's symptoms.

A89

Spoken Language Disorders in Children

A young child has been receiving speech-language therapy to remediate her language disorder. After many months of intervention, the speech-language pathologist (SLP) would like to assess the progress this child has made during intervention. What is the **MOST APPROPRIATE** method for assessing this child's progress?

Choices:
A. Review data collected during intervention sessions.
B. Elicit untrained exemplars during conversation.
C. Administer a standardized assessment and compare scores.
D. Implement dynamic assessment procedures.

Teaching Points

Correct Answer: B
Periodic measurement of client performance is a critical component of advancing clients through therapy. One way to assess progress is to utilize untrained exemplars when eliciting language. For example, if the client has been working on the third-person singular form of *come*, the clinician can probe for generalization to *walk*. Administration of standardized assessment is discouraged, as there may be a recall bias for assessment material. Dynamic assessment would reveal how the child is functioning currently, but may not probe generalization. Finally, reviewing data collected during intervention, while essential for steering the direction of treatment, will reveal when goals need to be updated, but does not probe for current level of progress.

A90

Spoken Language Disorders in Children

Greg is a child who demonstrates deficits in perspective taking during conversation. Specifically, Greg is struggling to infer other's feelings and thoughts, which has negatively impacted his ability to converse with others. In which form of perspective taking is Greg demonstrating deficits?

Choices:
A. Linguistic perspective taking.
B. Perceptual perspective taking.
C. Cognitive perspective taking.
D. Phonological perspective taking.

Teaching Points

Correct Answer: C

Cognitive perspective taking refers to a child's ability to make inferences about other people's thoughts, feelings, beliefs, and/or intentions, and involves making judgments about the internal psychological states of another person. In contrast to this, perceptual perspective taking refers to a child's ability to determine what and how another person sees an object. Finally, linguistic perspective taking refers to a child's ability to modify the form, content and/or use of language in relation to the child's listener's needs.

A91

Research, Evidence-Based Practice and Tests and Measurements

A speech scientist is performing a research study on a particular treatment program for childhood language disorders and has decided to utilize effect size as a measure of data outcome. What would be the **BEST** measure for this scientist to use in the study?

Choices:
A. Cohen's d.
B. Chi-square.
C. Cochran Q test.
D. Analysis of variance (ANOVA).

Teaching Points

Correct Answer: A

Cohen's *d* is one of the most common measurements of effect size and would be the most appropriate selection for this scientist. If the scientist was interested in measuring the level of significance between any relationships among nominal variables, chi-square would be the most appropriate selection. The Cochran Q test is a nonparametric procedure used to assess nominal level data from related samples and would not be appropriate for measuring effect size. Finally, the ANOVA would be the most appropriate selection if the scientist was interested in simultaneous comparison of several means.

A92
Motor Speech Disorders

Slowing speaking rate as a treatment method for individuals with dysarthria is contraindicated when the patient:

Choices:
A. Exhibits a clinically significant reduction in speech intelligibility.
B. Does not exhibit improvements in speech intelligibility when speaking rate is decreased.
C. Presents with a greater reduction in sentence intelligibility compared to word intelligibility.
D. Exhibits a 25% reduction in vital capacity.

Teaching Points

Correct Answer: B

Slowing the rate of a person's speech should result in immediate improvement in intelligibility, which can be targeted in further sessions. If patients with severe disorders do not exhibit improvements in intelligibility with a slowed rate of speech, this treatment method should not be targeted. If there is not an immediate effect on intelligibility, other treatment methods should be explored, which can lead to greater overall communicative effectiveness for the patient.

A93
Written Language Disorders in the School-Age Population

A fourth-grade child on a speech-language pathologist's (SLP's) caseload at a local public school has difficulty with phonological/orthographic associations, automaticity and fluency and underlying language abilities. Which impairment would the child **MOST LIKELY** demonstrate?

Choices:
A. Ability to learn spelling rules.
B. Articulation of alveolar fricatives.
C. Spoken language capabilities.
D. Reading comprehension.

Teaching Points

Correct Answer: D

If a student has impaired phonological/orthographic associated and impaired automaticity/fluency, the child will present with word recognition deficits and slow, labored reading. When these deficits are coupled with deficits in underlying language abilities, the cognitive load needed to complete reading is greatly increased. This leads to very little cognitive ability for the student to comprehend written material and will present as reading comprehension deficits.

A94
Written Language Disorders in the School-Age Population

Which approach has been found to have small to moderate effects on enhancing students' text level reading fluency?

Choices:
A. Diadochokinetic exercises.
B. Practice with repeated reading.
C. Vocabulary instruction.
D. Teaching oral sentence formulation skills.

Teaching Points

Correct Answer: B

The National Reading Panel indicates multiple approaches to intervention for improving children's reading skills. Small to moderate effects have been found for repeated reading, whereas moderate to large effects have been found for phonological awareness intervention and word attack/work identification instruction. Positive effects for systematical vocabulary and summary-writing instruction have also been found.

A95

Research, Evidence-Based Practice and Tests and Measurements

A speech scientist has begun a research study, utilizing a between-subjects treatment design. In order to reduce the effect of an extraneous variable, which of the following procedures should the scientist implement?

Choices:
A. Randomly assign participants to a particular treatment condition.
B. Establish a reliable baseline performance for each participant.
C. Match research participants across treatment groups.
D. Randomize the order of treatment conditions for participants.

Teaching Points

Correct Answer: C

Between-subjects research designs involve comparing two or more groups of subjects. For this type of research design, it is critical that extraneous variables are controlled as much as possible to minimize their effect on the dependent variable. One way that the researcher from this scenario could control extraneous variables is to match participants across groups, either by averages (i.e., average age) or through pairwise matching based on the extraneous variable (i.e., gender, education level, etc.).

A96

Speech Sound Disorders in Children

A speech-language pathologist (SLP) in private practice has been referred to work with a new client who recently moved into the area. After reviewing the client's transfer notes, the previous SLP has made comments that the client demonstrates significant difficulty with producing the "late eight sounds." Which of the following speech sounds would this child **MOST LIKELY** have difficulty producing?

Choices:
A. /m/.
B. /t/.
C. /ʃ/.
D. /f/.

Teaching Points

Correct Answer: C

The /ʃ/ is considered one of the "late eight" developing sounds, along with [ʒ, ð, θ, s, z, l, r]. The sound /m/ is considered one of the "early eight" developing sounds, and /t/ and /f/ are both considered two of the "mid-eight" developing sounds.

A97

Cleft Palate and Other Craniofacial Anomalies

A speech-language pathologist (SLP) has been assigned to provide therapy to a child with a documented history of velopharyngeal insufficiency (VPI). Which activity would be the most appropriate method of therapy for the SLP to utilize with this particular client?

Choices:
A. Blowing exercises.
B. Oral-motor exercises.
C. Articulation therapy.
D. Increasing oral activity.

Teaching Points

Correct Answer: C
When working with individuals who have velopharyngeal insufficiency, speech therapy may be appropriate to address the client's compensatory articulation errors. For this reason, articulation therapy is the most appropriate selection for use with this child. Blowing exercises, oral-motor exercises and increasing oral activity are not effective at ameliorating any of the speech deficits present in individuals with VPI and are not indicated for use with this population.

A98

Speech Sound Disorders in Children

A speech-language pathologist (SLP) is working with a young child and suspects the child is unable to tell correct from incorrect productions of errored sounds. The SLP administers Locke's SPPT procedure to the child, and his suspicions are confirmed. Which of the following statements best describes this client?

Choices:
A. The child demonstrates poor intelligibility.
B. The child demonstrates poor perception.
C. The child demonstrates poor phonation.
D. The child demonstrates poor coarticulation.

Teaching Points

Correct Answer: B
The SPPT is an informal procedure that helps determine if the errored production is produced that way because of how it is stored in the mental lexicon. In contrast to this, discrimination is the ability to determine if dissimilar sounds are thought to be the same or different. Intelligibility refers to how well a listener understands the speech of the speaker, which is not the case in this scenario. Phonation refers to the production of sound from the vocal folds, and coarticulation is the influence of phonetic context on speech production.

A99

Written Language Disorders in the School-Age Population

On a speech-language pathologist's (SLP's) caseload, there is a client who is a typically developing second grader. However, the client shows specific impairments in both word recognition and spelling. In which component abilities would you expect this client to **MOST LIKELY** show deficits?

Choices:
A. Phonological processing and phonological memory.
B. Receptive vocabulary and orthographic processing.
C. Pragmatics and receptive vocabulary.
D. Phonological and orthographic processing.

Teaching Points

Correct Answer: D
With regards to word recognition, success is contingent on the ability to break words down into corresponding graphemes while understanding the relationship between these graphemes and their associated phonemes. This corresponds to appropriate phonological processing. Orthographic processing, as it relates to spelling, is the ability of students to associate spoken sounds (i.e., phonemes) with the appropriate graphemes. Therefore, if a student has deficits in both orthographic and phonological processing, the student would have difficulty with word recognition and spelling.

A100

Cleft Palate and Other Craniofacial Anomalies

A young child with developmental dysarthria exhibits hypernasality and nasal emissions on pressure consonants. Examination of the hard palate failed to note any structural deviations while range of motion for elevation of the soft palate appeared limited. Occlusion of the nose via a nose clip normalized breath group length and improved clarity of speech sound production. What step should the speech-language pathologist (SLP) take next in order to proceed appropriately?

Choices:
A. The speaker should be immediately fitted with a palatal lift.
B. Complete a thorough evaluation of the velopharyngeal system prior to initiating treatment.
C. Treatment should target the respiratory system in order to improve breath group length.
D. Refer the child for reconstruction of the velopharyngeal system.

Teaching Points

Correct Answer: B
The fact that this pediatric client is experiencing improvements in speech clarity with occlusion of the nose is an indicator that further assessment is warranted. Further assessment would allow the SLP working with this client to determine the extent of weakness that this patient is experiencing and allow the SLP to determine what changes can be made in order to aid in reduction of nasal emission and hypernasality.

A101
Spoken Language Disorders in Children

Following a very successful intervention session, in which Annie produced 95% of targeted utterances correctly, her speech-language pathologist (SLP) implements a subsequent motivational event. Which therapy component **BEST** describes this situation?

Choices:
A. The SLP delivers feedback to Annie regarding her productions.
B. The SLP models appropriate productions for Annie.
C. The SLP presents Annie with a sticker for appropriate productions.
D. The SLP allows Annie to play with a board game before therapy.

Teaching Points

Correct Answer: C
A subsequent motivational event (SME) is reinforcement that occurs following a child's attempt at the language targets, which is likely to foster continued success and attention. Because Annie was given a sticker, this is likely to cause her to be motivated for continued participation in language therapy services. In contrast to this, antecedent instructional events (AIEs) include whatever methods the SLP employs before the child's attempt to use the language target (i.e., modeling, sequence pictures, etc.) Subsequent instruction events (SIEs) include the feedback the SLP provides to the child following an attempt to use the language target. Finally, antecedent motivational events (AMEs) are activities not directly related to the learning of the language target, which fosters the child's attention (i.e., playing with a board game).

A102
Acquired Language Disorders

A person with aphasia and acquired alexia was assessed for reading abilities and found to display a pattern consistent with letter-by-letter (LBL) reading. LBL readers:

Choices:
A. Are unable to read through the visual modality, but can read from kinesthetic input such as writing on the skin or tracing letters with their fingers.
B. Are able to access only the whole-word reading route, but cannot use the grapheme-phoneme reading route; therefore, a phonics-based approach works best for this person to strengthen this route.
C. Respond to the treatment method called multiple oral rereading.
D. Usually exhibit nonfluent forms of aphasia.

Teaching Points

Correct Answer: C
The treatment method called multiple oral rereading works well for LBL readers because the multiple readings of a given passage allow readers to use the context of remembered words to move away from their tendency to read each word in a letter-by-letter fashion. None of the other response choices in the question are true of LBL readers.

A103
Acoustics

What would the speech-language pathologist (SLP) expect to observe if comparing amplitude spectra for a sinusoid and a periodic complex sound?

Choices:
A. The sinusoid has evenly spaced lines, whereas the periodic complex sound has irregularly spaced lines.
B. The sinusoid has irregularly spaced lines, whereas the periodic complex sound has evenly spaced lines.
C. The sinusoid has only one line, whereas the complex periodic sound has more than one line.
D. The sinusoid has lines that are all the same amplitude, whereas the complex periodic sound has lines of different amplitudes.

Teaching Points

Correct Answer: C
A sinusoid contains only one frequency. It therefore has only a single line on a spectrum. A complex sound contains multiple frequencies and therefore has more than one line. Since this is a complex periodic sound, the lines are evenly spaced.

A104
Augmentative and Alternative Communication (AAC)

A speech-language pathologist (SLP) has been working with a patient, in order to implement an aided means of augmentative and alternative communication (AAC) device for communicative purposes. Which means of AAC would be of **GREATEST BENEFIT** for use with this patient?

Choices:
A. Head movements.
B. Pantomiming.
C. Labeled symbols.
D. Manual signs.

Teaching Points

Correct Answer: C
Aided AAC refers to any means of AAC that utilizes external aids or equipment to improve the communicative effectiveness of the user. As a labeled system requires external equipment in order to use it, this would be the most appropriate selection for use with this patient. In contrast to this, head movements, pantomiming and manual signs do not require the use of external aids and would be considered nonaided AAC. These methods would be inappropriate for use with the patient from this scenario.

A105
Language Acquisition

A speech and language researcher is performing research to determine the underlying method of child language learning. The researcher has accepted a stance that supports information-processing models of learning. This researcher believes that child language learning is:

Choices:
A. Dependent on strengthening of relationships between co-occurring events.
B. Dependent on short- and long-term memory stores.
C. Dependent on the amount of input provided.
D. Most prevalent in the preschool age group.

Teaching Points

Correct Answer: B

Information-processing models of learning focus on the role played by memory stores. Specifically, short-term and long-term memory play a large role in a child's language-learning ability. In contrast to this, connectionist models focus on strengthening of relationships between frequently co-occurring events, in addition to language forms. While the amount of linguistic input is important in a child's language-learning ability, this is not congruent with an established model of language-learning. Additionally, it is true that children experience language spurts during the preschool years, but again, this is not part of an established language-learning model.

A106

Speech Sound Disorders in Children

After performing a comprehensive speech evaluation on a pediatric client, a speech-language pathologist (SLP) has determined that although the child produces the /s/ phoneme, he demonstrates the phonological process of final consonant deletion for this phoneme, consistent with a phonemic error. Which method of intervention would be an appropriate selection for the SLP to utilize with this child?

Choices:
A. Van Riper traditional approach.
B. Multiple phoneme approach.
C. Paired stimuli approach.
D. Minimal contrast approach.

Teaching Points

Correct Answer: D

The minimal contrast approach is an intervention method used for phonemic speech errors and is utilized to eliminate excessive homonymy in children's speech. In contrast, the Van Riper traditional approach, multiple phoneme approach and paired stimuli approach are all intervention methods used for children with phonetic speech errors and would not be helpful in remediating this particular child's speech sound disorder as this child already knows the motor pattern for the /s/ phoneme and requires help to generalize production to new word positions.

A107

Cleft Palate and Other Craniofacial Anomalies

A speech-language pathologist (SLP) has been working with a patient to improve the hypernasality of their speech. The child has been diagnosed with a cleft palate, but also demonstrates a Pierre Robin sequence, mid-face hypoplasia and a mild sensorineural hearing loss. Given these specific characteristics, this child **MOST LIKELY** demonstrates which disorder?

Choices:
A. Fetal alcohol syndrome.
B. Trisomy 13.
C. Stickler syndrome.
D. Orofaciodigital syndrome type I.

Teaching Points

Correct Answer: C

Stickler syndrome includes cleft palate, specific craniofacial features (i.e., Pierre Robin sequence, midface hypoplasia, epicanthic folds, etc.) and a function concern for sensorineural hearing loss. Fetal alcohol syndrome, trisomy 13 and orofaciodigital syndrome type I include specific craniofacial features, but do not include sensorineural hearing loss as a functional concern. Sensorineural hearing loss is a functional concern in individuals with Stickler syndrome, so when this type of hearing loss is present, it is highly indicative of Stickler syndrome.

A108

Audiology and Hearing Impairment

An audiologist is evaluating a child who is hard of hearing by obtaining a speech recognition threshold (SRT). What type of speech stimuli should be used to elicit this test?

Choices:
A. Monosyllabic words.
B. Sentences.
C. Spondees.
D. Trochees.

Teaching Points

Correct Answer: C

As part of the comprehensive audiologic evaluation, the audiologist will obtain a speech recognition threshold (SRT). The SRT us used to validate pure-tone testing and should be within 6 dB of the pure-tone average. SRTs are assessed using spondees. These are bisyllabic words with equal stress on each syllable. Examples of spondees are baseball, ice cream, playground, railroad and sidewalk. Word recognition testing uses monosyllabic words that are phonetically balanced. Sentences may also be used for word recognition testing. Trochees are two-syllable words, but the stress is unequal, such as lemon, coffee, finger and trailer.

A109

Voice Disorders

A 1-month-old infant is brought to a speech and language clinic, with parent complaints of an "unnatural cry and loud sounds when the child is breathing." This problem has been present since birth and has remained stable since that time. Which of the following disorders is this child **MOST LIKELY** experiencing?

Choices:
A. Subglottic stenosis.
B. Laryngomalacia.
C. Laryngeal web.
D. Vocal fold nodules.

Teaching Points

Correct Answer: B
This child is most likely experiencing laryngomalacia, or immature development of laryngeal cartilages. This disorder is the most common congenital disorder and results in stridor and respiratory distress. As this child is experiencing "loud sounds when breathing," the child is experiencing the typical stridor associated with this condition. Additionally, as the laryngeal cartilages are underdeveloped and collapse inward, there would most likely be co-occurring vocal problems, such as hoarse or raspy cries. Alternatively, if the child was experiencing subglottal stenosis and laryngeal web, they may cause respiratory problems but would not cause an unnatural cry. Lastly, vocal fold nodules would cause a change in vocal quality but would not cause respiratory problems.

A110

Stuttering and Other Fluency Disorders

With children who stutter, a variety of indirect treatments have been developed. Indirect treatments are those that:

Choices:
A. Employ counseling on attitudes and fears to improve stuttering and ignore speech production.
B. Model easy, slow speech; reduce social and linguistic demands; and help parents to reduce speech pressure.
C. Use extensive practice in teaching others to provide treatment and eliminating the clinical role.
D. Delay the initiating of treatment until the parent indicates readiness and encourage annual reevaluations.

Teaching Points

Correct Answer: B
Indirect treatments are frequently used with young children as a less-intrusive approach to treatment. With these methods, children are engaged in social interactions with the clinician and the clinician models speech that is less complex and slower, with no direct response expected from the child. It has been observed that as the speech and language environment of the child is simplified, fluency is often facilitated.

A111

Augmentative and Alternative Communication (AAC)

A speaker with cerebral palsy can utter only a few words and phrases understood by unfamiliar listeners. Evaluation of the speech production system indicated severe impairment, with a limited ability to compensate. In order to maximize comprehensibility, the **BEST** course of therapy should focus on:

Choices:
A. Alternative forms of communication such as an alphabet board.
B. Modifying speaking patterns such as slowing the speaking rate.
C. Reducing impairment through pharmacological therapies.
D. Training communication partners to adopt the use of signal-independent strategies when communicating with the speaker.

Teaching Points

Correct Answer: A

Because the patient has a significant disorder and minimal ability to compensate on his/her own, augmentative and alternative communication modalities (AAC) should be explored in an effort to increase this patient's ability to communicate effectively with conversational partners.

A112

Motor Speech Disorders

A clinician working with the speaker wants to adopt the use of a pacing board to slow rate and improve speech intelligibility. The clinician is concerned about adversely influencing the naturalness of the speaker's speech. Pacing boards can reduce naturalness of speech because:

Choices:
A. They reduce vocal flexibility and stability.
B. They are used often in the acquisition of the earliest speech sounds for some speakers.
C. Speakers breathe in too much air prior to speaking.
D. Their use leads to placement of pauses in linguistically inappropriate locations.

Teaching Points

Correct Answer: D

A pacing board is a method to use when patients exhibit deficits that would benefit from a slowed or altered rate/rhythm of speech. A pacing board usually contains specific areas, differentiated by some type of visual (i.e., wooden slots, tape, etc.), during which a patient is allowed to speak a predetermined amount of words. Because pacing boards are utilized in a way to limit the amount of speech output (i.e., one word per differentiated space on the board) this can lead to longer pauses between words and pauses in linguistically inappropriate places.

A113

Spoken Language Disorders in Children

Eddie is a 5-year-old child who has been receiving language therapy at his school. Recently, Eddie has greatly enjoyed going to see his speech-language pathologist (SLP) because Eddie is able to bring in all his favorite toys and the SLP will play along with him and ask him questions. What type of language intervention is Eddie **MOST LIKELY** receiving?

Choices:
A. Hybrid approach intervention.
B. Clinician-centered intervention.
C. Experiential intervention.
D. Client-centered intervention.

Teaching Points

Correct Answer: D

Client-centered intervention occurs when the client interacts with the clinician and the clinician uses the interests of the child to direct the order and substance of the language intervention session. Because Eddie's SLP is following Eddie's lead and utilizing Eddie's interests, this is most likely a client-centered approach to intervention. In contrast to this, a clinician-centered approach occurs when the clinician chooses the targets and sets the agenda for the therapy session. Hybrid approaches draw aspects from both clinician- and client-centered therapy approaches. Finally, experiential intervention occurs in a conversational context and highlights appropriate conversational practices.

A114

Autism Spectrum Disorders

Stephanie is a speech-language pathologist (SLP) who is working with a child with autism spectrum disorder. This child demonstrates significant difficulty in understanding perception and beliefs from others' perspectives, which has negatively impacted her social relationships. Which method of intervention is **MOST APPROPRIATE** for Stephanie to utilize in this child's intervention sessions?

Choices:
A. Picture Exchange Communication System.
B. Social stories.
C. Theory of Mind.
D. Peer and play mediation.

Teaching Points

Correct Answer: C

This child's significant difficulty in understanding perception and beliefs from others' perspectives, which has negatively impacted her social relationships, is a deficit known as mindblindness. The Theory of Mind method of intervention is targeted at improving mindblindness through teaching the individual to understand mental states. In contrast to this intervention, Picture Exchange Communication System, social stories and peer and play mediation are forms of intervention targeted at deficits in social communication.

A115

Written Language Disorders in the School-Age Population

A fifth grader makes the following spelling errors: spliting/splitting, pated/patted, glanceing/glancing. These errors indicate difficulties with what type of spelling words?

Choices:
A. Semiphonetic.
B. Irregular.
C. Regular.
D. Rule based.

Teaching Points

Correct Answer: D

Rule-based spelling includes words that rely on systematic instruction of spelling rules, such as the doubling rule (i.e., splitting, patted) and the drop-e rule (i.e., glancing), which this child demonstrated in his/her spelling errors. The spelling mistakes exhibited by this child do not follow regular word spellings (i.e., *bat* spelled as *bet*), irregular word spellings (i.e., *yacht* spelled as *yat*), or semiphonetic spelling patterns (i.e., *are* spelled as *R*).

A116
Acoustics

The supralaryngeal vocal tract (SLVT) is a broadly tuned filter. This means that:

Choices:
A. The SLVT has an infinite number of resonant frequencies.
B. As the shape of the SLVT changes, the resonant frequencies also change.
C. Sinusoids will resonate if they are near a resonant frequency.
D. Sound output dies away immediately when the sound source stops.

Teaching Points

Correct Answer: C

A broadly tuned filter is one in which a sinusoid's frequency does not have to exactly equal the frequency of a filter peak in order to resonate. Frequencies that are near the filter peak will also resonate. When the resonant frequencies of a filter are changeable, it is called a variable filter. When sound output dies away immediately, it is called a heavily damped filter.

A117
Language Acquisition

What are three key language milestones that children meet between 18 and 24 months of age?

Choices:
A. Embedding sentences, expanding sentence types, conjoining sentences.
B. Showing objects, giving objects, pointing to objects.
C. Fifty-word vocabulary size, word spurt, combining words.
D. Increase in verb vocabulary, mastery of copula and auxiliary morphemes, phonological awareness skills.

Teaching Points

Correct Answer: C

It is well documented that young children at around 18 months of age show a period of rapid growth in vocabulary and making two-word combinations. The other choices in this answer are either seen much earlier (showing objects) or later in development.

A118

Augmentative and Alternative Communication (AAC)

A speech-language pathologist (SLP) has been working with a nonverbal teenaged client to program the client's augmentative and alternative communication (AAC) device with speech output. The SLP determines that the client would benefit from prerecorded phrases and other stimuli to increase communicative effectiveness, as the client shows poor initiation in generating novel utterances. What type of speech output should the SLP implement for this client's AAC device?

Choices:
A. Computerized speech.
B. Synthesized speech.
C. Digitized speech.
D. Hybrid speech.

Teaching Points

Correct Answer: C

Digitized speech is human speech that has been recorded, stored and reproduced for use in an AAC system. Additionally, this form of speech cannot be used to generate novel utterances due to its prerecorded nature. As the patient from this scenario demonstrates poor initiation in developing novel utterances and would benefit from prerecorded speech, the SLP will most likely utilize digitized speech. In contrast to this, synthesized speech and computer-generated speech constitute a form of communication in which words/messages are entered via text. Stored speech data may be used in this form of communication, but it is more likely to be used with individuals who have the ability to formulate novel utterances. Finally, hybrid speech utilizes both synthesized and digitized speech to aid in communication for the AAC user.

A119

Augmentative and Alternative Communication (AAC)

A speech-language pathologist (SLP) is working with a patient with severe global aphasia, for whom they are utilizing an augmentative and alternative communication (AAC) device to promote communicative effectiveness. The SLP believes that this patient would benefit from an organization strategy that utilizes individual pictures to capture both environmental and interactional aspects of the communicative context. What type of organizational strategy should the SLP implement with this patient

Choices:
A. Visual scene display.
B. Alphabet display.
C. Pragmatic organization dynamic display.
D. Grid display.

Teaching Points

Correct Answer: A

A visual scene display (VSD) is an image or picture that captures both environmental and action/interaction aspects of the communicative contexts. As the patient from this scenario would best benefit from a picture-based approach to AAC, the SLP would most likely implement a VSD. In contrast to this, alphabet display is a literacy-based approach in which letters are used for easy access. As this patient has global aphasia, they would demonstrate significant difficulty with reading comprehension, and this approach would be ineffective. Pragmatic organization dynamic display is a form of AAC in which pragmatic functions are purposefully added to every page in the AAC user's device. Finally, grid displays are those in which symbols, words and messages are arranged in a grid pattern.

A120

Anatomy and Physiology of Communication and Swallowing

Cranial nerves can include motor functions, sensory functions, or a mix of both. Which of the following cranial nerves (CNs) serve both motor and sensory functions:

Choices:
A. CN V, CN IX, CN X.
B. CN V, CN XI, CN XII.
C. CN III, CN IX, CN X.
D. CN III, CN X, CN XII.

Teaching Points

Correct Answer: A

The cranial nerves that are responsible for both motor movements and sensory information are V (trigeminal), VII (facial), IX (glossopharyngeal) and X (vagus). The other cranial nerves are responsible for either sensory information or motor movement, but not both.

A121

Acquired Language Disorders

A speech-language pathologist (SLP) in a home health service has been working with an individual who has right hemisphere brain damage and is exhibiting a significant left neglect. Which of the following is an appropriate treatment approach for the SLP to take with this client?

Choices:
A. Targeting reading comprehension by having the client match written words with pictures.
B. Targeting alternative and augmentative means of communication through computerized programs such as CSpeak Aphasia.
C. Targeting the client's written expression abilities by training phoneme-grapheme conversion rules.
D. Targeting the client's attention by using a brightly colored border on the edge of pen and paper tasks.

Teaching Points

Correct Answer: D

Left neglect is an attention deficit in which those affected do not attend to stimuli on the left side of their world. By using a treatment method in which brightly colored borders are added to the left edge of paper tasks, the person with left neglect may be "cued" to continue looking until the border is found, thus targeting their attention.

A122

Language Acquisition

Phonotactic probability, neighborhood density and semantic representation influence what aspect of language use and learning?

Choices:
A. Morphemes.
B. Phonemes.
C. Word intentions.
D. Words.

Teaching Points

Correct Answer: D

The characteristics described are all factors for word production as opposed to syllable forms of individual sounds or social rules.

A123

Spoken Language Disorders in Children

Michael is a speech-language pathologist (SLP) who has been asked to evaluate a child who recently moved from a different part of the country. During the evaluation, the child produces the following utterances: /hæn/ for /hænd/, /dɪs/ for /ðɪs/ and /æks/ for /æsk/. What should be the next step in Michael's assessment of this child?

Choices:
A. Determine if the productions are appropriate for the child's dialect.
B. Diagnose the child with a language disorder.
C. Perform a standardized childhood language assessment.
D. Perform in-depth research regarding the child's cultural background.

Teaching Points

Correct Answer: A

Because this child has recently moved from a different part of the country, there is a chance that the child may speak a dialect different from the typical one for the area that Michael lives in. Dialectal differences must be distinguished from language disorders in order to prevent misdiagnosis, inappropriate labeling and inappropriate referral for therapy. If the child's productions are appropriate for the dialect in which the child was raised, this would not constitute a language disorder, but a language difference, and therapy would not be an appropriate recommendation.

A124

Voice Disorders

A patient has undergone phonosurgery to remove lesions associated with polypoid degeneration. After a period of vocal rest, the patient returns to the hospital's voice center to begin treatment with the speech-language pathologist (SLP). Which of the following options is an appropriate first step in this patient's treatment?

Choices:
A. Vocal hygiene information, in order to reduce high-fat foods.
B. Use of hard glottal attack, in order to improve vocal fold closure.
C. Vocal hygiene information, in order to reduce smoking.
D. Recommendations for periodic, repeated phonosurgery as necessary.

Teaching Points

Correct Answer: C

Polypoid degeneration, or Reinke's edema, is a condition caused by a combination of vocal abuse and excessive smoking. Following phonosurgery, a patient with polypoid degeneration should be educated regarding the effects of smoking on the vocal folds and chances of reoccurrence with continued smoking. Hard glottal attacks to improve vocal fold closure are not recommended, as this could cause further phonotraumatic lesions to occur. Additionally, repeated surgeries are not recommended unless the lesion continues to reappear.

A125

Spoken Language Disorders in Children

Martin is a child who has demonstrated mastery of simple sentence structure, but who continues to present with difficulties in complex syntax. As such, it has been determined that Martin is an appropriate candidate for speech-language pathology services. Which of the following is the **BEST** choice of treatment target for Martin?

Choices:
A. Wh- questions.
B. Full propositional complements.
C. Conjoined sentences.
D. Embedded sentences.

Teaching Points

Correct Answer: D

Working on complex syntax is an appropriate intervention for children over the age of 4 years who have mastered simple syntactical structures. Appropriate targets include multiple embedding, embedding and conjoining, infinitive clauses with different subjects, relative clauses, gerunds, wh- infinitives and unmarked infinitives. In contrast to this full propositional complements, wh- questions, and conjoined sentences are simple syntactical structures and would not be an appropriate treatment target for this particular child.

A126

Augmentative and Alternative Communication (AAC)

A speech-language pathologist (SLP) in an acute care hospital has begun working with a patient with severe dysarthria, who they believe would benefit from the use of an augmentative and alternative communication (AAC) device. When the SLP approaches the director of rehabilitation, however, the director states that they are uninterested in providing the device for this patient and that the SLP needs to attempt other treatment methods. The SLP could provide evidence from which of the following legislative acts in order to procure the AAC device for this patient?

Choices:
A. Assistive Technology Act Amendments of 2004 (PL-108-364).
B. Americans with Disabilities Act (ADA).
C. Joint Commission's *Advancing Effective Communication*.
D. Rehabilitation Act of 1973.

Teaching Points

Correct Answer: B

According to the Americans with Disabilities Act (ADA), hospitals must provide effective means of communication for patients, family members and hospital visitors who are deaf or hard of hearing. As the SLP has deemed an AAC device the most effective means of communication for this patient, the hospital must acknowledge this and provide some form of AAC device for the patient to communicate. In contrast to this, PL-108-364 mandates that assistive technology centers must be present in each state and United States territory. The Joint Commission's *Advancing Effective Communication* is a resource to help health care providers learn to communicate with patients. Finally, the Rehabilitation Act of 1973 was a precursor to the Free Appropriate Public Education of 1975.

A127

Anatomy and Physiology of Communication and Swallowing

A patient who is experiencing nonfluent aphasia **MOST LIKELY** has some degree of cortical damage in Broca's area. This brain region is in which lobe?

Choices:
A. Frontal.
B. Temporal.
C. Parietal.
D. Occipital.

Teaching Points

Correct Answer: A

Broca's area can be found in the frontal lobes of the brain, in the inferior frontal gyrus. Refer to "Neuroanatomy and Neurophysiology for Speech, Language, and Swallowing" from Chapter 1 of this text for more information and visualization of this structure.

A128

Cleft Palate and Other Craniofacial Anomalies

A speech and language researcher is interested in compiling a data bank regarding objective measures of the acoustic characteristics of cleft palate speech. Which of the following instrumental procedures would be most helpful to this researcher?

Choices:
A. Nasopharyngoscopy.
B. Aerodynamic instrumentation.
C. Videofluoroscopy.
D. Nasometry.

Teaching Points

Correct Answer: D

Nasometry utilizes a nasometer to give acoustic data regarding the presence of nasality in speech production (i.e., nasalance). As this researcher is interested in gathering acoustic data for this population, nasometry would be the most appropriate choice. On the other hand, aerodynamic instrumentation measures air pressure and airflow during speech production, videofluoroscopy provides a radiographic view of the velopharyngeal valve and nasopharyngoscopy allows the examiner to view the velopharyngeal port during speech. As such, these instruments do not provide acoustic data and are not appropriate selections.

A129

Anatomy and Physiology of Communication and Swallowing

During the transmission of an action potential, after a neuron has fired there is an absolute refractory period. This is a delay during which a neuron is unable to transmit further action potentials. This delay must expire before that neuron can fire again because:

Choices:
A. Sodium (Na+) ions continue to flow out of the cell after an action potential spike.
B. Potassium ions (K+) continue to flow out of the cell after an action potential spike.
C. Voltage-gated sodium (Na+) channels are periodically inactivated after opening.
D. Voltage-gated potassium (K+) channels are periodically inactivated after opening.

Teaching Points

Correct Answer: C

During the refractory period, the sodium-gated channels are deactivated, so sodium is unable to flow through the neuron's cellular membrane. After a short period, these gates become activated and are able to help with the propagation of an action potential.

A130

Anatomy and Physiology of Communication and Swallowing

A person experiences weakness on the right side of the face resulting in right facial droop. Initial evaluation suggests cranial nerve damage. If verified, which cranial nerve is **MOST LIKELY** damaged?

Choices:
A. Trochlear.
B. Trigeminal.
C. Facial.
D. Vagus.

Teaching Points

Correct Answer: C

The facial nerve (CN VII) controls motor innervations to the muscles of facial expression. Damage to the lower motor neurons would cause ipsilateral (same-sided) weakness, which could result in the facial droop this patient is experiencing.

A131

Autism Spectrum Disorders

Cameron is a speech-language pathologist (SLP) who is working with a young child recently diagnosed with autism spectrum disorder (ASD). Cameron believes that this child would benefit from the use of a Floortime approach to intervention. In order to best implement this treatment approach, Cameron should:

Choices:
A. Teach the child social skills through a story-time format.
B. Establish a reciprocal communication system for the child.
C. Engage in a play-based activity with the child and an age-matched peer.
D. Engage in a semistructured play activity that interests the child.

Teaching Points

Correct Answer: D
When utilizing the Floortime approach of intervention for autism spectrum disorder, the SLP would engage the child in a spontaneous, interactive, pleasurable activity with the child, while following the child's leads and interests. This would be completed in a semistructured play scenario. In contrast to this, teaching children with ASD social skills through stories would be utilized in the social stories intervention approach. Picture Exchange Communication System (PECS) is a reciprocal communication system, in which the child exchanges pictures for desired objects. Finally, matching the child with ASD with an age-matched peer would be utilized in the peer and play mediation intervention approach.

A132

Written Language Disorders in the School-Age Population

Amanda is a 4-year-old, typically developing preschool student, who has begun to realize that words can be broken down into sounds and that some words "sound the same." Amanda is demonstrating phonological:

Choices:
A. Awareness.
B. Memory.
C. Processes.
D. Development.

Teaching Points

Correct Answer: A
Phonological awareness refers to the knowledge that words can be deconstructed into phonological parts (i.e., sounds and syllables) and includes knowledge of phoneme blending, segregation and rhyming. In contrast to this, phonological memory refers to the process of receiving, analyzing and processing of sound elements in a language. Phonological processes are patterns of speech production in which a child simplifies the adult form of a production. Finally, phonological development refers to the process a child undergoes in learning the phonology of a language.

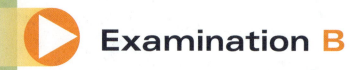

Examination B

B1

Spoken Language Disorders in Children

A child has been referred to a speech-language pathologist (SLP) for a comprehensive language evaluation, with reports of "global language problems." Following evaluation, the SLP determines that the child is demonstrating word-finding difficulties, comprehension deficits and disorganized language, in addition to deficits in attention and executive functioning. Which of the following disorders does the child MOST LIKELY demonstrate?

Choices:
A. Traumatic brain injury.
B. Cerebral palsy.
C. Autism spectrum disorder.
D. Down syndrome.

Teaching Points

Correct Answer: A

Language difficulties associated with traumatic brain injury include comprehension difficulties, telegraphic speech, word-finding deficits, disorganized language and potential pragmatic difficulties. In contrast to this, children with cerebral palsy may demonstrate general difficulties in both receptive and expressive language. Children with autism spectrum disorder demonstrate significant impairments in pragmatic language, as well as restricted interests and behaviors. Finally, children with Down syndrome demonstrate deficits in syntax, rather than semantics, and have a greater difficulty with language production over comprehension.

B2

Spoken Language Disorders in Children

A speech-language pathologist (SLP) has been working on narrative structure with a middle school student on the SLPs caseload. Recently, the child wrote a story about her weekend, which reads "My family was going to a friend's birthday party. We were late to the birthday party." Using this information, the SLP would like to assign a narrative episode level to this child's story. Which of the following narrative levels BEST describes the child's story.

Choices:
A. Abbreviated episode.
B. Incomplete episode.
C. Complete episode.
D. Action sequence.

Teaching Points

Correct Answer: B

An incomplete episode is a narrative episode level in which the child includes two out of three of initiating event, action and consequence. For this child's story, there is an initiating event (i.e., family members going to a birthday party) and a consequence (i.e., being late for the party), but no action event. If the child would have included an action, such as the care of getting a flat tire on the way to the party, this would constitute a complete episode, which includes an initiating event, an action, and a consequence all related to the initiating event. An action sequence consists of a series of actions that follow a chronological order, but are not causally linked. Finally, an abbreviated episode is one that contains causally related actions that are not associated with an initiating event or specific, goal-directed behavior.

B3

The Practice of Speech-Language Pathology

Andy is a speech-language pathologist who has recently branched out into providing telepractice services to in-state clients who are unable to be treated at his private practice center. Joseph is a friend of Andy's who lives in another state in which Andy does not have licensure and has just heard about Andy's new service delivery. Joseph asks Andy to treat his mother, who has Wernicke's aphasia, as Joseph would like his mother to receive more treatment than she is currently. How should Andy proceed in the treatment of Joseph's mother?

Choices:
A. Recommend against treatment, as telepractice has not been proven in treating Wernicke's aphasia.
B. Recommend against treatment, as Joseph's mother is already receiving services.
C. Share the mother's case information with a fellow SLP in the state in which Joseph lives.
D. Refer the friend to another SLP who has licensure in the state in which Joseph lives.

Teaching Points

Correct Answer: D

Currently, SLPs are required to maintain licensure in any state that they perform telepractice in (i.e., the state in which the client lives). As Andy does not live in the same state as Joseph, he is legally not able to provide services for Joseph's mother, and he should recommend a licensed SLP in that state. While there is currently limited efficacy regarding telepractice, it is regarded as a promising method of intervention and can lead to patient progress for all forms of communication disorders, including Wernicke's aphasia. Individuals who receive telepractice are always eligible for further in-person sessions. Lastly, all rules for privacy and confidentiality apply to all patients, and for this reason, Andy is unable to share the mother's case information without prior consent.

B4

Spoken Language Disorders in Children

During an intervention session, a child produces the utterance "Mommy go run." The child's speech-language pathologist (SLP) uses an expansion approach to increase the complexity of the child's utterance. Which of the following statements could this SLP use in response to the child?

Choices:
A. "Mommy's going to run."
B. "Mommy's going to run to the house."
C. "Where is Mommy going?"
D. "Say 'mommy is going to run.'"

Teaching Points

Correct Answer: A

An expansion (also known as recast) is a form of experiential instruction in which the SLP provides a corrected version of a child's word or utterance. Because the SLP from this scenario is utilizing an expansion for this child, the practitioner would provide only the corrected utterance (i.e., "Mommy's going to run."). In contrast to this, an expatiation is when the SLP provides a corrected version of a child's word or utterance and goes beyond the child's original meaning (i.e., "Mommy's going to run to the house"). Questioning occurs when the SLP asks follow-up questions to the child's original utterance (i.e., "Where is Mommy running?"). Finally, imitation occurs when the SLP provides a model and expects the child to replicate it (i.e., "Say 'Mommy's going to run.'").

B5

Speech Sound Disorders in Children

A speech-language pathologist (SLP) is attempting to perform an evaluation on a new pediatric client and would like to perform an analysis to compare the client's correct consonant productions to the entire speech sample. Which means of assessment would be the **MOST APPROPRIATE** choice for this SLP to make?

Choices:
A. Percent consonants correct.
B. Phonological mean length of utterance.
C. Phonological error patterns analysis.
D. Traditional analysis.

Teaching Points

Correct Answer: A

Percent consonants correct (PCC) is an analysis procedure that compares the number of consonants produced correctly to the total number of consonants that should have been produced. It gives the clinician a percentage of correct use, which is then corresponded to a severity rating for the child's disorder. In contrast, the phonological error pattern analysis allows the clinician to understand the error patterns that the child produces and provides a means of categorizing the errors into syllable structure, substitution and assimilation errors. Phonological mean length of utterance attempts to determine the length and complexity of words the child attempts to say and how well the child matches the target word. Finally, traditional analysis displays the child's errors across word or syllable positions, records the types of errors, and is most useful for those children with few errors.

B6

Spoken Language Disorders in Children

Erica is a young child who demonstrates pragmatic difficulties. Specifically, Erica has difficulties with presupposition skills, which her speech-language pathologist has been targeting in order to improve Erica's conversational abilities. Which of the following would be the **MOST APPROPRIATE** goal for Erica's intervention?

Choices:
A. The child will utilize gestures in conversation to reinforce engaging topics of conversation.
B. The child will understand that communication partners have perspectives and feelings different from her own.
C. The child will modify communicative attempts based on the needs of their communication partner.
D. The child will understand that communicative partners engage in conversation with certain expectations for communication.

Teaching Points

Correct Answer: C

Presupposition is a skill that involves judging what the listener already knows and making appropriate accommodations to facilitate successful communication. By targeting this ability, the child may have a better understanding of what the child's conversation partner requires for successful intervention. In contrast to this, Theory of Mind deals with understanding conversation partners have differing perspectives and feelings. Joint action routine is a skill that aids in establishing predictable roles and expectations for conversation. Finally, using gestures to reinforce topics of conversation may engage speakers more in conversation, but does not necessarily equate to a change in conversation based on the needs of the communicative partner.

B7

Speech Sound Disorders in Children

Andy is an infant being evaluated by a speech-language pathologist (SLP) during an early intervention home visit. The SLP notes that Andy demonstrates vocal play, raspberries, trills and marginal babbling during the evaluation. Using this information, which stage of linguistic development does Andy fall within?

Choices:
A. Exploration/expansion stage.
B. Coo and goo stage.
C. Canonical babbling stage.
D. Phonation stage.

Teaching Points

Correct Answer: A

Hallmark characteristics of the exploration/expansion stage include vocal play, squeals, raspberries, trills, frication noises, fully resonated vowels, marginal babbling and great variation in pitch and loudness. As the child from this scenario demonstrates several of these characteristics, it is appropriate to say that he is in the exploration/expansion stage. In contrast, during the phonation stage, a child would demonstrate predominantly reflexive and vegetative sounds. If the child was in the coo and goo stage, he would demonstrate quasi-resonant nuclei, sounds similar to back consonants and vowels, and possible self-imitations. Finally, if the child was in the canonical babbling stage he would demonstrate reduplicated and nonreduplicated babbling, in addition to producing stops, nasals, glides and some vowels.

B8

Anatomy and Physiology of Communication and Swallowing

During the transmission of an action potential, after a neuron has fired, there is an absolute refractory period. This is a delay during which a neuron is unable to transmit further action potentials. This delay must expire before that neuron can fire again because:

Choices:
A. Sodium (Na+) ions continue to flow out of the cell after an action potential spike.
B. Potassium ions (K+) continue to flow out of the cell after an action potential spike.
C. Voltage-gated Na+ channels are periodically inactivated after opening.
D. Voltage-gated potassium (K+) channels are periodically inactivated after opening.

Teaching Points

Correct Answer: C

During the refractory period, the sodium-gated channels are deactivated, so sodium is unable to flow through the neuron's cellular membrane. After a short period, these gates become activated and are able to help with the propagation of an action potential.

B9

Acoustics

An audiologist has recently completed a full audiometric evaluation on a patient with complaints of hearing loss with the following pure-tone average of 78 dB hearing loss (HL) in the right ear and 23 dB HL in the left ear. Which of the following statements **BEST** describes this patient?

Choices:
A. The patient demonstrates a severe right hearing loss and a minimal left hearing loss.
B. The patient demonstrates a profound right hearing loss and a mild left hearing loss.
C. The patient demonstrates a moderately severe right hearing loss and normal left hearing.
D. The patient demonstrates a severe right hearing loss and a mild left hearing loss.

Teaching Points

Correct Answer: A

When discussing range of hearing loss, 71–90 dB HL would be classified as a severe hearing loss, and 16–25 dB HL would be classified as a minimal hearing loss. As this patient fits these diagnostic markers, the patient would be diagnosed with a severe right hearing loss and a minimal left hearing loss.

B10

Cleft Palate and Other Craniofacial Anomalies

A client arrives at the speech-language pathology clinic at an acute care hospital with complaints of "a change in voice." After comprehensive endoscopic evaluation, the speech-language pathologist (SLP) notes that the deficit is most likely not one of resonance due to problems of velopharyngeal closure, as this client exhibits "the most common pattern of velopharyngeal closure." Which of the following **BEST** describes this client's pattern of closure?

Choices:
A. Circular pattern with approximately equal activity of the velum, lateral pharyngeal walls and posterior pharyngeal wall.
B. Coronal pattern with the velum contacting the pharyngeal wall.
C. Sagittal pattern with medial lateral pharyngeal wall motion as the primary contributor to closure.
D. Circular pattern with a Passavant's ridge.

Teaching Points

Correct Answer: B
The coronal pattern of velopharyngeal closure is the most common pattern in normal speakers and involves posterior movement of the soft palate against the posterior pharyngeal wall. If the SLP from this scenario noted "the most common closure pattern," this would be the most appropriate choice. Circular and sagittal closure patterns are the second most and third most common velopharyngeal closure pattern, respectively. For this reason, these answers would not be the most appropriate selection for the client from this scenario.

B11
Anatomy and Physiology of Communication and Swallowing

A person places a hand on a hot surface and experiences the sensation of heat. The feeling of heat is conveyed up to the primary somatosensory cortex in the parietal lobe. In order for this information to be received in this cortical area, it must first travel up the spinal column, via the:

Choices:
A. Lateral corticospinal tract.
B. Anterior corticospinal tract.
C. Anterolateral system.
D. Posterior column-medial lemniscal system.

Teaching Points

Correct Answer: C
If a person places a hand on a hot stove, this would cause pain and temperature sensation, which would be conveyed through the anterolateral system (pain, temperature and crude touch). The posterior column-medial lemniscus system is responsible for transmission of vibration, pressure and fine touch information. The lateral corticospinal tract and anterior corticospinal tract are both motor tracts, which control limb movement and girdle movement, respectively.

B12
Acoustics

If pitch contour for a vowel shows a frequency of 150 hertz (Hz) at the midpoint, the frequency of the fifth harmonic at the same location will be:

Choices:
A. 500 Hz.
B. 750 Hz.
C. 1000 Hz.
D. 1250 Hz.

Teaching Points

Correct Answer: B
All harmonics are integer multiples of F0. If F0 = 150 Hz, then H5 = 5 × 150 Hz or 750 Hz.

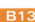

B13

The Practice of Speech-Language Pathology

A speech-language pathologist (SLP) has been asked to evaluate a patient recently admitted to the SLP's acute care hospital. When the SLP arrives to perform the evaluation, the SLP discovers through informal conversation that the patient is of a sexual orientation different from their own, and is uncomfortable working with the patient. What step should the SLP take in the treatment of this patient?

Choices:
A. The SLP must provide treatment to this patient.
B. The SLP should request another SLP work with this patient.
C. The SLP should formulate treatment plans and delegate the patient to an SLPA.
D. The SLP should discharge this patient from the SLP's services.

Teaching Points

Correct Answer: A

According to the ASHA Code of Ethics, Principle of Ethics I, Rule of Ethics C, "Individuals shall not discriminate in the delivery of professional services . . . on the basis of race or ethnicity, gender, gender identity/gender expression, age, religion, national origin, sexual orientation, or disability." Regardless of personal feelings toward the patient's sexual orientation, the SLP from this scenario is ethically bound to provide services competently to the patient. It is considered unethical for the SLP to discriminate against this patient in service delivery, refer the patient to another SLP simply for being uncomfortable, refer the patient to an SLPA, or discharge the patient prematurely.

B14

Cleft Palate and Other Craniofacial Anomalies

A child has been recently born with a complete cleft of the secondary palate. Given this diagnosis, which structure would most likely **NOT** be affected?

Choices:
A. Hard palate.
B. Velum.
C. Alveolar ridge.
D. Uvula.

Teaching Points

Correct Answer: C

Secondary palate structures include the hard palate, velum and uvula. If this child was experiencing a complete cleft of the secondary palate, there would be a full cleft extending from the uvula to the incisive foramen. As such, the alveolar ridge would remain intact with this type of cleft.

B15

Motor Speech Disorders

A 5-year-old child with a diagnosis of moderate childhood apraxia of speech (CAS) has been participating in speech therapy for the past month, with the speech-language pathologist (SLP) utilizing a motor-based approach to treatment. The SLP has determined that the child is not making satisfactory progress within the treatment sessions. The **BEST** course of action by the therapist is to:

Choices:
A. Evaluate if motor-learning principles have been applied appropriately and adjusted as needed.
B. Switch treatment to a phonologically based approach from the previously used motor-based approach.
C. Begin treatment at the isolated phoneme level to ensure all phonemes can be produced accurately before increasing length and complexity.
D. Apply maximal cueing.

Teaching Points

Correct Answer: A

Children with childhood apraxia of speech (CAS) exhibit a motor speech disorder that would not respond appropriately to a phonologically based approach to treatment. Additionally, children with CAS are often able to produce individual phonemes with ease and experience difficulty making the transitions between speech sounds during connected speech. The best approach in this type of situation would be to evaluate the treatment protocol to see if properties of motor-learning approaches (i.e., practice schedule, type of feedback, amount of feedback, learning, specificity of training, intensive practice, etc.) are effectively being utilized.

B16

Acquired Language Disorders

Which scenario BEST describes application of the Boston classification system for a person diagnosed with aphasia?

Choices:
A. Expressive aphasia was evident because problems in verbal expression were greater than problems in the comprehension of language.
B. Broca's aphasia was evident because the CT scan indicated that the cerebrovascular accident had damaged Broca's area in the frontal lobe.
C. Aphasia was evident because performance was poor on a picture description task and there was trouble following commands.
D. Conduction aphasia was evident because of a pattern of fluent output and comprehension and an impairment in the ability to repeat.

Teaching Points

Correct Answer: D

The Boston classification system involves assessment of three key areas: fluency of spontaneous verbal output, auditory comprehension and verbal repetition. Aphasia type is determined by the unique profile of skills in these areas and is not based on lesion location.

B17

Anatomy and Physiology of Communication and Swallowing

When forming the vowel /u/ in *boot*, which muscle **MOST LIKELY** contracts?

Choices:
A. Orbicularis oris.
B. Levator labii superioris.
C. Zygomatic major.
D. Risorius.

Teaching Points

Correct Answer: A

The orbicularis oris muscle is the sphincter-like muscle that surrounds the lips. Contraction of this muscle can lead to the lip-rounding associated with production of the /u/ phoneme in the word *boot*. In contrast to this, the levator labii superioris muscle contributes to elevation and everting of the upper lip. The zygomatic major contracts the corners of the mouth backward by simultaneously lifting and pulling the corners of the mouth sideways. Finally, the risorius muscle retracts the angle of the mouth upon contraction.

B18

Anatomy and Physiology of Communication and Swallowing

The spinal column is organized with respect to motor/sensory function, as well as upper and lower extremities. Cell bodies of lower motor neurons that control movement of the legs are generally found in:

Choices:
A. The precentral gyrus.
B. The postcentral gyrus.
C. The ventral horn of the spinal column.
D. The dorsal horn of the spinal column.

Teaching Points

Correct Answer: C

The ventral horns of the spinal column house the lower motor neurons responsible for movement, whereas the dorsal horns house neurons responsible for transmission of sensory information. The precentral and postcentral gyri are structures located in the cerebral hemispheres, which house the primary motor cortex and primary somatosensory cortices.

B19

Research, Evidence-Based Practice and Tests and Measurements

A speech-language pathologist (SLP) is interested in starting a research study to determine the effect of a particular treatment approach in alleviating symptoms of voice disorders. However, while the SLP believes that this treatment will be beneficial to persons with voice disorders of varying etiology, he only has access to persons with voice disorders caused by muscle tension dysphonia. If the SLP proceeds with this research study, he needs to be aware of the potential threat to which of the following principles?

Choices:
A. Internal validity.
B. External validity.
C. Reliability.
D. Content validity.

Teaching Points

Correct Answer: B

External validity is the amount of generalizability of results to real-life situations. This SLP needs to be aware of the external validity to those with other etiologies of the voice disorder, as he only has participants with muscle tension dysphonia in his study. His external validity would be strengthened further if he had participants with other etiologies.

B20
Spoken Language Disorders in Children

A young child has been receiving speech-language therapy to remediate her language disorder. After many months of intervention, the speech-language pathologist would like to assess the progress this child has made during intervention. What is the **MOST APPROPRIATE** method for assessing this child's progress?

Choices:
A. Review data collected during intervention sessions.
B. Elicit untrained exemplars during conversations.
C. Administer a standardized assessment and compare scores.
D. Implement dynamic assessment procedures.

Teaching Points

Correct Answer: B

Periodic measurement of client performance is a critical component of advancing clients through therapy. One way to assess progress is to utilize untrained exemplars when eliciting language. For example, if the client has been working on the third-person singular form of *come*, the clinician can probe for generalization to *walk*. Administration of standardized assessment is discouraged, as there may be a recall bias for assessment material. Dynamic assessment would reveal how the child is functioning currently, but may not probe generalization. Finally, reviewing data collected during intervention, while essential for steering the direction of treatment, will reveal when goals need to be updated, but does not probe for current level of progress.

B21
Stuttering and Other Fluency Disorders

Mary is a junior high student who has been working with a speech-language pathologist (SLP) in therapy for the past 6 months. Mary's therapy has focused on fluency-shaping activities primarily. Which of the following techniques was probably used during these sessions?

Choices:
A. Cancellation.
B. Avoidance treatment.
C. Counseling.
D. Operant conditioning to reinforce moments of fluency.

Teaching Points

Correct Answer: D

In fluency-shaping approaches to treatment, the goal is for the client to replace stuttered speech with fluent speech. These techniques are often delivered through modeling in an exaggerated manner, then the behavior is shaped toward a more standard production. Operant conditioning techniques are often used to promote this generalization and would most likely be used in Mary's treatment sessions.

B22

Stuttering and Other Fluency Disorders

The Lidcombe program is an evidence-based approach to stuttering treatment in which parents are trained to deliver fluency-shaping therapy daily and to measure fluency performance. Progress is monitored by the speech-language pathologist (SLP). This is an example of which type of approach to treatment:

Choices:
A. Direct treatment.
B. Indirect treatment.
C. Counseling approach.
D. Stuttering modification.

Teaching Points

Correct Answer: A

Direct treatment for stuttering includes a direct focus on speech (fluency-shaping approach). As the Lidcombe Program provides a direct focus on speech through fluency-shaping techniques, it can be considered a form of direct treatment for stuttering.

B23

Audiology and Hearing Impairment

American Sign Language (ASL) is a visual-spatial language used by persons who are deaf/Deaf in the United States and has several unique characteristics. Which of the following statements **BEST** describes ASL?

Choices:
A. ASL is completely dependent on hand movements only.
B. ASL is dependent on direction, but not speed, of movement.
C. ASL utilizes facial expression to mark idioms.
D. ASL utilizes its own grammar and syntax.

Teaching Points

Correct Answer: D

American Sign Language (ASL) is a visual-spatial language used by people who are deaf/Deaf in the United States and English-speaking parts of Canada. Unique features of this language include its own grammar, syntax, idioms and vocabulary. Additionally, ASL uses space, direction and speech of movement, and facial expression to mark grammar and convey meaning.

B24

Audiology and Hearing Impairment

A speech-language pathologist (SLP) is working in a rural outpatient setting, with no audiologist present. A patient arrives at the center with complaints that the behind-the-ear hearing aid has stopped functioning. The SLP knows that hearing aid troubleshooting is a process that falls under his scope of practice and begins helping the patient. What should be the first step the SLP takes in troubleshooting this hearing aid?

Choices:
A. Check the tonehook for blockages.
B. Check the earmold for blockages.
C. Check the status of the battery.
D. Check the status of the microphone.

Teaching Points

Correct Answer: C

In troubleshooting hearing aid problems, there are several steps that a speech-language pathologist can take. Battery problems (i.e., dead batteries, batteries being placed into the unit incorrectly, etc.) comprise the largest group of problems experienced by hearing aid users. By checking the status of the battery first, the SLP may quickly fix the problem and help the hearing aid user. If this does not work, the SLP can follow a chain and check for debris in the earmold, tonehook and microphone. If problems persist, the SLP may need to refer the patient to his/her audiologist for further troubleshooting of the device.

B25

Anatomy and Physiology of Communication and Swallowing

Contraction of the tensor veli palatini and levator veli palatini will **NOT** occur during the production of which of the following sounds?

Choices:
A. /f/.
B. /s/.
C. /m/.
D. /t/.

Teaching Points

Correct Answer: C

The tensor veli palatini and levator veli palatini muscles contract to raise the soft palate during speech, in order to block off the nasal cavity. The /m/ is a nasal phoneme, which means that the nasal cavity remains open during phonation. For this reason, the tensor veli palatini and levator veli palatini do not contract during production of /m/.

B26

Spoken Language Disorders in Children

Eddie is a 5-year-old child who has been receiving language therapy at his school. Recently, Eddie has greatly enjoyed going to see his speech-language pathologist (SLP) because Eddie is able to bring in all his favorite toys, and the SLP will play along with him and ask him questions. What type of language intervention is Eddie **MOST LIKELY** receiving?

Choices:
A. Hybrid approach intervention.
B. Clinician-centered intervention.
C. Experiential intervention.
D. Client-centered intervention.

Teaching Points

Correct Answer: D

Client-centered intervention occurs when the client interacts with the clinician and the clinician uses the interests of the child to direct the order and substance of the language intervention session. Because Eddie's SLP is following Eddie's lead and utilizing Eddie's interests, this is most likely a client-centered approach to intervention. In contrast to this, a clinician-centered approach occurs when the clinician chooses the targets and sets the agenda for the therapy session. Hybrid approaches draw aspects from both clinician- and client-centered therapy approaches. Finally, experiential intervention occurs in a conversational context and highlights appropriate conversational practices.

B27

Acquired Language Disorders

A person was given the diagnosis of primary progressive aphasia (PPA) about 3 months ago. What is most likely to be true about this person?

Choices:
A. The person had a history of progressive impairment of language, with no evidence of a global dementia or sign of an acute stroke on neuroimaging.
B. The person had a dementia syndrome characterized by progressive loss of language functioning and a significant memory impairment, with relative preservation of social graces.
C. The person experienced acute onset of a language disorder that was getting progressively worse over at least the past 2 years.
D. The CT scan showed atrophy in the frontal and temporal lobes and an infarct in the language zone of the left hemisphere.

Teaching Points

Correct Answer: A

A person diagnosed with PPA has a history of at least a 2-year period of decline in language functioning, without displaying a more global dementia syndrome. The onset was not acute, and there is no obvious infarct on neuroimaging. Atrophy may be present in the frontal and temporal lobes. Only the patient with neither global aphasia nor evidence of a stroke meets these criteria.

B28

Dysphagia

During a modified barium swallow (MBS) study, the patient demonstrates penetration to the level of the vocal folds, but does not spontaneously clear the material. In order to give the patient a grade that will be widely understood by other speech-language pathologists (SLPs), the SLP who completed the MBS uses the penetration-aspiration scale. Which of the following would be the appropriate scoring?

Choices:
A. Level 3.
B. Level 4.
C. Level 5.
D. Level 6.

Teaching Points

Correct Answer: C
Level 5 of the penetration-aspiration scale states "Material enters the airway, contacts the vocal folds, and is NOT ejected from the airway." If bolus material reaches the vocal folds and the patient does not clear the material, that person would be a PAS Level 5. In contrast, Level 3 of the PAS Scale states "Material enters the airway, remains above the vocal folds, and is NOT ejected from the airway." Level 4 states "Material enters the airway, contacts the vocal folds, and is ejected from the airway." Finally, Level 6 states "Material enters the airway, passes the glottis, and is ejected from the airway."

B29

Stuttering and Other Fluency Disorders

Mike is a 7-year-old who has demonstrated prolongations and repetitions during speech, as well as evident tension prior to these occurrences. Several of his classmates have noticed his speech differences and have begun teasing him. Due to the tension he feels in anticipation of his speech differences and the anxiety he feels toward his classmates' teasing, Mike has begun to fear speaking in public, and avoids doing so at all opportunities. Which of the following statements is the **MOST APPROPRIATE** description of this child?

Choices:
A. Mike is at the advanced stuttering stage and would benefit from an in-depth assessment to determine the effect of stuttering on his quality of life.
B. Mike is at the borderline stuttering stage and would benefit from assessment to determine if he exhibits a speech disorder.
C. Mike is at the intermediate stuttering stage and would benefit from assessment to determine the effect of stuttering on his class work.
D. Mike is not demonstrating behaviors congruent with stuttering and would benefit from teacher intervention to reduce the occurrence of bullying.

Teaching Points

Correct Answer: C
Because Mike is highly aware of his disfluencies and has begun demonstrating fear of his speech in addition to avoidance behaviors, he would fall into the intermediate level of stuttering. Those individuals at this level benefit from assessment to determine the type and severity of disfluencies and secondary behaviors, identify early risk facts and determine any effect on school performance.

B30

Spoken Language Disorders in Children

Amanda is a child who demonstrates relatively intact language comprehension skills, but significant impairments in language production and syntax. Which disorder does Amanda **MOST LIKELY** demonstrate?

Choices:
A. Attention deficit/hyperactivity disorder (ADHD).
B. Down syndrome.
C. Specific learning disability (SLD).
D. Traumatic brain injury (TBI).

Teaching Points

Correct Answer: B

A child with Down syndrome will most likely demonstrate intact language comprehension skills, with significant impairments in language production. Children in this population often demonstrate particular difficulty with expressive syntax and vocabulary acquisition. In contrast to this, children with ADHD present with difficulties in concentration, organization, impulse control, planning and pragmatic language secondary to distractibility. Children with SLD present with deficits in executive functions (i.e., planning, organization and problem solving), dysgraphia and social skills. Finally children with TBI present with deficits of telegraphic speech, comprehension difficulties, semantic difficulty, word finding and disorganized language.

B31

Voice Disorders

A patient has overcome a lengthy sickness with resultant voice difficulties. Following a voice evaluation at an acute care hospital, the patient is diagnosed with viral-induced superior laryngeal nerve damage. With which of the following difficulties would this patient **MOST LIKELY** present?

Choices:
A. Maintaining phonation.
B. Controlling respiration.
C. Changing pitch.
D. Valving the nasal cavity.

Teaching Points

Correct Answer: C

The superior laryngeal nerve (SLN) is the nerve that innervates the cricothyroid muscle, which assists in altering pitch. When this muscle contracts, the thyroid cartilage is tilted forward, lengthening the vocal folds and elevating pitch. If a patient experiences damage to this nerve, he/she would have difficulty elevating pitch. As this nerve only innervates the cricothyroid muscle, damage would not affect a patient's ability to maintain phonation, effectively control respiration or effectively valve the nasal cavity.

B32

Spoken Language Disorders in Children

A speech-language pathologist (SLP) is considered dismissing a child from therapy services, as the SLP believes the child has made the maximum amount of progress possible. What is the **MOST IMPORTANT** factor to consider when dismissing a child from language therapy from a SLP perspEktive?

Choices:
A. The child has met all measurable goals and objectives set for him through language therapy.
B. The child is refusing to participate in further language treatment sessions.
C. The child's family has become tired of receiving language intervention.
D. The child is able to meet all communication demands for activities of daily living.

Teaching Points

Correct Answer: D

There are multiple factors that are interrelated when considering dismissal from therapy for language disorders. Among these factors is whether the child is able to meet all of the communication demands imposed through activities of daily living. From a SLP perspective, being able to demonstrate adequate language skills for daily life is the ultimate goal of treatment. Once a client has demonstrated this ability, this may be indicative of dismissal from therapy. In contrast, if the child has met all language goals, but is unable to meet the communicative needs of the activities of daily living, the child may benefit from further therapy sessions. Finally, if the child and family would not like to receive language intervention, this is also an important factor to consider as SLPs are ethically bound to provide services that the family would like to receive; however, this is not a factor from a speech and language perspective.

B33

Research, Evidence-Based Practice and Tests and Measurements

A speech scientist has wrongfully interpreted data collected during a recent study and has claimed that the treatment method leads to participant progress when no progress was actually made. Which of the following **BEST** describes the scientist's situation?

Choices:
A. A type II error.
B. An order effect.
C. A type I error.
D. A treatment effect.

Teaching Points

Correct Answer: C

A type I error occurs when a true null hypothesis is rejected (i.e., a researcher rejects results showing that no improvement was made). Because this scientist has incorrectly claimed participant improvement, a type I error has been committed. On the other hand, if there was actual participant improvement, but the scientist dismissed this as no improvement, a type II error would have occurred.

B34

Motor Speech Disorders

A patient with a diagnosis of flaccid dysarthria exhibits mild hypernasality. It was noted during visualization of the velopharyngeal system that the patient was able to achieve closure of the velopharyngeal port, but not consistently. The therapy of **GREATEST BENEFIT** in this case would be to:

Choices:
A. Fit the patient with a palatal lift.
B. Teach the patient to speak with increased effort.
C. Strengthen the velopharyngeal muscles as a group through nonspeech strengthening exercises.
D. Improve velopharyngeal port closure through pharyngeal flap surgery.

Teaching Points

Correct Answer: B

Because this patient exhibits mild hypernasality, effortful speech production would be the most appropriate treatment route. Palatal lifts and pharyngeal flap approaches are appropriate for those dysarthric speakers who exhibit significant velopharyngeal weakness, whereas velopharyngeal strengthening regimens are more appropriate for those individuals with moderate impairments leading to hypernasality. Speaking with an increased effort may be effective as a compensatory technique for patients with mild deficits.

B35
Cleft Palate and Other Craniofacial Anomalies

A 6-year-old child is referred to a speech language pathologist (SLP) by an otolaryngologist (ENT) physician, in order to receive speech therapy. According to the child's mother, the child had normal speech until 2 years ago, when he underwent adenoidectomy. Following this surgery, the child demonstrated severe hypernasality, which has slightly improved over the past year. The SLP performs a full evaluation, which reveals normal articulation and significant hypernasality. What is the **FIRST** treatment option that should be instituted for this child?

Choices:
A. Speech and voice therapy for better sound control and airflow.
B. Exercises to strengthen the velopharyngeal musculature.
C. Discuss the inappropriateness of speech therapy, at this time, for the child with the physician.
D. Auditory training to improve awareness of the hypernasality.

Teaching Points

Correct Answer: D

The child in this scenario had a change in speech quality following a surgery. While there has been some noted improvement, the child continues to present with significant hypernasality, possibly due to lack of awareness. By bringing the deficit to the level of awareness, the child will be able to participate more fully in treatment efforts to reduce the perception of hypernasality. Following this step in treatment, other treatment options and speech therapy techniques may be utilized with this child.

B36
Research, Evidence-Based Practice and Tests and Measurements

A speech-language pathologist (SLP) is preparing to perform a language assessment on a child who comes from a cultural background with which the SLP is unfamiliar. In order to accurately gauge this child's linguistic skills, the SLP needs to be aware of the potential bias that assessment materials reflect because of the assumption that all cultural populations have the same life experiences. What type of bias is this SLP experiencing with the assessment materials?

Choices:
A. Content.
B. Linguistic.
C. Material.
D. Cultural.

Teaching Points

Correct Answer: A

Content bias refers to test stimuli, methods or procedures reflecting the assumption that all populations have the same life experiences and have learned similar concepts and vocabulary. If the child from this scenario has not been exposed to the material covered in this test, there may be an inaccurate diagnosis of a language disorder. In contrast to this, linguistic bias is the disparity between the language or dialect used by the examiner, the child, and/or the language or dialect expected in the child's response. Material bias and cultural bias are not forms of bias that are applicable in the evaluation of children from culturally diverse backgrounds.

B37

Acoustics

In examining a spectrogram of the phrase *Say sheep* produced by a male speaker, you notice that the lower limit of high-amplitude energy noise for both /s/ and /ʃ/ is near 2500 hertz (Hz). This **MOST LIKELY** indicates that:

Choices:
A. /s/ is being produced too far back in the mouth.
B. /s/ is being produced too far forward in the mouth.
C. /ʃ/ is being produced too far back in the mouth.
D. /ʃ/ is being produced too far forward in the mouth.

Teaching Points

Correct Answer: A

The cutoff of high-amplitude energy for sibilant fricatives is related to the size of the oral cavity in front of the obstruction. For /s/, the obstruction should be further forward than for /ʃ/, resulting in a smaller air pocket and a higher cutoff frequency. The /ʃ/ is expected to have a cutoff frequency around 2500 Hz. If /s/ has a similar cutoff frequency, then /s/ is being produced too far back in the mouth.

B38

The Practice of Speech-Language Pathology

A speech-language pathologist (SLP) is providing a social language group for a group of students with pragmatic language difficulties. The SLP wants to utilize means of intervention that provide the most good to all the members and is not willing to accept less progress by any member. Which philosophical approach **BEST** fits this SLP's approach to practice?

Choices:
A. Utilitarian approach.
B. Common good approach.
C. Fairness/justice approach.
D. The rights approach.

Teaching Points

Correct Answer: B

The common good approach seeks to find the action that best serves the whole community and not just some members. As this SLP seeks to find a means of intervention that is best for all the children in the social language group, the SLP is utilizing principles of the common good approach. In contrast, the utilitarian approach seeks to find the action that will do the most good and the least harm to the most people. The rights approach seeks to find the action that best respect the rights of all stakeholders. Finally, the fairness/justice approach seeks to find the option that treats people equally.

B39

Anatomy and Physiology of Communication and Swallowing

When producing the voiceless fricative /f/, the muscle that **MOST LIKELY** contracts is the

Choices:
A. Lateral cricoarytenoid.
B. Transverse interarytenoid.
C. Oblique interarytenoid.
D. Posterior cricoarytenoid.

Teaching Points

Correct Answer: D

As /f/ is a voiceless phoneme, it is important that the vocal folds are not contracted during production. In order for this to occur, the vocal folds needs to be abducted, invoking contraction of the posterior cricoarytenoid muscle, the sole vocal fold abductor. The other muscles listed function as vocal fold adductors and close the vocal folds for production as voiced phonemes. As /f/ is a voiceless phoneme, it would require no activation in these muscles.

B40

Autism Spectrum Disorders

A speech-language pathologist (SLP) is evaluating the communication skills of a child with autism spectrum disorder. Following the evaluation, the SLP notes that during communicative exchanges, this child demonstrates immediate and delayed repetition of utterances spoken by others. Which deficit is this child demonstrating?

Choices:
A. Jargon.
B. Verbal perseveration.
C. Childhood apraxia of speech.
D. Echolalia.

Teaching Points

Correct Answer: D

Echolalia is a communication deficit often present in autism spectrum disorder and is defined by repetition of utterances spoken by others. These repetitions may be immediate (i.e., immediately after being spoken) or delayed (i.e., following a long delay after initial production). In contrast to this, childhood apraxia of speech is an inability to voluntarily program neurological sequences for verbal speech production. Verbal perseveration is the continuous repetition of a sound, word or phrase. Finally, jargon is idiosyncratic speech production that is nonmeaningful to others.

B41

Voice Disorders

A patient arrives at the local voice center, and completes the patient intake form. There is a history of vocal fold surgeries and routine surgeon visits every couple of months for the past few years. The patient presents with frequent throat-clearing and inhalatory stridor. Without having an opportunity to use laryngoscopic evaluation, the speech-language pathologist reasons that this patient is **MOST LIKELY** experiencing which of the following disorders?

Choices:
A. Vocal fold nodules.
B. Laryngitis.
C. Reinke's edema.
D. Human papilloma virus.

Teaching Points

Correct Answer: D
Human papilloma virus can affect the laryngeal tissues and cause excessive, wart-like lesions throughout the larynx. A hallmark characteristic of this disorder is the need for frequent surgical interventions to remove affected tissue, as the virus causes continual growth of warty lesions. Additionally, perceptual characteristics of a patient experiencing HPV include frequent throat-clearing, restriction in breathing and stridor. In contrast, laryngitis does not require surgical intervention, and a history of interventions would contraindicate this diagnosis. While vocal fold nodules and Reinke's edema may require surgical intervention, if the patient follows an appropriate vocal hygiene regimen, there would most likely be no need for repeat surgeries.

B42

Voice Disorders

After undergoing open heart surgery, a patient emerges from anesthesia to find that the patient is presenting with a significantly hypophonic, breathy voice. After a few days in recovery, the patient's vocal quality has not improved, and a referral for otolaryngology and speech-language pathology consult is made. Based on the information given, what condition will most likely be discovered upon endoscopy?

Choices:
A. Vocal fold polyps.
B. Presbylaryngeus.
C. Vocal fold paralysis.
D. Arytenoid granuloma.

Teaching Points

Correct Answer: C
The left recurrent laryngeal nerve loops under the aortic arch, prior to innervating the muscles of the larynx. Patients who undergo open heart surgery may experience voice problems resulting from damage to the left recurrent laryngeal nerve. If the recurrent laryngeal nerve is significantly damaged, it could result in complete vocal fold paralysis, as this patient is experiencing. Vocal fold polyps occur due to phonotrauma, such as excessive screaming or cheering, and would not arise due to nerve damage. Similarly, arytenoid granulomas arise from direct vocal fold trauma from intubation or reflux, and are not neurological in origin. Finally, *presbylaryngeus* is the term for voice disorders in the elderly and is caused by normal aging.

B43

Dysphagia

A patient who exhibits reduced lip closure, reduced tongue grooving and reduced tongue-to-palate contact is **MOST LIKELY** experiencing a dysphagia in which phase of the swallow?

Choices:
A. Esophageal phase.
B. Oral phase.
C. Oral preparatory phase.
D. Pharyngeal phase.

Teaching Points

Correct Answer: B

During the oral phase, the bolus is contained in a central groove on the tongue surface and moves posteriorly until the swallow is triggered. The lips close, the tongue tip elevates and the floor of mouth muscles (FOM) contract during this phase as well. Deficits with any of these acts would qualify as an oral stage dysphagia.

B44

Autism Spectrum Disorders

A physician is evaluating a young child suspected of having autism spectrum disorder and has determined that the child demonstrates signs of hyperlexia. Which of the following **BEST** describes the condition of this child?

Choices:
A. The child demonstrates difficulty modulating vocal volume.
B. The child demonstrates negative reactions to loud noises.
C. The child demonstrates a fascination with letters and numbers.
D. The child demonstrates a disdain for certain clothing textures.

Teaching Points

Correct Answer: C

Hyperlexia is a condition often seen in children with autism spectrum disorder in which there is an extreme fascination with letters, numbers and words, which often begins at a young age. Additionally, these children demonstrate precocious decoding skills in the absence of comprehension. In contrast to this, the failure to modulate vocal volume is considered a problem of self-regulation. Negative reaction to loud noises or noisy environments is known as *hyperacusis*. Finally, disdain for particular clothing items may be considered tactile defensiveness.

B45

Written Language Disorders in the School-Age Population

A speech-language pathologist (SLP) in a high school is working with an adolescent student who has been struggling with generating detailed essay-length material. One of several research-based methods for enhancing quantity and quality of text produced by struggling writers that this SLP could employ with this student is:

Choices:
A. Sentence combining practice.
B. Repeated copying of sentences.
C. Decontextualized vocabulary instruction.
D. Incidental exposure to authentic texts.

Teaching Points

Correct Answer: A

Sentence combining practice is an efficacious approach to writing intervention that enhances the quantity and quality of text produced. With this type of practice, students gain experience combining different types of sentence structure in order to build their writing skills. The other types of interventions posed in this question are general bottom-up and top-down approaches to reading and writing instruction.

B46
Augmentative and Alternative Communication (AAC)

Mary is a 47-year-old with progressive amyotrophic lateral sclerosis. Her disease has progressed significantly enough to affect verbal communication; however, she maintains limited use of the fingers on her left hand. Her speech-language pathologist (SLP) has been updating Mary's augmentative and alternative communication (AAC) device so it utilizes alternate access to aid in Mary's communication. Mary's device now highlights each item in the first row of a selection set, followed by the second row, etc., until Mary makes a selection. What type of access has the SLP begun utilizing with Mary's device?

Choices:
A. Linear scanning.
B. Circular scanning.
C. Row-column scanning.
D. Group item scanning.

Teaching Points

Correct Answer: A

Linear scanning refers to a scanning pattern in which the device highlights each item in the first row of the selection set, followed by each item in the second row, etc., until the user makes a selection. As this matches the description of the method utilized by the SLP in this scenario, it is likely linear scanning is being implemented. In contrast to this, circular scanning occurs when the device presents the selections set in a circle and scans them item by item until a selection is made. Row-column scanning proceeds by highlighting each row until the user makes a selection, at which time items are then highlighted until the user makes a selection. Finally, group item scanning proceeds by presenting groups (i.e., semantically related items) until the user has made a selection, at which time items are presented until the user has made a selection.

B47
Autism Spectrum Disorders

A young child is brought to an outpatient clinic by the parents, with a chief complaint of "strange behaviors." After a thorough evaluation, the child is diagnosed with autism spectrum disorder, with significant impairments in syntactical aspects of language. Which of the following is **MOST LIKELY** a deficit exhibited by this child?

Choices:
A. The child cannot establish joint attention.
B. The child adds extraneous speech sounds.
C. The child omits past tense markers.
D. The child speaks telegraphically.

Teaching Points

Correct Answer: D

Children with autism spectrum disorder may demonstrate specific deficits in syntactic structure of language. Specifically, young children may speak telegraphically and omit articles, verb conjugations and small connective words. In contrast to this, failure to produce past tense markers would be considered a deficit in morphology, addition of excessive speech sound would be considered a deficit in phonology, and difficulty establishing joint attention would be considered a deficit in pragmatic language.

B48

Dysphagia

A speech-language pathologist (SLP) at a skilled nursing facility has been told that the facility is receiving a new patient this afternoon. The patient's paperwork has not yet been fully transferred. Only the results from a recent modified barium swallow (MBS) have been received, and the following is reported: "severe weakness throughout all phases of swallowing, which required a feeding tube be placed." However, by the time the SLP sees the patient, the reported weakness seems to have improved greatly. Which of the following disorders do you suspect is this patient's primary diagnosis?

Choices:
A. Multiple sclerosis.
B. Guillain-Barré.
C. Post-polio syndrome.
D. Parkinson's disease.

Teaching Points

Correct Answer: B

Guillain-Barré syndrome is an autoimmune disorder, which is characterized by demyelination and severe weakness, sometimes to the point of paralysis. However, the weakness is temporary, and there is spontaneous recovery observed in patients with the disorder. For the patient in this question, the spontaneous recovery could have occurred by the time they were transferred to their new facility.

B49

Spoken Language Disorders in Children

Judy is a young child who was brought into a speech and language center by her parents, who suspect that Judy may have a language disorder. However, when the speech-language pathologist (SLP) escorts Judy into her office, Judy begins playing by herself and will only interact with her mother. When the SLP brings out assessment measures, Judy runs into a corner to continue playing. What is the **MOST APPROPRIATE** means of assessing this child?

Choices:
A. Waiting until Judy is willing to participate and administer standardized measures.
B. Talking with Judy, to see what types of responses she will produce.
C. Administering a standardized case history to Judy's parents.
D. Collecting data through observation of Judy's interactions with parents.

Teaching Points

Correct Answer: D
When children become noncompliant during assessment, there are several methods that SLPs may implement to gather sufficient data. One such measure is watching the child's interactions, as a means of collecting language information. As the child may not become compliant during the session, waiting to administer standardized measures is not an efficient use of time. Additionally, administering a standard case history form may not deliver sufficient information regarding the child's language patterns. Finally, while it may be appropriate to attempt conversation with Judy, if she remains noncompliant, this method may not deliver appropriate information.

B50
Anatomy and Physiology of Communication and Swallowing

A person has a vital capacity of 5 liters and exchanges half a liter of air when typically breathing at rest. The person takes the biggest breath possible and inspires 3 liters of air. What is this person's expiratory reserve volume?

Choices:
A. 1.5 liters.
B. 2 liters.
C. 2.5 liters.
D. 3.5 liters.

Teaching Points

Correct Answer: A
A person's vital capacity is made of their inspiratory reserve volume, expiratory reserve volume, and their tidal volume. In the presented scenario, the patient has a tidal volume of 0.5 liters (the amount of air exchanged passively), and an inspiratory reserve volume (found from the largest inspiration) of 3 liters. The remaining volume needed to reach their vital capacity of 5 liters is 1.5 liters of expiratory reserve volume.

B51
Anatomy and Physiology of Communication and Swallowing

Neurotransmitters are chemicals in the brain that are important in sending neural signals between adjacent neurons. The **BEST** description of neurotransmitter release is that it:

Choices:
A. Excites neighboring cells.
B. Excites neighboring cells only if it binds with a receptor and causes a channel opening.
C. Excites or inhibits neighboring cells if it binds with a receptor and causes a channel opening.
D. Inhibits neighboring cells.

Teaching Points

Correct Answer: C
Neurotransmitters are chemicals that are released from neurons that help with neural signal transmission. Neurotransmitters can have one of two functions: excitatory or inhibitory. Excitatory neurotransmitters help continue the propagation of the neural signal, whereas inhibitory neurotransmitters slow or cancel the propagation of the neural signal.

B52

Acquired Language Disorders

The language zone has been described as a key region of the brain that, when damaged, is likely to result in some degree of aphasia. One characteristic of the language zone is that:

Choices:
A. It consists of two identical structures, found in each hemisphere.
B. It consists of key subcortical structures, including the basal ganglia and the thalamus.
C. It can be found on the dorsal portions of the frontal lobe.
D. It consists of portions of the frontal, temporal and parietal lobes.

Teaching Points

Correct Answer: D

The language zone is a left hemisphere brain region that is made up of parts of the frontal, temporal and parietal lobes that include Broca's area, Wernicke's area, the angular gyrus and the supramarginal gyrus.

B53

Stuttering and Other Fluency Disorders

Charles is a 3-year-old boy who has shown disfluencies in his speech since he began talking in sentences at about 2 years of age. Over time, his disfluencies have increased and now occur on about 12% of his words. He never comments about his stuttering moments and seems to be unaware when they occur. He has no other speech and language problems, is socially engaged and interactive, and has great motor skills. Charles' dad reports that he stuttered as a child, but grew out of it. Which of the following statements is **MOST ACCURATE**?

Choices:
A. He is showing normal disfluency, and the SLP should help his parents see if he "grows out of it."
B. He appears to be at the borderline stage of stuttering and is at risk because he is a male with a family history.
C. When preschoolers stutter, it is best to take a wait-and-see approach.
D. Direct therapy is indicated.

Teaching Points

Correct Answer: B

Charlie is showing signs of borderline stuttering in that his disfluencies exceed 10% and have lasted longer than 6 months. He also shows risk factors (gender, persistence and genetics) that increase the probability that he will need treatment to resolve his fluency problem.

B54

Acquired Language Disorders

A speech-language pathologist (SLP) in an acute rehabilitation setting has received a new patient on his/her case load. While reviewing notes from the patient's previous therapists, the SLP notices that this patient demonstrates anomia in discourse, impaired auditory comprehension, and impaired semantic memory, but has strengths in visuospatial skills, working memory and problem solving. The SLP decides that this patient may be experiencing which disorder?

Choices:
A. Primary progressive aphasia—nonfluent variety.
B. Primary progressive apraxia of speech.
C. Dementia with Lewy bodies (DLB).
D. Primary progressive aphasia—fluent variety.

Teaching Points

Correct Answer: D

Semantic dementia is an alternate term for the syndrome of primary progressive aphasia (PPA). It is characterized by fluent verbal output, word-finding problems, auditory comprehension deficit and difficulty with semantic memory. However, persons with semantic dementia demonstrate skills in visuospatial skills, problem solving, episodic memory and autobiographical memory.

B55

Research, Evidence-Based Practice and Tests and Measurements

A speech and language researcher has demonstrated the benefits of a newly developed treatment method through well-controlled studies that show internal validity, statistical significance and practical significance. This researcher's method demonstrates which of the following principles?

Choices:
A. Treatment efficacy.
B. Treatment effectiveness.
C. Treatment fidelity.
D. Treatment validity.

Teaching Points

Correct Answer: A

Research that demonstrates treatment efficacy shows the benefits of treatment through well-controlled studies with interval validity, statistical significance and practical significance. When a research study demonstrates all three of these principles, the study demonstrates good treatment efficacy. On the other hand, if research demonstrates clinical improvement when applied in real-life contexts, it demonstrates treatment effectiveness. When an application of a treatment in real-world context matches the controlled conditions of the original study, this demonstrates good treatment fidelity.

B56

Augmentative and Alternative Communication (AAC)

A speech-language pathologist (SLP) is administering an augmentative and alternative communication (AAC) evaluation to a patient with chronic, severe spastic dysarthria. In order to determine the most appropriate means of communication, the SLP engages in an assessment style that compares the skills of the patient with various AAC systems. Following the assessment, much has been learned about the patient's capabilities, and the SLP is able to recommend multiple AAC devices that the patient may be able to utilize. What type of assessment did this SLP engage in?

Choices:
A. Scanning.
B. Direct selection.
C. Feature matching.
D. System selection.

Teaching Points

Correct Answer: C

Feature matching is the process by which the skills and needs of the person with complex communication problems are matched with the features of various AAC systems. As the SLP from this scenario is engaging in an assessment to determine how the skills of the patient match the AAC devices present, he/she is utilizing a feature-matching approach. In contrast to this, direct selection is when the AAC user directly makes a choice on the system via touching, pointing, looking or speaking. Scanning is an indirect method of access in which choices are presented to the AAC user, and the person indicates when the desired target is reached through a predetermined signal. Finally, system selection is the final step of the assessment process in which an AAC user selects the AAC system through which he/she will communicate.

B57

Spoken Language Disorders in Children

A young child has recently been diagnosed with a language disorder, with particular deficits in the content and use of language. Which of the following areas of language **BEST** define this child's language disorder?

Choices:
A. Morphology and syntax.
B. Semantics and pragmatics.
C. Phonology and pragmatics.
D. Morphology and syntax.

Teaching Points

Correct Answer: B

According to Bloom and Lahey's 1978 model, language can be divided into form, content and use, in order to make more evident how language components interface during typical language learning. Language form can be divided into the components of syntax, morphology and phonology. Language content is constructed of semantics and associated vocabulary. Finally, language use consists of pragmatic language components. If this child is demonstrating deficits in language content and use, they would most likely have deficits in the areas of semantics and pragmatics.

B58

Stuttering and Other Fluency Disorders

Mr. Jones is a 56-year-old man who experienced a stroke and is now recovering in the rehabilitation unit at the hospital. He appears to have almost recovered from other stroke symptoms and has no aphasia. At first he was speaking more slowly than expected, but now he appears to have developed more disfluencies that occur during speech and reading. Which of the following is **MOST ACCURATE**?

Choices:
A. The patient's stroke unmasked an early developmental stuttering problem.
B. He needs an MRI before any conclusions could be made.
C. His stuttering is probably neurogenic in origin.
D. His stuttering is psychogenic.

Teaching Points

Correct Answer: C

Mr. Jones most likely is experiencing neurogenic stuttering because of the timing of onset with his stroke. While an MRI may help the neurologist determine if there is a lesion in the speech areas, the absence of a specific lesion would not rule out the probable etiology as neurogenic. If the patient's history or current state indicated extreme stress (more than typical for someone in this condition) or the presence of other acute psychiatric illness, then psychogenic etiology should also be considered.

B59

Speech Sound Disorders in Children

Following a comprehensive speech sound evaluation, a speech-language pathologist (SLP) is beginning to select specific sound error patterns to target in intervention with a pediatric client aged 3;4 years. The SLP understands that there are multiple factors to consider when choosing treatment targets. Which of the following selections is appropriate to utilize when selecting treatment targets for this client?

Choices:
A. The child has difficulty producing a speech sound that typically develops at age 6;0 years, so this sound should not be targeted as it is not age appropriate.
B. The child is not stimulable for a specific speech sound that is in error, so this speech sound should be targeted as it would likely not improve independently.
C. The child demonstrates "later occurring" phonological errors, so this child does not need to participate in speech therapy at this time.
D. The child is stimulable for specific speech sounds in error, so these speech sounds should be targeted as the child would likely not improve independently.

Teaching Points

Correct Answer: B

Several factors are important in choosing treatment targets for intervention. One such factor is stimulability. Sounds that are stimulable for production most often remediate on their own and do not require intervention. However, those that are unstimulable may be direct targets for intervention, as these sounds are not likely to remediate independently. In contrast, when discussing the factor of age, there has been work that shows targeting later-developing sounds (i.e., those more "age advanced" for children) may allow generalization to errored, age-appropriate sounds. Finally, as the child is demonstrating a speech sound error, the child is a candidate for speech therapy, which should begin as soon as possible and not when the child has matured.

B60

Language Acquisition

Obstruent sounds differ from resonant sounds in that obstruent sounds:

Choices:
A. Always include a quasi-periodic sound source.
B. Always include an aperiodic sound source.
C. Are always continuant sounds.
D. Are always noncontinuant sounds.

Teaching Points

Correct Answer: B

Obstruent sounds always involve a narrow constriction or blockage that results in an aperiodic sound source. If the obstruction is a blockage, airflow will be momentarily blocked, and the sound will be a noncontinuant. If the obstruction is a narrow constriction, airflow will never be completely blocked, and the sound will be a continuant.

B61

Spoken Language Disorders in Children

A speech-language pathologist (SLP) is working on conversation-level goals with a young child. However, the child continues to have significant difficulties with this form of communication. The SLP suspects that this child may have deficits in underlying skills needed for conversation, such as:

Choices:
A. Phonological memory span, turn-taking abilities and simple sentence structure.
B. Gestures, complex sentence structures and joint attention.
C. Intellectual functioning, morphosyntactic development and fluency.
D. Joint attention, following line of regard and joint action routines.

Teaching Points

Correct Answer: D

Successful development of conversational abilities, or any discourse type, depends on a child's skill in three areas. Joint attention (i.e., focusing on what the caregiver is focused on) skills set the stage for establishing a topic of conversation. Following line of regard (i.e., recognizing that the caregiver is attending to someone or something) is a prerequisite for seeking out a point of attention. Finally, joint action routines (i.e., repetitive, predictable patterns of interaction) aid in the learning of predictable roles and responsibilities for conversational partners.

B62

Spoken Language Disorders in Children

A speech-language pathologist (SLP) is working with a young child who has demonstrated significant difficulty with narrative generation. The SLP has decided that an initial target for this child is to produce recounts. Which of the following would be the **MOST BENEFICIAL** goal for this child?

Choices:
A. The child will produce narratives to relate a routine event or activity.
B. The child will spontaneously produce narratives about a specific weekend event.
C. The child will produce narratives about shared experiences when prompted.
D. The child will produce narratives about ongoing experiences during play activities.

Teaching Points

Correct Answer: C

A recount is a narrative that relates unique, shared experiences using past tense, which a child produces when prompted. In contrast to this, a personal narrative is a spontaneously given narrative, which relates specific experiences or events. An event cast is a type of narrative that is produced as a description of an ongoing activity, often during play. Finally, a script is a type of narrative that relates routine events or activities that occur with some degree of frequency.

B63

Speech Sound Disorders in Children

A speech-language pathologist (SLP) in private practice has been asked to perform a speech and language evaluation on a new client. After completing the evaluation, the SLP notices the following speech sound errors: /səpun/ for /spun/, /dzu/ for /zu/ and /tsɪt/ for /sɪt/. Which of the following BEST describes this child's speech sound errors?

Choices:
A. Epenthesis and affrication.
B. Tetism and deaffrication.
C. Backing and reduplication.
D. Fronting and stopping.

Teaching Points

Correct Answer: A

Epenthesis is the addition of a vowel sound in a consonant cluster, such as when the child from this scenario produces the word /səpun/. Affrication is the replacement of a fricative speech sound with an affricate-like speech sound, such as in the productions of /dzu/ and /tsɪt/. The other phonological processes collectively did not occur in this child's speech sample. Tetism is a phonological process that occurs when sounds are moved to the alveolar position, similar to consonant neutralization. Deaffrication occurs when a child replaces an affricate consonant with a fricative consonant. Backing is a phonological process that occurs when mid and front consonants are replaced with back consonants. Reduplication occurs when there is a repetition of a phoneme or syllable. Fronting occurs when back sounds are replaced by front or mid consonants. Finally, stopping occurs when continuant consonants are replaced by stop consonants.

B64

Language Acquisition

Brad is a typically developing 15-month-old toddler. How many words would Brad MOST LIKELY have in his expressive lexicon?

Choices:
A. 50 words.
B. 25 words.
C. 10 words.
D. 100 words.

Teaching Points

Correct Answer: C

By the time children are 15 months old, their expressive lexicon is around 10 words. By the time they are 19 months old, this expressive lexicon has steadily increased to around 100–300 words.

B65

Anatomy and Physiology of Communication and Swallowing

A patient presents to an acute care hospital, and imaging has revealed a hemorrhage localized to the left occipital lobe. Which deficit would **MOST LIKELY** result?

Choices:
A. Broca's aphasia.
B. Tardive dyskinesia.
C. Homonymous hemianopia.
D. Ataxic dysarthria.

Teaching Points

Correct Answer: C

The occipital lobe is the region of the brain that controls vision. Homonymous hemianopia occurs when one-half of a person's visual field is not functioning, secondary to brain damage. In this case, the patient would most likely present with a right homonymous hemianopia.

B66

Acoustics

The center of gravity for a sibilant fricative is expected to be:

Choices:
A. Higher than its skewness.
B. Lower than its skewness.
C. At the center of the spectrum.
D. Off-center in the spectrum.

Teaching Points

Correct Answer: D

Center of gravity for sibilant fricatives is expected to be off-center, whereas for nonsibilant fricatives, it should be at or near the center of the spectrum.

B67
Acoustics

In a narrowband spectrogram, the speech-language pathologist (SLP) can see that harmonic spacing becomes narrower throughout a vowel. When listening to the vowel, the SLP expects to hear that the vowel:

Choices:
A. Is a diphthong that shifts from a low vowel to a high vowel.
B. Is a diphthong that shifts from a front vowel to a back vowel.
C. Begins at a lower pitch and ends at a higher pitch.
D. Begins at a higher pitch and ends at a lower pitch.

Teaching Points

Correct Answer: D
The spacing between harmonics in the human voice is equal to F0. If harmonic spacing shifts from wider to narrower, the harmonics are getting closer together and F0 is getting lower.

B68
Acquired Language Disorders

Pragmatic treatment approaches for aphasia often adhere to the principles of Promoting Aphasics' Communicative Effectiveness (PACE). Which of the following is a good example of the PACE principles?

Choices:
A. Topics of conversation should be selected by the person with aphasia and should be personally relevant.
B. The person with aphasia should be encouraged to use spoken language expression when he/she communicates.
C. The conversational partner should avoid giving feedback to the person with aphasia about whether he/she understood the message or not.
D. The person with aphasia should dominate the conversation.

Teaching Points

Correct Answer: A
The four PACE principles include: the clinician and the person with aphasia (PWA) being equal conversational partners, exchanging new information by both parties, giving the PWA free choice of communication modality, and the clinician providing feedback to the PWA regarding how much of the communicative message was understood.

B69

Speech Sound Disorders in Children

A speech and language researcher is establishing a study to determine the effect of reinforcement on young children's phonological productions. One group of study participants will be given positive reinforcement for correct phonological productions, and the other group will participate in play sessions throughout the study. The researcher believes that the group receiving reinforcement for correct productions will learn the phonological pattern of their home language quicker than will the play session group. Which theory of phonological development **BEST** lines up with this researcher's views?

Choices:
A. Behavioral theory.
B. Prosodic theory.
C. Generative phonology theory.
D. Interactionist-discovery theory.

Teaching Points

Correct Answer: A

The behavioral theory postulates that children undergo phonological development when provided with contingent reinforcement. Because this researcher believes that the group of children that receive reinforcement for correct productions will develop quicker than children who undergo play scenarios, he is utilizing behaviorist principles to guide his research. On the other hand, the prosodic theory emphasizes the perception of whole words as early word productions and is not contingent upon reinforcement. The generative phonology theory is an expansion of the distinctive feature theory, and includes concepts such as underlying representations, surface forms and phonological rules. However, this theory also does not emphasize contingent reinforcement. Finally, the interactionist-discovery theory emphasizes that children discover their own rules as they develop and does not involve contingent reinforcement.

B70

Speech Sound Disorders in Children

Following a speech evaluation, a speech-language pathologist (SLP) has determined that the child he is working with demonstrates significant amounts of homonymy in his speech. For example, the child produces the word /bo/ for both /bot/ and /bo/. However, the child does produce the /t/ phoneme in other word positions. Which intervention approach would be of the **GREATEST BENEFIT** for the SLP to utilize in working with this particular child?

Choices:
A. Maximal contrast approach.
B. Integral stimulation.
C. Traditional approach.
D. Minimal pairs approach.

Teaching Points

Correct Answer: D

The goal of the minimal pairs method is to eliminate a child's creation of homonyms or a singular production for multiple words. In this case, the child is producing /bo/ for both /bot/ and /bo/, which could be directly targeted utilizing this approach. In contrast, the maximal opposition method focuses on contrasting a target word with a maximally distinct sound (i.e., one that varies across a variety of features). However, in this method reduction of homonymy is indirectly addressed, unlike in the minimal pairs method. Both the traditional method and integral stimulation method are used to treat phonetic errors and are utilized to establish a sound that is not present in a child's repertoire. Because this child is able to produce /t/ in other word positions, these methods would not help alleviate the homonymy being experienced.

B71

The Practice of Speech-Language Pathology

A speech-language pathologist (SLP) has recently been employed in a skilled nursing facility. The SLP knows that he is ethically responsible to provide services to patients, but is unsure of the specific roles he must fill. Which of the following is **NOT** a role of this SLP?

Choices:
A. Use of all modes of service delivery, including those that are technology based.
B. Participation in the evaluation, selection and use of assistive devices.
C. Counseling patients, families and caregivers regarding assessment and treatment.
D. Evaluation and determination of eligibility for special education and related services.

Teaching Points

Correct Answer: D
Speech-language pathologists (SLPs) that work in medical settings are required to use all modes of service delivery (including those that are technology based); participate in the evaluation, selection and use of assistive devices; and counsel patients, families and caregivers regarding assessment and treatment. In contrast, SLPs in educational settings are required to evaluate and determine eligibility for special education and related services.

B72

Autism Spectrum Disorders

A physician has been consulted by a couple who is hoping to have children. However, the couple has also expressed interest in learning about risk factors for children with autism spectrum disorder. Which is a risk factor associated with having a child with autism spectrum disorder?

Choices:
A. If a father uses antidepressants while trying to conceive.
B. If a mother uses antihistamines during pregnancy.
C. If a mother is over 30 years old.
D. If a father is over 40 years old.

Teaching Points

Correct Answer: D
Two main risk factors associated with having a child with autism spectrum disorder are paternal age and maternal drug use. Specifically, if a father is over 40 years of age, there is a six times greater chance of having a child with autism. Additionally, maternal use of antidepressants during pregnancy has also been linked to a greater chance of having a child with ASD. In contrast to this, there has been no established evidence of maternal age over 30, paternal use of antidepressants, or maternal use of antihistamines associated with having a child with autism spectrum disorder.

B73

Written Language Disorders in the School-Age Population

A speech-language pathologist (SLP) is called in to evaluate a new student in a ninth-grade English Language Arts class. The SLP notices that the student reads a single article quickly and accurately and reports knowledge gained directly from reading the article to classmates. The cluster of behaviors observed in this student is most closely associated with which of Chall's reading stages?

Choices:
A. Stage 1: Initial reading or decoding.
B. Stage 2: Confirmation, fluency, ungluing from print.
C. Stage 3: Reading for learning the new.
D. Stage 4: Multiple viewpoints.

Teaching Points

Correct Answer: C

The student has demonstrated the ability to read fluently, which is a skill that is developed in Chall's stage 2. Hallmarks of Chall's stage 3 include a predominance of expository text, such as the report that this student was reading, and identification/generation of the main idea of a text. This student would not fall into Chall's stage 4 as he/she is not utilizing multiple viewpoints in the report back to the class.

B74

Anatomy and Physiology of Communication and Swallowing

The telencephalon is the area of the brain that includes the cerebral hemispheres, and it receives its blood supply from a variety of different arteries. The artery that supplies most of the medial surfaces of the telencephalon is the:

Choices:
A. Anterior cerebral artery.
B. Middle cerebral artery.
C. Posterior artery.
D. Anterior cerebral artery.

Teaching Points

Correct Answer: A

The telencephalon includes the cerebral hemispheres, which receive blood from the anterior, middle and posterior cerebral arteries. The anterior cerebral artery branches off from the internal carotid artery and feeds the cerebral hemispheres, starting in the area of the optic chiasm, which can be found in the medial portions of the hemispheres. In contrast to this, the middle cerebral artery supplies blood to a majority of the lateral cerebral hemispheres. The posterior cerebral artery supplies blood to the posterior cerebral hemispheres, including the occipital lobes. Finally, the anterior spinal artery supplies blood to the anterior spinal cord and posterior cerebellum.

B75

Speech Sound Disorders in Children

After performing a comprehensive speech evaluation on a pediatric client, a speech-language pathologist (SLP) has determined that the child demonstrates difficulty producing the /l/ phoneme, consistent with a phonetic error. Which method of intervention would be an appropriate selection for the SLP to utilize with this child?

Choices:
A. Minimal contrast method.
B. Distinctive feature approach.
C. Integral stimulation approach.
D. Cycles remediation approach.

Teaching Points

Correct Answer: C

The integral stimulation approach is an intervention method used for phonetic speech errors in which emphasis on multiple input modes is used to help a child establish a speech sound into his/her repertoire. In contrast, the minimal contrast approach, distinctive features approach and cycles remediation approach are all intervention methods used for children with phonemic speech errors, and they would not be helpful in remediating this particular child's speech sound disorder as this child needs to learn the motor pattern to produce the /l/ phoneme.

B76

Motor Speech Disorders

A patient is in the emergency department of a hospital following a massive motorcycle accident. After receiving a computerized tomography (CT) scan, the patient is revealed to have sustained diffuse, bilateral hemispheric damage. Later results from a speech and language evaluation show that the patient has a strained-strangled vocal quality, hypernasality during speech activities and a slow, effortful rate of speech. Based on this information, the patient would MOST LIKELY be diagnosed with which motor speech disorder?

Choices:
A. Hypokinetic dysarthria.
B. Flaccid dysarthria.
C. Ataxic dysarthria.
D. Spastic dysarthria.

Teaching Points

Correct Answer: D

Spastic dysarthria arises from bilateral hemispheric damage, which leads to excessive spasticity during speech activities. Associated perceptual correlates include a strained-strangled vocal quality, hypernasality and effortful speech. Flaccid dysarthria arises from lower motor neuron damage (either unilateral or bilateral), ataxic dysarthria arises from cerebellar damage and hypokinetic dysarthria arises from basal ganglia damage.

B77

Spoken Language Disorders in Children

A speech-language pathologist (SLP) is working in a preschool class, targeting increasing the children's language skills. After the SLP reads a story to the class, she asks a student to describe the main character's feelings throughout the story. The student responds with "they were happy, because it was a good story," indicating her own personal feelings regarding the story. This child demonstrates difficulty with:

Choices:
A. Theory of Mind.
B. Pragmatic language.
C. Syntactical structure.
D. Semantic language.

Teaching Points

Correct Answer: A

Theory of Mind describes a child's ability to take another's point of view, including beliefs, knowledge or feelings. As this child describes his/her own, personal feelings in response to probing a different character's feelings, they are demonstrating difficulty with concepts that fall under Theory of Mind. Pragmatic language refers to social language use, such as joint attention, turn taking, or eye contact. Syntactic structure refers to grammatical structure of a language, of which this child appears to have some level of mastery. Finally, semantic language refers to the meaning of language, such as vocabulary, of which this child demonstrates competency.

B78

Autism Spectrum Disorders

Jamie is a speech-language pathologist (SLP) working with a child who has autism spectrum disorder. Jamie believes that this child would benefit from implementation of Picture Exchange Communication System (PECS) to enhance their communicative effectiveness. Which of the following goals is **BEST** for use with this child?

Choices:
A. The child will use pictures during play scenarios.
B. The child will perform desired acts in response to pictures.
C. The child will use images to obtain desired items.
D. The child is given pictures in response to desired motor acts.

Teaching Points

Correct Answer: C

The goal of the Picture Exchange Communication System (PECS) is to establish a functional, reciprocal picture communication system in a social context. In this method of intervention, the child exchanges a picture of a desired item with a communication partner in order to establish communication and receive the desired object. This method of intervention is a form of augmentative and alternative communication that focuses on teaching, motivation and reinforcement.

Examination B 555

B79

Speech Sound Disorders in Children

A speech-language pathologist (SLP) has been working with a child who demonstrates difficulty producing /k/ in the initial and final word positions. However, the child does correctly produce the following words: /ki/, /kæt/, /bæk/ and /baɪk/. The SLP decides to utilize a treatment method that capitalizes on these correct productions to aid in faulty productions. Which of these interventions is **MOST LIKELY** the method chosen by this SLP?

Choices:
A. Integral stimulation.
B. Multiple phoneme approach.
C. Sensory-motor approach.
D. Paired-stimuli approach.

Teaching Points

Correct Answer: D

The paired-stimuli approach utilizes four key words as a starting point, and 10 training words are then paired with the key words to aid in production. As the child from this scenario is able to produce the errored speech sound correctly in four separate words, these may act as the key words and aid further production of the /k/ phoneme. In contrast, the integral stimulation approach may be utilized to establish a speech sound that the child is unable to produce, and it would not be recommended for this client. The sensory-motor approach uses bisyllable productions of nonerrored phonemes as facilitating contexts to produce a target sound. As the child is able to produce the target /k/, this method of intervention is contraindicated. Finally, the multiple phoneme approach is utilized for children with multiple phoneme errors, and as this child only demonstrates errors on the /k/ phoneme, this method is also contraindicated for use in intervention.

B80

Research, Evidence-Based Practice and Tests and Measurements

A speech and language researcher has completed final analysis on a data set and has discovered a highly homogenous distribution of participant scores. Due to this homogeneity, the researcher is also likely to find a small:

Choices:
A. Mean.
B. Median.
C. Standard deviation.
D. Confidence interval.

Teaching Points

Correct Answer: C

The standard deviation is the average amount that all the scores in a particular distribution will deviate from the mean. When there is more homogeneity of data points in the set, there will be a smaller standard deviation, as there will be less deviation from the median.

B81

Dysphagia

During a patient's bedside swallowing evaluation, the speech-language pathologist (SLP) notices that there is copious amounts of lingual residue present in the patient's oral cavity following their swallow. Which of the following parts of the oral phase is the patient **MOST LIKELY** having difficulty with?

Choices:
A. Bolus formation.
B. Anterior-posterior movement.
C. Labial seal.
4 Mastication.

Teaching Points

Correct Answer: A

The patient would most likely be experiencing difficulty with bolus formation. If the patient is not able to form a cohesive bolus prior to swallowing, this would most likely lead to residue being left at any location in the oral cavity.

B82

Speech Sound Disorders in Children

A speech-language pathologist (SLP) has been providing speech therapy to a child with a speech sound disorder. As this child demonstrates errors on multiple phonemes, the SLP has selected the cycles remediation approach for intervention with this child. What could the SLP do to utilize this treatment approach?

Choices:
A. Target a different phoneme each treatment session.
B. Provide multiple input modes to establish productions of phonemes.
C. Target different areas of language for generalization to phonological impairments.
D. Target word pairs that are contrasted by a single phoneme.

Teaching Points

Correct Answer: A

The cycles remediation approach targets a single errored phoneme per treatment session, and once all errored phonemes have been targeted, a full cycle has been completed. A new cycle is then started, which builds on the work completed in the previous cycle. This intervention method would be the best match to the SLP's wishes for intervention. In contrast, the integral stimulation approach utilizes multiple input modes to help a child learn the motor pattern for speech sound production. The maximal opposition approach utilizes sound pairs that are maximally different (i.e., by more than one feature) to help with errored speech sound production. Finally, the whole-language treatment approach targets multiple areas of language simultaneously to help build a child's phonological skills.

B83

Stuttering and Other Fluency Disorders

A speech-language pathologist (SLP) report for a 4-year-old with a history of disfluencies stated that the child exhibited simple phrase repetitions and occasional grammatical interjections of one iteration. Occasionally, the child is observed to prolong speech sounds at the beginning of an utterance for up to 3 seconds and also to occasionally show tense lip posturing on certain sounds. Which of the following statements is the MOST ACCURATE regarding the behavior?

Choices:
A. The child is showing only core behaviors of stuttering.
B. The child's prolongations and tense posturing are insignificant.
C. The child is at low risk for advanced stuttering.
D. The child is showing core and secondary stuttering behaviors.

Teaching Points

Correct Answer: D

The child is showing the emergence of secondary stuttering behaviors (beginning stuttering) as evidenced by the presence of secondary behaviors as well as core behaviors. The presence of these secondary behaviors is significant in that they signal attempts to control the core elements of stuttering.

B84

Autism Spectrum Disorders

A speech-language pathologist (SLP) is working with a group of school-aged children diagnosed with autism spectrum disorder. The SLP would like to set appropriate pragmatic goals for the children, while utilizing a social communication group approach. Which of the following pragmatic goals is of GREATEST BENEFIT for use with these children?

Choices:
A. Sharing interests with other group members.
B. Generating polite requests and responses.
C. Determining appropriate questions for other group members.
D. Understanding other group members' feelings.

Teaching Points

Correct Answer: A

School-age children require pragmatic skills consistent with peer interaction. For this age group, pragmatic goals include considering others' feelings, sharing interests, expressing preferences politely and shared attention. In contrast to this, generating polite request would be an appropriate pragmatic goal for younger children, while determining appropriate questions and understanding others' feelings would be an appropriate pragmatic goal for adolescents and adults.

B85

Voice Disorders

A speech-language pathologist (SLP) at the local speech and language clinic has been assigned a patient presenting as completely aphonic. After comprehensive evaluation, the SLP finds nothing structurally or physiologically wrong with the patient's laryngeal mechanism; however, the patient continues to present with difficulties during speech-related activities. Which of the following is an appropriate approach for the SLP to take in treating this patient?

Choices:
A. Refer the patient to a gastroenterologist, in order to establish a potential diagnosis of laryngopharyngeal reflux.
B. Refer the patient to a pulmonologist, to determine the state of the patient's respiratory mechanism.
C. Refer the patient to a psychiatrist, in order to establish a potential diagnosis of psychogenic dysphonia.
D. Send the patient home with referral for 2 weeks of complete voice rest, at which point all problems should resolve.

Teaching Points

Correct Answer: C

Patients suspected of psychogenic dysphonia would present with normal vocal fold tissue and movement during evaluation; however, they would continue to present with difficulty during speech-related activities. As psychogenic dysphonia is often associated with emotional distress, a referral to a psychological professional may be warranted to help the patient understand and deal with any psychological underpinnings of the patient's voice disorder. As psychogenic dysphonia is not caused by gastric or pulmonary deficits, referrals to specialists in these areas would not help alleviate the symptoms of the disorder. Lastly, as the patient is unable to produce any voice at all, some form of immediate treatment or recommendation is required, so a period of vocal rest is contraindicated.

B86

Written Language Disorders in the School-Age Population

A 12-year-old student demonstrates fluent reading at the text level and shows average spelling for regular and irregular words; nevertheless, his reading comprehension is quite poor. This pattern of literacy behaviors is associated with deficits in which areas?

Choices:
A. Phonological awareness and grapheme-phoneme correspondence.
B. Word recognition and rapid automatic naming.
C. Oral vocabulary and sentence processing.
D. Sight word reading skills and structural analysis.

Teaching Points

Correct Answer: C

Although this student demonstrates adequate reading of sentence-level material, deficits in oral vocabulary and sentence processing would lead to deficits in reading comprehension. Because this student has difficulty with vocabulary, this child would most likely not understand the meaning behind multiple words encountered. Sentence-level processing deficits would lead to further difficulty with reading comprehension, as the student would not be able to hold the elements of the story in working memory or comprehend word-order patterns within the sentence.

B87

Motor Speech Disorders

What are the **KEY** attributes of a therapy session to be considered when treating a child with childhood apraxia of speech (CAS)?

Choices:
A. Number of sessions per week and amount of practice (i.e., number of productions) per session.
B. Adoption of nonspeech tasks and number of sessions per week.
C. Syllable shape and the number of cues provided by the clinician to achieve a correct production.
D. Number of suprasegmental facilitators and the number of sessions per week.

Teaching Points

Correct Answer: A

Session characteristics for clients with CAS include intensive and individualized treatment, maximization of production practice during each session, more frequent occurrence of treatment sessions and length of the session matched to the attention/learning abilities of the child. Focusing on the number of treatment sessions and maximizing the amount of productions for the client can promote improvements in the client's speech output capabilities.

B88

Research, Evidence-Based Practice and Tests and Measurements

A speech-language pathologist (SLP) is in the process of starting a study on autism and is selecting proper assessment measures. In order to select the most appropriate test, the SLP should be aware of how well specific tests measure the characteristics of autism. Which of the following best describes the need for an accurate description?

Choices:
A. Criterion validity.
B. Content validity.
C. Construct validity.
D. Internal validity.

Teaching Points

Correct Answer: B

Content validity refers to how well the test items measure the characteristics or behaviors of interest. As this SLP is interested in assessments for autism, the SLP should be primarily concerned with how well the selected test measurements describe the characteristics of autism. In contrast, criterion validity refers to how well the measure correlates with an outside criterion, and construct validity refers to how well the measure reflects a theoretical construct of the characteristic of interest.

B89

Acquired Language Disorders

A clinician evaluates a patient with a left cerebrovascular accident (CVA) and determines that the patient exhibits both aphasia and apraxia of speech (AOS). Which of the following choices is the **MOST IMPORTANT** consideration when planning treatment for this client?

Choices:
A. Adopting a linguistic approach to treatment.
B. Considering contributions of both disorders to the communication deficit.
C. Adopting a motor approach to treatment.
D. Identifying alternative forms of communication in order to compensate for both the linguistic and motoric deficits.

Teaching Points

Correct Answer: B

Considerations from both disorders should be taken into consideration when planning treatment for this particular patient. As aphasia is a language disorder, and AOS is a motor planning/programming deficit, the focus of treatment will be different for each disorder. Planning for these differences can lead to the greatest amount of improvement for this type of patient. Adopting approaches that target only one of the disorders leads to a lack of gains made in the untargeted disorder. Additionally, alternative and augmentative communication could be utilized during treatment to supplement SLP treatment. It should only be used as a complete compensation for both linguistic and motoric deficits if the patient persists with significant deficits in both areas after treatment.

B90

Motor Speech Disorders

Motor learning may be enhanced by introducing a delay between the time the speaker produces a targeted stimulus and the clinician provides feedback in the form of knowledge performance or knowledge of results. There should be:

Choices:
A. No delay in feedback in knowledge of performance in most cases.
B. A 1- to 2-second delay in all feedback.
C. A 3- to 5-second delay in all feedback.
D. A delay in feedback dependent upon the explicitness of the expected response by the clinician.

Teaching Points

Correct Answer: C

Allowing a 3- to 5-second delay before giving feedback to patients with apraxia allows for improved motor learning. If feedback is given immediately, the person with childhood apraxia of speech/apraxia of speech (CAS/AOS) is not able to evaluate his/her own performance and builds a reliance on the clinician for feedback on performance. Delays in feedback give persons with CAS/AOS time to process and reflect on the motor patterns associated with certain movements.

B91

Language Acquisition

A child is being seen by a speech-language pathologist (SLP) in an early intervention setting. The child is demonstrating deficits in foundational skills for social use of language, and these have been chosen as intervention targets. For which skills would this child **MOST LIKELY** have deficits?

Choices:
A. Gestures and vocalizations.
B. Vegetative sounds such as coughing and burping.
C. Eye contact, joint attention and taking turns.
D. Talking about objects and events.

Teaching Points

Correct Answer: C

Research has demonstrated that these behaviors are important precursors to the development of social communication in young children. In typical development, children who show these aspects of interaction are believed to be advancing in their communicative development. Gestures and vocalizations and naming behaviors are later-developing occurrences and may or may not signal social awareness.

B92

Spoken Language Disorders in Children

A young child is brought into a speech and language clinic by his parents, with primary complaints of "little language use." Upon initial evaluation, the speech-language pathologist determines that the child communicates appropriately through use of gestures for requests for actions and objects, but uses little verbal language. What would be of the **GREATEST BENEFIT** in the next step in this child's treatment?

Choices:
A. Expand the child's expressive syntax to include simple sentence structure.
B. Expand the child's expressive morphology to include plural markers.
C. Expand the child's receptive vocabulary to include more functional items.
D. Expend the child's repertoire to include vocalizations with gestures.

Teaching Points

Correct Answer: D

The child from this scenario demonstrates communicative intentions through use of gestures to request objects and actions. An appropriate next step would be to add vocalizations or words to the gestures, as a means of expanding the child's expressive repertoire. This sets a foundational skill, on which later-developing skills such as simple sentence structure and plural markers. As this child demonstrates the ability to request objects and actions successfully, the child will likely demonstrate age-appropriate receptive vocabulary skills and may not require intervention in this area.

B93

Dysphagia

A patient at an acute rehabilitation hospital is working with the speech-language pathologist (SLP) on therapy techniques to improve his/her symptoms of dysphagia, which primarily consist of decreased laryngeal elevation. Which of the following techniques would **BEST** be suited to this patient?

Choices:
A. Shaker head lifts and the Mendelsohn maneuver.
B. The supraglottic swallow and the super-supraglottic swallow.
C. The effortful swallow and the Masako maneuver.
D. VitalStim and thickened liquids.

Teaching Points

Correct Answer: A

The Shaker head-lift exercises involve the patient lying on the floor and lifting only the head until able to see his/her toes. This maneuver has been proven to increase upper esophageal sphincter opening through strengthening of the suprahyoid muscles. The Mendelsohn maneuver involves having the patient engage their suprahyoid muscles to hold the larynx at the height of the swallow, thus strengthening that muscle group. Both exercises would be good for a patient who has decreased laryngeal elevation because increased strength in the suprahyoids would help elevate the larynx.

B94

Cleft Palate and Other Craniofacial Anomalies

A speech-language pathologist (SLP) is scheduled to perform an evaluation on a child with a chief complaint of "nasality." After performing the evaluation, the SLP finds that the child demonstrates insufficient resonance on nasal consonants. What type of resonance does this child demonstrate?

Choices:
A. Hypernasality.
B. Hyponasality.
C. Oral cul de sac resonance.
D. Nasal cul de sac resonance.

Teaching Points

Correct Answer: B

Nasal consonants normally experience some level of nasality due to the way they are produced. Because this type of consonant is produced with an open velopharyngeal port, hypernasality would be highly difficulty to perceive without instrumental quantification. However, if the velopharyngeal port remains closed during articulation of nasal sounds, they would readily be perceived as misarticulated. This type of resonance is referred to as *hyponasality*, or lack of normal nasality on consonants.

B95

Written Language Disorders in the School-Age Population

A child who a speech-language pathologist (SLP) has just begun working with in a private practice clinic spells words semiphonetically. This would be **BEST** illustrated by which of the following choices:

Choices:
A. "I am watching TV" spelled as "I am waching TV."
B. "I am happy" spelled as "I m hap."
C. "I like cats" spelled as "I lik cats."
D. "I went to the game" spelled as "I goed to the game."

Teaching Points

Correct Answer: B

Semiphonetic spelling, also called letter-name spelling, occurs when the child uses letter names to convey the spelling of words. When the child uses "I M HAP" to spell the sentence "I am happy," the child is associating the letters as the appropriate spelling of those words. The other choice includes errors in rule-based spelling (watching/waching; like/lik) and past tense (went/goed).

B96

Audiology and Hearing Impairment

An audiologist is preparing to perform audiologic evaluation on a patient who recently arrived at the clinic. The patient presents with chief complaints of severe "ringing in the ears," problems hearing in only one ear, dizziness and a feeling of "fullness in the ear." Which disorder is this patient likely experiencing?

Choices:
A. Presbycusis.
B. Noise-induced hearing loss.
C. Cholesteatoma.
D. Ménière's disease.

Teaching Points

Correct Answer: D

Ménière's disease is an inner ear disorder that results from overproduction of endolymph. This leads to a triad of symptoms that include unilateral hearing loss, roaring tinnitus (i.e., ringing in the ears) and vertigo. There may also be a feeling of aural fullness. As this matches the description of the problems experienced by the patient from this scenario, he/she is likely experiencing Ménière's disease. In contrast to this, presbycusis is hearing loss associated with aging. Noise-induced hearing loss is hearing loss caused by overexposure to excessively loud sounds. Cholesteatoma is a nonmalignant growth in the middle ear that may interrupt transmission of sound.

B97

Anatomy and Physiology of Communication and Swallowing

Following a motor vehicle accident, an individual is experiencing complete paralysis of the upper and lower extremities. A magnetic resonance imaging (MRI) scan reveals damage to the lateral corticospinal tract in the spinal column. The lateral corticospinal tract is:

Choices:
A. An ascending pathway that conveys motor signals that control movement of the arms and legs.
B. A descending pathway that conveys motor signals that control movement of the arms and legs.
C. An ascending pathway that conveys motor signals that control movement of all trunk musculature.
D. A descending pathway that conveys motor signals that control movement of all trunk musculature.

Teaching Points

Correct Answer: B

The lateral corticospinal tract begins as a descending motor pathway (from the cerebral hemispheres into the spinal column) in the cerebral hemispheres. In the medulla, 85% of the fibers decussate and form the lateral corticospinal tract, which is responsible for control of the upper and lower extremities. The 15% that does not decussate forms the anterior corticospinal tract, which is responsible for motor control of trunk/girdle muscles.

B98

Voice Disorders

A patient has been experiencing essential tremor of the voice, and is roughly 65% intelligible in unfamiliar settings. This patient is highly motivated to participate in speech-language therapy in order to improve communicative effectiveness. Which of the following treatment options are the **BEST** for an SLP to take with this patient?

Choices:
A. Elevating pitch and shortening phrase length.
B. Lowering pitch and semioccluded vocal tract tasks.
C. Resonant voice therapy and shortening vowel durations.
D. Elevating pitch and optimizing breath groups.

Teaching Points

Correct Answer: A

Although there is limited evidence at this time, shortening phrase duration, shortening vowel length and slightly elevating pitch have been found to be effective in alleviating the symptoms of essential tremor. By utilizing these approaches to treatment, the rhythmic oscillations of the tremor are effectively "masked" and do not appear during phonation. No other specific treatment approaches are uniformly efficacious in the treatment of this disorder, including lowering pitch, semioccluded vocal tract tasks, resonant voice therapy and optimizing breath groups.

B99

Audiology and Hearing Impairment

A speech-language pathologist (SLP) has been working with a pediatric patient with a hearing loss. Currently, the patient has difficulty making same versus different judgments of presented phonemes. At which level of the auditory hierarchy of listening is this child demonstrating deficits?

Choices:
A. Comprehension.
B. Detection.
C. Discrimination.
D. Recognition.

Teaching Points

Correct Answer: C

The discrimination level of the auditory hierarchy of listening requires individuals to make same versus different judgments of sounds. As this child is demonstrating difficulty with making this type of judgment, he/she is exhibiting deficits in discrimination. In contrast, the detection level requires individuals to identify the presence of absence of sound and is the foundation of the auditory hierarchy of listening. The recognition level requires a listener to point to a picture in response to an auditorily presented sound. Finally, the comprehension level requires that listeners respond to linguistic information and provide a response that proves they have understood what was presented.

B100

Anatomy and Physiology of Communication and Swallowing

A person is experiencing ataxia. Which central nervous system structure is **MOST LIKELY** impaired?

Choices:
A. Midbrain.
B. Pons.
C. Medulla.
D. Cerebellum.

Teaching Points

Correct Answer: D

The cerebellum is the structure below the cerebral hemispheres that is highly responsible for coordination of movements. Damage to the cerebellum would result in ataxia, or uncoordinated movement, on the ipsilateral side of the body.

B101

Voice Disorders

A patient comes in for a consult at the local voice clinic with a primary complaint of rough vocal quality. Upon patient interview, the speech-language pathologist (SLP) notes that the patient complains of persistent bad breath and a globus sensation. Additionally, the patient reports that this has been occurring for the past month and has progressively worsened. While a medical diagnosis would need to confirm the findings, which of the following causes is **MOST LIKELY**?

Choices:
A. Vocal fold cyst.
B. Laryngeal papilloma.
C. Vocal fold atrophy.
D. Laryngeal cancer.

Teaching Points

Correct Answer: D

A hallmark characteristic of laryngeal cancer is hoarse or rough vocal quality. Additionally, patients suffering from laryngeal cancer may experience globus, as the tumor may invade other healthy tissue. As cancer is a progressive disorder, if left untreated, these symptoms may continue to worsen. While human papilloma virus (HPV) and cysts could cause hoarse/rough vocal quality, HPV, cysts and vocal fold atrophy are not all associated with persistent bad breath or globus. Thus, these disorders would not be the problem for this patient and may be effectively ruled out.

B102

Language Acquisition

A child has been brought to an early language learning clinic to receive speech and language intervention. The speech-language pathologist (SLP) has set goals to increase the child's understanding of vocabulary utilizing principles of neighborhood density. Which of the following vocabulary words would be easiest for this child to learn?

Choices:
A. Jump.
B. Cat.
C. Five.
D. Fruit.

Teaching Points

Correct Answer: B

Neighborhood density is a lexical representation variable that influences word learning. When words are in a high-density neighborhood, there are several neighbor words that differ by a single phoneme, which aids in word learning. *Cat* is a high-density neighborhood word, which includes neighbors such as *bat, fat, hat, coat, rat*, etc. Low-density neighborhood words have fewer neighbor words and are more difficult for children to learn initially. *Jump, five* and *fruit* are all low-density words, and while they would be harder for the child to learn, they would be easier for the child to retrieve after having learned the words.

B103

Research, Evidence-Based Practice and Tests and Measurements

A group of speech scientists is attempting to determine the treatment efficacy for a previously developed method of intervention for spastic dysarthria. In order to determine an accurate measure of treatment efficacy, which of the following measures should this group of scientists utilize?

Choices:
A. Test-retest measures and construct validity.
B. Content validity and interobserver agreement.
C. Randomization and effect size.
D. Meta-analysis and systematic review.

Teaching Points

Correct Answer: D

Treatment efficacy is aimed at demonstrating the benefits of treatment through well-controlled studies with internal validity, statistical significance and practical significance. The strongest evidence of this treatment efficacy comes from meta-analysis (i.e., statistical analysis of accumulated evidence from multiple studies) and systematic reviews (i.e., objective and comprehensive overviews of research focused on a particular clinical issue). The best way for this group of researchers to prove the treatment efficacy for the intervention for spastic dysarthria is to utilize both of these methods.

B104

Language Acquisition

At what age do a variety of word classes and sentence types emerge?

Choices:
A. Infancy.
B. Toddlerhood.
C. Preschool.
D. School age.

Teaching Points

Correct Answer: C

It is during the preschool years that more complex language is noted. Prior to this time, children express language through babbling, which gives way to first words. Children then build their expressive lexicon, and begin expressing language through simple sentences before reaching complex language structures.

B105

Augmentative and Alternative Communication (AAC)

A patient with amyotrophic lateral sclerosis has recently been administered an augmentative and alternative communication (AAC) assessment. Following the assessment, the speech-language pathologist (SLP) has made recommendations for devices that the patient might be able to use. The patient reviewed the selections and has chosen an AAC device that she believes best fits her skills and needs. What contributing factor is **MOST IMPORTANT** for this patient's AAC intervention?

Choices:
A. The patient will require multiple AAC systems in order to effectively communicate.
B. The patient will have frequent need for feature matching as the disorder progresses.
C. The patient will better benefit by more articulatory-based intervention methods.
D. The patient will require a nonlinguistic AAC system as her language deteriorates.

Teaching Points

Correct Answer: B

Because amyotrophic lateral sclerosis is a neurodegenerative disorder, patients will require frequent reassessment, utilizing feature matching, in order to pair them with an appropriate device that matches their level of functioning. Patients with ALS will most likely not require more than one device at a time to supplement their communication. Additionally, articulatory-based approaches are contraindicated with this population, secondary to the degenerative nature of the process. Finally, ALS is a motor speech disorder, not a language disorder. As such, patients' language skills will not deteriorate with the process.

B106

Acoustics

Two 150 hertz (Hz) sinusoids with a peak amplitude of 2 are added together. The sinusoids are 180° out of phase. The resulting sound will be a:

Choices:
A. 150 Hz sinusoid with a peak amplitude of 0.0.
B. 150 Hz sinusoid with a peak amplitude of 4.0.
C. 300 Hz sinusoid with a peak amplitude of 0.0.
D. 300 Hz sinusoid with a peak amplitude of 4.0.

Teaching Points

Correct Answer: A

When sinusoids of the same frequency are added together, the result is always another sinusoid with the same frequency (in this case, 150 Hz). Amplitudes also add together. Since these sinusoids are 180° out of phase, when one is at its peak of +2, the other is at −2; therefore, their amplitudes will sum to 0.

B107

Anatomy and Physiology of Communication and Swallowing

If a speaker has difficulty controlling vocal fold vibration it is **MOST LIKELY** manifested by:

Choices:
A. Voicing throughout the silence for /p/.
B. Voicing throughout the silence for /b/.
C. Lack of voicing throughout the continuant noise for /f/.
D. Lack of voicing throughout the continuant noise for /v/.

Teaching Points

Correct Answer: A

Voicing is expected during the silence for voiced stops but should not be seen during the silence for voiceless stops unless a speaker has difficulty controlling vocal fold vibration. However, voicing may be absent in both voiced and voiceless fricatives even for healthy speakers, since duration provides strong cues to fricative voicing.

B108

Anatomy and Physiology of Communication and Swallowing

A person experiences weakness on the right side of the face resulting in right facial droop. Initial evaluation suggests cranial nerve damage. If verified, which cranial nerve is **MOST LIKELY** damaged?

Choices:
A. Trochlear.
B. Trigeminal.
C. Facial.
D. Vagus.

Teaching Points

Correct Answer: C

The facial nerve (CN VII) controls motor innervations to the muscles of facial expression. Damage to the lower motor neurons would cause ipsilateral (same-sided) weakness, which could result in the facial droop that this patient is experiencing.

B109

Audiology and Hearing Impairment

A patient with a cochlear implant (CI) arrives at an audiology clinic with complaints of his/her cochlear implant malfunctioning. After performing troubleshooting of the CI, the audiologist has decided that the malfunctioning component is the part of the CI that converts the sounds into a digital signal. Which part of this patient's cochlear implant is malfunctioning?

Choices:
A. Microphone.
B. External sound processor.
C. Internal unit.
D. Electrode array.

Teaching Points

Correct Answer: B

The external sound processor is the portion of a CI that filters and processes the sound (i.e., convert sound into a digital signal). As this fits the description given by the audiologist in this scenario, it is likely the external sound processor that is experiencing difficulties. In contrast to this, the microphone is the portion of a CI that picks up sound, the internal unit is the portion of a CI that converts the digital signal into electrical signals, and the electrode array is the portion of a CI that stimulates CN VIII for sound perception.

B110

Written Language Disorders in the School-Age Population

Two grade-school children are referred to a speech-language pathologist (SLP) for a comprehensive diagnostic assessment of their literacy abilities. A basic literacy assessment should consider the children's:

Choices:
A. Reading/writing skills, cultural context and articulation abilities.
B. Underlying spoken language skills, vocal quality and reading/writing skills.
C. Reading/writing skills, underlying cognitive processing skills and cultural context.
D. Underlying spoken language skills, reading/writing skills, and cultural context.

Teaching Points

Correct Answer: D

Key areas that should be addressed during a literacy assessment include underlying spoken language skills (i.e., skills and metalinguistic awareness in morphology, syntax, semantics and discourse), reading and writing skills (i.e., accuracy and automaticity in these skill areas) and cultural context (i.e., extrinsic factors associated with literacy learning). Additionally, underlying processing skills should be assessed, which includes phonological awareness, phonological short-term memory, working memory, rapid naming, visual/orthographic processing, attention and executive functioning.

B111

The Practice of Speech-Language Pathology

A speech-language pathologist (SLP) working in an acute rehabilitation hospital is asked to work with a patient with severe flaccid dysarthria. When the SLP arrives at the patient's room, the patient expresses that the change in communication has significantly affected his/her self-image and that he/she is depressed. The SLP delivers treatment to the patient, which does not lead to improvements in the patient's state of mind. What should the SLP do in order to ensure the **BEST** treatment of this patient?

Choices:
A. Continue targeting the patient's intelligibility for improvements in psychological outlook.
B. Refer the patient to another SLP who has more experience in working with persons with dysarthria.
C. Refer the patient for a psychological consult to assess the patient's state of mind.
D. Discuss the impact of communication disorders on psychological outlook with the patient.

Teaching Points

Correct Answer: C

According to the ASHA Code of Ethics, Principle of Ethics I, Rule of Ethics B, "Individuals shall use every resource, including referral when appropriate, to ensure that high-quality service is provided." As this patient is showing obvious signs of difficulty coping with the change in communication, referral to a psychological professional is warranted. While improvements in intelligibility may lead to an improved psychological outlook, the need for a referral is warranted and should be capitalized on in this scenario.

B112

Research, Evidence-Based Practice and Tests and Measurements

A speech-language pathologist (SLP) is researching if the amount of time spent undergoing a new treatment under study will make an impact on intelligibility in dysarthric speakers. Specifically, the SLP has one group participating for 30 minutes a day, while another group participates for 60 minutes a day. In order to determine the effect of the differing amounts of time on intelligibility, which means of analysis would be **MOST BENEFICIAL** to this SLP?

Choices:
A. A Cochran Q test.
B. An analysis of variance (ANOVA).
C. A *t*-test.
D. A multivariate analysis of variance (MANOVA).

Teaching Points

Correct Answer: C

In this situation, the independent variable is the time spent in treatment, while the dependent variable is the amount of participant progress made in treatment. A *t*-test is a means of analysis that can be utilized when there is a single dependent variable. Specifically, an independent *t*-test would be utilized in this situation because there is a single dependent variable, but a comparison between two different groups (i.e., 30 minutes vs. 60 minutes) needs to be made.

B113

The Practice of Speech-Language Pathology

A graduate student in speech-language pathology is preparing to submit final paperwork to the American Speech-Language-Hearing Association (ASHA) before beginning his/her clinical fellowship experience. Which of the following is a requirement that must be met by graduate student clinicians?

Choices:
A. Clinical experience during the educational program of at least 400 clock hours.
B. Thirty semester credit hours of study focused on the knowledge pertinent to speech-language pathology.
C. Graduate coursework and clinical practicum completed in an advanced level program.
D. Knowledge of the "big 10" areas of speech-language pathology practice.

Teaching Points

Correct Answer: A

Graduate student clinicians are required to gather 400 direct hours of clinical experience with persons who have communication and swallowing disorders during their education. Additionally, graduate students are required to maintain a minimum of 36 semester credit hours at the graduate level, must complete graduate coursework and clinical practicum in a CAA-accredited program, and gain knowledge in the "big 9" areas of speech-language pathology practice.

B114

Cleft Palate and Other Craniofacial Anomalies

After receiving surgical correction of velopharyngeal insufficiency, a child is referred to a speech-language pathologist (SLP) to receive speech therapy. Which activity is appropriate for correction of compensatory errors following the child's surgical procedure?

Choices:
A. Articulation placement procedures.
B. Velopharyngeal exercises.
C. Blowing exercises.
D. Further surgical management.

Teaching Points

Correct Answer: A

Following correction of velopharyngeal insufficiency, speech therapy may be indicated to improve any remaining speech errors. VPI often requires only one instance of surgical management to fix the problem, and blowing exercises and velopharyngeal exercises are not effective as treatment methods for this population. Therefore, the best selection would be articulation placement to help the client learn proper placement of the articulators following the surgical change.

B115

Cleft Palate and Other Craniofacial Anomalies

A neonate was diagnosed with cleft palate, micrognathia and airway obstruction. Given these characteristics, which of the following disorders is this infant **MOST LIKELY** experiencing?

Choices:
A. Pierre Robin sequence.
B. Velocardiofacial syndrome.
C. Down syndrome.
D. Pfeiffer syndrome.

Teaching Points

Correct Answer: A

The Pierre Robin sequence includes the characteristics of micrognathia (small lower jaw), glossoptosis (downward displacement of the tongue), and airway obstruction. While these characteristics may be individually present in velocardiofacial syndrome, Down syndrome and Pfeiffer syndrome, when they are collectively present, this indicates a diagnosis of Pierre Robin sequence.

B116

Motor Speech Disorders

A patient incurred a hemorrhagic infarct with a resulting diagnosis of apraxia of speech (AOS). The speaker exhibits right-sided hemiplegia, and the left arm has been immobilized in a cast. Verbal communication consists of a few automatic words and phrases. When speech sound errors occurred, they were distorted. Reading and receptive language skills are intact. Adaptive techniques were used to suggest writing skills appear to be intact. The **BEST** treatment targeting verbal expression should involve:

Choices:
A. A linguistic approach to treatment targeting increased length of utterance.
B. Adoption of melodic intonation therapy (MIT).
C. An articulatory kinematic approach.
D. Training communication partners in the use of repair strategies when communication breakdowns occurred.

Teaching Points

Correct Answer: C

Because this patient demonstrates relatively intact receptive language skills and has a moderate-to-severe AOS, he/she is a perfect candidate for an articulatory kinematic approach. Use of this approach focuses on improving spatial/temporal aspects of articulatory movement as a means to improve speech production. This would help improve the patient's distortion of phonemes, thus improving verbal expression.

B117

Spoken Language Disorders in Children

Alex is a speech-language pathologist (SLP) who has been working with a young child with a language disorder. Alex has recently begun utilizing clinician-directed approaches during intervention sessions with this child as a means of reducing the distracting stimuli. Which of the following methods of intervention is Alex **MOST LIKELY** utilizing in this child's intervention sessions?

Choices:
A. Demonstration.
B. Modeling.
C. Expansion.
D. Questioning.

Teaching Points

Correct Answer: B

Modeling is a form of clinician-directed (i.e., a means of intervention that allows the clinician to specify the materials that are used in intervention, how they are used, and the type and frequency of reinforcement) in which numerous examples of a target structure are provided during an interactive activity. The child is not required to produce the target during intervention sessions. In contrast to this, demonstration, expansion and questioning are all indirect language facilitation techniques. Demonstration occurs when repeated, but variable use of a sentence or text pattern is presented to a child. Expansion is a contingent verbal response that increases the length or complexity of the child's utterance. Finally, questioning (i.e., asking questions to a child) serves to extend what the child has said or written.

B118
Acoustics

The pitch contour of a vowel shows that the pitch begins at 200 hertz (Hz). If the pitch contour is accurate, the period at the beginning of the vowel will be:

Choices:
A. 0.005 sec.
B. 0.05 sec.
C. 0.005 Hz.
D. 0.05 Hz.

Teaching Points

Correct Answer: A

Frequency and period are in an inverse relationship. Period is a time measurement. If F0 = 200 Hz, the period will be 1/200 = 0.005 sec.

B119
Spoken Language Disorders in Children

A speech-language pathologist (SLP) working in an elementary school has been asked to perform a comprehensive language evaluation on a new student. The SLP determines the most appropriate assessment for the child and begins administration. However, the SLP utilizes a more dynamic approach to assessment in order to better understand the child's language skills. This change to assessment **MOST LIKELY** determined how well the child performed:

Choices:
A. On tasks of daily living.
B. On a classroom assignment.
C. With modeling techniques.
D. With no comparison to peers.

Teaching Points

Correct Answer: C

In a dynamic assessment, the assessment is designed to measure the extent to which a child's performance in a specific task may be modified or extended with contextual support. Because this SLP offered modeling techniques in order to see how the child responded, the SLP engaged in a dynamic assessment of the child's learning abilities. In contrast to this, a curriculum-based assessment measures how well the child would perform on a classroom assignment, a functional assessment measures the extent to which a language disorder impacts daily living, and a criterion-referenced assessment measures the child's capabilities with no comparison to peers.

B120

Augmentative and Alternative Communication (AAC)

A speech-language pathologist (SLP) has been working with a severely dysarthric patient in an acute rehabilitation setting, targeting improved functional communication. The patient was nonliterate at baseline and has conveyed that literacy is not a focal area of communication. The SLP decides to utilize topic supplementation to aid in the comprehension of communicative partners. Which approach best matches this SLP's choice for intervention?

Choices:
A. Training the patient to utilize an AAC device by modeling and explaining the process.
B. Training the patient's spouse to expand upon their topic of conversation.
C. Providing the patient with a list of letters to utilize in conversation.
D. Providing the patient with a list of pictures to utilize in conversation.

Teaching Points

Correct Answer: D

Topic supplementation may be used for people with complex communication needs who have severely dysarthric speech, and it utilizes a communication board with lists of commonly discussed topics (either pictorial or written). As the user from this scenario is employing pictures to supply context clues about the topic of communication, he/she is engaging in topic supplementation. In contrast to this, alphabet supplementation allows users to select the initial letter of words to provide context clues and improve intelligibility at the word level. Message co-construction occurs when the person with complex communication needs (CCN) supplies the content words of his/her message, a facilitator confirms these words, and then expands the person with CCN's message. Finally, augmented input occurs when a facilitator models how a system is used by providing both input and speech.

B121

Acoustics

In order to accurately measure voice onset time (VOT) in a series of stop consonants, the speech-language pathologist (SLP) should work from:

Choices:
A. Shorter VOT.
B. Longer VOT.
C. More compact spectrum.
D. More diffuse spectrum.

Teaching Points

Correct Answer: B

VOT is a time measurement. Time measurements should be made from broadband spectrograms or waveforms. Narrowband spectrograms have poor time resolution and should never be used for time measurements. Amplitude spectra have no time axes.

B122

Spoken Language Disorders in Children

Michael is a speech-language pathologist (SLP) who has been asked to evaluate a child who recently moved from a different part of the country. During the evaluation, the child produces the following utterances: /hæn/ for /hænd/, /dɪs/ for /ðɪs/ and /æks/ for /æsk/. What should be the next step in Michael's assessment of this child?

Choices:
A. Determine if the productions are appropriate for the child's dialect.
B. Diagnose the child with a language disorder.
C. Perform a standardized childhood language assessment.
D. Perform in-depth research regarding the child's cultural background.

Teaching Points

Correct Answer: A

Because this child has recently moved from a different part of the country, there is a chance that the child speaks a different dialect from the typical one for the area in which Michael lives. Dialectal differences must be distinguished from language disorders in order to prevent misdiagnosis, inappropriate labeling and inappropriate referral for therapy. If the child's productions are appropriate for the dialect in which he/she was raised, this would not constitute a language disorder, but a language difference, and therapy would not be an appropriate recommendation.

B123

Voice Disorders

A young child is brought into a local voice clinic by the child's parents for a full voice assessment battery. After completing and reviewing all test measures, the speech-language pathologist (SLP) and otolaryngologist (ENT) have decided that the child is presenting with early-stage, bilateral vocal fold nodules, most likely due to phonotraumatic behaviors (i.e., yelling for siblings, making funny voices, etc.). Which of the following approaches to treatment would be appropriate for this particular client?

Choices:
A. Use of confidential voice.
B. Utilization of laryngeal massage.
C. Use of pushing/pulling exercises.
D. Surgical intervention.

Teaching Points

Correct Answer: A

Confidential voice therapy is a treatment approach that has the participant engage in low-volume phonation, which effectively reduces contact between the vocal folds. Reducing vocal fold contact reduces the chances of increasing phonotraumatic lesions, such as this pediatric patient is experiencing. Surgical intervention is not recommended in the pediatric nodule population, as their nodules often spontaneously improve as the patient improves. Use of laryngeal massage would not provide benefit to this patient, as it is not excessive laryngeal tension causing their problems. Pushing and pulling exercises would increase the contact between the vocal folds and exacerbate the child's problem.

B124

Language Acquisition

During a language evaluation, a child produces the utterance, "The boy pushed the cars." How many free morphemes are there in this child's utterance?

Choices:
A. 2.
B. 3.
C. 4.
D. 5.

Teaching Points

Correct Answer: D

Free or unbound morphemes are those units of meaning that can stand alone in an utterance. In the sentence given, the additional morphemes (-s after car and -ed after push) cannot stand alone.

B125

Augmentative and Alternative Communication (AAC)

Rebecca is a speech-language pathologist (SLP) working in a rehabilitation hospital. She has recently begun working with a patient who developed severe spastic dysarthria following a significant motor vehicle accident. Rebecca believes that this patient is a candidate for an augmentative and alternative communication (AAC) device while in the hospital and wishes to prioritize essential messages for recording on the device. Specifically, Rebecca wishes to record words such as *hungry*, *thirsty*, and *bathroom*. What type of vocabulary does Rebecca wish to record for this patient?

Choices:
A. Fringe vocabulary.
B. Developmental vocabulary.
C. Inventory vocabulary.
D. Coverage vocabulary.

Teaching Points

Correct Answer: D

Coverage vocabulary includes words/phrases that the person with complex communication needs (CCN) requires to communicate essential messages that typically relate to basic needs. As the SLP would like to program the patient's AAC device with vocabulary relating to basic needs, the SLP is interested in using coverage vocabulary. In contrast to this, fringe vocabulary includes words and phrases that are specific to a particular topic/activity/individual, which are often content rich and not used frequently. Developmental vocabulary includes words/phrases that the person with CCN does not yet know, but are included on the system to encourage vocabulary growth. Finally, inventory vocabulary includes all the vocabulary in the AAC user's inventory.

B126

Augmentative and Alternative Communication

Anthony has recently been admitted to a skilled nursing facility, following a large left middle cerebral artery infarction. He was previously diagnosed with severe Broca's aphasia and verbal apraxia, and his verbal expression is characterized by content words, paraphasias and overly stereotyped utterances. However, Anthony has relatively preserved cognitive skills, including memory and attention. The speech-language pathologist assigned to work with Anthony believes he would benefit from augmentative and alternative communication (AAC) intervention. Which of the following approaches would Anthony **MOST LIKELY** benefit from?

Choices:
A. Supplemental verbal expression with an eye gaze system.
B. Provision of a speech-generating device.
C. Supplemental verbal expression with writing.
D. Supplemental verbal expression with a picture board.

Teaching Points

Correct Answer: D
As the patient demonstrates agrammatical speech and paraphasias, the patient's verbal expression is significantly compromised. However, as the patient demonstrates intact cognitive skills, he/she may be taught to utilize a picture board to improve communicative effectiveness by using picture symbols to supplement verbal expression. In contrast, patients with Broca's aphasia demonstrate writing that typically mirrors their verbal expression, making writing an inappropriate selection for use with this patient. For the same reason, selection of a speech-generating device would be inappropriate for this patient, as his/her written expression is compromised, and the patient would demonstrate difficulty formulating messages. Finally, as the patient is able to produce some means of verbal expression and is ambulatory, utilizing only eye gaze would not improve the communicative effectiveness for this patient.

B127

Autism Spectrum Disorders

A speech-language pathologist (SLP) is providing language intervention for an adolescent student with autism spectrum disorder, and is targeting improved semantic language use. Which of the following is an appropriate treatment goal for the SLP to use in treatment with this student?

Choices:
A. Reading conversation partners' intentions.
B. Understanding sarcastic comments made by conversation partners.
C. Understanding idiomatic expressions mentioned by conversation partners.
D. Determining when to make appropriate decisions.

Teaching Points

Correct Answer: B
Semantic goals for adolescents with autism spectrum disorder could entail comprehending semantic nuances, such as inferred meaning, humor, discourse/conversational rules and sarcasm. In contrast to this, reading others' intentions and making appropriate decisions are pragmatic language goals for adolescents, while understanding of idiomatic expressions is a semantic language goal for school-aged children.

B128

Stuttering and Other Fluency Disorders

Paul is a successful architect who has stuttered throughout life. His disfluencies are notable in complicated social situations, but most people say that they rarely notice it. Paul reports significant struggle in many communication situations and says he is tired of using avoidance as his main tool to deal with stuttering. He finds himself refusing to answer the phone when others are present and feeling the need to substitute words all the time. Which of the following descriptions is **MOST** accurate?

Choices:
A. Paul exhibits hysterical stuttering.
B. Paul should have had behaviorally focused therapy.
C. Paul should be advised to maintain his current level of fluency and learn better avoidance strategies.
D. Paul is a covert stutterer.

Teaching Points

Correct Answer: D
This pattern of "covert" stuttering is not unusual in individuals who have stuttered throughout life and have used avoidance as a primary method for dealing with stuttering.

B129

Acquired Language Disorders

The Life Participation Approach to Aphasia (LPAA) can **BEST** be exemplified by which of the following scenarios?

Choices:
A. Encouraging a person with aphasia (PWA) to remain in the home, to work on home-based communication.
B. Hiring a gardener for a PWA with hemiparesis, in order to keep their garden in adequate condition.
C. Providing emotional support services to only the PWA, in order to keep their psychological outlook positive.
D. Providing audiobooks at the local library, to aid PWA who have reading deficits.

Teaching Points

Correct Answer: D
The LPAA is an approach to intervention that has five core values and seeks to improve the life participation of people with aphasia by focusing on intervention at all stages and for all people affected by aphasia; that requires documentation of life participation enhancement as the outcome measure. By providing audiobooks to PWA who have reading deficits, this encourages these individuals to continue a hobby they had prior to their stroke. In contrast to this, the PWA should be encouraged to participate fully in the community and not be restricted to the home. Additionally, gardening could be adapted to allow the PWA to tend to the garden, rather than have another person do this completely. Finally, according to LPAA principles, all people affected by aphasia, including family members and caretakers, are entitled to services.

B130

Dysphagia

A patient has just completed a bedside swallow evaluation and has been placed on a basic soft solid/nectar thick liquid diet for an oropharyngeal dysphagia. No significant weakness was found during the bedside evaluation. Knowing this information, which of the following treatment approaches is appropriate to treat this patient's dysphagia?

Choices:
A. Meals of basic soft solids and nectar thick liquids.
B. Therapeutic trials of advanced soft solids and thin liquids.
C. Therapeutic trials of advanced soft solids and nectar thick liquids.
D. Oral motor exercises and compensatory maneuvers.

Teaching Points

Correct Answer: B
Because the patient does not demonstrate significant amounts of weakness, oral motor exercises to improve the strength of the muscles involved in swallowing are not appropriate. Because swallowing is often the best approach to treating swallowing disorders (as evidenced by the principle of "use it or lose it"), having the patient engage in swallowing-based activities would be the best approach. Trying more advanced textures with this patient would be the most appropriate approach, before advancing them to meals.

B131

Written Language Disorders in the School-Age Population

A speech-language pathologist (SLP) at a local speech and language clinic has an adolescent client with dyslexia on the SLP's caseload. During an evaluation, the client writes "I went to the zu" after being prompted with the cue "write about something you did over the weekend." This mistake suggests that the client has difficulties primarily in what aspect of literacy?

Choices:
A. Phonological memory span.
B. Syntax.
C. Orthography.
D. Discourse.

Teaching Points

Correct Answer: C
Orthography is a symbolic system that is superimposed over an oral language system, which lends itself to writing. Because the student demonstrates impairments in the spelling of particular words (i.e., zoo) they are experiencing orthographic errors. As the sentence is written with correct grammar, the student does not demonstrate syntactic errors. Phonological memory span is measured using oral means (i.e., nonword repetition or digit span) and discourse includes more involved writing processes, both of which do not apply to this particular student.

B132

The Practice of Speech-Language Pathology

A speech-language pathologist (SLP) working in a hospital setting has implemented a breakfast group for individuals with cognitive-communication deficits. For a specific group meeting, the SLP has decided to implement a method of intervention that is a good fit for 12 out of 15 members. The other three members will benefit from this method of intervention, but not as much as the others. The SLP has decided that since most of the group members will maximally benefit from this method it is an appropriate choice. Which philosophical approach best matches this SLP's approach to treatment?

Choices:
A. The Rights Approach.
B. Fairness/Justice Approach.
C. Utilitarian Approach.
D. Common Good Approach.

Teaching Points

Correct Answer: C
The utilitarian approach seeks to find the action that will do the most good and the least harm to the most amount of people. As the SLP in this scenario is selecting a method of intervention that will provide the maximum amount of gain for the most patients, without causing harm to the other patients, the SLP is utilizing utilitarian views. In contrast to this, the rights approach seeks to find the action that best respects the rights of all stakeholders, the fairness/justice approach seeks to find the option that treats people equally, and the common good approach seeks to find the action that best serves the whole community and not just some members.

Examination C

C1

Acoustics

The frequency of a periodic sound is increased by 100 hertz (Hz). What effect would this change in frequency have on the wavelength of the sound?

Choices:
A. There would be no change in wavelength.
B. There would be an increase in wavelength.
C. There would be a decrease in wavelength.
D. There would be a dampening of the sound.

Teaching Points

Correct Answer: C
Wavelength is the distance traveled by a sound during a single period. This measure has an inverse relationship with frequency. This means that higher frequency sounds would have a shorter wavelength, whereas lower frequency sounds would have a longer wavelength. Therefore, if the frequency of a sound was increased, its wavelength would decrease accordingly.

C2

Spoken Language Disorders in Children

Sydney is a speech-language pathologist (SLP) working in a local public school. She has been asked to evaluate a child to better understand her current level of linguistic functioning. Sydney decides to use a curriculum-based assessment to evaluate this child's linguistic competency. Which of the following statements BEST describes the design of this type of assessment?

Choices:
A. Measures linguistic skill with modifications or support put in place.
B. Measures linguistic skill in order to select targets to improve daily living.
C. Measures the impact of a linguistic disorder on daily living.
D. Measures linguistic skill with no comparison to other students.

Teaching Points

Correct Answer: B
A curriculum-based assessment is designed to measure the extent to which a child's communication disorder impacts academic functioning in order to select linguistic targets that improve daily functioning. Progress on these targets should be monitored over the course of instruction. In contrast to this, dynamic assessment is designed to assess a child's linguistic skills with modifications or supports put in place. Ecological assessment is designed to measure the extent to which a child's communication disorder impacts daily living. Finally, criterion-referenced assessment is designed to measure a specific linguistic skill with no comparison to other students.

C3

Acoustics

In a narrowband spectrogram, the speech-language pathologist (SLP) can see that harmonic spacing becomes narrower throughout a vowel. When listening to the vowel, the SLP expects to hear that the vowel:

Choices:
A. Is a diphthong that shifts from a low vowel to a high vowel.
B. Is a diphthong that shifts from a front vowel to a back vowel.
C. Begins at a lower pitch and ends at a higher pitch.
D. Begins at a higher pitch and ends at a lower pitch.

Teaching Points

Correct Answer: D

The spacing between harmonics in the human voice is equal to F0. If harmonic spacing shifts from wider to narrower, then the harmonics are getting closer together and F0 is getting lower.

C4

Spoken Language Disorders in Children

During an intervention session, a child produces the utterance "Mommy go run." The child's speech-language pathologist (SLP) uses an expansion approach to increase the complexity of the child's utterance. Which of the following statements could this SLP use in response to the child?

Choices:
A. "Mommy's going to run."
B. "Mommy's going to run to the house."
C. "Where is Mommy going?"
D. "Say 'mommy is going to run.'"

Teaching Points

Correct Answer: A

An expansion (also known as recast) is a form of experiential instruction in which the SLP provides a corrected version of a child's word or utterance. Because the SLP from this scenario is utilizing an expansion for this child, the SLP would provide only the corrected utterance (i.e., "Mommy's going to run"). In contrast to this, an expatiation is when the SLP provides a corrected version of a child's word or utterance and goes beyond the child's original meaning (i.e., "Mommy's going to run to the house"). Questioning occurs when the SLP asks follow up questions to the child's original utterance (i.e., "Where is Mommy running?"). Finally, imitation occurs when the SLP provides a model and expects the child to replicate it (i.e., "Say 'Mommy's going to run' ").

C5

Acquired Language Disorders

A speech-language pathologist (SLP) is addressing the agrammatism of a person with aphasia in the treatment plan. A treatment goal to address this aspect of the disorder would be:

Choices:
A. Working on lexical retrieval of single nouns.
B. Assessing writing abilities to dictation.
C. Working on correct noun-verb agreement.
D. Addressing the motor speech difficulties associated with apraxia of speech.

Teaching Points

Correct Answer: C
Agrammatism refers to difficulty producing and comprehending the grammatical aspects of language inherent in word morphology and syntax. Therefore, treatment of agrammatism addresses grammatical abilities such as noun-verb agreement and the use of functor words like prepositions, articles and auxiliary verbs.

C6

Anatomy and Physiology of Communication and Swallowing

The telencephalon is the area of the brain that includes the cerebral hemispheres and receives its blood supply from a variety of different arteries. The artery that supplies most of the medial surfaces of the telencephalon is the:

Choices:
A. Anterior cerebral artery.
B. Middle cerebral artery.
C. Posterior cerebral artery.
D. Anterior spinal artery.

Teaching Points

Correct Answer: A
The telencephalon includes the cerebral hemispheres, which receive blood from the anterior, middle and posterior cerebral arteries. The anterior cerebral artery branches off from the internal carotid artery and feeds the cerebral hemispheres starting in the area of the optic chiasm, which can be found in the medial portions of the hemispheres. In contrast to this, the middle cerebral artery supplies blood to a majority of the lateral cerebral hemispheres. The posterior cerebral artery supplies blood to the posterior cerebral hemispheres, including the occipital lobes. Finally, the anterior spinal artery supplies blood to the anterior spinal cord and posterior cerebellum.

C7

Research, Evidence-Based Practice and Tests and Measurements

A speech-language pathologist (SLP) is completing a study to prove that two different treatment approaches provide differing amounts of progress in persons with aphasia. She would like to utilize a strict statistical test in order to prove significance between the amounts of progress. Which of the following would be the **BEST** method for this SLP to utilize in the data analysis?

Choices:
A. One-tailed test.
B. Meta-analysis.
C. Two-tailed test.
D. Cochran Q test.

Teaching Points

Correct Answer: C

Because this SLP has developed a nondirectional hypothesis (i.e., there will be differing amounts of progress between the two interventions), she may utilize a two-tailed statistical test. Additionally, two-tailed statistical tests are stricter than one-tailed statistical tests, and most researchers utilize these tests to help prove significance.

C8

Spoken Language Disorders in Children

A child has been diagnosed with a cognitive disability, with "expected associated language difficulties." Using this information, what should be targeted in this child's intervention sessions?

Choices:
A. Complex sentence structure and increasing relative clauses.
B. Pragmatic communication and increasing vocabulary.
C. Phonological memory and increasing attention span.
D. Simple sentence structure and increasing sight word recognition.

Teaching Points

Correct Answer: A

Children with cognitive disabilities generally show delayed morphological development due to their tendency to use less complex sentences and fewer relative clauses. By targeting these language structures through intervention, these children can make improvements in both syntax and morphology. While there are semantic deficits associated with cognitive disability, they tend to be deficits in understanding abstract vocabulary, rather than vocabulary acquisition. Additionally, pragmatic communication is generally commensurate with cognitive age and is not the most appropriate treatment target for this population. Phonological combinations would be appropriate if the child demonstrated an associated speech sound disorder, and attention span would be appropriate with associated attention deficits (i.e., ADHD). Finally, children with cognitive disability often use simple sentence structure, thus more advanced skills should be targeted.

C9

Stuttering and Other Fluency Disorders

Micah is a 4-year-old child who is beginning preschool. He stutters on about 8% of words and his language is mildly delayed. His pediatrician advised against early referral for assessment by the speech-language pathologist (SLP) because she is concerned that labeling the problem will make it worse. The mother is concerned about Micah's stuttering problem and calls the school-based SLP for advice. Which of the following points is **LEAST LIKELY** to be helpful in discussion with Micah's mother?

Choices:
A. Assessment of the child's speech will not make it worse and should be completed if there is concern.
B. There might be some benefit in providing the parent with some evidence-based materials that clarify the purpose of early assessment.
C. Explain the various goals of early stuttering assessment and treatment.
D. Explain that the pediatrician is in error.

Teaching Points

Correct Answer: D

These are all points that might be helpful in dealing with this common concern. Many individuals in health care and education have been taught that delaying evaluation is a good idea, so as not to label symptoms as "stuttering." There is no evidence that identification and differential diagnosis of stuttering causes stuttering to worsen or persist.

C10
Anatomy and Physiology of Communication and Swallowing

Which muscle contributes to hyolaryngeal depression?

Choices:
A. Stylohyoid.
B. Geniohyoid.
C. Mylohyoid.
D. Sternohyoid.

Teaching Points

Correct Answer: D

The muscles most responsible for laryngeal depression are the infrahyoids, which include the sternohyoid, sternothyroid, omohyoid and thyrohyoid. The stylohyoid, geniohyoid and mylohyoid muscles are suprahyoid muscles and contribute to laryngeal elevation.

C11
Motor Speech Disorders

A speech-language pathologist (SLP) at an acute rehabilitation hospital is scheduled to evaluate a newly admitted patient with a diagnosis of flaccid dysarthria. Following a comprehensive speech evaluation, the SLP notes that the patient demonstrates significant hypernasality secondary to poor velum mobility and makes recommendations for prosthodontist consult. Which of the following prosthetic devices would be **MOST APPROPRIATE** for use with this patient?

Choices:
A. Speech bulb.
B. Palatal lift.
C. Palatal obturator.
D. Palatal expander.

Teaching Points

Correct Answer: B

The palatal lift device is recommended for use with patients who have poor velar mobility, such as the patient in this scenario. The palatal obturator (used to close/occlude an open cleft or fistula) and speech bulb (used to occlude the nasopharynx when the velum is short) would not be an appropriate choice for this patient, due to the nature of their disorder.

C12

Cleft Palate and Other Craniofacial Anomalies

A child is referred to a speech-language pathologist (SLP) in order to receive speech therapy for problems associated with velopharyngeal insufficiency (VPI). In the referral notes, the SLP notices that this child demonstrates several common speech characteristics associated with VPI. Which of this child's speech characteristics would be most responsive to speech therapy?

Choices:
A. Hypernasality.
B. Compensatory productions.
C. Obligatory errors.
D. Nasal emission.

Teaching Points

Correct Answer: B

Compensatory production errors are those that occur as a response to altered anatomy (i.e., velopharyngeal insufficiency, abnormal dental occlusion, etc.). This type of error can be improved through participation in speech therapy, specifically utilizing articulatory placement strategies. Hypernasality, nasal emission and obligatory errors are all problems that require surgical intervention for improvement, as no speech therapy technique will lead to a change in these conditions.

C13

Acquired Language Disorders

A speech-language pathologist (SLP) in an outpatient clinic has recently been given a new patient to his/her caseload. The patient's medical records reveal that the patient is experiencing aphasia with limb apraxia. Which treatment scenario would be MOST helpful for this patient?

Choices:
A. The SLP will work on nonverbal communication using Amerind.
B. The SLP will focus on reducing paraphasias and improving word-finding.
C. The focus of the treatment program is to improve agrammatism.
D. The person being treated has mixed nonfluent aphasia and the treatment plan will include a trial of voluntary control of involuntary utterances.

Teaching Points

Correct Answer: A

Limb apraxia is likely to affect an individual's ability to perform manual gestures to command. Of the scenarios presented, only working on nonverbal communication requires the production of manual gestures using the treatment method Amerind. While limb apraxia might affect performance within the other treatment programs, the plans are all focused on the remediation of verbal expression which is less likely to be affected by limb apraxia.

C14

Anatomy and Physiology of Communication and Swallowing

Inspiration during quiet breathing involves contraction of the diaphragm which:

Choices:
A. Increases the volume of the thoracic cavity and causes pressure in the lungs to increase.
B. Increases the volume of the thoracic cavity and causes pressure in the lungs to decrease.
C. Decreases the volume of the thoracic cavity and causes pressure in the lungs to increase.
D. Decreases the volume of the thoracic cavity and causes pressure in the lungs to decrease.

Teaching Points

Correct Answer: B
When the diaphragm contracts, it pulls downward toward the abdominal cavity, increasing the volume of the thoracic cavity, where the lungs are housed. According to Boyle's law, as volume increases, pressure decreases. Thus, if the volume of the thoracic cavity increases, the pressure in the lungs decreases, which is the main drive behind inspiration.

C15

Research, Evidence-Based Practice and Tests and Measurements

Two researchers are analyzing the data collected from a recently completed research study. The researchers have found that their measurements are in good agreement, thus demonstrating adequate interobserver agreement. This finding is a good estimate of measurement:

Choices:
A. Accuracy.
B. Agreement.
C. Precision.
D. Consistency.

Teaching Points

Correct Answer: D
Interobserver agreement is a measurement of how consistent two or more researchers are in making a particular measurement. As the two researchers from this scenario demonstrate good interobserver agreement, it is safe to say that they are being consistent in their measurements.

C16

Anatomy and Physiology of Communication and Swallowing

Neurotransmitters are chemicals in the brain that are important in sending neural signals between adjacent neurons. The **BEST** description of neurotransmitter release is that it:

Choices:
A. Excites neighboring cells.
B. Excites neighboring cells only if it binds with a receptor and causes a channel opening.
C. Excites or inhibits neighboring cells if it binds with a receptor and causes a channel opening.
D. Inhibits neighboring cells.

Teaching Points

Correct Answer: C

Neurotransmitters are chemicals that are released from neurons that help with neural signal transmission. Neurotransmitters can have one of two functions: excitatory or inhibitory. Excitatory neurotransmitters help continue the propagation of the neural signal, whereas inhibitory neurotransmitters slow or cancel the propagation of the neural signal.

C17

Dysphagia

While performing a modified barium swallow (MBS) study, the speech-language pathologist (SLP) discovers that the patient is experiencing premature spillage into the pharyngeal cavity, where the bolus sits for many seconds before being swallowed. Which part of the swallow is this patient having difficulty with?

Choices:
A. Hyolaryngeal elevation.
B. Initiation of the swallow.
C. Anterior-posterior movement.
D. Bolus formation.

Teaching Points

Correct Answer: B

The swallow is typically initiated when the bolus head reaches the faucial pillars (in younger adults) or the back of the tongue (in older adults). If the bolus is spilling into the patient's pharyngeal cavity prior to hyolaryngeal elevation and excursion, the patient is experiencing difficulty with initiating swallowing.

C18

Spoken Language Disorders in Children

An infant is being raised in a home with English-speaking parents, one of whom also speaks German. The parents have decided that they would like to expose their child to both the English and German language while the child grows up. Which of the following **BEST** describes this scenario?

Choices:
A. Successive bilingualism.
B. Simultaneous biculturalism.
C. Simultaneous bilingualism.
D. Generative biculturalism.

Teaching Points

Correct Answer: C

Simultaneous bilingualism occurs when two or more languages are learned at the same time. Because this child is being exposed to both English and German at the same time, the child is experiencing simultaneous bilingualism. This typically begins shortly after birth and continues to be a feature of the care-giving environment. In contrast to this, successive bilingualism occurs when a second language (or more) is learned after the acquisition of a first language. If the child from this scenario learned English first, and then his parents taught him German, this would constitute successive bilingualism. Finally, simultaneous biculturalism technically refers to being raised in two cultures at the same time. While language is intertwined with a culture, the child's language learning does not have to include learning about the associated culture.

C19

Motor Speech Disorders

When planning treatment for individuals with childhood apraxia of speech (CAS), a clinician needs to be cognizant of deficits beyond speech sound production. Other frequently occurring deficit areas include:

Choices:
A. Fluency, feeding/swallowing and literacy.
B. Hearing, metalinguistic/phonemic awareness and syllable shapes.
C. Language, metalinguistic/phonemic awareness and syllable shapes.
D. Prosody, phonation and feeding/swallowing.

Teaching Points

Correct Answer: C
Children with CAS often have co-occurring deficits in nonspeech motor behaviors, motor speech behaviors, speech sounds/structures (i.e., words and syllable shapes), prosody, language, metalinguistic/phonemic awareness and literacy. However, these children do not have problems with fluency, hearing or feeding/swallowing skills.

C20

Speech Sound Disorders in Children

A child is brought to a speech and language clinic by the child's parents, who provide a chief complaint of "being hard to understand." The speech-language pathologist (SLP) administers a comprehensive speech evaluation and reveals the following errors: /bu/ for /blu/, /gin/ for /grin/, and /sar/ for /star/. Which phonological process does this child demonstrate?

Choices:
A. Nasal assimilation.
B. Affrication.
C. Metathesis.
D. Cluster simplification.

Teaching Points

Correct Answer: D
The child from this scenario is eliminating one consonant from a consonant cluster (i.e., two or more consonants not separated by a vowel), which is known as the phonological process of cluster simplification. This occurs in this child's speech sample when he removes the /l/ phoneme from the /bl/ cluster or the /r/ phoneme from the /gr/ cluster. In contrast, nasal assimilation occurs when produce of a phoneme is more like a nasal phoneme in the target word. Affrication occurs when a fricative consonant is replaced with an affricate consonant. Finally, metathesis occurs when there is transposition of phonemes or syllables in a target word.

C21

Voice Disorders

A patient recently admitted to an acute rehabilitation hospital is presenting with hoarse vocal quality following spinal surgery. After a speech-language pathologist (SLP) consult, the patient reports he believes his vocal quality has changed since the surgery and that it is beginning to affect his self-perception. Following comprehensive voice assessment, the SLP notes that the patient is presenting with mild vocal fold edema, most likely caused by intubation during surgery. Which of the following approaches is the most appropriate for the SLP to take with this patient?

Choices:
A. Introduce a vocal function exercise regimen.
B. Introduce vocal hygiene principles.
C. Introduce Lee Silverman Voice Treatment (LSVT).
D. Introduce augmentative communication.

Teaching Points

Correct Answer: B
Vocal fold edema arises from phonotrauma, such as being intubated. This patient has no previous history of voice problems and has recently undergone intubation during surgery, suggesting that the voice problem is still relatively acute. Introducing vocal hygiene information to this patient can help them reduce the trauma to their vocal folds and reduce the amount of swelling that is present. As the edema resolves, the patient's vocal quality should return to baseline. Vocal function exercises and LSVT require excessive vocal fold movements and could cause further damage to the patient's vocal folds. Additionally, as the patient is able to communicate vocally, augmentative and alternative communication approaches are not recommended.

C22

Motor Speech Disorders

A speech-language pathologist (SLP) at an acute rehabilitation hospital has just received a patient with flaccid dysarthria on his/her caseload. After the first session, the SLP decides that the patient may benefit from abdominal trussing. Which of the following rationales for adopting this method for this particular patient would be appropriate for the SLP to use?

Choices:
A. To counter inspiratory weakness and assist in creation of inspiratory force for the generation of subglottal pressure during inspiration.
B. To increase vocal fold tension leading to increased loudness and improved vocal quality.
C. To counter expiratory weakness and assist in creation of expiratory force for the generation of subglottal pressure during expiration.
D. To improve functioning of both the direct and indirect upper motor neuron pathways.

Teaching Points

Correct Answer: C
Use of abdominal trussing would most likely be used with patient who has impairments in the respiratory subsystem. This method would be used to counter expiratory weakness and assist in the creation of expiratory force for increased subglottal pressures. Depending upon the needs of the specific patient, abdominal trussing can be used on a short-term or long-term basis.

C23

Language Acquisition

Zach's parent speaks to him with exaggerated speech, short utterances and heightened inflections. They are showing:

Choices:
A. Motherese.
B. Bootstrapping.
C. Word-learning biases.
D. Frequent exposure to television.

Teaching Points

Correct Answer: A

Motherese refers to the universally observed style of adjusting speech patterns in interacting with very young children. In contrast to this, *bootstrapping* refers to use of language to infer the meaning of unknown vocabulary words. Finally, *word-learning biases* help children determine what referent is being labeled during early word learning.

C24

Speech Sound Disorders in Children

A parent arrives at a local speech and language clinic with his young son, with complaints of "difficulty speaking." A speech-language pathologist (SLP) provides a comprehensive speech evaluation and determines that the child is exhibiting the phonological processes of affrication, epenthesis and reduplication. The SLP decides to target only the child's reduplication, as she believes the child has not reached an age where he should suppress affrication and epenthesis. Which theory of phonological development best matches this SLP's approach to treatment?

Choices:
A. Prosodic theory.
B. Generative phonology.
C. Behavioral theory.
D. Natural phonology.

Teaching Points

Correct Answer: D

The natural phonology theory emphasizes that children are born with a set of natural phonological processes that they need to suppress as they age. These phonological processes are suppressed as the child develops. Because this SLP believes that the child has not developed enough to suppress specific phonological processes, she utilizes principles from the natural phonology theory. In contrast to this, the generative phonology theory is an expansion of the distinctive feature theory and includes concepts such as underlying representations, surface forms and phonological rules, but does not include suppression of phonological processes. The prosodic theory emphasizes the perception of whole words as early word productions, but, again, does not emphasize suppression of phonological patterns. Finally, behavioral theory posits that phonological development is contingent upon reinforcement, not suppression of phonological processes.

C25

Voice Disorders

To check jitter and shimmer in a voice, the speech-language pathologist (SLP) should record the speaker:

Choices:
A. In a brief natural conversation.
B. Reading a short, phonetically balanced passage.
C. Producing a vowel with sustained pitch.
D. Producing a vowel with a rising and falling pitch contour.

Teaching Points

Correct Answer: C

Jitter and shimmer are cycle-to-cycle variations in frequency and amplitude that reflect the degree of regularity of vocal fold vibration. To examine jitter and shimmer the recording should be a sustained vowel, so that voluntary changes in frequency and amplitude are not misinterpreted as jitter and shimmer.

C26

Written Language Disorders in the School-Age Population

A student reads seven research articles regarding recycling challenges and methods. He summarizes and critiques the articles and then, based on his synthesis, proposes a novel strategy to solve urban recycling efforts. This cluster of behaviors is **MOST CLOSELY** associated with which of Chall's reading stages?

Choices:
A. Stage 2: Confirmation, fluency, ungluing from print.
B. Stage 3: Reading for learning the new.
C. Stage 4: Multiple viewpoints.
D. Stage 5: Construction and reconstruction.

Teaching Points

Correct Answer: D

This student would fall into Chall's stage 5 as the student synthesized multiple viewpoints in order to generate a novel hypothesis. The hallmark characteristics of Chall's stage 5 include creation of new theories based on analysis, synthesis and evaluation of existing sources of information, which this student has demonstrated. Because the student has generated his/her own hypothesis regarding the material, the student has advanced past Chall's stage 4.

C27

Stuttering and Other Fluency Disorders

Pediatricians, preschool teachers and parents often wonder if a child who is showing disfluencies should be evaluated and when. The usual rule of thumb about speech-language pathology assessment for stuttering is "the earlier the better." Evaluation should **NOT** be delayed if the:

Choices:
A. Child is totally unaware of his disfluencies.
B. Parent reports that someone in the family stuttered.
C. Child is evidencing secondary behaviors of stuttering.
D. Child is ready to begin preschool.

Teaching Points

Correct Answer: C

If the child is beginning to exhibit secondary behaviors that evidence struggle, then it is a good time for referral. The SLP can help the family and referral source determine the appropriate course of treatment, if indicated. While family history is a risk factor, it is less critical for determining need for referral than are secondary behaviors or the child's educational or social situation.

C28
Audiology and Hearing Impairment

An audiologist has recently completed an audiologic evaluation on a patient. During the evaluation, the audiologist utilized instrumentation that allowed determination of the severity of the patient's hearing loss as well as the type of hearing loss the patient is experiencing. Which means of evaluation did this audiologist utilize in working with this patient?

Choices:
A. Pure-tone audiometry.
B. Tympanometry.
C. Acoustic reflex testing.
D. Speech audiometry.

Teaching Points

Correct Answer: A

Pure-tone audiometry refers to a form of evaluation that determines the severity of a hearing loss and provides information to help diagnose the type of hearing loss (i.e., conductive, sensorineural or mixed). In contrast to this, tympanometry evaluates middle ear integrity, specifically, tympanic membrane mobility and middle ear pressure. Acoustic reflex testing assesses the neural pathways. Finally, speech audiometry crosschecks the validity of pure-tone threshold results and quantifies suprathreshold speech recognition abilities.

C29
Written Language Disorders in the School-Age Population

Which teaching strategies are **MOST** consistent with a so-called top-down approach to reading instruction?

Choices:
A. Teaching of grapheme-phoneme skills.
B. Instruction in decoding and spelling words containing the six syllable types.
C. Teaching children how to use context to infer the pronunciation of words that they cannot decode.
D. Teaching children how to recognize and pronounce high-frequency roots and affixes.

Teaching Points

Correct Answer: C

In top-down instruction, approaches to reading and/or writing emphasize exposure to authentic literature and leveraging of discourse contexts. By having the student engage in reading unfamiliar words through contextual guessing, the student is gaining experience with reading through authentic means. The other answers for this question include portions of a bottom-up instruction progression, which includes phonological awareness, grapheme-phoneme relationships, syllable structure recognition, morphological analysis and text-level decoding fluency.

C30

Audiology and Hearing Impairment

An elderly man arrives at an audiology clinic with complaints of hearing loss. After complete evaluation, the audiologist diagnoses the patient with a symmetric mild to moderate sensorineural hearing loss. Which of the following conditions is affecting this patient?

Choices:
A. Otosclerosis.
B. Presbycusis.
C. Ototoxicity.
D. Otitis media.

Teaching Points

Correct Answer: B

Presbycusis refers to hearing loss associated with aging. As this patient is an elderly man complaining of hearing loss, and the audiologist did not discover another organic cause of this patient's loss, he is likely experiencing presbycusis. In contrast to this, otosclerosis refers to stiffening of the ossicles in the middle ear, ototoxicity refers to environmental toxins or pharmaceutical agents causing hearing impairment, and otitis media refers to a middle ear effusion.

C31

Speech Sound Disorders in Children

A child with speech sound problems has recently been diagnosed with a speech sound disorder, characterized by difficulty producing interdental and alveolar fricatives. Which of the following speech sounds would this child demonstrate difficulty producing?

Choices:
A. /f/ and /h/.
B. /ð/ and /s/.
C. /z/ and /tʃ/.
D. /θ/ and /b/.

Teaching Points

Correct Answer: B

The interdental fricatives include /ð/ and /θ/, and the alveolar fricatives include /s/ and /z/. As this child demonstrates speech sound errors on the /ð/ and /s/. In contrast, /f/ and /h/ are labiodental and glottal fricatives. While /z/ is an alveolar fricative, /tʃ/ is a palatal affricate. Similarly, while /θ/ is an interdental fricative, /b/ is a bilabial stop. There is no mention of the child's ability to produce affricates or stops, so these answers are not the most appropriate.

C32
Acoustics

If pitch contour for a vowel shows a frequency of 150 hertz (Hz) at the midpoint, the frequency of the fifth harmonic at the same location will be:

Choices:
A. 500 Hz.
B. 750 Hz.
C. 1000 Hz.
D. 1250 Hz.

Teaching Points

Correct Answer: B
All harmonics are integer multiples of F0. If F0 = 150 Hz, then H5 = 5 × 150 Hz or 750 Hz.

C33
Spoken Language Disorders in Children

Following a very successful intervention session, in which Annie produced 95% of targeted utterances correctly, her speech-language pathologist (SLP) implements a subsequent motivational event. Which therapy component BEST describes this situation?

Choices:
A. The SLP delivers feedback to Annie regarding her productions.
B. The SLP models appropriate productions for Annie.
C. The SLP presents Annie with a sticker for appropriate productions.
D. The SLP allows Annie to play with a board game before therapy.

Teaching Points

Correct Answer: C
A subsequent motivational event (SME) is reinforcement that occurs following a child's attempt at the language targets, which is likely to foster continued success and attention. Because Annie was given a sticker, this is likely to cause her to be motivated for continued participation in language therapy services. In contrast to this, antecedent instructional events (AIEs) include whatever methods the SLP employs before the child's attempt to use the language target (i.e., modeling, sequence pictures, etc.) Subsequent instruction events (SIEs) include the feedback the SLP provides to the child following an attempt to use the language target. Finally, antecedent motivational events (AMEs) are activities not directly related to the learning of the language target, which fosters the child's attention (i.e., playing with a board game).

C34

Spoken Language Disorders in Children

Amy is a paraprofessional who has been working with a young child with autism spectrum disorder. Recently, Amy has found that the child's language skills have been lagging behind those of his peers. Amy has contacted the school's speech-language pathologist (SLP) in order to procure expert advice on what she can do to aid the child's linguistic development in the classroom. What role has the SLP taken in an endeavor to help Amy?

Choices:
A. Instructor.
B. Interventionist.
C. Consultant.
D. Collaborator.

Teaching Points

Correct Answer: C

When a speech-language pathologist acts as a consultant, the SLP provides indirect services through giving expert advice to teachers, parents and paraprofessionals regarding the speech or language needs of a child. In contrast to this, when an SLP acts as a collaborator, he/she is working with teachers, parents and paraprofessionals to assess and provide intervention to a student with speech or language needs. Although SLPs may act as educators or interventionists, these are not specific roles they would assume in working with paraprofessionals or teachers.

C35

Spoken Language Disorders in Children

A child in an elementary school is currently producing one-word utterances and has demonstrated difficulty producing more advanced utterances. The speech-language pathologist (SLP) who is working with this child has decided to use expatiations during play activities as a means of increasing utterance length. If the child produces the utterance "kitty," which of the following is an appropriate response for this SLP to use?

Choices:
A. "What does the kitty like to do?"
B. "That is a kitty."
C. "What's the kitty's name?"
D. "That is a soft kitty."

Teaching Points

Correct Answer: D

Expatiations are contingent verbal responses that add new but relevant information to a child's utterance and can be used to indirectly target language facilitation. By adding the information that the kitty is "soft," the SLP is offering new information and vocabulary to the child. In contrast to this, an expansion is a contingent verbal response that increases the length or complexity of the child's utterance. The response "That is a kitty" is an example of expansion. The response "What does the kitty like to do?" is an example of a prompt, which is a comment or question that serves to extend what the child has said. Finally, the response of "What's the kitty's name?" utilizes the vertical structure method, where the SLP asks questions in order to construct a syntactically correct sentence.

C36
Voice Disorders

A 34-year-old male has been referred to an outpatient voice center with a presenting problem of excessively high pitch. After complete evaluation, the speech-language pathologist (SLP) is unable to find any structural or physiological deficits in this patient's voice mechanism, and the patient is diagnosed with puberphonia. Which of the following are appropriate treatment methods to use with this patient in order to establish a more appropriate voice?

Choices:
A. Vocal function exercises and resonant voice therapy.
B. Circumlaryngeal massage and hard glottal attacks.
C. Pitch glides and psychological referral.
D. Straw phonation and tongue trills.

Teaching Points

Correct Answer: B
When a patient is experiencing puberphonia, treatment is focused on production and maintenance of a habitually lower pitch. Utilization of circumlaryngeal massage and/or hard glottal attacks have been found to be effective in lowering pitch in puberphonic patients. Continued practice with the newly established lower pitch is critical for these patients, as they may not immediately identify with their voices. While a psychological referral may be necessary for patients who demonstrate puberphonia, vocal function exercises, resonant voice therapy, pitch glides and semioccluded vocal tract tasks (i.e., straw phonation and tongue trills) do not help the presenting problem of excessively high pitch. As such, these intervention methods are contraindicated in this population.

C37
Anatomy and Physiology of Communication and Swallowing

A person is experiencing ataxia. Which central nervous system structure is MOST LIKELY impaired?

Choices:
A. Midbrain.
B. Pons.
C. Medulla.
D. Cerebellum.

Teaching Points

Correct Answer: D
The cerebellum is the structure below the cerebral hemispheres that is responsible for coordination of movements. Damage to the cerebellum would result in ataxia, or uncoordinated movement, on the ipsilateral side of the body.

C38

Autism Spectrum Disorders

A child is brought into a physician's (MDs) office for a comprehensive evaluation, with parental suspicions of autism spectrum disorder. Following the evaluation, the child is diagnosed with autism spectrum disorder, with level 1 severity in repetitive behaviors. Which of the following **BEST** describes the behaviors exhibited by this child?

Choices:
A. The child demonstrates difficulty switching between tasks.
B. The child becomes distressed when changing focus or activity.
C. The child's behaviors markedly interfere with functioning.
D. The child's inflexible behavior is obvious to observers.

Teaching Points

Correct Answer: A

Level 1 severity of restricted, repetitive behaviors reflect inflexible behaviors that cause interference with functioning, difficulty switching between tasks, and problems with organization and planning. In contrast to this, Level 2 severity reflects inflexible behaviors that are obvious to the casual observer and distressed behavior noted when changing focus. Finally, level 3 severity reflects difficulty in coping with change, repetitive behaviors markedly interfering with functioning, and significant distress upon changing focus.

C39

Spoken Language Disorders in Children

Gus is a speech-language pathologist (SLP) working in an early childhood education setting. Recently, he has begun working with a child who has a significant language disorder. For this child, Gus has chosen to utilize induction teaching to facilitate the child's learning of language. Which of the following statements BEST describes this approach to intervention?

Choices:
A. Providing an enriched language-learning environment with no specific targets.
B. Targeting of specific forms and functions through repetition and modeling.
C. Increasing the rate at which a targeted form or function is learned.
D. Using a more explicit and systematic set of teaching steps.

Teaching Points

Correct Answer: D

Induction teaching refers to use a more explicit and systematic set of teaching steps, beyond modeling. When this form of instruction is utilized, it is not assumed the targeted form would have been learned without intervention, or learned to the same degree. Use of induction teaching also leads to concomitant achievements in academic and/or social contexts. In contrast to this, facilitation refers to increasing the rate at which a targeted form or function is learned, focused stimulation refers to the targeting of specific forms and functions by the SLP through repetition or modeling, and general stimulation refers to a provision of an enriched language-learning environment with no specific target for learning.

C40

Augmentative and Alternative Communication (AAC)

Sean is an elderly gentleman with severe flaccid dysarthria and right hemiparesis caused by a large left hemispheric infarction. Prior to sustaining his stroke, Sean was declared legally blind, secondary to macular degeneration. Sean has been experiencing difficulty with verbal expression and has made few gains in treatment. His speech-language pathologist (SLP) has decided to implement an augmentative and alternative communication (AAC) approach to treatment in order to increase Sean's communicative effectiveness. Which intervention would be of the MOST benefit?

Choices:
A. Augmentative device utilizing line drawings.
B. Augmentative device with auditory scanning.
C. Alphabet board supplementation.
D. Augmentative device utilizing eye gaze system.

Teaching Points

Correct Answer: B

As the patient from this scenario was declared legally blind prior to his stroke, he will most likely not benefit from use of a visual AAC system to improve communication. In a system that utilizes auditory scanning, choices are presented to the user auditorily until the user makes a selection. This would be the most appropriate selection for this patient. In contrast to this, line drawings, eye gaze systems and alphabet board supplementation all require some level of visual acuity and would not be recommended for a patient who is legally blind.

C41

Speech Sound Disorders in Children

A speech-language pathologist (SLP) has been working with a child who demonstrates difficulty producing /k/ in the initial and final word positions. However, the child does correctly produce the following words: /ki/, /kæt/, /bæk/ and /baɪk/. The SLP decides to utilize a treatment method that capitalizes on these correct productions to aid in faulty productions. Which of these interventions is MOST LIKELY the method chosen by this SLP?

Choices:
A. Integral stimulation.
B. Multiple phoneme approach.
C. Sensory-motor approach.
D. Paired-stimuli approach.

Teaching Points

Correct Answer: D

The paired-stimuli approach utilizes four key words as a starting point, and ten training words are then paired with the key words to aid in production. As the child from this scenario is able to produce the errored speech sound correctly in four separate words, these may act as the key words and aid further production of the /k/ phoneme. In contrast, the integral stimulation approach may be utilized to establish a speech sound that the child is unable to produce and would not be recommended for this client. The sensory-motor approach uses bisyllable productions of nonerrored phonemes used as facilitating contexts to produce a target sound. As the child is able to produce the target /k/, this method of intervention is contraindicated. Finally, the multiple phoneme approach is utilized for children with multiple phoneme errors, and as this child only demonstrates errors on the /k/ phoneme, this method is also contraindicated for use in intervention.

C42

Spoken Language Disorders in Children

Barbara is a young child with a severe cognitive deficit. Barbara's speech-language pathologist (SLP) is beginning to formulate a treatment plan for intervention and would like to focus on the **MOST** functional treatment targets during intervention. What should be targeted during Barbara's intervention sessions?

Choices:
A. Complex sentence structure.
B. Recreational vocabulary.
C. Phonological memory.
D. Joint attention skills.

Teaching Points

Correct Answer: B

Most children with cognitive deficits will learn some language, although normalization of language skills may not be the most appropriate expectation in these cases. For this population, functional language goals are the most appropriate treatment target, which may include focusing intervention on a limited language repertoire. For this child, as she is still relatively young, the most functional goal may be initially targeting vocabulary surrounding her favorite recreational activities as a means of improving her means of communication. Other functional tasks for this population include understanding of different syntactic structures and understanding useful vocabulary for the child's activities of daily living.

C43

Acoustics

What would the speech-language pathologist (SLP) expect to observe if comparing amplitude spectra for a sinusoid and a periodic complex sound?

Choices:
A. The sinusoid has evenly spaced lines, while the periodic complex sound has irregularly spaced lines.
B. The sinusoid has irregularly spaced lines, while the periodic complex sound has evenly spaced lines.
C. The sinusoid has only one line, while the complex periodic sound has more than one line.
D. The sinusoid has lines that are all the same amplitude, while the complex periodic sound has lines of different amplitudes.

Teaching Points

Correct Answer: C

A sinusoid contains only one frequency. It therefore has only a single line on a spectrum. A complex sound contains multiple frequencies, and therefore contains more than one line. Since this is a complex periodic sound, the lines are evenly spaced.

C44

Spoken Language Disorders in Children

Caitlin is a typically developing 2-year-old girl. Which of the following semantic structures would she **MOST LIKELY** demonstrate?

Choices:
A. Declarative sentences and contracted forms.
B. Gestures and phonological process suppression.
C. Relational terms and interrogative terms.
D. Derivational affixes and bound morphemes.

Teaching Points

Correct Answer: C

Relational (i.e., on, under, next, to) and interrogative (i.e., what, who, how, why) terms are semantic structures that are typically developed by 24 months of age. Additional terms that are developed include temporal relationship terms (when, before), physical relations (big, little, wide, narrow), and kinship terms (son, parent, aunt, nephew). Declarative sentences and contracted forms are syntactic structures, gestures are pragmatic constructs, phonological process suppression deals with phonology, and derivational affixes and bound morphemes are morphological structures.

C45

Dysphagia

A speech-language pathologist (SLP) at a skilled nursing facility has been asked by a nurse to perform a swallowing evaluation on an elderly patient with whom they have been working. The SLP knows that there are multiple, typical changes to the swallow as one ages, but which of the following would still be considered an **ABNORMAL** result from the examination?

Choices:
A. Increased duration of the swallow.
B. Reduction in smell and taste.
C. Increased presence of aspiration.
D. Lower salivary flow.

Teaching Points

Correct Answer: C

Because of decreased muscle tone with aging, there are typical amounts of associated increased duration of swallowing, delayed hyoid elevation and longer opening of the upper esophageal sphincter. Additionally, while it does not occur with everyone, there is a typical decrease in smell and taste abilities in the elderly population. However, any presence of aspiration is considered a deficit in the swallow, regardless of the age group.

C46

Written Language Disorders in the School-Age Population

A typically developing fourth-grade girl reads grade-level single words accurately and promptly. Her spelling is appropriate for her grade level. When she reads aloud a passage from her English language arts textbook, her reading, while accurate, is extremely slow and halting. When the speech-language pathologist (SLP) asks this client questions that assess her understanding of what she has read, she formulates her responses clearly and accurately. The client's text-level reading difficulty suggests problems with:

Choices:
A. Reading fluency.
B. Orthographic memory for letter patterns.
C. Rules for orthographic-phonological association.
D. Underlying vocabulary skills.

Teaching Points

Correct Answer: A

This student is demonstrating adequate automaticity, as she is able to accurately and quickly read individual words. However, because she has difficulty with reading of connected text, she is presenting with problems in reading fluency. Fluent reading reflects appropriate rhythm, intonation and syntactic chunking, all of which would be affected in this student's slow, halting, oral reading.

C47

Speech Sound Disorders in Children

A 5-year-old client is brought by his parents to the local speech-language pathologist clinic for a full speech and language evaluation. After completion of the evaluation, the speech-language pathologist (SLP) reviews the results and notices that the child produces the words /bo/ (*boat*), /fɪʃ/ (*fish*), /kʌ/ (*cup*), /sʌn/ (*sun*) and /dɔ/ (*dog*). Which of the following best describes this child's speech pattern?

Choices:
A. Affrication of medial fricatives.
B. Fronting of initial fricatives.
C. Final consonant deletion of stops.
D. Initial consonant deletion of nasals.

Teaching Points

Correct Answer: C

When evaluating the child's errors, it is important to note that the child omits some, but not all of the final consonants of the words produced. Of those omitted, all consonants are stop consonants (i.e., /g/, /t/, /p/). Therefore, the most appropriate phonological pattern that this child demonstrates is final consonant deletion of stop consonants. If the child deleted the first phoneme of each word (i.e., /ot/ for /bot/), then the child would demonstrate initial consonant deletion. As the child appropriately produces all of the initial consonants in the sample, the child is also not demonstrating fronting. Finally, as the child is producing consonant-vowel-consonant (CVC) words, there is not an opportunity for the child to affricate medial consonants, making this selection incorrect.

C48

Voice Disorders

A speech-language pathologist (SLP) in an acute care hospital has been preparing a patient to undergo a total laryngectomy following diagnosis of malignant laryngeal cancer. After being educated regarding the various forms of alaryngeal communication, the patient decides that he/she would like to utilize a form of communication that allows the most natural vocal quality that also restores spoken communication as quickly as possible. Which of the following treatment options would be the **BEST** to introduce to this patient, keeping in mind the patient's particular communicative wishes?

Choices:
A. Electrolarynx with neck placement.
B. Tracheoesophageal speech.
C. Esophageal speech.
D. Intraoral electrolarynx.

Teaching Points

Correct Answer: B

Tracheoesophageal speech involves inserting a prosthesis through the tissue wall separating the trachea from the esophagus in a laryngectomee. This prosthesis diverts air from the trachea in order to vibrate the pharyngoesophageal segment, producing voice. Tracheoesophageal speech produces the most natural sounding voice for alaryngeal speakers, and following insertion of the prosthesis, there may be immediate restoration of oral communication. Thus, this method of communication may prove the best match for this patient's wishes. Both forms of electrolarynx (i.e., neck placement and with intraoral adapter) produce a very unnatural, robotic sounding voice. This is in direct contrast with the patient's wishes for a natural vocal quality. Lastly, while esophageal speech offers a more natural vocal quality than the electrolarynx, it takes lengthy periods of time for patients to learn and has a high fail rate. As such, this goes against the patient's wishes for immediate restoration of voice.

C49

Autism Spectrum Disorders

Allison is a speech-language pathologist (SLP) working in an elementary school, with a caseload comprising predominantly children with autism spectrum disorder. How should Allison structure her intervention sessions to maximize gains made by these children?

Choices:
A. She should provide parenting training once behaviors have been established.
B. She should provide intervention sessions that are lengthy in duration.
C. She should provide intervention that utilizes a group format.
D. She should provide intervention that promotes active engagement.

Teaching Points

Correct Answer: D

According to the National Research Council's review of intervention evidence for autism spectrum disorder, intervention should be provided intensively and in a way that promotes active engagement through collaboration with family and teachers. Additionally, individualized intervention (as opposed to group treatment), which is brief and focused in nature (as opposed to lengthy treatment) shows greater efficacy. Finally, family members should be trained to implement teaching strategies as a means of reinforcing learning while it is occurring (as opposed to after learning has been established).

C50

Anatomy and Physiology of Communication and Swallowing

When producing the voiceless fricative /f/, the muscle that MOST LIKELY contracts is the:

Choices:
A. Lateral cricoarytenoid.
B. Transverse interarytenoid.
C. Oblique interarytenoid.
D. Posterior cricoarytenoid.

Teaching Points

Correct Answer: D

As /f/ is a voiceless phoneme, it is important that the vocal folds are not contracted during production. In order for this to occur, the vocal folds need to be abducted, invoking contraction of the posterior cricoarytenoid muscle, the sole vocal fold abductor. The other muscles listed function as vocal fold adductors and close the vocal folds for production as voiced phonemes. As /f/ is a voiceless phoneme, it would require no activation in these muscles.

C51

Audiology and Hearing Impairment

An audiologist has been consulted by the local school system in order to make the classrooms more acoustically appropriate for students who are hard of hearing. Which of the following accommodations could the audiologist recommend to augment the classroom?

Choices:
A. High ceilings.
B. Floor carpeting.
C. Remove window shades.
D. Reverberating ceiling tiles.

Teaching Points

Correct Answer: B

There are several means of acoustic treatment for an audiologist to perform in a classroom setting. Such accommodations include recommending a low ceiling with acoustic tiles, providing floor carpeting, and utilizing shades or curtains on windows and covers for other hard surfaces. In contrast to this, reverberating tiles would be tiles that encourage echoing of sound, which would not be recommended for use with children with hearing loss.

C52

Language Acquisition

A speech-language pathologist (SLP) has been consulted to perform a comprehensive language evaluation on a young child. Following the evaluation, the SLP determines that the child is functioning at Brown's stage II of morphological development. Which structure would this child MOST LIKELY be producing?

Choices:
A. Auxiliary *am*.
B. Auxiliary *do*.
C. Auxiliary *have*.
D. Auxiliary *be*.

Teaching Points

Correct Answer: D
At Brown's stage II, children develop copula *be*, auxiliary *be*, modals and irregular past tense. Auxiliary *am* is developed during Brown's stage III, auxiliary *do* is developed during Brown's stage IV, and auxiliary *have* is developed during Brown's stage V.

C53

Research, Evidence-Based Practice and Tests and Measurements

A clinician in private practice is looking to purchase speech and language evaluations. She is interested in tests that will correctly rule out children who do not have speech and language disorders. This clinician should look up information in the evaluation manuals regarding test:

Choices:
A. Sample size.
B. Specificity.
C. Evidence.
D. Sensitivity.

Teaching Points

Correct Answer: B
Specificity refers to how well a test detects that a condition is not present when it is actually not present. If the clinician wanted to know information about how well evaluations rule out children who do not actually have speech and language disorders, the clinician should refer to the test manuals' sections on test specificity. Contrary to this, test sensitivity refers to how well the test detects a condition that is actually present. Sample size and test evidence would not help this clinician find information about how well the test detects disorders or lack of disorders.

C54

Language Acquisition

Jonathon is a typically developing 4-year-old preschooler. Which of the following structures would **MOST LIKELY** be in his language repertoire?

Choices:
A. Suggesting intention, emerging mastery of copula *to be*, identifies the first sound in a word.
B. Predominantly nouns, calling and requesting action intentions, ritual request gestures.
C. Spurts in word learning, combining two to three words, deletion of possessive –s.
D. Combining single words with pointing, 50 words in his expressive vocabulary, words composed of open syllables.

Teaching Points

Correct Answer: A
A typical 4-year-old child usually exhibits more sophisticated pragmatic, metalinguistic and grammatical forms. The other items in this question all occur earlier in development.

C55

Voice Disorders

After taking a patient's measurements, a speech-language pathologist (SLP) has discovered that the patient exhibits increased jitter and shimmer, most likely from bilateral vocal fold nodules. However the patient's glottal pressure and airflow volumes are considered within the typical range. This patient is exhibiting deficits in which aspects of voice assessment?

Choices:
A. Resonatory.
B. Acoustic.
C. Aerodynamic.
D. Perceptual.

Teaching Points

Correct Answer: B

Jitter is the average cycle-to-cycle change in frequency, and shimmer is the average cycle-to-cycle change in amplitude from one cycle to the next. Both of these measures are included in acoustic evaluation of the voice. If a patient's jitter and shimmer values are higher than expected, they would present with acoustic deficits. Other acoustic measurements include fundamental frequency, intensity and noise-to-harmonic ratio. Aerodynamic instrumentation measures transglottal airflow and subglottal pressure, which was noted in this scenario to be normal. Perceptual and resonatory measures include distinctions such as "hoarse," "breathy," or "hypernasal," of which there is no true standard of measurement.

C56

Language Acquisition

A child is brought into a speech and language clinic for a language evaluation. After performing the evaluation, the speech-language pathologist (SLP) reveals the following utterances: "look doggy," "more cookie," "no bed," and "mommy good." Which of the following statements **BEST** describes this child's speech sample?

Choices:
A. The child is producing babbling.
B. The child is producing narratives.
C. The child is producing simple sentences.
D. The child is producing telegraphic speech.

Teaching Points

Correct Answer: D

Telegraphic speech is characterized by content word combinations that often contain a pivot word or phrase. As this child is producing two-word utterances that contain content words, they are demonstrating telegraphic speech. In contrast, babbling is an early form of communication consisting of consonant-vowel (CV) syllables, such as "bababa." Narratives include decontextualized monologues that convey a story, personal recount or retelling of a book or movie. Finally, simple sentences are a characteristic of Brown's stages II and III and include some form of grammatical structure, such as "I am walking."

C57 Language Acquisition

Jake is a typically developing 13-month-old toddler, and is demonstrating several common forms of communicative intention for his age group. Which type of communicative intention would Jake **MOST LIKELY NOT** demonstrate?

Choices:
A. Requesting action.
B. Requesting permission.
C. Repeating.
D. Practicing.

Teaching Points

Correct Answer: B

Requesting permission is a form of communicative intent often expressed by preschoolers. As Jake has not reached preschool age, it is unlikely that he would be demonstrating this form of communicative intention. However, as he is a typically developing toddler, he would most likely demonstrate the communicative intentions of requesting an action, repeating and practicing.

C58 Research, Evidence-Based Practice and Tests and Measurements

A speech and language researcher has completed treatment tasks selected for a study and is preparing to administer a posttest to the study participants. However, this posttest is the same used as the pretest the study participants previously completed. As the study participants have already seen this test, the researcher needs to be aware of the potential threat to which of the following principles?

Choices:
A. Internal validity.
B. External validity.
C. Reliability.
D. Content validity.

Teaching Points

Correct Answer: A

Internal validity is how well the study is testing or describing what it purports to be testing or describing and is dependent on the methods and procedures used to answer the research questions. As the participants have already seen the posttest material, this may cause their performance to improve more than it actually did. If this were the case, the internal validity would be reduced, as the study would not accurately describe improvement, but would describe the participant's ability to recall pretest materials.

C59

Speech Sound Disorders in Children

After performing a comprehensive speech evaluation on a pediatric client, a speech-language pathologist (SLP) has determined that although the child produces the /s/ phoneme, he demonstrates the phonological process of final consonant deletion for this phoneme, consistent with a phonemic error. Which method of intervention would be an appropriate selection for the SLP to utilize with this child?

Choices:
A. Van Riper traditional approach.
B. Multiple phoneme approach.
C. Paired stimulus approach.
D. Minimal contrast approach.

Teaching Points

Correct Answer: D

The minimal contrast approach is an intervention method used for phonemic speech errors and is utilized to eliminate excessive homonymy in children's speech. In contrast, the Van Riper traditional approach, multiple phoneme approach and paired-stimuli approach are all intervention methods used for children with phonetic speech errors and would not be helpful in remediating this particular child's speech sound disorder as this child already knows the motor pattern for the /s/ phoneme and requires help to generalize production to new word positions.

C60

The Practice of Speech-Language Pathology

A speech-language pathologist (SLP) in an acute care hospital is interested in starting a research project, but is unsure of what direction to take. A large pharmaceutical company that works with the hospital discusses their new pill that will treat the hypokinetic dysarthria aspects of Parkinson's disease with the SLP and reveal that it still needs to be tested. The company representatives offer the SLP 10% of total profit if they are able to prove through a controlled study that this pill is more effective than just treatment alone. What course of action should this SLP take?

Choices:
A. Deny participation in the research study, as this is a conflict of interest.
B. Accept participation in the research study, as this could be beneficial to many people.
C. Deny participation in the research study, but offer to recommend patients to the company.
D. Reduce their earnings to 2% profit, to minimize any conflict of interest.

Teaching Points

Correct Answer: A

According to the American Speech-Language-Hearing Association Code of Ethics, Principle of Ethics III, Rule of Ethics B, "Individuals shall not participate in professional activities that constitute a conflict of interest." The SLP from this scenario is bound by the Code of Ethics to deny participation in this research study, as their receiving profit from the successful pill is a conflict of interest. For this reason, it would also be unethical for the SLP to recommend participants for the research study, as they are still participating in the project in a minimal degree. Finally, receiving any amount of profit (i.e., 2%–10%) still represents a conflict of interest and should be denied, regardless.

C61

Motor Speech Disorders

A clinician notices the speaker fails to take a breath to replenish his air supply, talking into his reserve volume. The speaker exhibits loudness decay when this occurs and breath group lengths are a little longer than age- and gender-matched controls. Therapy should focus on:

Choices:
A. A thorough assessment of respiratory shape.
B. Improving coordination of the respiratory and phonatory system.
C. Reducing maladaptive respiratory behaviors.
D. Adopting the Lee Silverman Voice Treatment.

Teaching Points

Correct Answer: C

The type of breathing patterns that this particular speaker is exhibiting is not efficient from a communicative perspective. Focusing on reduction of the maladaptive respiratory behaviors can lead to reduction in loudness decay and age- and gender-appropriate breath groups. The speaker should be instructed in optimal breath groups and to replenish air supply at appropriate conversation junctures.

C62

Spoken Language Disorders in Children

A 3-year-old child is brought to a speech and language clinic and is suspected of having a language disorder. Upon initial interview, the child's parents reveal that the child first learned to speak English, and they have now begun to teach the child Spanish. Following the evaluation, the speech-language pathologist (SLP) determines that the child demonstrates age-appropriate linguistic skill with English, but presents with significant difficulty with Spanish. Which of the following **BEST** describes this child?

Choices:
A. The child does not present with a language disorder.
B. The child presents with a language disorder for Spanish only.
C. The child presents with a language disorder for both languages.
D. The child presents with a language delay for Spanish only.

Teaching Points

Correct Answer: A

For children who are bilingual, determination of the first language (L_1) is critical, because a language disorder can only be diagnosed if the child presents with difficulties in only their L_1. If the child presents with difficulties in L_2, this may be a sign of difficulty learning a new language, but it is not indicative of a language disorder.

C63

Research, Evidence-Based Practice and Tests and Measurements

A speech and language researcher is designing a research study to determine the effects of time spent in intervention, dosage of intervention and type of feedback on the amount of progress made in children with phonological disorders. Which of the following methods should this research utilize in the study?

Choices:
A. Nonparametric experiment.
B. Parametric experiment.
C. Within-subjects experiment.
D. Between-subjects experiment.

Teaching Points

Correct Answer: B
A parametric experiment is one that is designed to study the simultaneous effects of more than one independent variable on the dependent variable. In this scenario, the researcher is studying the effect of the independent variables of time in intervention, dosage of intervention and type of feedback on the dependent variable of progress made in intervention. As there are three separate independent variables, a parametric experiment would be the best selection for this researcher.

C64

Dysphagia

A patient has just been admitted to an acute care hospital after having a right middle cerebral artery (MCA) cerebrovascular accident (CVA). The initial symptoms appear to be left-sided pharyngeal weakness and reduced vocal fold closure. The SLP is consulted to perform an evaluation on the patient, and in order to maximize the limited time spent with the patient, which of the following compensatory maneuvers should be used during the modified barium swallow (MBS), based on the patient's symptoms?

Choices:
A. Chin-tuck maneuver.
B. Head rotation toward the left.
C. Head tilt toward the left.
D. Head back.

Teaching Points

Correct Answer: B
A head rotation toward the weak side closes off the weak side of the pharynx and allows the bolus to be directed down the strong half of the pharynx. Additionally, when the pharynx is turned toward the side of damage, the airway is narrowed, which would help with the patient's reduced vocal fold closure.

C65

Research, Evidence-Based Practice and Tests and Measurements

A speech-language pathologist (SLP) has begun a research study, utilizing a within-subject experimental design. However, the research participant has demonstrated significant fatigue from beginning to the end of the study. Any potential change in data due to this fatigue is known as a:

Choices:
A. Treatment effect.
B. Carryover effect.
C. Hawthorne effect.
D. Order effect.

Teaching Points

Correct Answer: D

An order effect is a potential change in data that occurs sometime from the beginning to the end of an experiment. These changes can arise due to factors such as participant fatigue or familiarity with assessment and/or intervention materials. Alternatively, a carryover effect would occur if a first treatment condition affected participant performance on a second treatment condition. Lastly, a Hawthorne effect would occur if a research participant's performance in the study was influenced by their awareness of being in a research study.

C66

Spoken Language Disorders in Children

Richard is a speech-language pathologist (SLP) in a preschool setting. Currently, he is working with a child who has specific deficits in morphological developments. Richard wants to establish that morphemes he has targeted in this child's intervention sessions are being used consistently. What level of use is appropriate for establishing acquisition of morphological structures?

Choices:
A. 85% of use in obligatory contexts.
B. 90% of use in obligatory contexts.
C. 95% of use in obligatory contexts.
D. 100% of use in obligatory contexts.

Teaching Points

Correct Answer: B

The consistency of morpheme use in obligatory contexts is the most appropriate measure for establishing the acquisition of a morpheme. This consistency can be calculated as the number of times the child correctly produced a specific morpheme (in obligatory context) divided by the total number of opportunities for that specific morpheme to have been produced in a spoken or written passage. Traditionally, 90% of use in obligatory contexts has been used as the standard for establishing morpheme acquisition.

C67

Acoustics

Tongue position is related to F1 frequency in that, when the tongue is:

Choices:
A. Low in the mouth, F1 is low.
B. Low in the mouth, F1 is high.
C. At the front of the mouth, F1 is low.
D. At the front of the mouth, F1 is high.

Teaching Points

Correct Answer: B

Tongue position determines the size of the pharynx and oral cavity. The pharynx is larger than the oral cavity and is therefore associated with F1. Tongue height is most strongly associated with pharynx size: When the tongue is pulled up toward the roof of the mouth, the air cavity in the pharynx is large and F1 is low; when the tongue is low in the mouth it occupies most of the space in the pharynx, leaving a small air pocket and resulting in a high F1.

C68

Augmentative and Alternative Communication (AAC)

A school-aged, pediatric patient with cerebral palsy has been brought to an outpatient augmentative communication clinic by their parents, in order to participate in a comprehensive augmentative and alternative communication (AAC) evaluation. According to the child's parents, the patient had been working with a Go Pro AAC system at school, but now that the school is on summer vacation, the school has mandated that the device be returned. The parents are now hoping to receive a device for use at home, in order to promote their child's communication. Which barrier to communication is this patient experiencing?

Choices:
A. Policy barrier.
B. Skill barrier.
C. Practice barrier.
D. Access barrier.

Teaching Points

Correct Answer: C

A practice barrier is a type of opportunity barrier (i.e., a barrier that is imposed by forces external to the AAC user) that has become commonplace in the environment. As the school district is preventing this pediatric client from utilizing the AAC device during the summer, this child is experiencing a practice barrier to communication. In contrast, a policy barrier is based on legislative decisions that govern specific environments, and a skill barrier is caused by facilitator difficulty implementing an AAC technique or strategy. Finally an access barrier is different from an opportunity barrier in that it is imposed by the limitations of the AAC user.

C69

The Practice of Speech-Language Pathology

A pharmaceutical company has approach a group of speech-language pathologists (SLPs) working in the school system regarding their new product "Speak Easy!" pills. The company claims that these pills are a cure for childhood apraxia of speech (CAS) and would like the SLPs to represent the products at the upcoming American Speech-Language-Hearing Association (ASHA) Convention. One of the SLPs is interested, as the SLP would like to earn extra money by representing the product. The SLP should first:

Choices:
A. Ask to see the research supporting the pill's effectiveness.
B. Try the pills with clients with CAS.
C. Approach his/her director for permission to be the representative.
D. Accept the position as representative for this product.

Teaching Points

Correct Answer: A

According to the ASHA Code of Ethics, Principle of Ethics III, Rule of Ethics G, "Individuals' statements to the public when advertising, announcing, and marketing their professional services; reporting research results; and promoting products shall adhere to professional standards and shall not contain misrepresentations." As the SLP does not know the research evidence behind the pills, the SLP's immediate promotion of the pills may constitute an unethical misrepresentation. If the research shows that the pills are effective, and do in fact cure CAS, the SLP can then make an appropriate informed decision about whether to promote the product or not. Trying the pills on their clients would also prove to be unethical, as the SLP does not have any information on the product.

C70

Cleft Palate and Other Craniofacial Anomalies

Following a complete otolaryngology (ENT) and speech-language pathology (SLP) evaluation after complaints of hypernasal speech, a child is diagnosed with a complete cleft of the primary palate. Which of the following structures would most likely **NOT** be affected by this type of cleft?

Choices:
A. Lip.
B. Hard palate.
C. Alveolar ridge.
D. Nasal sill.

Teaching Points

Correct Answer: B

Primary palate structures are those that are located anterior to the incisive foramen, including the lips, alveolar ridge and nasal sill. If this child was experiencing a complete cleft of the primary palate, there would be a full cleft extending from the lips to the incisive foramen. As such, the hard palate would remain intact with this type of cleft.

C71

Motor Speech Disorders

In working with a client with a diagnosis of apraxia of speech, the speech-language pathologist (SLP) acquires the following percentage of correct scores for spontaneous (without cueing) productions for one-, two- and three-syllable words targeting a specific transition involving the /s/: 98%, 68% and 15%. Using integral stimulation, the percentage correct for the same stimuli was 100%, 84% and 42%. Treatment should begin:

Choices:
A. With three-syllable words in the absence of any cueing, followed by the addition of tactile, visual and auditory cueing.
B. With one-syllable words in the absence of any cueing, followed by two-syllable words without cueing.
C. With two-syllable words in the presence of integral stimulation while gradually decreasing cueing.
D. With two-syllable words in the presence of integral stimulation.

Teaching Points

Correct Answer: C

Because this patient is highly intelligible at the spontaneous one-syllable level, beginning treatment at this level may lead to lower motivation for the participant, as there is not much room for improvement. However, as the patient has significantly reduced intelligibility at the two-syllable level and is stimulable to the use of cues at this level, they are an appropriate candidate to begin treatment by focusing on production of two-syllable words. As this skill builds and the patient is able to spontaneously produce intelligible utterances at the two-syllable level, treatment focus may transition to the three-syllable level.

C72

Dysphagia

A patient is in the later stages of amyotrophic lateral sclerosis (ALS). Which of the following treatment approaches is most appropriate for an individual at this stage of the disease?

Choices:
A. Enhancing the sensory capacities of the bolus.
B. Using postural adjustments.
C. Introduction of a percutaneous endoscopic gastrostomy (PEG) tube.
D. Oral range of motion exercises.

Teaching Points

Correct Answer: C

Amyotrophic lateral sclerosis is a neurodegenerative disease that affects both upper and lower motor neurons. Over the course of the disease, patients gradually lose their ability to engage in motor acts, such as walking, speaking and swallowing. In the later stages of the disease, there may be such a great loss of swallowing ability that patients may not be able to receive their nutrition and hydration orally, indicating the need for a PEG tube to be placed.

C73

Dysphagia

A speech-language pathologist (SLP) is working with a patient and observes signs at a bedside examination of potential penetration or aspiration. In order to accurately diagnose the presence of penetration or aspiration, which of the following instrumental assessment measures should be consulted?

Choices:
A. Modified barium swallow/video fluoroscopic swallow study (MBS/VFSS).
B. Esophageal manometry.
C. Cervical auscultation.
D. Ultrasound.

Teaching Points

Correct Answer: A

The MBS/VFSS is a radiographic assessment measure that allows an SLP to determine the presence of either penetration or aspiration. Additionally, the MBS allows the SLP to determine the depth of infiltrate using such measures as the Penetration-Aspiration Scale and can alert the SLP to when penetration or aspiration occurs (i.e., before, during or after the swallow).

C74

Spoken Language Disorders in Children

A speech-language pathologist (SLP) is considering dismissing a child from therapy services, as the SLP believes the child has made the maximum amount of progress possible. What is the MOST IMPORTANT factor to consider when dismissing a child from language therapy from a SLP perspective?

Choices:
A. The child has met all measurable goals and objectives set for him through language therapy.
B. The child is refusing to participate in further language treatment sessions.
C. The child's family has become tired of receiving language intervention.
D. The child is able to meet all communication demands for activities of daily living.

Teaching Points

Correct Answer: D

There are multiple factors that are interrelated when considering dismissal from therapy for language disorders. Among these factors is whether the child is able to meet all of the communication demands imposed through activities of daily living. From an SLP perspective, being able to demonstrate adequate language skills for daily life is the ultimate goal of treatment. Once a client has demonstrated this ability, this may be indicative of dismissal from therapy. In contrast, if the child has met all language goals, but is unable to meet the communicative needs of the activities of daily living, the child may benefit from further therapy sessions. Finally, if the child and family would not like to receive language intervention, this is also an important factor to consider, as SLPs are ethically bound to provide services that the family would like to receive, but this is not a factor from a speech and language perspective.

C75

Anatomy and Physiology of Communication and Swallowing

A patient who is experiencing nonfluent aphasia **MOST LIKELY** has some degree of cortical damage in Broca's area. This brain region is in which lobe?

Choices:
A. Frontal.
B. Temporal.
C. Parietal.
D. Occipital.

Teaching Points

Correct Answer: A

Broca's area can be found in the frontal lobes of the brain, in the inferior frontal gyrus. Refer to "Neuroanatomy and Neurophysiology for Speech, Language and Swallowing" from Chapter 1 of this text for more information and visualization of this structure.

C76

Spoken Language Disorders in Children

A speech-language pathologist (SLP) is working in a school setting and has many students that come from culturally and linguistically diverse (CLD) backgrounds. The SLP knows that there are many issues associated with CLD populations, including which of the following issues?

Choices:
A. The SLP should try to use English as much as possible in intervention.
B. There are no cultural difference that influence perception of gender.
C. Using English-language assessments predict language performance in other languages.
D. The SLP must respect the home culture and assist acculturation in the school.

Teaching Points

Correct Answer: D

An issue that arises for SLPs working with CLD populations includes respecting the home culture of any client and assisting with acculturation as needed. In contrast, SLPs should utilize interpreters as needed, which includes providing intervention in a client's language (i.e., one that may be different from English). Finally, English-language test instruments should not always be utilized and do not predict performance in any of the client's other languages.

C77

Cleft Palate and Other Craniofacial Anomalies

A speech-language pathologist (SLP) in an outpatient clinic had a child referred to them by an otolaryngologist (ENT). In the client's notes, the physician states that the client demonstrates problems that are not able to be corrected medically or surgically and that speech therapy is indicated for this child. Given this information, which deficit is this child **MOST LIKELY** demonstrating?

Choices:
A. Cul de sac resonance.
B. Nasal emission.
C. Pharyngeal fricative.
D. Hypernasality.

Teaching Points

Correct Answer: C

A production of a pharyngeal fricative is a type of compensatory articulation error often seen in individuals with velopharyngeal insufficiency. This type of articulatory error is an appropriate target for intervention through speech therapy. In contrast to this, speech therapy alone cannot improve hypernasality or nasal emission, and these problems require surgical intervention. Cul de sac resonance occurs due to a blockage in the pharyngeal or nasal cavity, which traps sound energy. No speech therapy technique can change the quality of resonance for this type of deficit, and surgery is required to remove the blockage (i.e., enlarged tonsils).

C78

Speech Sound Disorders in Children

A speech-language pathologist (SLP) is starting to work with a young child with a speech sound disorder. After reviewing the child's evaluation results, the SLP determines that the child is demonstrating errors in all word positions for the following phonemes: [l, t, g, a, v, w]. The SLP would like to utilize a treatment method that will simultaneously target the child's speech sound errors. Which intervention would this SLP **MOST LIKELY** implement?

Choices:
A. Sensory-motor approach.
B. Integral stimulation.
C. Minimal pairs approach.
D. Multiple phonemes approach.

Teaching Points

Correct Answer: D

The multiple phoneme approach was developed for children with multiple phoneme errors, such as the child in this scenario. The child is given simultaneous instruction on errored phonemes, although the child may be at different phase of learning for each errored phoneme. In contrast to this, integral stimulation is an intervention method that helps establish a single phoneme at a time and concentrates on productions of that phoneme. The sensory-motor approach stresses the production of bisyllable units and facilitative phonetic contexts to help in production of errored phonemes, but does not aid in simultaneous instruction of these phonemes. Finally, the minimal pairs method may be utilized when the child demonstrates homonymy in speech, but does not focus on establishment of errored speech sounds.

C79

Stuttering and Other Fluency Disorders

Zach, a 25-year-old man who stutters, has been in therapy off and on over the years. His therapist has consistently used a fluency shaping approach. In these sessions, Zach is able to make improvement in therapy but has trouble generalizing his fluent speech to his work and social settings. Together they decide to try an approach that uses more focus on stuttering modification. Which techniques are they likely to emphasize in this new treatment?

Choices:
A. Relationship focused therapy that addresses feelings and attitudes about communication and speaking.
B. Cancellation, speech modification.
C. Avoidance reduction.
D. All of the above.

Teaching Points

Correct Answer: D

All of the items listed are most often associated with traditional or stuttering modification approaches and less so with fluency shaping.

C80

The Practice of Speech-Language Pathology

Shannon and Stephanie are two speech-language pathologists (SLPs) who work in an outpatient speech and language clinic and are very close friends. Recently, Stephanie overheard Shannon discussing a client with another client's wife and is very distressed by what has happened. However, she is unsure how to handle the situation with her friend. What is the **BEST** way for Stephanie to handle the situation with Shannon?

Choices:
A. Give Shannon one more chance.
B. Report Shannon to the Board of Ethics.
C. Report Shannon to the client being discussed.
D. Discuss the incident directly with Shannon.

Teaching Points

Correct Answer: B

According to the ASHA Code of Ethics, Principle of Ethics IV, Rule of Ethics M, "Individuals who have reason to believe that the Code of Ethics has been violated shall inform the Board of Ethics." Because Shannon has violated the Code of Ethics and has shared client information without appropriate consent, Stephanie is ethically bound to report her friend to the Board of Ethics. At that time, the Board of Ethics will choose an appropriate sanction. While it is important that Stephanie also tell the client and discuss the violation with Shannon directly, she MUST tell the Board of Ethics, thus making this the most appropriate course of action.

C81

Acquired Language Disorders

A speech-language pathologist (SLP) in an outpatient aphasia clinic has decided to use constraint-induced language therapy (CILT) in a group session format. Why would this choice of treatment method, in theory, lead to improvements in a PWA's (person with aphasia's) language?

Choices:
A. The PWA is not allowed to use his/her "good," unimpaired limb when making a gestural response to describe pictures, thus forcing the person to learn gestures with the impaired limb.
B. The PWA is not allowed to use nonverbal means of communication, such as drawing, gesturing, or augmentative communication devices, when performing language tasks, thus forcing the person to use spoken language output.
C. The PWA is not allowed to use augmentative communication devices, but is allowed to use other nonverbal means of expression when performing language tasks, thus increasing the likelihood his/her message will be understood.
D. The PWA is not allowed to respond immediately, but is constrained to respond after delays of increasing length, starting with a 5-second delay, thus increasing the likelihood of the ability to respond appropriately at various times during conversation.

Teaching Points

Correct Answer: B

In constraint-induced language therapy, PWA must respond verbally when performing treatment tasks. Any nonverbal means of expression is not permitted, and a barrier is used to prevent the communication partner from seeing the PWA.

C82

Autism Spectrum Disorders

A speech-language pathologist (SLP) working in a preschool setting has been working with several children with autism spectrum disorder. This SLP believes the children would individually benefit from a social stories approach to intervention. The SLP develops individual stories for each child and is proceeding to implement the stories during intervention sessions. What is the next step that should be taken by this SLP?

Choices:
A. Read the stories only during the first intervention session to model an appropriate social response.
B. Read the stories repetitively during intervention sessions, to establish a social response.
C. Read the stories when the child demonstrates pragmatic difficulty to model an appropriate social response.
D. Send the stories home with the children, to allow their parents to model appropriate social responses.

Teaching Points

Correct Answer: B

In the social stories method of intervention, social skills are taught through a story format. Each story must be specific to the child and the child's problem situation. Once the stories are developed, it is important that they are read repetitively until it becomes a routine for the child. Following repetitive reading, the story may be sent home with the child for carryover purposes, but this should occur only after the child has been read the story multiple times.

C83

Language Acquisition

During a language evaluation, a child produces the utterance "The boy pushed the cars." How many free morphemes are there in this child's utterance?

Choices:
A. 2.
B. 3.
C. 4.
D. 5.

Teaching Points

Correct Answer: D

Free or unbound morphemes are those units of meaning that can stand alone in an utterance. In the sentence given, the additional morphemes ("-s" after car and "-ed" after push) cannot stand alone.

C84

Autism Spectrum Disorders

A 24-month-old male child has been brought into an outpatient speech and language clinic for a comprehensive evaluation. According to the parents, the child has recently begun demonstrating "strange" behaviors, and the parents believe the child may have autism spectrum disorder. Which of the following is **MOST LIKELY** a warning sign these parents witnessed?

Choices:
A. Unusual prosody in speech.
B. Lack of pointing to share interest.
C. Repetitive movement with objects.
D. Lack of response to his name.

Teaching Points

Correct Answer: B

There are several social communication warning signs for autism spectrum disorder, which can be observed at varying points in development. At 24 months, if children demonstrate a lack of pointing to share interest, this could be a warning sign of ASD. In contrast to this, unusual prosody in speech and repetitive movement with objects are warning signs for ASD often seen at 18 months. Finally, lack of response to a child's own name is a warning sign for ASD seen at 9–12 months.

C85

Acoustics

Nasal consonants have a low-frequency nasal formant because the nasal cavity acts as:

Choices:
A. A side cavity, resulting in a zero between F1 and F2.
B. A side cavity, resulting in a low-frequency F1.
C. The largest resonating cavity, resulting in a zero between F1 and F2.
D. The largest resonating cavity, resulting in a low-frequency F1.

Teaching Points

Correct Answer: D

In nasal consonants, the oral cavity acts as a side cavity (i.e., a resonating cavity with no direct connection to the outer air). The nasal cavity is the largest of the three resonating cavities in the supralaryngeal vocal tract (the pharynx, oral cavity and nasal cavity) so it has the lowest resonating frequency. Since air resonates in the nasal cavity during nasal consonants, F1 is at its lowest for nasal sounds.

C86

Acquired Language Disorders

A person with acute onset of aphasia whose first language is Spanish and who knows only a few words of English has been assigned to the caseload of a monolingual English-speaking speech-language pathologist (SLP) in a large urban medical center. The SLP should:

Choices:
A. Proceed as usual with the evaluation and use English-language tests and any Spanish-language tests available in the department.
B. Conduct an informal evaluation with the help of a multilingual friend or family member present who can translate what the SLP says and what the patient says.
C. Arrange to have a professional interpreter to be present during the evaluation and use the English-language tests he/she usually uses with the interpreter translating the items.
D. Explain to the patient and family that she or he must delay the evaluation until arrangements can be made to have another SLP who speaks Spanish conduct the evaluation.

Teaching Points

Correct Answer: C

It is recommended that SLPs use interpreter services whenever they are needed in conducting evaluations of people whose native language is not the same as the SLP's native language. Use of family members or friends as translators should be avoided, and the SLP should not attempt to use a test written in a language with which the patient is not proficient. The SLP should not delay the evaluation just because the native language of the patient is different. Timely and culturally appropriate assessment is important to quality patient care.

C87

Cleft Palate and Other Craniofacial Anomalies

A speech-language pathologist (SLP) in private practice has been working with a child for the past 6 months in order to correct the child's speech distortions. However, the child has made no progress over the course of treatment, and the SLP prepares a referral for otolaryngology (ENT) intervention. With which of the following distortions does this child **MOST LIKELY** present?

Choices:
A. Glottal stop.
B. Compensatory production.
C. Phoneme-specific nasality.
D. Obligatory distortion.

Teaching Points

Correct Answer: D

Obligatory distortions occur when there is normal articulatory placement but an abnormal structure (i.e., velopharyngeal insufficiency). It is likely that this child is experiencing obligatory distortions, as this type of error does not respond to speech therapy. However, compensatory articulation productions, phoneme-specific nasal emission and glottal stop are all forms of error that would see improvement through speech therapy. Therefore, it is unlikely that this child is demonstrating any of these error types.

C88

Augmentative and Alternative Communication (AAC)

Jessica is a patient who was recently admitted to an acute rehabilitation hospital. Her physician has requested a referral for speech-language pathology, for reasons of "communicative difficulties." After the speech-language pathologist performs an evaluation, he determines that while Jessica is a candidate for augmentative and alternative communication (AAC), she will likely require only temporary use of AAC. Which of the following conditions is Jessica **MOST LIKELY** experiencing?

Choices:
A. Intubation-induced vocal fold edema.
B. Severe Broca's aphasia.
C. Total glossectomy.
D. Amyotrophic lateral sclerosis.

Teaching Points

Correct Answer: A

Temporary use of AAC may be implemented for patients with conditions that are likely to alleviate or improve drastically. In intubation-induced vocal fold edema, the patient may present as aphonic, which may reduce the patient's communicative effectiveness. However, this condition typically improves within a few weeks and would require temporary means of AAC. In contrast to this, patients with severe Broca's aphasia, total glossectomy and ALS have chronic and/or degenerative communication problems and would likely benefit from permanent means of AAC to aid their communicative effectiveness.

C89

Motor Speech Disorders

A speech-language pathologist (SLP) has been working with a patient who has flaccid dysarthria. After many weeks of therapy, the SLP has decided to refer the patient for a palatal lift fitting. Adequate fitting of a palatal lift should result in which of the following outcomes for this patient?

Choices:
A. Occlusion of the nares during tidal breathing.
B. Improvements in phonation for sustained vowels.
C. Production of perceptually distinct nasal consonants.
D. Increase in nasal emissions during running speech.

Teaching Points

Correct Answer: C

Use of a palatal lift is a compensatory maneuver for weakness in the soft palate, which allows for the reduction of hypernasality and perception of distinct nasal and non-nasal phonemes. Use of a palatal lift does not fully occlude the nares during tidal breathing and allows for appropriate nasal breathing. Nasal emission should be decreased, due to the decrease in size of the velopharyngeal port. As a palatal lift does not directly affect the vocal folds, improvements in phonation would not occur from use of a lift alone.

C90

Autism Spectrum Disorders

Megan is a young child who demonstrates behaviors consistent with the triad of deficits seen in autism spectrum disorder. Specifically, Megan demonstrates severely restricted, repetitive behaviors. Which of the following is a behavior **MOST LIKELY** demonstrated by this child?

Choices:
A. Exaggerated gestures that accompany speech, to the point of interrupting communicative attempts from her parents.
B. Aversion of eye contact with parents and siblings to a degree that prohibits communication.
C. Prolonged sustained attention on a stuffed toy tiger, to the point of blocking out all communicative attempts from her parents.
D. Verbal perseveration of a favorite phrase, with very little other spontaneous verbal output.

Teaching Points

Correct Answer: C

Restricted, repetitive behaviors exhibited by children with autism spectrum disorder may come in the form of stereotyped or repetitive motor movement, insistence on sameness, inflexible adherence to routines, highly restricted interests and hypo-/hyper-reactivity to sensory input. Megan's prolonged sustained attention toward her stuffed tiger would be classified as a restricted, repetitive behavior as it is a highly restricted, fixated interest on a single item. This could be considered abnormal in intensity or focus. In contrast to this, exaggerated gestures accompanying speech and aversion of eye contact are considered deficits in social communication, whereas verbal perseveration is considered a language deficit.

C91

Language Acquisition

Following a comprehensive language evaluation, a 2-year-old child has been diagnosed as a "late talker." The characteristic that **BEST** describes this child is that she does not use at least:

Choices:
A. 25 different expressive vocabulary words.
B. 30 different expressive vocabulary words.
C. 45 different expressive vocabulary words.
D. 50 different expressive vocabulary words.

Teaching Points

Correct Answer: D

A child who is classified as a "late talker" is traditionally defined as child who has not demonstrated the use of 50 different expressive vocabulary words by the time the child has reached 24 months of age. As this child is 2 years old, the child fits the diagnosis of a late talker. If the child demonstrated less than 50 different words, this may be indicative of a language disorder.

C92

Dysphagia

A speech-language pathologist (SLP) is working with a patient with myasthenia gravis (MG) for the patient's presenting dysphagia. Knowing the symptoms of myasthenia gravis, what would be the **MOST LIKELY** effective method of intervention?

Choices:
A. A diet consisting of purees and thickened liquids.
B. Smaller meals eaten more frequently throughout the day.
C. Sensory stimulation (i.e., cold and sour bolus).
D. VitalStim therapy.

Teaching Points

Correct Answer: B

Myasthenia gravis is a lower motor neuron disorder characterized by exacerbated weakness with use and improvement with rest. Giving patients with MG smaller meals can reduce their fatigue, and increasing the amount of meals throughout the day ensures that these patients will receive the proper amount of nutrition and hydration.

C93

Spoken Language Disorders in Children

Adam is a child enrolled in a local preschool who has a language disorder. Adam's speech-language pathologist (SLP) has been targeting appropriate use of present progressive tense. During their sessions together, Adam has maintained 100% accuracy for trained targets, but has recently produced an appropriate form for an untrained target. Which form of generalization is Adam demonstrating with this type of production?

Choices:
A. Stimulus generalization.
B. Production generalization.
C. Response generalization.
D. Treatment generalization.

Teaching Points

Correct Answer: C

Response generalization refers to a child's production of untrained targets at the same or different linguistic level. As Adam from this scenario demonstrated the ability to produce untrained verbs using the present progressive tense, he is demonstrating response generalization. In contrast to this, stimulus generalization refers to a child's production of the same level of accuracy in an untrained setting, with new stimuli, or with a new clinician. If Adam's productions of trained stimuli would have occurred in his classroom, this could be considered stimulus generalization. Production generalization and treatment generalization are not forms of generalization associated with language disorder intervention.

C94

The Practice of Speech-Language Pathology

A speech-language pathologist (SLP) in private practice was recently reported for violating the American Speech-Language-Hearing Association (ASHA) Code of Ethics. ASHA has provided a sanction in which the SLP was officially rebuked, which was published to the membership of ASHA. Which sanction was leveled against this SLP?

Choices:
A. Reprimand.
B. Revocation.
C. Censure.
D. Withholding.

Teaching Points

Correct Answer: C

When an SLP has been censured, they have been sanctioned with a public reprimand, which is published to the membership of ASHA, such as the SLP in this scenario. If the SLP had received a private rebuke, this is known as a reprimand. Revocation occurs for serious violations, and membership/certification can be revoked for a year, years or life. Finally, withholding may be sanctioned to clinical fellows in violation and their ability to apply for the Certificate of Clinical Competence may be withheld for a period of years, up to life.

C95

Stuttering and Other Fluency Disorders

Katie is a 4-year-old girl. Her parents are concerned about her speech because she increasingly is hesitant to respond in preschool. She has shown disfluencies for the past year or so, although they never seemed to interfere with communication. Now, though, she seems to be holding her breath and closing her eyes when she has a moment of stuttering. Some of these blocks last more than 10 seconds. Her older sisters have begun to tease Katie. Which of the following statements is MOST ACCURATE?

Choices:
A. Katie and her parents should see a psychologist to help them cope with this problem.
B. Katie's secondary behaviors indicate that she is trying to control her stuttering.
C. Katie would definitely benefit from a more direct approach to treatment.
D. Because she is a girl, her risk for chronic stuttering is less. Therefore she doesn't need to be seen for treatment. Watch and wait is best.

Teaching Points

Correct Answer: B

Katie's secondary behaviors indicate that her stuttering is advancing and is a serious concern. Whenever a child has secondary behaviors it is important to think about the intervention needed. Regardless of the risk factors present, the stuttering behaviors (core and secondary) indicate the need for more careful evaluation and treatment by a SLP.

C96

Speech Sound Disorders in Children

After a speech and language evaluation, a speech-language pathologist (SLP) has diagnosed a 3-year-old client with an articulation disorder, characterized by difficulty producing the phonemes /l/, /r/, and /θ/. However, due to the client's young age, the SLP decides that this is an age-appropriate finding, as the child hasn't learned many sounds that "come before" the problem sounds. Which theory of development is this SLP MOST LIKELY using in their practice?

Choices:
A. Natural phonology theory.
B. Distinctive features theory.
C. Behavioral theory.
D. Interactionist-discovery theory.

Teaching Points

Correct Answer: B

According to the distinctive features theory, articulatory aspects of speech sounds are defined as binary feature contrasts (i.e., + or –) that are learned in hierarchical development. Because the SLP in the scenario has determined that earlier developing sounds have not yet been learned, it then follows that the child would not have learned later developing sounds, according to this theory. In contrast to this, the natural phonology theory dictates that children learn to repress the use of specific phonological processes. Behavioral theory views verbal development as learned using the processes of contingent reinforcement and stimulus-response, and as there is no mention of lack of reinforcement for this child, this would not be an appropriate selection. Finally, according to Interactionist-discovery theory, the child is an active learner in phonological development and discovers phonological patterns at any point in development.

C97

Audiology and Hearing Impairment

A patient arrives at an audiology clinic with complaints of difficulty hearing. The audiologist wishes to use a means of audiologic evaluation that allows a systematic visual inspection of the outer ear, surrounding tissue, external auditory meatus and tympanic membrane, in order to rule out problems with this portion of the hearing mechanism. Which means of evaluation should this audiologist utilize?

Choices:
A. Hearing screening.
B. Otoscopy.
C. Tympanometry.
D. Pure-tone audiometry.

Teaching Points

Correct Answer: B

Otoscopy is a type of audiologic evaluation that allows for a systematic inspection of the outer ear and surrounding tissue, external auditory meatus and tympanic membrane. This matches the wishes of the audiologist from this scenario and would likely be selected for evaluation of this patient. In contrast to this, a hearing screening is a tool utilized to assess if a patient may have a hearing loss and thus needs a full audiologic evaluation. Tympanometry assesses the integrity of the middle ear system. Finally, pure-tone (air and bone conduction) audiometry evaluates types, severity and configuration of the hearing loss.

C98

Augmentative and Alternative Communication (AAC)

A speech-language pathologist (SLP) has been asked to perform an evaluation on a patient with a neurodegenerative communication disorder with very limited verbal output. Following assessment, it is also revealed that the patient is not literate and greatly struggles with any literacy-based material. Which approach to intervention would be **BEST** for this patient's needs?

Choices:
A. The patient will benefit from intervention targeting cognitive, rather than communicative, skills.
B. The patient will not be an appropriate candidate for AAC due to deficits in literacy.
C. The patient can use alphabet supplementation following intense instruction in phoneme/grapheme association.
D. The patient can use an AAC device that utilizes symbolic representations of words and phrases.

Teaching Points

Correct Answer: D

Persons with complex communication needs (CCN) do not need to be literate in order to be eligible for AAC use. If a patient is not literate, a speech-language pathologist may utilize symbolic representations that aid in the person's communicative effectiveness, similar to this scenario. As this patient was not interested in literacy-based approaches, direct instruction in phoneme-grapheme association would be contraindicated. Lastly, if a patient is referred for AAC, communication should be directly targeted and cognitive skills may also be targeted during intervention sessions.

C99

Acoustics

The speech-language pathologist (SLP) is examining a spectrogram and waveform for the initial sounds in a child's production of the word *spaghetti*. The waveform begins with a silence followed by a transient noise. In the spectrogram, the transient noise is followed by formants, then by high-amplitude, high-frequency continuant noise. When listening to the word, the SLP expects to hear that the child:

Choices:
A. Produced the initial part of the word normally.
B. Metathesized /s/ and /p/.
C. Produced /s/ as /f/.
D. Produced /p/ as /m/.

Teaching Points

Correct Answer: B

A silence followed by a transient noise indicates a stop manner of articulation; therefore, the word begins with a stop. Formants indicate a resonant sound such as a vowel. Continuant noise is a characteristic of fricatives, and high-amplitude, high-frequency continuant noise is characteristic of /s/. Therefore, the sequence in the child's production is stop-vowel-/s/, while the expected sequence is /s/-stop-vowel. If /s/ were produced as /f/, then the frication noise would be low amplitude with no high-frequency peak. If /p/ were produced as /m/, then there would be no silence or transient noise.

C100

Anatomy and Physiology of Communication and Swallowing

Cranial nerves can include motor functions, sensory functions, or a mix of both. Which of the following cranial nerves (CN) serve both motor and sensory functions?

Choices:
A. CN V, CN IX, CN X.
B. CN V, CN XI, CN XII.
C. CN III, CN IX, CN X.
D. CN III, CN X, CN XII.

Teaching Points

Correct Answer: A

The cranial nerves that are responsible for both motor movements and sensory information are V (trigeminal), VII (facial), IX (glossopharyngeal) and X (vagus). The other cranial nerves are responsible for either sensory information or motor movement, but not both.

C101

The Practice of Speech-Language Pathology

Speech-language pathologists (SLPs) are required to gain knowledge of the nature of communication disorders, differences and swallowing disorders in the "big 9" areas of practice. Which of the following is not one of the big 9?

Choices:
A. Voice and resonance.
B. Communication modalities.
C. Research and research methods.
D. Hearing.

Teaching Points

Correct Answer: C

The big 9 areas of speech-language pathology practice include: articulation, fluency, voice and resonance (including respiration and phonation); receptive and expressive language (phonology, morphology, syntax, semantics and pragmatics) in speaking/listening/reading/writing/and manual modalities; hearing (including impact on speech and language); swallowing (including all phases of the swallow, oral function for feeding and orofacial myofunction); cognitive aspects of communication (attention, memory, sequencing, problem-solving and executive functioning); social aspects of communication (challenging behavior, ineffective social skills, lack of communication opportunities); and communication modalities (oral, manual, augmentative and alternative communication techniques and assistive technologies).

C102

Dysphagia

A patient has arrived at an acute rehabilitation hospital having been made "non per os" (NPO) at the acute care setting. Following the patient's bedside examination, the speech-language pathologist (SLP) decides to continue keeping the patient NPO. Which of the following is the **MOST APPROPRIATE** treatment approach for the SLP to engage in?

Choices:
A. Therapeutic trials of ice chips.
B. Aggressive oral hygiene.
C. Therapeutic trials of honey-thick liquids.
D. Administration of parenteral nutrition.

Teaching Points

Correct Answer: A

While working with patients who have PEG tubes falls within the SLP's scope of practice, administering parenteral nutrition is not a treatment approach that an SLP would take. While providing aggressive oral hygiene is an important precaution, it is not a treatment method and does not improve the symptoms of dysphagia. Finally, patients who are made NPO are at a significant risk for aspirating food and drink items. While honey-thick liquids may eventually be an appropriate goal, treatment for NPO patients should begin with administration of ice chips in order to minimize the chances of aspiration pneumonia if aspiration does occur.

C103

Acquired Language Disorders

A patient who had a stroke was referred for a language and cognitive evaluation. The referral specifically mentioned that the man had trouble with "Theory of Mind" tasks, indicating he had difficulty understanding what another person's beliefs or thoughts might be. In which adult diagnostic groups would deficits of Theory of Mind be categorized?

Choices:
A. Alzheimer's disease in the early stage.
B. Wernicke's or conduction aphasia.
C. Parkinson's disease and dementia.
D. Right-hemisphere strokes.

Teaching Points

Correct Answer: D

Deficits in Theory of Mind are associated with damage to the right hemisphere in adult stroke patients. None of the other diagnostic groups listed are known to display difficulties with Theory of Mind tasks to the same extent as right-hemisphere stroke patients.

C104

Acquired Language Disorders

A speech-language pathologist (SLP) is asked to evaluate a newly admitted patient, who has suffered from a diagnosed left middle cerebral artery (MCA) stroke. Knowing that assessment of auditory comprehension in adults with acquired disorders is an important part of any comprehensive language evaluation, the SLP wants to get a detailed profile of the patient's auditory comprehension abilities. In order to develop results for an assessment of auditory comprehension, the SLP could use which of the following methods?

Choices:
A. Asking the person to respond to yes/no questions presented in pairs, such as "Is your name Alice?" followed later by "Is your name Amy?"
B. Asking the person to answer open-ended autobiographical questions about the person's name and address, such as "Where do you live?"
C. Asking the person to follow commands that include naming objects, such as "Tell me what this is called."
D. Asking the person to produce automatic spoken sequences, such as "Count from 1 to 10."

Teaching Points

Correct Answer: A

When assessing auditory comprehension, the SLP should avoid tasks that are also dependent on other language abilities such as verbal expression that might be impaired as well. Therefore, the scenario most likely to yield reliable information about auditory comprehension is one in which the individual does not have to respond verbally.

C105

Voice Disorders

A patient arrives at the hospital, with complaints of sudden onset of voice loss. During the intake interview, the patient utilizes writing to convey to the speech-language pathologist (SLP) that she was cheering at her son's high school football game when suddenly she was not able to phonate above a whisper. Which diagnosis is the **MOST LIKELY** presenting problem?

Choices:
A. Vocal fold hemorrhage.
B. Laryngitis.
C. Vocal fold ectasia.
D. Vocal fold bowing.

Teaching Points

Correct Answer: A

Vocal fold hemorrhage, or bleeding into the vocal fold tissues, is often associated with a single, phonotraumatic episode. When the person experiencing the hemorrhage participates in excessive vocally abusive behaviors, a blood vessel in the vocal fold tissues may rupture, causing the hemorrhage. Vocal fold varices and ectasias may predispose the patient to experience vocal fold hemorrhage, as these are vascular structures not normally present on the vocal fold tissues. Laryngitis, vocal fold ectasias and vocal fold bowing would not occur after a single, isolated incident and are not the appropriate diagnosis for this patient.

C106

Spoken Language Disorders in Children

James is a high school student who has been referred to a speech-language pathologist (SLP) for assessment of language and executive functioning skills. During the initial interview, James tells the SLP that he has significant difficulties making friends and has not been able to hold down a job. Following the assessment, the SLP notes that James presents with significant impairments in recognizing safe and unsafe behaviors. Utilizing this information, James **MOST LIKELY** presents with which of the following difficulties?

Choices:
A. Cognitive disability.
B. Autism spectrum disorder.
C. Spina bifida.
D. Cerebral palsy.

Teaching Points

Correct Answer: A

The American Association on Intellectual and Developmental Disabilities defines a cognitive disability as a limitation in at least two of the following areas: communication, self-care, home living, social skills, community use, self-direction, health and safety, functional academics, leisure and work. As James has stated that he has difficulty making friends (i.e., social skills) and has difficulty holding down a job (i.e., difficulty with work), he most likely presents with a cognitive disability. In contrast to this, there is no strict association of work difficulties or safety deficits in the populations of autism spectrum disorder, spina bifida, or cerebral palsy.

C107
Language Acquisition

Charlie is a 3-year-old boy who is having trouble communicating with others. At school he has a habit of interrupting and seems rude. His mother says his speech is clear, but he has trouble getting to the point of his message, making his intentions hard to understand. Which of the following BEST describes the language area in which he is having the most problems?

Choices:
A. Morphology.
B. Semantics.
C. Gestural.
D. Pragmatics.

Teaching Points

Correct Answer: D

Charlie's behaviors indicate difficulty using the social rules of communication, rather than trouble with the grammar (syntax) or meaning (semantic) levels of language. There was no description of gesturing in this question.

C108
Audiology and Hearing Impairment

A person in the community with hearing loss refers to herself as being culturally deaf and uses American Sign Language (ASL) as the primary means of communication. Which of the following statements BEST describes this person?

Choices:
A. The person is capital *D* Deaf.
B. The person is audiometrically deaf.
C. The person is hard of hearing.
D. The person is hearing impaired.

Teaching Points

Correct Answer: A

Capital "D" Deaf refers to persons who identify as culturally deaf, who would typically make use of ASL and are proud to be deaf, such as the person from this scenario. In contrast to this, audiometrically deaf refers to the most significant hearing sensitivity challenge based solely on audiologic testing (profound hearing loss). Hard of hearing and hearing impairment are terms currently used in U.S. federal legislation to describe children and adults with any degree of hearing sensitivity deficits/differences.

C109
Autism Spectrum Disorders

A speech-language pathologist (SLP) is working with a group of school-aged children diagnosed with autism spectrum disorder. The SLP would like to set appropriate pragmatic goals for the children, while utilizing a social communication group approach. Which of the following pragmatic goals is of **GREATEST BENEFIT** for use with these children?

Choices:
A. Sharing interests with other group members.
B. Generating polite requests and responses.
C. Determining appropriate questions for other group members.
D. Understanding other group members' feelings.

Teaching Points

Correct Answer: A

School-age children require pragmatic skills consistent with peer interaction. For this age group, pragmatic goals include considering others' feelings, sharing interests, expressing preferences politely and shared attention. In contrast to this, generating polite requests would be an appropriate pragmatic goal for younger children, while determining appropriate questions and understanding others' feelings would be an appropriate pragmatic goal for adolescents and adults.

C110
Acquired Language Disorders

A speech-language pathologist (SLP) in an inpatient rehabilitation hospital is working with a patient who displays the following symptoms: poor ability to explain the meaning of metaphorical language, inability to produce a melody when asked to sing, hemiplegia, tendency to bump into items on the patient's left side when using a wheelchair. These are diagnostic characteristics of:

Choices:
A. A large brainstem stroke.
B. A left-hemisphere cerebrovascular accident (CVA).
C. Dementia with Lewy bodies.
D. A right-hemisphere CVA.

Teaching Points

Correct Answer: D

The constellation of symptoms described in the patient profile is characteristic of someone with damage to the right hemisphere, i.e., difficulty with metaphorical language, poor ability to produce and comprehend melodies and visual neglect of items in the left visual field. While hemiplegia may be the result of a right- or left-hemisphere CVA, the other symptoms are more likely only in a right-hemisphere CVA.

C111

Acquired Language Disorders

A speech-language pathologist (SLP) at an acute rehabilitation hospital has completed an evaluation on a recently admitted patient who had sustained a stroke a week earlier. According to the SLP's findings, this patient is exhibiting symptoms associated with deep dyslexia. This patient would display which of the following symptoms?

Choices:
A. Verbal production of semantically related words in oral reading (e.g., reading aloud the word *vehicle* as "car") and inability to read nonwords.
B. Production of phonologically relayed words in oral reading (e.g., reading aloud the word *carpet* as "carpenter").
C. Inability to read words presented visually, with intact ability to read through other modalities such as traced letters on the skin.
D. Severe agraphia and difficulty reading any written material.

Teaching Points

Correct Answer: A

Deep dyslexia is characterized by inability to use the grapheme-phoneme conversion rules when reading text; rather, only the "whole word" recognition route is available. People tend to make semantically related paragraphic errors when reading text aloud and cannot read nonwords at all.

C112

Stuttering and Other Fluency Disorders

Mrs. Lyons is a 55-year-old teacher in a large urban school district. She was recently forced to transfer to a different school because of reorganization. The new school has a history of conflict with parents and students, takes an extra hour of commute time for Mrs. Lyons, and she is sad about leaving her friends at the former school. While teaching, Mrs. Lyons notes that she is starting to stutter and she is frustrated and angry. When students laugh, she notes that it gets worse. When she comes for an evaluation, she responds immediately to cues provided by the speech-language pathologist (SLP) and her speech is fluent. Which of the following is **MOST ACCURATE**?

Choices:
A. Mrs. Jones probably is exhibiting psychogenic stuttering.
B. Mrs. Jones is a developmental stutterer.
C. The SLP should help advocate for Mrs. Jones to return to her old school.
D. Mrs. Jones should be referred to a psychiatrist right away.

Teaching Points

Correct Answer: A

The onset of disfluency associated with significant stress is most likely psychogenic. Because the onset is in adulthood, it rules out developmental stuttering. The focus in SLP should be on helping Mrs. Jones recover her fluent speech. If her psychological difficulties were significant, ideally, Mrs. Jones might benefit from a referral and some coordination of treatment between the mental health professional and the SLP.

C113

Voice Disorders

A patient is admitted to an acute care hospital after having a cerebrovascular accident (CVA). Imaging shows that the stroke affected function of the pharyngeal nerve. Which of the following voice problems would this patient **MOST LIKELY** experience?

Choices:
A. Strained vocal quality.
B. Aphonia.
C. Breathy vocal quality.
D. Hypernasal vocal quality.

Teaching Points

Correct Answer: D

The pharyngeal nerve is a branch of the vagus nerve that innervates the soft palate. If this nerve is damaged, the soft palate would become weak and would not effectively close off the nasal cavity during phonation. The effect would be air escape through the nasal cavity during phonation, causing hypernasal vocal quality. As the pharyngeal nerve does not innervate the vocal folds (i.e., the vocal folds are innervated by the recurrent and superior laryngeal nerves), breathy vocal quality, strained vocal quality and aphonia would not result from lesions of this nerve.

C114

Cleft Palate and Other Craniofacial Anomalies

A speech-language pathologist (SLP) in private practice is receiving a new client in the clinic for treatment of a speech sound disorder. Upon reading the child's intake forms, the SLP notes that the child has previously been diagnosed with pronounced micrognathia, glossoptosis and hearing loss. Given these specific characteristics, this child **MOST LIKELY** demonstrates which disorder?

Choices:
A. Treacher Collins syndrome.
B. Beckwith-Wiedemann syndrome.
C. Van der Woude syndrome.
D. Opitz G syndrome.

Teaching Points

Correct Answer: A

Treacher Collins syndrome includes lack of clefts, specific craniofacial features (i.e., micrognathia, glossoptosis, etc.) and a functional concern of hearing loss. Beckwith-Wiedemann syndrome, Van der Woude syndrome and Optiz G syndrome include specific craniofacial features, but do not include hearing loss as a functional concern. When hearing loss is present, this is highly indicative of Treacher Collins syndrome.

C115

Augmentative and Alternative Communication (AAC)

An elderly patient with primary progressive aphasia and his wife have been working with a speech-language pathologist in order to implement an appropriate augmentative and alternative communication (AAC) system to facilitate the patient's communication. However, the patient's wife does not understand AAC and has not been able to adequately perform partner-assisted scanning, despite large amounts of training. What type of barrier is this patient facing?

Choices:
A. Access barrier.
B. Skill barrier.
C. Knowledge barrier.
D. Attitude barrier.

Teaching Points

Correct Answer: B
A skill barrier is a form of opportunity barrier (i.e., one caused by forces external to the AAC user) that is caused by facilitator difficulty implementing an AAC technique. As the patient's wife is demonstrating significant difficulty with implementing her husband's AAC strategies, the patient is experiencing a skill barrier to communication. In contrast to this, a knowledge barrier is caused by a lack of information on the part of the facilitator for person with complex communication needs (CCN), and an attitude barrier is caused by incorrect, outdated, outmoded, or discriminatory attitudes regarding the abilities of people with CCN. Finally, an access barrier is a communicative barrier caused by limitations of the person with CCN.

C116

Acoustics

Compared to voiced stops, word-initial voiceless stops in English are expected to have a:

Choices:
A. Shorter voice onset time (VOT).
B. Longer VOT.
C. More compact spectrum.
D. More diffuse spectrum.

Teaching Points

Correct Answer: B
VOT duration distinguishes voiced and voiceless stops, with voiceless stops having longer VOTs, especially in word-initial position. A compact vs. diffuse spectrum distinguishes stop place of articulation, with bilabial stops having diffuse falling spectra, alveolar stops having diffuse rising spectra, and velar stops having compact spectra.

C117

Anatomy and Physiology of Communication and Swallowing

Following a motor vehicle accident, an individual is experiencing complete paralysis of the upper and lower extremities. A magnetic resonance imaging (MRI) scan reveals damage to the lateral corticospinal tract in the spinal column. The lateral corticospinal tract is:

Choices:
A. An ascending pathway that conveys motor signals that control movement of the arms and legs.
B. A descending pathway that conveys motor signals that control movement of the arms and legs.
C. An ascending pathway that conveys motor signals that control movement of all trunk musculature.
D. A descending pathway that conveys motor signals that control movement of all trunk musculature.

Teaching Points

Correct Answer: B

The lateral corticospinal tract begins as a descending motor pathway (from the cerebral hemispheres into the spinal column) in the cerebral hemispheres. Eighty-five percent of the fibers decussate in the medulla and form the lateral corticospinal tract, which is responsible for control of the upper and lower extremities. The 15% that does not decussate forms the anterior corticospinal tract, which is responsible for motor control of trunk/girdle muscles.

C118

Written Language Disorders in the School-Age Population

Two grade-school children are referred to a speech-language pathologist (SLP) for a comprehensive diagnostic assessment of their literacy abilities. A basic literacy assessment should consider the children's:

Choices:
A. Reading/writing skills, cultural context and articulation abilities.
B. Underlying spoken language skills, vocal quality and reading/writing skills.
C. Reading/writing skills, underlying cognitive processing skills and cultural context.
D. Underlying spoken language skills, reading/writing skills and cultural context.

Teaching Points

Correct Answer: D

Key areas that should be addressed during a literacy assessment include underlying spoken language skills (i.e., skills and metalinguistic awareness in morphology, syntax, semantics and discourse), reading and writing skills (i.e., accuracy and automaticity in these skill areas) and cultural context (i.e., extrinsic factors associated with literacy learning). Additionally, underlying processing skills should be assessed, which includes phonological awareness, phonological short-term memory, working memory, rapid naming, visual/orthographic processing, attention and executive functioning.

C119

Stuttering and Other Fluency Disorders

In evaluating an adult who stutters, a speech-language pathologist (SLP) uses a conversational speech sample and an attitudinal survey about communication. She decides not to record the session so as not to make the client more nervous. What's wrong with this approach?

Choices:
A. It would have been better to use a standardized test to assess this person's speech.
B. Attitudinal surveys are not helpful communication assessment measures.
C. There is nothing wrong with this approach; recording isn't really necessary.
D. Failure to record the sample makes reliability assessment and further analysis impossible.

Teaching Points

Correct Answer: D
Recording speech samples allows for determination of the types of disfluencies present and their frequency (i.e., per 100 words), units of repetition and prolongation, and any secondary behaviors or word avoidances. As the SLP from this case did not utilize recording devices during the assessment of the adult from this scenario, the SLP is unable to perform a reliable assessment of the disfluencies present.

C120

Motor Speech Disorders

To facilitate performance in the speech of a 4-year-old with childhood apraxia of speech (CAS), the clinician instructs the child to produce a word produced incorrectly a second time. Before the clinician had the child repeat the word again, specific feedback was provided regarding how to produce the movement more successfully. What type of feedback was provided?

Choices:
A. Blocked practice.
B. Knowledge of performance.
C. Variable practice.
D. Knowledge of results.

Teaching Points

Correct Answer: B
Knowledge of performance (KP) consists of specific feedback provided to the patient following practice (i.e., the production of a sound) regarding the quality of the motor behavior. Because this patient was given specific feedback on how to improve the speech sound from the faulty production, this constitutes feedback to the quality of the motor movements. This is in contrast to knowledge of results (KR) in which feedback is given to the degree of success in achieving a motor behavior.

C121

Written Language Disorders in the School-Age Population

A speech-language pathologist (SLP) is tutoring a teenager who is writing a report for her science class. The student's difficulties with setting her goals and organizing an approach to her writing are consistent with deficits in which component area of writing?

Choices:
A. Translating.
B. Planning.
C. Reviewing.
D. Spelling.

Teaching Points

Correct Answer: B

Planning includes the ability to set goals for the writing product, organize a plan, and monitor plans being formulated. As this child demonstrates difficulties with setting goals and organizing plans for her report, she is exhibiting deficits in planning for writing.

C122

Anatomy and Physiology of Communication and Swallowing

Contraction of the tensor veli palatini and levator veli palatini will **NOT** occur during the production of which of the following sounds?

Choices:
A. /f/.
B. /s/.
C. /m/.
D. /t/.

Teaching Points

Correct Answer: C

The tensor veli palatini and levator veli palatini muscles contract to raise the soft palate during speech in order to block off the nasal cavity. The /m/ is a nasal phoneme, which means that the nasal cavity remains open during phonation. For this reason, the tensor veli palatini and levator veli palatini do not contract during production of /m/.

C123

Cleft Palate and Other Craniofacial Anomalies

A child is referred to an otolaryngology (ENT) and speech-language pathology (SLP) clinic at an acute care hospital after experiencing multiple episodes of nasal regurgitation in addition to significantly hypernasal speech. Upon full evaluation, it is found that the child has difficulty with elevation and retraction of the velum. Given these problems, this child is **MOST LIKELY** experiencing deficits in which of the following muscles?

Choices:
A. Tensor veli palatini.
B. Musculus uvulae.
C. Palatoglossus.
D. Levator veli palatini.

Teaching Points

Correct Answer: D
The levator veli palatini is the muscle that provides the main muscle mass of the velum. Its functions include velar elevation and retraction in a 45-degree angle and formation of the velar dimple. If the child was experiencing deficits within this muscle, he/she would have problems with velar elevation and retraction. Contrary to this muscle, the tensor veli palatini opens the eustachian tubes, the palatoglossus depresses the velum, and the musculus uvulae contracts during phonation to create a superior velar bulge.

C124

Research, Evidence-Based Practice, and Tests and Measurements

A speech-language pathologist (SLP) has finished analyzing the data collected during his research study and has found that the p value is 0.04. Due to this level of statistical significance, the SLP may decide to reject which of the following?

Choices:
A. Hypothesis.
B. Null hypothesis.
C. Means of analysis.
D. Conclusion.

Teaching Points

Correct Answer: B
The null hypothesis is a statement that expresses belief that no change will occur. Because this SLP has found statistical significance (i.e., $p < 0.05$), the SLP is able to demonstrate that some amount of change has occurred. As this is a direct contrast to "no change will occur," the SLP may confidently reject the null hypothesis for his/her research. In contrast, if the SLP did not demonstrate statistical significance, he/she would have to reject the hypothesis, as there truly would be no change made.

C125

Spoken Language Disorders in Children

A speech-language pathologist (SLP) working in an outpatient speech and language clinic has been asked to evaluate a new client who was referred with a language disorder. However, when the SLP reads the client's intake forms, he notices that the child comes from a culturally diverse background. The SLP has never worked with someone from this cultural background and would like to take an alternative route in assessment. Which is the **BEST** method of assessment for this SLP to utilize?

Choices:
A. Processing-dependent assessment.
B. Curriculum-based assessment.
C. Diadochokinetic assessment.
D. Standardized assessment.

Teaching Points

Correct Answer: A

Many standardized assessment measures are inappropriate to administer to children from these populations, as there may be content bias (i.e., the assessment reflects the assumption that all populations have the same life experiences, concepts and vocabulary), linguistic bias (i.e., disparity between the language used by the examiner and child), or a disproportionate representation in the normative sample. Processing-dependent assessment includes methods such as testing digit span, working memory or nonword repetition and is most appropriate because it is minimally dependent on prior knowledge. In contrast to this, curriculum-based assessment may require a level of background knowledge that the child does not have to perform at his/her true potential. Finally, diadochokinetic assessment is a form of assessment for speech sound intervention and measures the rate of syllable repetition.

C126

Augmentative and Alternative Communication (AAC)

A speech-language pathologist (SLP) in private practice has been assigned to evaluate a new patient, who has recently moved into the area. After reading the patient's intake file, the SLP realizes that the patient has been utilizing an augmentative and alternative communication (AAC) device for communicative purposes for the last few years. The description of the patient's AAC device is as follows "a functional computer that utilizes communicative software. The patient is also able to utilize the Internet on their device and has few gaming apps for personal enjoyment." Which statement **BEST** describes this patient's AAC device?

Choices:
A. The patient is utilizing a mid-tech, nondedicated AAC device.
B. The patient is utilizing a no-tech, dedicated AAC device.
C. The patient is utilizing a high-tech, nondedicated AAC device.
D. The patient is utilizing a low-tech, dedicated AAC device.

Teaching Points

Correct Answer: C

High-tech AAC refers to more sophisticated electronic devices that support speech and/or written output. As the patient from this scenario is utilizing a functional computer for communicative purposes, the patient is most likely utilizing high-tech AAC. Additionally, nondedicated AAC refers to devices that support a range of functions in addition to speech output. As this patient utilizes their AAC device for the Internet and for gaming apps, they are utilizing a nondedicated device.

C127

Spoken Language Disorders in Children

Jennifer is a middle-school student who was diagnosed with Fragile-X syndrome at birth and presents with language difficulties typically associated with Fragile-X syndrome. Which of the following treatment areas would be of **GREATEST BENEFIT** for the SLP to target in working with Jennifer?

Choices:
A. Executive functions and semantic skills.
B. Semantic skills and syntactic skills.
C. Auditory skills and pragmatic skills.
D. Pragmatic skills and reading skills.

Teaching Points

Correct Answer: C

Children with Fragile-X syndrome present with language difficulties in syntactic development, organization, auditory memory, fluency and prosody. For this reason, the most appropriate targets for the SLP to choose in working with Jennifer would be auditory skills (i.e., targeting auditory memory) and pragmatic skills (i.e., fluency and prosody). In contrast to this, semantic skills, receptive language and visual skills are a relative strength for this population and would not be most appropriate for target selection.

C128

Anatomy and Physiology of Communication and Swallowing

There are several parts of a neuron that are important in the transmission of neural signals throughout the body. Which of the following components is **MOST IMPORTANT** for receiving signals from other neurons?

Choices:
A. Soma.
B. Dendrite.
C. Axon.
D. Phospholipid bilayer.

Teaching Points

Correct Answer: B

Dendrites are the part of the neuron that are important in receiving action potentials from other neurons. The soma is the term for the cell body of the neuron, whereas the axon is the portion of the neuron that is important for propagation of action potentials to future neurons.

C129

Speech Sound Disorders in Children

Following a comprehensive speech sound evaluation, a speech-language pathologist (SLP) is beginning to select specific sound error patterns to target in intervention with a pediatric client aged 3;4 years. The SLP understands that there are multiple factors to consider when choosing treatment targets. Which of the following selections is appropriate to utilize when selecting treatment targets for this client?

Choices:
A. The child has difficulty producing a speech sound that typically develops at age 6;0 years, so this sound should not be targeted as it is not age appropriate.
B. The child is not stimulable for a specific speech sound that is in error, so this speech sound should be targeted as it would likely not improve independently.
C. The child demonstrates "later occurring" phonological errors, so this child does not need to participate in speech therapy at this time.
D. The child is stimulable for specific speech sounds in error, so these speech sounds should be targeted as the child would likely not improve independently.

Teaching Points

Correct Answer: B

Several factors are important in choosing treatment targets for intervention. One such factor is stimulability. Sounds that are stimulable for production most often remediate on their own and do not require intervention. However, those that are unstimulable may be direct targets for intervention, as these sounds are not likely to remediate independently. In contrast, when discussing the factor of age, there has been work that shows targeting later developing sounds (i.e., those more "age advanced" for children) may allow generalization to errored, age-appropriate sounds. Finally, as the child is demonstrating a speech sound error, they are a candidate for speech therapy, which should begin as soon as possible and not when the child has matured.

C130

Spoken Language Disorders in Children

Erica is a young child who demonstrates pragmatic difficulties. Specifically, Erica has difficulties with presupposition skills, which her speech-language pathologist (SLP) has been targeting in order to improve Erica's conversational abilities. Which of the following would be the MOST APPROPRIATE goal for Erica's intervention?

Choices:
A. The child will utilize gestures in conversation to reinforce engaging topics of conversation.
B. The child will understand that communication partners have perspectives and feelings different from her own.
C. The child will modify communicative attempts based on the needs of her communication partner.
D. The child will understand that communicative partners engage in conversation with certain expectation for communication.

Teaching Points

Correct Answer: C

Presupposition is a skill that involves judging what the listener already knows and making appropriate accommodations to facilitate successful communication. By targeting this ability, the child may have a better understanding of what her conversation partner requires for successful intervention. In contrast to this, Theory of Mind deals with understanding conversation partners have differing perspectives and feelings. Joint action routine is a skill that aids in establishing predictable roles and expectations for conversation. Finally, using gestures to reinforce topics of conversation may engage speakers more in conversation, but does not necessarily equate to a change in conversation based on the needs of the communicative partner.

C131

Autism Spectrum Disorders

Cameron is a speech-language pathologist (SLP) who is working with a young child recently diagnosed with autism spectrum disorder (ASD). Cameron believes that this child would benefit from the use of a Floortime approach to intervention. In order to **BEST** implement this treatment approach, Cameron should:

Choices:
A. Teach the child social skills through a story-time format.
B. Establish a reciprocal communication system for the child.
C. Engage in a play-based activity with the child and an age-matched peer.
D. Engage in a semistructured play activity that interests the child.

Teaching Points

Correct Answer: D
When utilizing the Floortime approach of intervention for ASD, the SLP would engage the child in a spontaneous, interactive, pleasurable activity with the child, while following the child's leads and interests. This would be completed in a semistructured play scenario. In contrast to this, teaching children with ASD social skills through stories would be utilized in the social stories intervention approach. Picture Exchange Communication System (PECS) is a reciprocal communication system, in which the child exchanges pictures for desired objects. Finally, matching the child with ASD with an age-matched peer would be utilized in the peer and play mediation intervention approach.

C132

Anatomy and Physiology of Communication and Swallowing

Dopamine is a neurotransmitter that plays an important role in neural signals involved in motor movement. Lack of dopamine in the substantia nigra has been associated with disease processes such as Parkinson's disease. What **BEST** describes the role of dopamine on basal ganglia circuits?

Choices:
A. Dopamine is excitatory to the direct and indirect pathways of the basal ganglia.
B. The net result of dopamine release to direct and indirect pathways of the basal ganglia is a facilitation of movement.
C. The net result of dopamine release to the direct pathway facilitates movement while release to the indirect pathway inhibits movement.
D. Dopamine is inhibitory to the direct and indirect pathways of the basal ganglia.

Teaching Points

Correct Answer: B
The net result of dopamine release into the basal ganglia control circuits is facilitation of movement, although the effect is different depending on which pathway is activated. Activation of the direct activation pathway assists with excitation of movement, whereas activation of the indirect activation pathway assists with inhibition of movement.

Index

Note: *b* indicates box; *f*, figure; and *t*, table.

A

AAC. *See* Augmentative and alternative communication (AAC)
Abdominal cavity, 5, 5*f*
Achalasia, 380
Acoustic assessment, in voice disorders, 357
Acoustic measures, of voice production, 346–347
Acoustic reflex testing, in auditory function assessment, 422
Acoustics, 47–77
Acoustic theory, of speech production, 57–59, 57*f*, 58*f*, 59*f*
Action potentials (APs), 10–11, 10*f*
Activity limitation, WHO definition of, 431
AD. *See* Alzheimer's dementia (AD)
Adenoids, 333
ADHD. *See* Attention deficit/hyperactivity disorder (ADHD)
Adipose tissue, 6
ADMET theory of phonation, 348–349
Admission criteria, resources on, 123
Adolescents, stuttering in, approaches to, 250–251, 251*t*
Adults, stuttering in, approaches to, 250–251, 251*t*
Advancing Effective Communication, Cultural Competence, and Patient- and Family-Center Care: A Roadmap for Hospitals (TJC, 2010), augmentative and alternative communication and, 395
Aerodynamic assessment, in voice disorders, 357
Aerodynamic measures, of voice production, 347
Affordable Care Act of 2010, 111
Affricates
  in consonant production, 141, 141*t*
  voiced and voiceless pairs for, comparison of, 67*t*
Age, changes in vocal mechanism related to, 348
Aging, normal
  language and cognition in, 286–287
  swallowing and, 367, 371

Agnosias, in aphasia, 257–258
Agrammatism, in aphasia, treatments for, 274–276
Agraphia, in aphasia, 257
  treatments for, 279–280
Airflow rate, as measure of voice production, 347
Alexia
  in aphasia, 256–257
  aphasic, treatments for, 279–280
Allophone, definition of, 143
Alternative communication treatments. *See also* Augmentative and alternative communication (AAC)
  for aphasia, 281
Alzheimer's dementia (AD)
  characteristics of, 288–289
  medications for, 293
  warning signs of, 289*t*
American Sign Language (ASL), 432
American Speech Correction Association (ASCA), 104
American Speech-Language-Hearing Association (ASHA), 107
  cardinal documents of, 123–124
  Code of Ethics of, 92, 109, 132–135
    violations of, 109
  in credentialing, 440
  history of, 104
  Scope of Practice in Speech-Language Pathology of, 117–128 (*See also Scope of Practice in Speech-Language Pathology* [ASHA])
Americans with Disabilities Act (ADA), augmentative and alternative communication and, 395
Amer-Ind Gestural Training, for aphasia, 281
Amplitude
  as measure of voice production, 347
  of sound, 48
Amplitude gain, of sinusoids in vocal tract, 60–61, 61*f*
Amplitude modulated noise, 57, 57*f*
Amplitude spectrum(a)
  of aperiodic complex sound, 55, 55*f*
  of periodic complex sounds, 54, 54*f*

  of sinusoid, 52, 53*f*
  of sound, 51–52, 51*f*
Amyotrophic lateral sclerosis (ALS), dysphagia in, 373
Anagram Copy and Recall Treatment, for aphasic agraphia, 280
Anatomy, 4
Anesthetics, resources on, 127
Anomia, treatments for, 277–278
Anosognosia, in aphasia, 258
Antecedent instructional events, 188
Antecedent motivational events, 188
Anterior communicating arteries, 31, 32*f*
Anterolateral system, 26–27, 27*f*
AOS. *See* Apraxia of speech (AOS)
Aperiodic complex sounds, characteristics of, 55*t*
Aperiodic noise, 65
  waveforms and spectrograms of, 66, 66*f*
Apert syndrome, 337
Aphasia, 256–285
  assessment of, 261–266
    cognitive assessment in, 264–265
    examination of all language components in, 261–262
    limb and oral-facial praxis assessment in, 265
    multicultural considerations for, 265–266
    standardized language examination components in, 262–264
  classification of, 266–268, 266*t*, 267*t*, 268*t*, 269*f*
    Boston system for, 266–267, 266*t*, 267*t*
    neuropsychological models for, 268, 269*f*
  crossed, 259
  definition of, 256
  disorders accompanying, 257–258
  dysarthria from, differential diagnosis of, 308
  etiologies of, common, 259–261
  expressive, 268
  havoc wrought by, alleviating, 269–270
  language components affected by, 256–257
  logopenic, 291, 292*t*

645

Aphasia (*continued*)
  neuroanatomical bases of, 258–261
  neuroanatomy and, 259
  nonfluent progressive, 291, 292*t*
  person with, psychological state of, assessment of, 270
  phonological, 291, 292*t*
  primary progressive, 291–292
  psychosocial effects of, on individual and family, 269–270
  reactions to, 270
  receptive, 268
  recovery from, 284–285
  study of, modern, history of, 258
  treatment of, 270–284
    efficacy of, 283–284
    general considerations for, 270–272
    for improving verbal expression, 273–278
    multicultural considerations for, 272–273
    for other language modalities, 279–284
  Wernicke's, treatment of, 279
Aphasia Diagnostic Profiles (ADP), 261
AphasiaScripts, 277
Aphasic alexia, treatments for, 279–280
Aphonia, psychogenic, etiologies and characteristics of, 351–352
Applied behavioral analysis (ABA), in autism spectrum disorders, 239
Approximants, in consonant production, 141, 141*t*
Apraxia
  in aphasia, 257
  of speech (AOS), 301–303, 302*t*
    in aphasia, 257
    assessment in, 306
    childhood (*See* Childhood apraxia of speech [CAS])
    definition of, 301
    dysarthria from, differential diagnosis of, 308
    general features of, 301–302
    resources on, 124
    treatment of, in adults, 321–323
Apraxia Battery for Adults-2 (ABA-2), 306
Apraxia Profile, 306–307
Arachnoid mater, 15, 16*f*
Arizona Battery for Communication Disorders of Dementia (ABCD), 288, 288*t*
Artery(ies)
  carotid, 30
  cerebral, 30
    middle, language zone of brain and, 258, 259*f*
    communicating, 31, 32*f*
    posterior cerebral, 30, 32*f*
    subclavian, 30, 31*f*, 32*f*
    vertebral, 30, 31*f*, 32*f*
Articulation
  impaired, in autism spectrum disorders, 236
  manner of, in consonant production, 140–141, 140*t*, 141*t*
  place of, in consonant production, 140, 140*f*, 140*t*
    acoustic cues to, 68–73

Articulators, integrity of, in speech sound disorder assessment, 153
Articulatory kinematic treatment, of apraxia of speech, 322
Articulatory phonology theory, of speech sound acquisition and disorders, 147
Articulatory subsystem, treatment of, for dysarthrias, 316–317
Arytenoid cartilages, 36–37
Ascending pathways, 26–29
ASD. *See* Autism spectrum disorders (ASD)
ASHA *See* American Speech-Language-Hearing Association (ASHA)
Asperger's Disorder, characteristics of, 229, 229*f*
Aspiration, 378–379
Aspiration-penetration scale, 378–379
Aspiration underscore noise, 66
Assessment of Children with Developmental Apraxia of Speech, 307
Assistive Technology Act Amendments of 2004 (PL 108-364), augmentative and alternative communication and, 395
Ataxic dysarthria, perceptual features of, 301*t*
Attention, in reading, 214
Attention deficit/hyperactivity disorder (ADHD), 218
  school-age language disorders in, 204
Audiogram
  interpretation of, 416–418, 417*f*, 417*t*, 418*f*, 419*f*
  speech sounds and, 420, 420*f*
Audiologic evaluation, 415–423
Audiology, 409–435
Audiometrically deaf, definition of, 431
Audiometry
  in audiologic evaluation, 416–421
  clinical masking in, 419–420
  pediatric strategies for, 420
  pure tone, 416, 417*f*, 417*t*
  speech, 418–419, 419*t*
  test findings with, implications of, on auditory perception, 420–421
Auditory brainstem response (ABR), 423, 423*f*
Auditory comprehension
  aphasia affecting, 256
  in aphasia assessment, 263–264
  impairments of, treatment of, 279
Auditory-evoked potentials (AEPs), in auditory function assessment, 422–423
Auditory function
  assessment of
    behavioral, 415–421, 417*f*, 417*t*, 418*f*, 419*f*, 419*t*, 420*f*, 420*t*
    physiologic, 421–423, 421*f*, 421*t*, 422*f*, 423*f*
  of outer ear, 410–411
Auditory implants, bone-anchored, 430–431
Auditory late responses, 423
Auditory meatus, external, 410
Auditory neuropathy spectrum disorder (ANSD), 426–427
Auditory processing, resources on, 124

Auditory rehabilitation, 431–434
  assessment tools for, 423–433
  auditory hierarchy of listening in, 433
  communication options, opportunities and modalities for, 432
  educational audiology issues in, 433–434
Auditory steady state response (ASSR), 423
Auditory system
  anatomy and physiology of, 410–415, 410*f*, 412*f*, 413*f*
  ear in, 410–414 (*See also* Ear[s])
Augmentative & Alternative Communication Profile: A Continuum of Learning (Kovach, 2009), 402
Augmentative and alternative communication (AAC), 393–408
  access to, 397–398
    law and, 395
  across lifespan, 394
  aided
    symbols for, types of, 396
    systems for
      additional features of, 397
      physical characteristics of, 396–397
    types of, 396
    vs. unaided, 395–396
  apps and, 406, 407*t*
  assessment in, 401–403
    feature matching for, 403
    models of, 401–402
    phases of, 401
    skills/status/domains in, 401
    system selection for, 403
    team, importance of, 401
    tools for, 402–403
  in autism spectrum disorders, 239
  candidacy for, 394, 401
  communication displays/devices in, organization and layout of, 400–401
  communicator in, type of, 398
  core concepts in, 395–401
  definition of, 394
  for dementia, 293–294
  devices for
    anatomy of, 405–406
    characteristics of, 405
    commercially available *vs.* dedicated, 405
    dedicated *vs.* nondedicated, 396, 396*f*
  facilitator training requirements for, 404
  in improving phonatory coordination, 315
  intervention in, 403–404
  issues in, 406
  mobile tablets and, 407
  need for
    communication disorders associated with, 394
    temporary *vs.* permanent, 394
  person characteristics for, 405
  purpose of, identification of, 401
  rate enhancement in, 399–400
  reasons for, 399
  resources on, 124
  strategies and techniques for, sample, 404
  switch site assessment in, 398
  systems for
    funding of, 403

646

symbol selection and placement on, refinement of, 404
use of, training person with complex communication needs in, 404
in treatment
of apraxia of speech, 323
of childhood apraxia of speech, 325
users of, communicative competence for, 399
Aural rehabilitation, resources on, 124
Auricle, 410, 410f
Autism spectrum disorders (ASD), 225–240
assessment of, 233–235, 234f, 234t
characteristics of
behavioral, 231–232
DSM-5, 226–228, 227f
definition of, 177–178
diagnostic procedures in, 235
educational definition of, 229, 230f
environmental theories of, 230–231
etiology of, 230–231
genetic basis for, 226
research on, 230
goal prioritization for, guidelines for, 236–237, 237f
incidence and prevalence of, 226
interdisciplinary approach to, 230t, 239
intervention for
ASHA guidelines for, 236
classification system for, 237, 238t
goals of, 235–236
methodologies of, 237–239, 238t
language impairments in, 236
neurochemical research on, 230
related services for, 239, 240t
resources on, 125
risk factors for, 231
school-age language disorders in, 205–206
screening for, 234
severity levels of, 228–229, 228t
social-communication warning signs for, 234t
speech-language pathologist role in, 232–233, 233t
symptoms of, 226
treatment of, 235–237, 237f
Automaticity, in reading, 212
Autonomic nervous system, 12–13
Axons, 8, 9, 9f
PNS, 12
of spinal cord, 17

B

Balanced Budget Act of 1997, 111
Barium swallow, modified, in dysphagia evaluation, 381–382, 382t, 383t
Basal ganglia, 21
control circuits of, 24t, 25–26, 25f
Basilar artery, 30, 32f
Basilar membrane, 413, 413f
Beckwith-Wiedemann syndrome, 337
Behavioral management, for dysarthrias, 315–316
Behavioral observation audiometry, 420

Behavioral theory, of speech sound acquisition and disorders, 143–144
Behaviors, communicative, 80
Bilingual-bicultural manual communication, 432
Bilingualism, 169
Biological factors
influencing word learning, 85–86
in language disorders, 178
Bite block, for dysarthrias, 317
Blood, 7
Blood flow
cerebral, 30–32, 31f, 32f
from heart to brain, 30, 31f
Blood supply, brain and, 32
Body
anatomy of, 4
cavities of, 5, 5f
directional nomenclature for, 4–5, 4f
parts of, 4–5
planes of section of, 4, 4f
tissue types in, 5–8, 6f, 7f
Bone, 7
Bone-anchored auditory implants, 430–431
Boston Assessment of Severe Aphasia (BASA), 262
Boston classification system, for aphasia, 266–267, 266t, 267t
Boston Diagnostic Aphasia Examination (BDAE-3), 261
Boston Naming Test (BNT), 261
Botox, in voice treatment, 358
Bound morphemes, 86
Brain
blood flow from heart to, 30, 31f
blood supply and, 32
directional nomenclature for, 5, 5f
injury to (See also Brain damage)
traumatic (See Traumatic brain injury [TBI])
language zone region of, 258–259, 258f
tumors of, aphasia from, 251
ventricular system of, 16–17, 17f
Brain damage
aphasia from, 256 (See also Aphasia)
right-hemisphere, communication disorders with, 285–286
Brainstem, 17–18
in central auditory pathway, 414f, 415
disorder of, audiometric test findings in, 421
Breathing
after total laryngectomy, 359
nasal, velum during, 333, 333f
quiet, 33–34
speech, 34, 35, 345
Breathy voice, 76t, 77, 346
Broadband spectrogram, 51, 51f
Broca, Paul, in aphasiology, 258
Brodmann's areas, 19
Brown, Roger, grammatical morphemes of, 88, 88t
Brown's stages, mean length of utterance an, 87t
Brown vs. the Board of Education, 112
Buccinator muscle, 45
Business practices in health care settings, resource on, 127

C

Cancer, head and neck
classification of tumors in, 376–377
dysphagia and, 375–378
management of, 359–361
surgical procedures for, 377–378
swallowing recovery after, 376
tumor staging in, 376
CAPE-V, 357
Cardiac muscle, 8
Caregiver-Administered Active Cognitive Stimulation, for dementia, 294
Carotid arteries, 30
Cartilage(s), 6–7
arytenoid, 36–37
cricoid, 35
laryngeal, 35–37
thyroid, 35
CAS. See Childhood apraxia of speech (CAS)
Cavities, body, 5, 5f
Central nervous system (CNS), 12, 13f, 14–22
dysphagia and, 375
meninges of, 14–16, 16f
Central tendency, in data measurement, 97
Cerebellum, 18–19
Cerebral artery, middle, language zone of brain and, 258, 259f
Cerebral blood flow, 30–32, 31f, 32f
Cerebral cortex, 19, 20f
in central auditory pathway, 414f, 415
Cerebral dominance, for language, 259
Cerebral hemispheres, 19, 21f
Cerebral palsy, school-age language disorders in, 204–205
Cerebrospinal fluid (CSF), 16
Cerebrovascular accident (CVA, stroke)
aphasia from, 260
dysphagia in, 372–373
Cerebrovascular disease, aphasia from, 259–260
Certificate of Clinical Competence (CCC), 105–106
Chall's Stage Theory, of reading acquisition, 215
CHARGE syndrome, 337
Checklist for Autism in Toddlers (CHAT), 234
Chemically gated sodium channels, 10
Chemotherapy, for head and neck cancer, voice disorders form, 359
Chest, 32
Childhood apraxia of speech (CAS), 302–303
articulation and phonologic disorders differentiated from, 309t
assessment in, 306–307
childhood dysarthria differentiated from, 309t
definition of, 302
dysarthria and speech sound disorders distinguished from, 156–158, 157t
general features of, 302–303
treatment of, 323–325
Childhood dysarthria (CD), definition of, 300

647

Childhood motor speech disorders, definition of, 300
Children
  audiometric testing in, 420
  communicative intentions of, 81
  dysarthrias in (See Dysarthria[s], childhood)
  gesture use by, 81
  with motor speech disorders, assessment of, 405–406
  motor speech disorders in, differential diagnosis of, 308–309
  school-age (See School-age children)
  speech sound disorders in, 139–165
  voice disorders in, 354–355
  young
    language disorders in, 167–191 (See also Language disorders, in young children)
    stuttering in, approaches to, 248–249, 249t
CHL See Conductive hearing loss (CHL)
Chromosomal syndromes, school-age language disorders in, 202
Circle of Willis, 31, 32f
Classroom, acoustics in, 433–434
CLD populations. See Culturally and linguistically diverse (CLD) populations
Cleft lip, 335
  syndromes associated with, 336
Cleft palate, 335
  Pierre Robin sequence with, 335 336
  syndromes associated with, 336
Client-centered approaches, to language therapy, 187
Clinical masking, in audiometry, 419–420
Clinical practice, framework for, in Scope of Practice in Speech-Language Pathology, 118–119
Clinical practice guidelines (CPGs), for evidence-based practice, 99
Clinical services and populations, resources on, 124–125
Clinician-centered approaches, to language therapy, 187
Closed pattern, as measure of voice production, 347
Cluttering, 244, 245t
CNS. See Central nervous system (CNS)
Coarticulation, definition of, 143
Cochlea, 412, 412f
  disorders of, hearing loss from, 424–425, 424t
Cochlear implants, 429–430, 430f
Code of ethics, of American Speech-Language-Hearing Association, 92, 109, 132–135
  violations of, 109
Cognate(s)
  definition of, 143
  voiced and voiceless, 66, 67t
Cognitive aspects of communication, resources on, 125
Cognitive assessment, of person with aphasia, 264–265
Cognitive competencies
  in language development, 171
  in normal aging, 286–287

Cognitive disability
  with right-hemisphere brain damage, 285–286
  school-age language disorders in, 202–203
Cognitive factors
  in language disorders, 178
  in reading, 214–215
Cognitive Linguistic Quick Test (CLQT), 262, 288
Combinations, word, 87
Communicating arteries, 31, 32f
Communication
  augmentative and alternative (See Augmentative and alternative communication [AAC])
  disorders of
    associated with augmentative and alternative communication, 394
    with right-hemisphere brain damage, 285–286
    face-to-face, definition of, 394
    manual, 432
    written, definition of, 394
Communication Activities of Daily Living, 2nd edition (CADL-2), 262
Communication and Symbolic Behavior Scales Developmental Profile (CSBS DP), 234
Communication notebooks, for aphasia, 282, 282t
Communicative behaviors, 80
Communicative Drawing Program, for aphasia, 281–282
Communicative Effectiveness Index (CETI), 262
Communicative intention, in language development, 172
Community-based treatment approaches, for persons with aphasia, 282–283
Community settings, augmentative and alternative communication in, 395
Compounding, 87
Comprehension
  auditory
    in aphasia assessment, 263–264
    impairments of, treatment of, 279
    reading, in aphasia assessment, 264
Computer-Assisted Cognitive Interventions (CACIs), for dementia, 295
Computer-assisted communication, for persons with aphasia, 281
Conditioned play audiometry, 420
Conductive hearing loss (CHL), 417, 418f
  audiometric test findings in, 420
Congenital syndromes, school-age language disorders in, 202
Congenital voice disorders, 354–355
Connectionist model, of language development, 170
Connective tissue, 6–7
Consonants
  nasal, 63–64, 64f
  production of, dimensions of, 140t
  stop, 71t, 73
  three dimensions of, 140–141
Constraint-Induced Language Therapy (CILT), 276–277

Contextual testing, in speech sound disorder assessment, 154
Continuant noise, 66
Conversational areas, in curriculum-based language disorder assessment, 197
Core Vocabulary Intervention, for phonemic errors, 164–165
Correlational statistics, in research results, 97–98
Cortical control, of swallowing, 366
Cortical stroke, dysphagia in, 373
Corticobulbar tract, 23–24
Corticospinal tract, 22–23, 23f
Council of Clinical Certification in Audiology and Speech-Language Pathology (CFCC), 440
Cover-body theory of phonation, 349
Cranial nerves, 13–14, 14t
  auditory function of, 414–415
  input of, to larynx, 345
  swallowing and, 364–366, 367
Craniosynostosis syndromes, 337
Creaky voice, 76t, 77, 346
Credentialing, 105–107
  agencies for, 440
Cricoarytenoid muscles, lateral, 38, 38t
Cricoid cartilage, 35
Cricothyroid muscles, 38, 38t
Crouzon syndrome, 337
Cul-de-sac resonance, 339
Cultural diversity, in evidence-based practice, 100
Culturally and linguistically diverse (CLD) populations
  aphasia in
    assessment of, 265–266
    treatment of, 272–273
  dementia in, working with, 295
  issues associated with, 114
  providing services for, 114
  school-age language disorders in, 198–199
  speech sound disorder assessment in, 156
Culturally appropriate services, resources on, 123
Cultural values, beliefs and customs, in evidence-based practice, 100
Culture, language development and, 170–171
Cuneate fasciculus, 28
CVA See Cerebrovascular accident (CVA, stroke)
Cycles Remediation Approach, for phonemic errors, 163
Cysts, vocal fold, etiologies and characteristics of, 350

D

Data analysis
  in research articles, 96–87
  techniques of, 97–98
Dax, Marc, in aphasiology, 258
Deaf. See also Hearing loss
  audiometrically, definition of, 431
  definition of, 431
  resources on, 125

Deep brain stimulation (DBS), for
    Parkinson's disease, 293
Deixis, 81
Deletion 22q11.2 syndrome, 336
Dementia, 287
    Alzheimer's, 288–289 (See also
        Alzheimer's dementia [AD])
    aphasia in, 251
    cognitive-communicative interventions
        for, 293–294
    dysphagia in, 375
    frontal, 290
    frontotemporal, 290–292
    with Lewy Bodies (DLB), 292
        treatment of, 293
    multicultural considerations for, 295
    resources on, 125
    semantic, 291, 292t
    vascular, characteristics of, 289–290
Dendrites, 8, 9, 9f
Depressor anguli oris muscle, 45
Depressor labii inferioris muscle, 45
Dermatomyositis, dysphagia in, 374
Descriptive research, 95
Developmental disabilities, resources on,
    126
Developmental dysarthria (DD), definition
    of, 300
Developmental stuttering, 242–244
Diacritics, definition of, 143
Diadochokinesis (DDK), measurement of,
    in speech sound disorder assessment,
    153
*Diagnostic and Statistical Manual of Mental
    Disorders*-5th Edition (DSM-5),
    definition of
    of Asperger's Disorder, 229, 229f
    of autism spectrum disorders, 226–228,
        227f
Diagnostic assessments, of literacy skills,
    215–216
Dialect, definition of, 143
Dialectal differences, in language,
    168–169
Diencephalon, 21–22
Diet modifications, for dysphagia, 386
Digastric muscle, 39, 41t
Diphthongs, 141t, 142
Direct motor pathway, 22–24
Discharge criteria, resources on, 123
Discourse, in curriculum-based language
    disorder assessments, 195–197
Discourse management, in language
    development, 172–173
Discrete trial teaching (DTT), in autism
    spectrum disorders, 239
Disfluency, definition of, 242
Distinctive Feature Analysis, in assessment
    data analysis, 155
Distinctive Features Approach, for
    phonemic errors, 162
Distinctive features theory, of speech
    sound acquisition and disorders,
    144
Divergent therapies, for aphasia, 271–272
Diversity, cultural, in evidence-based
    practice, 100
Dorsal cavity, 5, 5f

Double-function words, acquisition of, 85
Down syndrome, school-age language
    disorders in, 203
Drill play, in language therapy, 189
Drills, in language therapy, 188–189
Dura mater, 15–16, 16f
Duration, of sound, 49
Dysarthria(s), 300
    from aphasia, differential diagnosis of,
        308
    from apraxia of speech, differential
        diagnosis of, 308
    childhood
        articulation and phonological
            disorders differentiated from,
            308–309, 308t
        childhood apraxia of speech
            differentiated from, 156–158, 157t,
            309t
        considerations for, 312
        definition of, 300
    definition of, 300
    developmental, definition of, 300
    general features of, 300
    perceptual features of, 301t
    treatment of, 311–321
        articulatory subsystem management in,
            316–317
        global management techniques in,
            318–319
        participation strategies in, 319–321,
            320f
        principles of, 311–312
        prosody treatment in, 318
        for respiratory/phonatory subsystem,
            312–315
        velopharyngeal subsystem management
            in, 315–316
Dyslexia, 218
    in aphasia, 256–257
Dysphagia, 363–389, 371–375
    definition of, 364, 371
    diagnostic procedures for, 380–381
    instrumental evaluation of, 381–384,
        382t, 383t
        fiberoptic endoscopic, 382–383
        functional magnetic resonance imaging
            in, 384
        manometry in, 383
        modified barium swallow in, 381–382,
            382t, 383t
        scintigraphy in, 384
        surface electromyography in, 384
        ultrasound imaging in, 383
    neurological conditions causing,
        371–375
        amyotrophic lateral sclerosis as, 373
        cerebrovascular accident as, 372–373
        classification of, 372
        dementia as, 375
        dermatomyositis as, 374
        dystonias as, 374
        Guillain-Barré syndrome as, 374
        Huntington's disease as, 374
        multiple sclerosis as, 373–374
        myasthenia gravis as, 374
        Parkinson's disease as, 373
        postpolio syndrome as, 374

        progressive supranuclear palsy as, 373
        traumatic brain injury as, 374–375
    signs and symptoms of, 371f, 372, 372t
    treatments of, 384–387
        diet modifications as, 386
        direct or indirect, 384
        effortful swallow as, 385
        for geriatric patients, 385
        Masako maneuver as, 385
        McNeill dysphagia therapy program
            as, 387
        mealtime strategies as, 387
        Mendelsohn maneuver as, 385
        neuromuscular electrical stimulation
            as, 387
        postural changes as, 385–386
        Shaker exercise as, 385
        supraglottic swallow as, 384
        surgical, 387
        thermal tactile stimulation as, 385
Dysphonia
    muscle tension, etiologies and
        characteristics of, 351
    psychogenic, etiologies and characteristics
        of, 351–352
    spasmodic, etiologies and characteristics
        of, 353–354
Dystonias, dysphagia in, 374

E

Ear(s)
    inner
        anatomy and physiology of, 411–414,
            412f, 413f
        disorders of, hearing loss from, 424–
            425, 424t
    middle
        anatomy and physiology of, 411
        disorders of, hearing loss from, 424,
            424t
    outer
        anatomy and physiology of, 410–411,
            410f
        disorders of, hearing loss from, 424,
            424t
Early development, morphemes in, 87–88,
    88t
Early intervention
    for language disorders, 186–187
    resources on, 125
    speech-language pathology in, 113
Educating Caregivers on Alzheimer's Disease
    and Training Communication
    Strategies, for dementia, 294–295
Educational audiology issues, 433–434
Educational service delivery, 111–112
Educational settings, augmentative and
    alternative communication in, 395
Education for All Handicapped Children Act
    of 1972 (PL 94-142), 112, 199
    Amendments of 1986, 112
Education Testing Services, in credentialing,
    440
Effect size estimates, in research results,
    98–99
Egressive sounds, definition of, 143

Elastic cartilage, 7
Elderly, dysphagia in
    hiatal hernia and, 367
    treatment for, 385
    xerostomia and, 370
Electrocochleography, 423
Electromyography, surface, in dysphagia evaluation, 384
Ellipsis, 81
Employment, in speech-language pathology, 110
End-plate potentials, 11–12
Enhancing Stimulability, in approach to phonetic errors, 162
Environment, gas exchange with, 32
Environmental factors
    influencing word learning, 85–86
    in language disorders, 178
Environmental theories, of autism spectrum disorder etiology, 230–231
Epiglottis, 37
Epithelial layers, 5–6, 6f
Error patterns, in assessment data analysis, 155
Errors in judgment, 113
Esophageal disorders, 379–380
Esophagitis, pill-induced, 380
Ethical issues, in speech-language pathology, 108–109
Ethics, code of, of American Speech-Language-Hearing Association, 92, 109, 132–135
    violations of, 109
Ethnic minority groups, evidence-based practice and, 100
Eustachian tube, 333, 411
Evidence-based practice (EBP), 92–93
    cultural diversity in, 100
    definition of, 92
    evidence for
        collecting best available, 93
        external, evaluating, 93
    interpreting tests and measurements in, 100
    process of, 92–93
    research applied to, 92
    resources on, 124
    for school-age language disorders, 201
    speech-language pathology in, 116
    treatment efficacy studies and, 99
Evidence-based voice treatment approaches, 358
Executive functioning, in reading, 214
Exocytosis, 11–12
Expansion/recast techniques, 188
Expatiation techniques, 188
Experiential language interventions techniques, 187–189
Experimental research, 95
Expiration
    during quiet breathing, 33–34
    during speech breathing, 34
Expiratory reserve volume (ERV), 34, 34f
Expository, in curriculum-based language disorder assessment, 197
Expressive aphasia, 268
Extrapyramidal system control circuits, 24–26, 24t

F

Face
    anatomy of, 332
    lower, muscles of, 369t
Face-to-face communication, definition of, 394
Facial (VII) nerve, swallowing and, 364, 366, 367, 368t, 369t
Facilitation techniques, in language therapy, 185
Falsetto, mutational, etiologies and characteristics of, 352
Family, psychosocial effects of aphasia on, 269–270
F.A.S.T. acronym, 260
Faucial pillars, 332
Feature geometry theory, of speech sound acquisition and disorders, 146
Feedback, in treatment of motor speech disorders, 310
Feeding
    cleft lip and palate and, 335
    definition of, 364
Fetal alcohol syndrome (FAS), 336
Fiberoptic endoscopic evaluation of swallowing (FEES), 382
    with sensory testing (FEEST), 382–383
Fibrocartilage, 6
First Year Inventory (FYI), 234
Flaccid dysarthria, perceptual features of, 301t
Flap, definition of, 143
Floor time, in autism spectrum disorders, 239
Fluency
    definition of, 242
    in reading, 212
    resources on, 125
Fluency disorders, 241–252
    cluttering as, 244, 245t
    neurogenic stuttering as, 244, 245t
    psychogenic stuttering as, 244–245, 245t
    stuttering as, 242 (See also Stuttering)
Focused stimulation techniques, in language therapy, 185
Forebrain, 19–22
Formant frequencies, 61–62, 63f
Formant transitions, 68, 68f
Fragile-X syndrome, school-age language disorders in, 203
Free Appropriate Public Education, 395
Free morphemes, 86
Frequency
    of sound, 48 48t
    of vocal fold vibration (F_0), 73, 74f, 75f
    summary statistics on, 73, 75t
Frequency-modulated hearing-assistive devices, 431
Frication noise, 66
    acoustic characteristics of, 69–71, 70t
Fricatives
    in consonant production, 140–141, 141t
    interdental, spectral moment characteristics of, 69, 70t
    labiodental, spectral moment characteristics of, 69, 70t
    place of articulation for, 68–69, 69f
    sibilant
        place of articulation for, 68
        spectral moment characteristics of, 69, 70t
    voiced and voiceless pairs for, comparison of, 67t
Frontal dementia, 290
Frontal lobe, 19
Frontotemporal dementia (FTD), 290–292
    treatment of, 293
Functional Assessment of Communication Skills for Adults (ASHA FACS), 262
Functional Communication Measure (FCM), 356
Functional hearing loss, audiometric test findings in, 421
Functional magnetic resonance imaging, in dysphagia evaluation, 384
Fundamental frequency, as measure of voice production, 346–347

G

Gas exchange, with environment, 32
Gastroesophageal reflux disease (GERD)
    in elderly, 367
    esophageal motility disorders and, 379–380
Generalization, in language therapy, 185
General phonology theory, of speech sound acquisition and disorders, 147
General stimulation techniques, in language therapy, 185
Generative phonology theory, of speech sound acquisition and disorders, 144–145
Genetic basis, for autism spectrum disorders, 226
Genetic features, of language disorders, 178
Genetic syndromes, school-age language disorders in, 202
Genioglossus muscle, 44, 44t
Geniohyoid muscle, 39, 41f
GERD. See Gastroesophageal reflux disease (GERD)
Geriatric patients. See Elderly
Glia, 9
    CNS, 12
    PNS, 12
Glides, 64
    in consonant production, 141, 141t
    vowels compared with, 65t
Globus pallidus, 21
Glossectomy, speech and swallowing after, 361
Glossopharyngeal (IX) nerve, swallowing and, 364–365, 366, 367, 368t
Glottal fry voice, 346
Glottal resistance, as measure of voice production, 347
Glottal source, of periodic complex sounds, 55–56, 56f
Glottal stop voice, 346
Glottic tumors, 377
Golgi tendon organs, in proprioception, 29
Gracile fasciculus, 28

Gradual Release of Responsibility Model (GRRM), for literacy learning, 219–220
Grammatical competence, aphasia affecting, 256
Grapheme-phoneme correspondence, 211
Gravelly voice, 346
Gray matter, of spinal cord, 17 18f
GRBAS, 356
Group reminiscence therapy, for dementia, 294
Group research design, 95–96
Guillain-Barré syndrome, dysphagia in, 374
Guitar's model, of stuttering experience, 245–247

H

Hair cells, sensory, 412–413, 413f
Harmonics, in sound, frequency of, 53–54, 53t
Head
  and neck, cancer of (See Cancer, head and neck)
    management of, 359–361
    special senses of, 29
Health care environment, speech-language pathology in, 110–111
Health care services, resources on, 127
Health Insurance Portability and Accountability Act (HIPAA) of 1996, 111
Hearing
  behavioral assessment of, 415–421, 417f, 417t, 418f, 419f, 419t, 420f, 420t
  differences in, variables associated with, 432
  hard of
    definition of, 431, 432
    resources on, 125
  screening of
    resources on, 125
    in speech sound disorder assessment, 153
Hearing aids (HA/s), 427–429, 427f, 428f
Hearing assessment, in voice disorders, 357
Hearing-assistive technology, 431
Hearing disorders, 423–427. See also Hearing loss
Hearing impaired/impairment, definition of, 432
Hearing loss. See also Deaf
  audiometric test findings in, 420–421
  in auditory neuropathy spectrum disorder, 426–427
  bone-anchored auditory implants for, 430–431
  cochlear implants for, 429–430, 430f
  definition of, 432
  general factors causing, 423–424
  hearing aids for, 427–429, 427f, 428f
  from inner ear disorders, 424–425, 424t
  from middle ear disorders, 424, 424t
  noise-induced, 425, 425t
  from outer ear disorders, 424, 424t
  from retrocochlear disorders, 425–426, 426t

  sensory technology for, 427–431
  types of, 417, 418f
  voice problems in persons with, 356
Heart, blood flow to brain from, 30, 31f
Hemifacial microsomia, 337
Hemilaryngectomy, 377
Hemorrhagic CVA, aphasia from, 260
Hernia, hiatal, in elderly, 367
Hertz, in sound measurement, 48, 48t
Heschl's gyrus, 20, 414f, 415
Hiatal hernia, in elderly, 367
Homorganic, definition of, 143
Homunculus, 19, 21f
Hospitals, augmentative and alternative communication in, 395
Human papilloma virus (HPV), laryngeal infection from, etiologies and characteristics of, 350–351
Huntington's disease, dysphagia in, 374
Hyaline cartilage, 6–7
Hyoglossus muscle, 44, 44t
Hyoid bone, 38
Hyperadduction, in dysarthrias, treating, 314–314
Hyperfunctional dysphonia, etiologies and characteristics of, 351
Hyperkinetic dysarthria, perceptual features of, 301t
Hyperlexia, 218
Hypernasality, 339
Hypoadduction, in dysarthrias, treating, 314
Hypoglossal (XII) nerve, swallowing and, 366, 368t, 369t
Hypokinetic dysarthria, perceptual features of, 301t
Hyponasality, 339
Hypopharyngeal tumors, 377
Hypothalamus, 22

I

Ideomotor apraxia, in aphasia, 257
Imitation techniques, 188
Immittance measurement, in auditory function assessment, 421
Impairment, WHO definition of, 431
Impulse noises, 56, 56f
Incisivus labii inferioris muscle, 45
Incisivus labii superioris muscle, 45
Inclusive practices, resources on, 128
Incus, 411
Indirect motor pathways, 24, 24t
Individual Educational Plans (IEPs), 199
Individuals with Disabilities Education Act (IDEA, 1990), (PL 101-476), 112, 113
  augmentative and alternative communication and, 395
  autism spectrum disorders defined by, 229, 230f
  as support for persons with reading/writing disabilities, 220–221
Induction techniques, in language therapy, 185
Infancy, pragmatic skills in, 80
Inferential statistics, in research results, 98
Inferior laryngeal nerve paralysis, 353
Inferior longitudinal muscles, 43, 44t

Information processing model, of language development, 170
Infrahyoid muscles, 39–41, 41t
Ingressive sounds, definition of, 143
Inner ear (IE)
  anatomy and physiology of, 411–414, 412f, 413f
  disorders of, hearing loss from, 424–425, 424t
Inspiration
  during quiet breathing, 33
  during speech breathing, 34
Inspiratory reserve volume (IRV), 34, 34f
Insufflation testing, in alaryngeal voice assessment, 360
Insurance, liability, 113
Integral Stimulation, in approach to phonetic errors, 162
Intellectual disability, school-age language disorders in, 202–203
Intelligibility
  development of, 152
  informal measure of, in speech sound disorder assessment, 154
  reduced, in dysarthrias, treatment of, 320
  in voice evaluation, 357
Intensity
  as measure of voice production, 347
  of sound, 49
Interactionist-discovery (cognitive) theory, of speech sound acquisition and disorders, 146
Interdental fricatives, place of articulation for, 68
International Association of Logopedics and Phoniatrics (IALP), 108
International Classification of Functioning, Disability, and Health (ICF), 356
Intersystemic reorganization, in aphasia treatment, 271
Interval measurement data, 97

J

Jitter, as measure of voice production, 347
Judgment errors, 113

K

Kanner, Leo, autistic disturbances and, 226
Kaufman Speech Praxis Test for Children (KSPT), 306
Kurtosis, in data measurement, 97

L

Labiodental fricatives, place of articulation for, 68
Labyrinth
  membranous, 412, 412f
  osseous, 411–412
Language
  acquisition of, 79–90
    morphology in, 86–88
    phonology in, 82–83
    pragmatics in, 80–82

Language (*continued*)
    semantics in, 83–86
    syntax in, 89–90
  cerebral dominance for, 259
  characteristics of, 168–170
  formulation of, in writing skill development, 213–214
  neuroanatomy and neurophysiology of, 8–29
  resources on, 125
  spoken, acquisition of, 84–85
  study of, 4–8
  understanding and use of, techniques to modify, 184–185
  written (*See* Written language)
Language Acquisition Device (LAD), in syntactic development, 89
Language comprehension, assessment of, tasks for, 180
Language development
  communication competence as goal of, 168
  early sound production in, 173–174
  gestures in, 174
  meaning/language content in, 174–175
  milestones component of, 172–176
  models of, 170–172
  morphology development in, 175–176
  pragmatic, 172–173
  receptive *vs.* expressive vocabulary in, 174
  semantic relations in, 174–175
  syntactic development in, 175
  vocabulary development in, 174
Language disorders
  acquired, 255–297
    aphasia as, 256–285 (*See also* Aphasia)
    with neurodegenerative syndromes, 286–295 (*See also* Neurodegenerative syndromes)
    with right-hemisphere brain damage, 285–286
  assessment of, 179–184
    creating test battery and appointment for, 182–183
    data for
      focus and pre-assessment, 179–180
      interpreting, 183–184
      resources for, 180–182
    dynamic, 184
    material selection for, 182
    standardized *versus* nonstandardized, 181–182
  in autism spectrum disorders, 236
  definitions of, 176–178, 194
  models of, 176–178
  potential causal factors for, 178
  spoken, in school-age populations, 193–207 (*See also* School-age spoken language disorders)
  written, in school-age populations, 209–224 (*See also* School-age written language disorders)
  in young children, 167–191
    intervention for, 184–190
      dismissal from, 190
      early, 186–187
      measuring progress in, 189–190
      success of, factors for, 185–186
      techniques used in, 187–189

Language-learning disability, definition of, 177
Language-Learning Disability (LLD), 218
Language production, assessment of, tasks for, 180–181
Language zone region of brain, 258–259, 258*f*
Laryngeal cartilages, 35–37
Laryngeal dystonia, dysphagia in, 374
Laryngeal system, in speech production, 45
Laryngeal web, 355
Laryngectomy
  partial, 377
    swallowing after, 361
  total, 377
    anatomical and physiologic changes after, 359
Laryngitis, etiologies and characteristics of, 351
Laryngologic assessment, of vocal fold vibration, 357
Laryngologic/stroboscopic assessment, in voice disorders, 357
Laryngomalacia, 354
Laryngopharyngeal reflux (LPR), 379–380
Larynx
  anatomy of, 36*f*
  cranial nerve input to, 345
  extrinsic muscles of, 39–41, 41*t*
  human papilloma virus infection of, etiologies and characteristics of, 350–351
  intrinsic muscles of, 38–39, 38*t*
    motor innervation of, 39, 40*f*
  muscles of, 368*t*, 369*t*
  in phonation, 35
  removal of
    partial, 360–361
    total, 359–360
  tumors of, classification of, 377
Lateral cricoarytenoid muscles, 38, 38*t*
Lateral pterygoid muscles, 42, 43*f*
Late talkers, 86
  definition of, 177
Laws
  access to augmentative and alternative communication and, 395
  on nondiscriminatory employment and practice, 110
Learning, implicit and explicit, in treatment of motor speech disorders, 310–311
Learning disability, definition of, 177
Lee Silverman Voice Treatment (LSVT), 314
Legislation
  health care, 110–111
  on SLP services in schools, 112, 199
Letter-by-letter reading, in aphasia, 257
Letters, acoustic characteristics of, 61–62
Levator anguli oris muscle, 45
Levator labii superioris alaque nasi muscle, 45
Levator labii superioris muscle, 45
Lewy Bodies, dementia with, 292
  treatment of, 293
Lexical representations, of word, 83–84
Lexical retrieval
  aphasia affecting, 256
  in normal aging, 286–287

Liability, professional, 113
Ligaments, of middle ear, 411
Limbic cortex, 21
Limb praxis, in aphasia assessment, 265
Lingual dystonia, dysphagia in, 374
Linguistically appropriate services, resources on, 123
Linguistic units, longer, in language acquisition, 81–82
Lip
  cleft, 335
    syndromes associated with, 336
  upper, anatomy of, 332
Liquids, 64
  in consonant production, 141, 141*t*
  vowels compared with, 65*t*
Listening, auditory hierarchy of, 433
Literacy
  in curriculum-based language disorder assessment, 198
  definition of, 210
  nature of, 210–215
  resources on, 125
Literacy instruction, effective practices in, 219–220
Literacy skills, assessment of, 215–217
Logopenic aphasia, 291, 292*t*
Loudness, 49
Lungs, 32, 33*f*

M

Magnetic resonance imaging, functional (fMRI), in dysphagia evaluation, 384
Malleus, 411
Manofluorography, in dysphagia evaluation, 383
Manometry, in dysphagia evaluation, 383
Manually Coded English, 432
Masako maneuver, for dysphagia, 385
Masseter muscles, 42, 43*f*
Mastication, muscles of, 42–43, 43*f*, 369*t*
Maximum phonation time, as measure of voice production, 347
Mayo Clinic speech dimensions summary, 304*t*
McNeill dysphagia therapy program, 387
Mealtime strategies, for dysphagia, 387
Mean Length of Utterance (MLU), in early development, 87–88, 87*t*
Measurement, in research articles, 94–95
Medial pterygoid muscles, 42, 43*f*
Medicaid, legislation on, 110–111
Medicare, legislation on, 110
Medications, swallowing and, 380
Medulla oblongata, 18
Medullary stroke, dysphagia in, 372
Meissner's corpuscles, 28
Melodic Intonation Therapy (MIT), in aphasia treatment, 271, 273–274, 274*t*–275*t*
Mels, in sound measurement, 48, 48*t*
Memory functions, in reading, 214–215
Mendelsohn maneuver, for dysphagia, 385
Mendelson's syndrome, 378
Ménière's disease, management strategies for, 425

Meninges, 14–16, 16f
Mentalis muscle, 45
Mental retardation, resources on, 126
Merkel receptors, 28
Meta-analyses, treatment efficacy evidence from, 99
Metalinguistics, in language development, 173
Metaphon, for phonemic errors, 164
Metaphonological Intervention, for phonemic errors, 165
Metrical phonology theory, of speech sound acquisition and disorders, 146
Microsomia, hemifacial, 337
Midbrain, 18
Middle cerebral artery (MCA), language zone of brain and, 258, 259f
Middle ear (ME)
　anatomy and physiology of, 411
　disorders of, hearing loss from, 424, 424t
Middle latency response, in auditory function assessment, 423
Mild cognitive impairment (MCI), 287
Mini-Mental State Exam (MMSE), 287
Minnesota Test for the Differential Diagnosis of Aphasia (MTDDA), 262
Mixed hearing loss, 417, 418f
MLU. See Mean Length of Utterance (MLU)
Modal voice, 76t, 77
Modified barium swallow (MBS), in dysphagia evaluation, 381–382, 382t, 383t
Monophthongs, 141, 141t, 142
Morpheme(s), 86
　definition of, 143
　in early development, 87–88, 88t
　grammatical
　　age of acquisition order for, 88t
　　Brown's, 88
　　mastering, 88
Morphological construction, 86–87
Morphology
　in curriculum-based language disorder assessment, 198t
　in language acquisition, 86–88
Morphology development, in language development, 175–176
Morphosyntax Approach, for phonemic errors, 164
Motherese, word learning and, 85–86
Motility disorders, esophageal, 379–380
Motor learning principles, in treatment of motor speech disorders, 310–311
Motor speech disorders (MSDs), 29–327
　assessment of, 303–309
　　in developing direction of therapy, 308
　　differential diagnosis in, 308–309, 308t, 309t
　　historical information in, 303
　　identify presence of MSD and other related disorders in, 304
　　motor speech examination in, 304–307, 304t, 305t
　　neuromuscular impairment detection in, 307
　　reasons for, 303t
　　speech activity in, 307
　prosodic impairments of, 305t
　terminology for, 3070
　treatment of, general principles of, 310–311
Motor Speech Examination, 304–307, 304t, 305t
　for Children, 307
Motor speech production, in voice evaluation, 357
Mouth, floor of, tumors of, 376–377
MSD. See Motor speech disorders (MSDs)
Mucosal wave behavior, as measure of voice production, 348
Multicultural populations. See also Culturally and linguistically diverse (CLD) populations
　serving, 114
Multiethnic society. See also Culturally and linguistically diverse (CLD) populations
　providing services in, 114
Multi-modality approaches, to aphasia treatment, 271
Multiple Oral Re-reading, for aphasic alexia, 280
Multiple Phoneme Approach, for phonetic errors, 161
Multiple sclerosis (MS), dysphagia in, 373–374
Multisensory Structured Language (MSL) Principles, for struggling readers/writers, 219
Multiskilling, resources on, 127
Muscle(s)
　buccinator, 45
　cricothyroid, 38, 38t
　depressor anguli oris, 45
　depressor labii inferioris, 45
　digastric, 39, 41t
　facial, 44–45
　genioglossus, 44, 44t
　geniohyoid, 39, 41t
　hyoglossus, 44, 44t
　incisivus labii inferioris, 45
　incisivus labii superioris, 45
　inferior longitudinal, 43, 44t
　infrahyoid, 39–41, 41t
　intrinsic, of larynx, 38–39, 38t
　　motor innervation of, 39, 40f
　lateral cricoarytenoid, 38, 38t
　lateral pterygoid, 42, 43f
　levator anguli oris, 45
　levator labii superioris, 45
　levator labii superioris alaque nasi, 45
　masseter, 42, 43f
　of mastication, 42–43, 43f
　medial pterygoid, 42, 43f
　mentalis, 45
　of middle ear, 411
　mylohyoid, 39, 41t
　omohyoid, 40, 41t
　orbicularis, 44
　palatoglossus, 44, 44t
　platysma, 45
　posterior cricoarytenoid, 38t, 39
　risorius, 45
　sternohyoid, 39, 41t
　sternothyroid, 41, 41t
　styloglossus, 44, 44t
　superior longitudinal, 43, 44t
　suprahyoid, 39, 41t
　in swallow
　　oral phase, 366–367, 368t
　　oral preparatory phase, 366
　　pharyngeal phase, 367
　temporal, 42, 43f
　thyroarytenoid, 38, 38t
　thyrohyoid, 40–41, 41t
　tongue, 43–44, 44t
　transverse, 43, 44t
　transverse and oblique interarytenoid, 38–39, 38t
　vertical, 43–44, 44t
　zygomatic major, 45
　zygomatic minor, 45
Muscle spindles, in proprioception, 29
Muscle tension dysphonia, etiologies and characteristics of, 351
Muscular tissue, 7–8, 7f
Mutational falsetto, etiologies and characteristics of, 352
Myasthenia gravis (MG), dysphagia in, 373
Mylohyoid muscle, 39, 41t
Myoelastic aerodynamic theory, of vocal fold vibration, 41–42

N

Narratives, in curriculum-based language disorder assessments, 195–197
Narrowband spectrogram, 51, 52f
　of periodic complex sound, 54
Nasal cavity, 45f, 46
　anatomy of, 332
Nasal consonants, 63–64, 64f
Nasal obturator, for dysarthrias, 315
Nasals, in consonant production, 140, 140t
National Association of Teachers of Speech (NATS), 104
National Outcomes Measurement System (NOMS), 99
National Research Council (NRC), recommendations of, for autism spectrum disorder treatment, 235
National Student Speech-Language-Hearing Association (NSSLHA), 108
Naturalistic Speech, for phonemic errors, 163
Natural phonology theory, of speech sound acquisition and disorders, 145
Neck
　and head, cancer of (See Cancer, head and neck)
　muscles of, 368t
Neck dystonia, dysphagia in, 374
Neighborhood density, in word learning, 84
Neonatal intensive care unit, resources on, 127
Nerve(s)
　cranial, 13–14, 14t (See also Cranial nerves)
　motor, of intrinsic laryngeal muscles, 39, 40f
　spinal, 14, 15f
Nervous system, 8–29
　cell types in, 8–9, 9f

Index

Nervous system (continued)
  central, 12, 13f, 14-22 (See also Central nervous system [CNS])
  neural pathways of, 22-29
Nervous tissue, 8
Neural hearing loss, audiometric test findings in, 421
Neural pathways, 22-29
Neural signaling, 9-12
Neural tube defects (NTD), school-age language disorders in, 204
Neuroanatomy, of speech, language and swallowing, 8-29
Neurodegenerative syndromes, 286-295
  aphasia from, 251
  characteristics of, 288-293
  communication in, treatment of, 293-295
  dementia as, 287
  language and cognition in, assessment of, 287-288
  mild cognitive impairment as, 287
  normal aging as, 286-287
  Parkinson's disease as, 292-293
Neurogenic stuttering, 244, 245t
Neuromuscular electrical stimulation (NMES), for dysphagia, 387
Neuromuscular impairment, in motor speech disorders, evaluation for, 307
Neurons, 8-9, 9f
  CNS, 12
  PNS, 12
Neurophysiology, of speech, language and swallowing, 8-29
Neuroplasticity
  swallowing and, 375
  in treatment of motor speech disorders, 310
Neuropsychological models in aphasia classification, 268, 269f
Neurotransmitters, 11-12
No Child Left Behind Act of 2001 (PL 107-110), 112
Nodules, vocal
  bilateral, 355
  etiologies and characteristics of, 349-350
Noise-induced hearing loss, 425, 425t
Noise measures, of voice production, 347
Nondiscriminatory employment and practice, laws governing, 110
Nonfluent progressive aphasia, 291, 292t
Nonlinear Phonological Intervention, for phonemic errors, 165
Nonlinear theories, of speech sound acquisition and disorders, 146-147
Nonparametric statistics, 97
Non-specific language impairment, definition of, 177
Nonstandardized probes, in language disorder assessment, 181-182
Nose, anatomy of, 332
Nouns, acquisition of, 85

O

Obstruent, definition of, 143
Obstruent sounds, 57
  acoustic characteristics of, 65-66, 67t

Occipital lobe, 21
Occlusive stroke, aphasia from, 260
Octave, intervals in, 48, 49t
Oculoauriculovertebral dysplasia, 337
OMD-Meige syndrome, dysphagia in, 374
Omnibus Budget Reconciliation Acts, 111
Omohyoid muscle, 40, 41t
Opitz G syndrome, 336
Optimality theory, of speech sound acquisition and disorders, 146
Oral cavity, 45-46, 45f
Oral-facial praxis, in aphasia assessment, 365
Oral Reading for Language in Aphasia (ORLA), 277
Oral structures, 332, 332f
Orbicularis oris muscle, 44
Organ of Corti, 412-413, 413f
Orofacial myofunctional disorders, resources on, 126
Orofaciodigital syndrome Type I (OFD I), 336
Oromandibular dystonia, dysphagia in, 374
Orthography, definition of, 210
Ossicles, of middle ear, 411
Otoacoustic emissions, in auditory function assessment, 422, 422f
Otoscopy, 415
Outcomes assessments, of literacy skills, 216
Outer ear (OE)
  anatomy and physiology of, 410-411, 410f
  disorders of, hearing loss from, 424, 424t

P

Pacinian corpuscles, 28
  in proprioception, 29
Paired-Stimuli Approach, for phonetic errors, 161
Palatal lift, for dysarthrias, 315, 316t
Palate, cleft, 335
  syndromes associated with, 336
Palatoglossus muscle, 44, 44t
Paradoxical vocal fold motion, etiologies and characteristics of, 352-353
Parallel talk techniques, 188
Paralysis
  inferior laryngeal nerve, 353
  superior laryngeal nerve, 353
Parametric experiment, 95
Parametric statistics, 97
Parasympathetic division, of autonomic nervous system, 12
Parietal lobe, 19
Parkinson's disease (PD), 292-293
  dysphagia in, 373
  treatment of, 293
Participation restriction, WHO definition of, 431
Passavant's ridge, 334
Passy-Muir speaking valve, 377
Patient Protection and Affordable Care Act of 2010, 111
Peer and play remediation, in autism spectrum disorders, 239
Penetration, aspiration and, 378-379
Percentage Consonants Correct, in assessment data analysis, 154-155

Perceptual abilities, in language development, 171
Perceptual measures, of voice production, 347
Period, of sound, 48
Periodic complex sounds, 53-54, 53t
  amplitude spectrum of, 54, 54f
  characteristics of, 55t
  narrowband spectrogram of, 54
  in speech, glottal source of, 55-56, 56f
  waveforms of, 54, 54f
Periodicity, as measure of voice production, 347
Peripheral nervous system (PNS), 12
  major divisions of, 12-14, 13f
Perseveration, in aphasia, 257
Pfeiffer syndrome, 337
Pharyngeal cavity, 45, 45f
  structures of, 333
  wall movement in, in speech, 334
Pharynx, muscles of, 369t
Phase, of sound, 50, 50f
Phonation, 55
  anatomy of, 35-46
  neuroanatomy of, 345
  and respiration, coordination of, in dysarthrias, improving, 313-314
  theories and processes of, 348-349
  type of, 346
  ventricular, etiologies and characteristics of, 352
Phonatory function, improving, in dysarthrias, 314-315
Phoneme(s), 82
  definition of, 143
  formation of, phonological rules governing, 82
  omission of, in second language learning, 156
  overdifferentiated, in second language learning, 156
  substitution of, in second language learning, 156
  target, for speech sound disorders treatment, 158-159
  underdifferentiated, in second language learning, 156
Phoneme Intelligibility Test (PIT), 306
Phonemic awareness (PA)
  skills in
    assessment of, 154
    development of, by school-age children, 152
    in word recognition and spelling, 211
Phonemic errors, intervention approaches for, 162-165
Phonemic inventory, in assessment data analysis, 155
Phonetic Contrast Test (PCT), 306
Phonetic errors, intervention approaches for, 160-162
Phonetics, 140-143
  consonants in, 140-141, 140f, 140t, 141t
  vowels in, 141-143, 141t, 142f
Phonological aphasia, 291, 292t
Phonological awareness
  in curriculum-based language disorder assessment, 198

654

skills in, assessment of, 154
in word identification/spelling, 211
Phonological characteristics, of first 50 words, 148
Phonological Contrast Intervention, for phonemic errors, 162–163
Phonological Error Patterns Analysis, in assessment data analysis, 155
Phonological errors
patterns of, use and suppression of, 148, 152
in second language learning, 156
Phonological loop, 84
Phonological Mean Length of Utterance, in assessment data analysis, 155
Phonological patterns and definitions, 149t–152t
Phonological Processes Analysis, in assessment data analysis, 155
Phonological representation, of word, 83
Phonology
definition of, 143
development of, 82–83
impaired, in autism spectrum disorders, 236
in language acquisition, 82–83
rules of, 82
Phonotrauma, 358
Physiologic measures, of voice production, 348
Pia mater, 14–15, 16f
Picture exchange communication system (PECS), in autism spectrum disorders, 239
Piedgin Sign English, 432
Pierre Robin sequence, 335–336
Pinna, 410, 410f
Pitch, of sound, 48, 48t, 49t
Place-Manner-Voicing, in assessment data analysis, 155
Platysma muscle, 45
Play, in language therapy, 189
PL 94-142 - Education for All Handicapped Children Act of 1971, 112, 199
PL 99-457 - Education for the Handicapped Act Amendments of 1986, 112
PL 101-476 - Individuals with Disabilities Education Act (IDEA), 1990, 112, 113
PL 107-110 - The No Child Left Behind Act of 2001, 112
Plica ventricularis, etiologies and characteristics of, 352
Pneumonia, aspiration, 378
Pneumonitis, aspiration, 378
PNS. *See* Peripheral nervous system (PNS)
Polypoid degeneration, etiologies and characteristics of, 350
Polyps, vocal fold, etiologies and characteristics of, 350
Pons, 18
Pontine stroke, dysphagia in, 372
Porch Index of Communicative Abilities Revised (PICA-R), 262
Posterior cerebral arteries, 30, 32f
Posterior column-medial lemniscal system, 27–29, 28f
Posterior communicating arteries, 31, 32f
Posterior cricoarytenoid muscles, 38t, 39

Postpolio syndrome, dysphagia in, 374
Postural changes, in dysphagia management, 385–386
Postvocalic, definition of, 143
Potassium ion (K+) channels, 11
PPA *See* Primary progressive aphasia (PPA)
Practice, intensive, in treatment of motor speech disorders, 311
Pragmatic approaches, to aphasia treatment, 272
Pragmatic language, in autism spectrum disorders, 236
Pragmatics
developmental stages of, 80
in language acquisition, 80–82
Prelinguistic development, of speech sounds, 147–148
Preschool-age children
at risk for literacy disorders, identification of, 216–217
speech sound development in, 148
stuttering in, approaches to, 248–249, 249t
Pressure wave, 48
Presupposition, in language development, 172
Prevention, resources on, 126
Prevocalic, definition of, 143
Primary progressive aphasia (PPA), 291–292
augmentative and alternative communication approaches for, 293–294
Private practice, resources on, 124
Procedure, in research articles, 95
Processing speed, in reading, 214
Professional liability and responsibility, 113
Professional organizations, 107–108
Professional service programs, resources on, 124
Professional voice users, voice problems of, 355
Progressive supranuclear palsy (PSP), dysphagia in, 373
Progress monitoring assessments, of literacy skills, 216
Proportion of Whole-Word Proximity, in assessment data analysis, 155
Proprioception, 29
Prosodic impairments
in dysarthrias, treatment of, 318
of motor speech disorders, 305t
Prosodic theory, of speech sound acquisition and disorders, 145–146
Prosody, definition of, 143
Prosopagnosia, in aphasia, 258
Prosthetic devices
articulatory, for dysarthrias, 317
tracheoesophageal, voice production with, 359, 360
velopharyngeal, 340
for dysarthrias, 315, 316t
Psychogenic dysphonia/aphonia, etiologies and characteristics of, 351–352
Psychogenic stuttering, 244–245, 245t
Psychometric properties, of standardized assessments, 194–195

Puberphonia, etiologies and characteristics of, 352
Pyramidal tract, 22

Q

Qualitative research, 96
Quantitative research, 95–96
Quarter wave resonator, 60, 60f

R

Radiation, for head and neck cancer, voice disorders from, 359
Ratio measurement data, 97
Reading
aphasia affecting, 256
cognitive factors in, 214–215
component processes influencing, 211–215
instruction in, "top down" *versus* "bottom up" approaches to, 218–219
letter-by-letter, in aphasia, 257
sight-word, 211–212
Reading comprehension, 212–213
in aphasia assessment, 264
Reading disorders, school-age, 218
Receptive aphasia, 268
Rehabilitation, auditory, 431–434
Rehabilitation Act of 1973, 199
Section 504 of, 112
Reinke's edema, etiologies and characteristics of, 350
Reissner's membrane, 413
Relational terms, acquisition of, 85
Reliability
of measurement, 94
of standardized assessments, 194
Research, 91–100
application of, to evidence-based practice, 92
on autism spectrum disorder etiology, 230
framework for, in *Scope of Practice in Speech-Language Pathology*, 118–119
principles of, 92
process of, 92
Research articles
interpreting, 93–99
"Introduction" section of, 93
"Methods" section of, 93–97
"Results" section of, 97–99
Research design, in research articles, 95
Residual volume (RV), 34–35, 34f
Resonance
disorders of, velopharyngeal dysfunction and, 339
resources on, 127
in voice evaluation, 357
Resonance dysfunction
evaluation of, 339–340
treatment of, 340–341
Resonant voice therapy, 358
Resonation, of sounds, in vocal tract, 60–61, 61f
Respiration, 32–35
anatomy for, critical, 32–33, 33f
and phonation, coordination of, in dysarthrias, improving, 313–314

Respiratory system
  in speech production, 45
  support of, in dysarthrias, 312–313
Respiratory volumes/capacities, 34–35, 34f
Response Elaboration Therapy (RET), for aphasia, 271–272, 272t
Response generalization, in language therapy, 185
Response to Instruction (RTI) model, 219t
  challenges to, 219
Response to intervention (RTI), in school-age language disorders, 200
Resting potential, of neurons, 9
Reticular formation, 19
Reticulospinal tract, 24
Retrieval errors, 84
Retrocochlear disorders, 425–426, 426t
Rhotacization, definition of, 143
Rib cage, 32
Right-hemisphere brain damage (RBD), communication disorders with, 285–286
Risorius muscle, 45
RTI. *See* Response to Intervention (RTI)
RTI model. *See* Response to Instruction (RTI) model
Rubrospinal tract, 24, 24t
Ruffini endings/corpuscles, 28
  in proprioception, 29

S

Saethre-Chotzen syndrome, 337
Scala media, 412, 412f
Scala tympani, 412, 412f
Scala vestibuli, 412, 412f
School(s)
  role of speech-language pathologist in, 112
  SLP services in, legislation and legal decisions on, 112
School-age children
  definition of, 194
  hearing screening for, 433
  language disorders in
    spoken, 193–207 (*See also* School-age spoken language disorders)
      prevalence of, 194
    written, 209–224 (*See also* School-age written language disorders)
  phonemic awareness skills development in, 152
  speech sound development in, 148
  stuttering in, approaches to, 249–250, 250t
School-age spoken language disorders
  assessment of, 194–198
    criterion-referenced/curriculum-based, 195–198, 198t
    dynamic, 195
    functional/ecological, 195
    purpose of, 194
    standardized/formal, 194–195
      psychometric properties of, 194–195
  in attention deficit/hyperactivity disorder, 204
  in autism spectrum disorders, 205–206
  causal categories of, 202
  in cerebral palsy, 204–205
  in chromosomal syndromes, 202
  in cognitive/intellectual disability, 202–203
  in congenital syndromes, 202
  in culturally and linguistically diverse populations, 198–199
  in Down syndrome, 203
  in genetic syndromes, 202
  intervention for, 199–200
    approaches to, 199–200
    evidence-based practice in, 201
    legislation on, 199
    response to, 200
    service delivery models for, 199
  in neural tube defects, 204
  in specific learning disabilities, 204
  in traumatic brain injury, 205
  in X-linked syndromes, 203
School-age written language disorders, 209–224, 218
  Individuals with Disabilities Education Act (IDEA) for persons with, 220–221
  risk for, identification of, 216–217
School-based practitioners, roles and responsibilities for, resources on, 128
School services, resources on, 128
Scintigraphy, in dysphagia evaluation, 384
Scleroderma, GERD in, 380
Scope of Practice in Speech-Language Pathology (ASHA), 117–128
  clinical services in, 121–122
  education, administration, and research in, 122
  framework for research and clinical practice of, 118–119
  practice settings in, 122
  prevention and advocacy in, 122
  professional roles and activities in, 120–121
  qualifications for speech-language pathologist in, 120
  resources for, 123–128
  statement of purpose of, 118
Screening assessments, of literacy skills, 215
Screening Test for Developmental Apraxia of Speech (STDAS-2), 306
Sedation, resources on, 127
Self-talk techniques, 188
Semantic dementia, 291, 292t
Semantic hierarchy, 84
Semantic language, impaired, in autism spectrum disorders, 236
Semantic relations, in language development, 174–175
Semantic representations, of word, 84
Semantics
  in language acquisition, 83–86
  system of meanings in, 83
  word learning in, 83–84
Semicircular canals, 411–412
Semitones, 48, 49t
Sensorineural hearing loss, 417, 418f
  management strategies for, 425
Sensory hair cells, 412–413, 413f
Sensory hearing loss, audiometric test findings in, 420
Sensory-Motor Approach, for phonetic errors, 161
Sentence Production Program for Aphasia (SPPA), 276, 276t
Severe disabilities, resources on, 126
Shaker exercise, for dysphagia, 385
Shimmer, as measure of voice production, 347
Sibilant, definition of, 143
Sibilant fricatives
  place of articulation for, 68–69, 69f
  spectral moment characteristics of, 69, 70f
Simulated presence therapy, for dementia, 294
Single-subject research, 96
Sinusoid(s), 52–55
  characteristics of, 55t
  waveforms of, 52–53, 53f
Skeletal muscle, 7
Skewness, in data measurement, 97
SLP. *See* Speech-language pathologist (SLP); Speech-language pathology (SLP)
SLVT. *See* Supralaryngeal vocal tract (SLVT)
Smooth muscle, 8
Social aspects of communication, resources on, 126
Social Communication Questionnaire (SCQ), 234
Social Networks: A Communication Inventory for Individuals with Complex Communication Needs and Their Communication Partners (Blackstone & Hunt Berg, 2003), 402
Social Security Act
  Amendments of, 111
  Title XIX of, on Medicaid, 110–111
  Title XVIII of, on Medicare, 110
Social stories, in autism spectrum disorders, 239
Sodium (Na^+) channels, in neural signaling, 10
Somatic nervous system, 12
Somatosensory pathways, major, 26–29
Sound(s)
  complex
    aperiodic, 54–55, 55f, 56–5, 56f, 57f (*See also* Aperiodic complex sounds)
    periodic, 53–54, 53t, 55–56, 56f (*See also* Periodic complex sounds)
    waveforms of, 52–53, 53f
  graphical representation of, 50–52, 51f, 51t, 52f
  nature of, 48–50
  obstruent, 57
    acoustic characteristics of, 65–66, 67t
  resonant, acoustic characteristics of, 61–64, 62f, 63f, 64f, 65t
  resonation of, in vocal tract, 60–61, 61f
  system of, 82
  types of, graphical representations of, 52–55, 53f, 53t, 54, 54f, 55, 55f, 55t
Source-filter theory, of speech production, 57–59, 57f, 58f, 59f
Spaced-Retrieval Training (SRT), for dementia, 294
Spasmodic dysphonia, etiologies and characteristics of, 353–354
Spasmodic dystonia, dysphagia in, 374

Spastic dysarthria, perceptual features of, 301t
Specific language impairment, definition of, 177
Specific learning disabilities (SLD), school-age language disorders in, 204
Spectral moment characteristics, of nonsibilant and sibilant fricatives, 69, 70t
Spectrogram(s), 50–51, 51f, 51t, 52f
   of aperiodic noise, 66, 66f
   comparing liquids/glides and vowels, 65t
Speech
   after glossectomy, 361
   after partial laryngectomy, 361
   after total laryngectomy, 359
   apraxia of (See Apraxia of speech [AOS])
   breathing during, 34
   breathing for, 345
   cleft lip and palate and, 335
   cued, 432
   intelligibility of (See Intelligibility)
   neuroanatomy and neurophysiology of, 8–29
   periodic complex sounds in, glottal source of, 55–56, 56f
   production of, systems involved in, 45–46, 45f
   study of, 4–8
   velopharyngeal dysfunction and, 339
   velum during, 333, 333f
Speech audiometry, 418–419, 419t
Speech breathing, 34, 35
Speech detection threshold (SDT), 418
Speech discrimination skills, assessment of, in speech sound disorder assessment, 154
Speech disorders, motor, 299–327. See also Motor speech disorders (MSDs)
Speech-language pathologist (SLP)
   credentialing of, 105–107, 440
   role of
      in early intervention, 113
      in medical setting, 111
      in school setting, 112
   scope of practice of, 117–128
   state licensure of, 106
Speech-language pathology assistants, resources on, 124
Speech-Language Pathology Clinical Fellowship (SLPCF) Report and Rating Form, 129–131
Speech-language pathology examination
   analysis for, 450
   background on, 441
   content of, 441–442
   critical reasoning applied to, 442, 444t
   critical thinking and, 449–452
   day of, 447–448
   developing critical-thinking skills for, 452
   evaluation for, 450–451
   explanation for, 451
   format of, 442
   inference for, 450
   levels of questions on, 442, 443t
   preparation for, 442–447
      guidelines for, 442
      psychological outlook in, 442–443, 445t
      resources for, 447
   question answering strategies for, 448, 449t
   results of, waiting for and receiving, 453
   retaking, 453
   reviewing professional education for, 443–447
   scoring and reporting of, 452–453
   self-correction for, 452
   self-examination for, 451
   test center procedures and, 447–448
   test taker personalities and, 446, 446t
   time/time keeping for, 448
Speech-language pathology services, in schools, legislation and legal decisions on, 112
Speech-language pathology (SLP)
   in addressing literacy, 210
   in autism spectrum disorder, role of, 232–233, 233t
   ethical issues in, 108–109
   in evidence-based practice, 116
   examination on, preparing for, 439–454
   in health care environment, 110–111
   history of, 104
   international organizations for, 108
   with multicultural populations, 114
   policies and procedures on, 114
   practice of, 103–135
      scope of, 104–105
   professional development in, 104
   professional liability and responsibility in, 113
   professional organizations in, 107–108
   related professional organizations, 108
   research principles and, 92
   rules and regulations on, 114
   service delivery models for, 110
   specialty recognition in, 107
   state organizations for, 108
   supervision in, 115
   teacher licensure in, 106–107
   telepractice and, 115
   workforce issues/employment in, 110
Speech output, from augmentative and alternative communication device, 405–406
Speech production
   acoustic theory of, 57–59, 57f, 58f, 59f
   source-filter theory of, 57–59, 57f, 58f, 59f
Speech recognition threshold (SRT), 418
Speech sound disorders (SSDs)
   articulation, characteristics of, 155–156
   assessment of, 153–158
      in culturally and linguistically diverse clients, 156
      data analysis in, 154–156
      procedures for, 153–154
      purpose of, 153
   childhood apraxia of speech and dysarthria distinguished from, 156–158, 157t
   in children, 139–165
   diagnosis of, determining, 155
   phonological, characteristics of, 156
   treatment of, 158–165
      intervention approaches in, 159–165
         for phonemic errors, 162–165
         for phonetic errors, 160–162
      intervention targets selection in, 158–159
Speech sounds
   acquisition of
      articulatory phonology theory of, 147
      behavioral theory of, 143–144
      distinctive features theory of, 144
      feature geometry theory of, 146
      general phonology theory of, 147
      generative phonology theory of, 144–145
      interactionist-discovery (cognitive) theory of, 146
      metrical phonology theory of, 146
      models (theories) of, 143–147
      natural phonology theory of, 145
      nonlinear theories of, 146–147
      optimality theory of, 146
      prosodic theory of, 145–146
   audiogram and, 420, 420f
   development of, typical, 147–152
      development of physical structures of speech in, 147
      development of speech intelligibility in, 152
      in early/mid/late 8, 148
      first 50 words in, phonological characteristics of, 148
      prelinguistic, 147–148
      in preschool-age children, 148
      in school-age children, development of phonemic awareness skills in, 152
      in two-year-olds, 148
      use and suppression of phonological error patterns in, 148, 149t–152t, 152
   disorders of (See Speech sound disorders [SSDs])
   in error, stimulability of, in speech sound disorder assessment, 154
Speech therapy, for resonance and velopharyngeal dysfunction, 340–341
Speech/word recognition testing, 418–419, 419t
Spelling, in writing skill development, 213
Spinal accessory (XI) nerve, swallowing and, 365
Spinal cord, 17, 18f
Spinal nerves, 14, 15f
Spoken language
   acquisition of, 84–85
   disorders of, in school-age populations, 193–207 (See also School-age spoken language disorders)
SSDs. See Speech sound disorders (SSDs)
Standard error of measurement, 94
Standardized tests
   in assessment data analysis, 155
   in language disorder assessment, 181
Stapes, 411
State licensure, for speech-language pathologist, 106, 440
Statistical significance testing, 97

Statistics, in research results, 97–98
Sternohyoid muscle, 39–40, 41t
Sternothyroid muscle, 41, 41t
Stickler syndrome, 336
Stimulus generalization, in language therapy, 185
Stop bursts, 72t, 73
Stop consonants, 71t, 73
Stops
  in consonant production, 140, 140t
  voiced and voiceless pairs for, comparison of, 67t
Story-retelling tasks, in language disorder assessment, 181
Striatum, 21
Strident, definition of, 143
Stroboscopic assessment, of vocal fold vibration, 357
Stroboscopic measures, of voice production, 347–348
Stroke. See Cerebrovascular accident (CVA, stroke)
Structural analysis, in word identification, 211
Structured play, in language therapy, 189
Stuttering, 241–252. See also Fluency disorders
  assessment in, 245–247
  behaviors, feelings and attitudes about, 246t
  definition of, 242
  developmental, 242–244
  neurogenic, 244, 245t
  psychogenic, 244–245, 245t
  treatment of, 248–251
    approaches to, 248–251, 249t, 250t, 251t
    decisions on, 248
Styloglossus muscle, 44, 44t
Stylohyoid muscle, 39, 41t
Subclavian arteries, 30, 31f, 32f
Subcortical stroke, dysphagia in, 372–373
Subglottic pressure, as measure of voice production, 347
Subglottic stenosis, 355
Subglottic tumors, 377
Subjects, in research articles, 93–94
Subsequent instructional events, 188
Subsequent motivational events, 188
Substantia nigra, 21
Subthalamic nucleus, 21
Subthalamus, 22
Superior laryngeal nerve paralysis, 353
Superior longitudinal muscles, 43, 44t
Supervision
  resources on, 124
  of speech-language pathologist, 115
Supported Conversation for Adults with Aphasia (SCA), 283, 283t
Supraglottic swallow, for dysphagia, 384
Supraglottic tumors, 377
Suprahyoid muscles, 39, 41t
Supralaryngeal system, in speech production, 45–46, 45f
Supralaryngeal vocal tract (SLVT)
  acoustic characteristics of, 59–60, 60f
  in speech production, 57, 57f
Suprasegmental, definition of, 143

Surface electromyography (SEMG), in dysphagia evaluation, 384
Surgical options, for dysphagia, 387
Swallow
  effortful, for dysphagia, 385
  esophageal phase of, 367, 370f
  oral phase of, 366–367, 370f
  oral preparatory phase of, 367, 370f
  pharyngeal phase of, 367, 370f
  physiology of, 366–367
  supraglottic, for dysphagia, 384
Swallowing
  after glossectomy, 361
  after partial laryngectomy, 361
  after total laryngectomy, 359
  anatomy of, 35–46, 364, 365f
  aspiration and, 378–379
  cortical innervation and, 366
  cranial nerves and, 364–366
  definition of, 364
  disorders of, 363–389 (See also Dysphagia)
  evaluation of
    fiberoptic endoscopic, 382
      with sensory testing, 382–383
    modified barium swallow in, 381–382, 382t, 383t
  innervation of, 359t, 368t
  medications and, 380
  muscles of, 368t, 369t
  neuroanatomy and neurophysiology of, 8–29
  neuroplasticity and, 375
  normal, 364
  normal aging and, 367, 371
  penetration and, 378–379
  recovery of, after head and neck cancer, 376
  resources on, 126–127
  study of, 4–8
  subcortical innervation and, 366
Syllabication rules, 211
Syllable, definition of, 143
Syllable-type recognition skills, 211
Symmetry, as measure of voice production, 347
Sympathetic division, of autonomic nervous system, 12–13
Synaptic potentials, 11–12
Syntactic construction and combination, 89
Syntactic development, 89–90
  in language development, 175
Syntax
  in curriculum-based language disorder assessment, 197
  in language acquisition, 89–90
Systematic reviews, treatment efficacy evidence from, 99

T

Tangible Symbol Systems (Rowland & Schweigert, 2000), 402–403
TBI. See Traumatic brain injury (TBI)
Teacher licensure, for speech-language pathologist, 106–107

Technology-Related Assistance for Individuals with Disabilities Act of 1988, 111
Tectorial membrane, 413, 413f
Telencephalon, 19
Telepractice
  resources on, 127
  speech-language pathology and, 115
Temporal lobe, 19–20
Temporal muscles, 42, 43f
Temporomandibular joint (TMJ), 43
TEP (tracheoesophageal puncture), 377
  voice production with, 359, 360
Terminology, resources on, 124
Thalamus, 22
Theory of mind
  in autism spectrum disorders, 239
  in language acquisition, 82
Thermal tactile stimulation, for dysphagia, 385
Thoracic cavity, 5, 5f
Thyroarytenoid muscles, 38, 38t
Thyrohyoid muscle, 40–41, 41t
Thyroid cartilage, 35
Tidal volume (TV), 34, 34f
Timing measures, of voice production, 347
Tissue types, 5–8, 6f, 7f
TNM staging, of head and neck tumors, 376
Tongue, 43, 332
  anatomy of, 36f
  muscles of, 43–44, 44t, 369t
  surgical removal of, speech and swallowing after, 361
  tumors of, glossectomy and, 376
Tonsils, 332
  tumors of, 377
Trachea, 33
Tracheoesophageal puncture (TEP), 377
  voice production with, 359, 360
Transgender individuals, voice problems of, 355
Transient ischemic attack (TIA), 260
Transverse and oblique interarytenoid muscles, 38–39, 38t
Transverse muscles, 43, 44t
Traumatic brain injury (TBI)
  aphasia from, 260–261
  dysphagia in, 374–375
  school-age language disorders in, 205
Treacher Collins syndrome, 337
Treatment effectiveness, 99
Treatment efficacy research, 99
Treatment efficacy studies, evidence-based practice and, 99
Treatment fidelity, 99
Treatment for Aphasic Perseveration (TAP), 278
Treatment of Underlying Forms (TUF), for improving verbal expression, 274–276, 275t
Tremor
  voice, essential, etiologies and characteristics of, 354
  in voice evaluation, 357
Trigeminal (V) nerve, swallowing and, 364, 366, 367, 368t, 369t
Trisomy 13, cleft lip and palate in, 336

Vowel quadrilateral, 142, 142f
Vowels, compared with liquids and glides, 65t

W

Wallenberg's syndrome, dysphagia in, 372
Waveform(s), 49f, 50, 51f, 51t
   of amplitude modulated noise, 57f
   of aperiodic complex sound, 55
   of aperiodic noise, 66, 66f
   of complex sounds, 52–53, 53f
   of impulse noise, 56f
   of periodic complex sounds, 54, 54f
   of sinusoids, 52–53, 53f
   of turbulent noise, 57f
Wavelength, of sound, 49, 49f
Wernicke, Carl, in aphasiology, 258
Wernicke's aphasia, treatment of, 279
Western Aphasia Battery-Revised (WAB-R), 261
Whisper, 346
White matter, of spinal cord, 17, 18f
Whole-Language Treatment Approach, for phonemic errors, 163–164
Wolf-Hirschhorn syndrome, 336
Word identification, components of, 211
Word learning, 83–84
Words
   order and combination of, 89
   structure of, system of, 86
Workforce issues, in speech-language pathology, 110
Workload, resources on, 128
World Health Organization (WHO) International Classification of Functioning, Disability and Health, 431
Writing
   aphasia affecting, 256
   assessment of, in aphasia assessment, 264
   component processes influencing, 211–215
   instruction in, "top down" versus "bottom up" approaches to, 218–219
Writing skill, development of, 213–214
Written communication, definition of, 394
Written language
   characteristics of, 210
   disorders of, in school-age populations, 209–224 (*See also* School-age written language disorders)

X

Xerostomia, in elderly, 371
X-linked syndromes, school-age language disorders in, 203

Z

Zenker's diverticulum, 380
Zygomatic muscles, 45

Tumor(s)
    brain, aphasia from, 251
    esophageal, 380
    head and neck
        classification of, 376–377
        staging of, 376
Turbulent noises, 56, 57f
Two-year old children, speech sound development in, 148
Tympanic membrane (TM), 410
Tympanometry, in auditory function assessment, 421

U

Ultrasound (US) imaging, in dysphagia evaluation, 383
"Under the Direction of" rule, resources on, 128
Unilateral upper motor neuron dysarthria, perceptual features of, 301t

V

VaD. See Vascular dementia (VaD)
Vagus (X) nerve, swallowing and, 365, 367, 368t, 369t
Validity
    of measurement, 94–95
    of standardized assessments, 194–195
Van der Woude syndrome, 336
Van Riper Approach, for phonetic errors, 160–161
Variability, in data measurement, 97
Variables, in research articles, 94
Vascular dementia (VaD)
    characteristics of, 289–290
    treatment of, 293
Veins, cerebral, 30
Velocardiofacial syndrome, 336
Velopharyngeal closure, variations in, 334
Velopharyngeal dysfunction, 338–339
    evaluation of, 339–340
    resonance disorders and, 339
    treatment of, 340–341
Velopharyngeal function, normal resonance and, 338
Velopharyngeal incompetence, 338–339, 338f
    voice problems with, 355
Velopharyngeal insufficiency (VPI), 338, 338f
    surgery for, 340
    syndromes associated with, 336
Velopharyngeal mislearning, 339
Velopharyngeal subsystem, treatment of, for dysarthrias, 315–316
Velopharyngeal valve
    muscles of, 334, 368t
    physiology of, 333–335, 333f
Velum
    movement of, 333–334, 333f
    structures of, 332, 332f
Ventral cavity, 5, 5f
Ventricular phonation, etiologies and characteristics of, 352
Ventricular system of brain, 16–17, 17f
Verbal expression
    in aphasia assessment, 262–263
    by aphasia patient, treatments for improving, 273–278
Verbal Motor Production Assessment for Children (VMPAC), 306
Verbal repetition of words, aphasia affecting, 256
Verb Network Strengthening Treatment (VNeST), 278
Verbs, acquisition of, 85
Vertebral arteries, 30, 31f, 32f
Vertical muscles, 43–44, 44t
Vestibulocochlear (VIII) nerve, 414–415
Vestibulospinal tract, 24
Vibration
    sound and, 48
    vocal fold, 345–346
        acoustic measurement of, 73–77, 74f, 75f, 75t, 76t, 77f
        myoelastic aerodynamic theory of, 41–42
        stability of, 73, 76
Visual Action Therapy (VAT), for aphasia, 281
Visual agnosia, in aphasia, 257–258
Visual measures, of voice production, 347–348
Visual reinforcement audiometry, 420
Vital capacity (VC), 34f, 35
Vocabulary
    in curriculum-based language disorder assessment, 197
    development of, 174
    receptive vs. expressive, in language development, 174
Vocal cord dysfunction, etiologies and characteristics of, 352–353
Vocal fold(s), 41, 42f
    appearance of, as measure of voice production, 348
    cysts of, etiologies and characteristics of, 350
    histology of, 344–345
    polyps of, etiologies and characteristics of, 350
    vibration of, 345–346
        acoustic measurement of, 73–77, 74f, 75f, 75t, 76t, 77f
        frequency of, 73, 74f, 75f
        summary statistics on, 73, 75t
        myoelastic aerodynamic theory of, 41–42
        stability of, 73, 76
Vocal fold abductors, 39
Vocal fold adductors, 38–39, 38t
Vocal fold edge, as measure of voice production, 348
Vocal function exercises, 358
Vocal health, promotion of, 358
Vocal mechanism
    age-related changes in, 348
    anatomy of, 344
    development of, 348
        in children, 348
    neuroanatomy of, 345
    physiology of, 344–345
Vocal nodules
    bilateral, 355
    etiologies and characteristics of, 349–350
Vocal tract
    constriction of
        for obstruent sounds, 65
        for resonant sounds, 63, 63f
    sounds resonating in, 60–61, 61f
Voice
    after total laryngectomy, 359
    assessment of, after total laryngectomy, protocol for, 360
    essential tremor of, etiologies and characteristics of, 354
    registers of, 346
    resources on, 127
Voiced cognates, in obstruents, 66, 67t
Voice disorders, 343–361
    assessment of
        acoustic, 357
        aerodynamic, 357
        functional, 356
        hearing, 357
        laryngologic/stroboscopic, 357
        perceptual, 356–357
    etiologies and characteristics of, 349–354
    evaluation protocol for, 356–357
    functional, etiologies and characteristics of, 351–353
    from head and neck cancer, management of, 359–361
    high-risk populations for, 355–356
    management recommendations and referrals for, 358
    of neurologic origin, etiologies and characteristics of, 353
    pediatric, 354–355
    prevention of, 358
    treatment approaches to, evidence-based, 358
Voice Handicap Index (VHI), 356
Voiceless cognates, in obstruents, 66, 67t
Voiceless phonation, 346
Voice onset time (VOT), 66
    duration of, in stop consonants, 71t, 73
Voice production
    after partial laryngectomy, 360–361
    measures of, 346–348
        acoustic, 346–347
        aerodynamic, 347
        perceptual, 347
        physiologic, 348
        stroboscopic, 347–348
        timing, 347
        visual, 347–348
    TEP, 359, 360
Voice qualities, comparison of, 76t, 77, 77f
Voice-Related Quality of Life (VRQOL), 356
Voice therapy, 358
    alaryngeal, approaches to, 360
Voicing, 55
    in consonant production, 140, 140t
Voltage-gated sodium channels, 10, 11
Voluntary Control of Involuntary Utterances (VCIU), in improving verbal expression, 273, 273t
VOT. See Voice onset time (VOT)